GULF WAR and HEALTH

VOLUME 3

FUELS, COMBUSTION PRODUCTS, AND PROPELLANTS

Committee on Gulf War and Health: Literature Review of Selected Environmental Particulates, Pollutants, and Synthetic Chemical Compounds

Board on Health Promotion and Disease Prevention

INSTITUTE OF MEDICINE
OF THE NATIONAL ACADEMIES

THE NATIONAL ACADEMIES PRESS
Washington, D.C.
www.nap.edu

THE NATIONAL ACADEMIES PRESS • 500 Fifth Street, NW • Washington, DC 20001

NOTICE: The project that is the subject of this report was approved by the Governing Board of the National Research Council, whose members are drawn from the councils of the National Academy of Sciences, the National Academy of Engineering, and the Institute of Medicine. The members of the committee responsible for the report were chosen for their special competences and with regard for appropriate balance.

This study was supported by Contract No. V101(93)P-1637, Task Order No. 25 between the National Academy of Sciences and the Department of Veterans Affairs. Any opinions, findings, conclusions, or recommendations expressed in this publication are those of the author(s) and do not necessarily reflect the view of the organizations or agencies that provided support for this project.

International Standard Book Number 0-309-09527-1 (Book)
International Standard Book Number 0-309-54736-9 (PDF)
Library of Congress Control Number: 200109510

Additional copies of this report are available from the National Academies Press, 500 Fifth Street, NW, Lockbox 285, Washington, DC 20055; (800) 624-6242 or (202) 334-3313 (in the Washington metropolitan area); http://www.nap.edu.

For more information about the Institute of Medicine, visit the IOM home page at **www.iom.edu.**

Printed in the United States of America.

The serpent has been a symbol of long life, healing, and knowledge among almost all cultures and religions since the beginning of recorded history. The serpent adopted as a logotype by the Institute of Medicine is a relief carving from ancient Greece, now held by the Staatliche Museen in Berlin.

*"Knowing is not enough; we must apply.
Willing is not enough; we must do."*
—Goethe

INSTITUTE OF MEDICINE
OF THE NATIONAL ACADEMIES

Adviser to the Nation to Improve Health

THE NATIONAL ACADEMIES

Advisers to the Nation on Science, Engineering, and Medicine

The **National Academy of Sciences** is a private, nonprofit, self-perpetuating society of distinguished scholars engaged in scientific and engineering research, dedicated to the furtherance of science and technology and to their use for the general welfare. Upon the authority of the charter granted to it by the Congress in 1863, the Academy has a mandate that requires it to advise the federal government on scientific and technical matters. Dr. Bruce M. Alberts is president of the National Academy of Sciences.

The **National Academy of Engineering** was established in 1964, under the charter of the National Academy of Sciences, as a parallel organization of outstanding engineers. It is autonomous in its administration and in the selection of its members, sharing with the National Academy of Sciences the responsibility for advising the federal government. The National Academy of Engineering also sponsors engineering programs aimed at meeting national needs, encourages education and research, and recognizes the superior achievements of engineers. Dr. Wm. A. Wulf is president of the National Academy of Engineering.

The **Institute of Medicine** was established in 1970 by the National Academy of Sciences to secure the services of eminent members of appropriate professions in the examination of policy matters pertaining to the health of the public. The Institute acts under the responsibility given to the National Academy of Sciences by its congressional charter to be an adviser to the federal government and, upon its own initiative, to identify issues of medical care, research, and education. Dr. Harvey V. Fineberg is president of the Institute of Medicine.

The **National Research Council** was organized by the National Academy of Sciences in 1916 to associate the broad community of science and technology with the Academy's purposes of furthering knowledge and advising the federal government. Functioning in accordance with general policies determined by the Academy, the Council has become the principal operating agency of both the National Academy of Sciences and the National Academy of Engineering in providing services to the government, the public, and the scientific and engineering communities. The Council is administered jointly by both Academies and the Institute of Medicine. Dr. Bruce M. Alberts and Dr. Wm. A. Wulf are chair and vice chair, respectively, of the National Research Council.

www.national-academies.org

COMMITTEE ON GULF WAR AND HEALTH: LITERATURE REVIEW OF SELECTED ENVIRONMENTAL PARTICULATES, POLLUTANTS, AND SYNTHETIC CHEMICAL COMPOUNDS

LYNN R. GOLDMAN (*Chair*), Professor, Bloomberg School of Public Health, Johns Hopkins University, Baltimore, MD

MELVYN BRANCH, Joseph Negler Professor of Mechanical Engineering, Department of Mechanical Engineering, University of Colorado, Boulder, CO

MICHAEL BRAUER, Professor, School of Occupational and Environmental Hygiene, University of British Columbia, Vancouver, BC

DEBORAH A. CORY-SLECHTA, Director, Environmental and Occupational Health Sciences Institute, Piscataway, NJ (*Resigned January 22, 2004*)

MARK EISNER, Assistant Professor, Department of Medicine, University of California, San Francisco, CA

ERIC GARSHICK, Assistant Professor of Medicine, Pulmonary and Critical Care Medicine Section, VA Boston Healthcare System, Channing Laboratory, Brigham and Women's Hospital, and Harvard Medical School, Boston, MA

RUSS B. HAUSER, Associate Professor of Occupational Health, Department of Environmental Health, Harvard School of Public Health, Boston, MA

JOEL KAUFMAN, Associate Professor of Medicine, Environmental and Occupational Health Sciences, Departments of Medicine and Environmental and Occupational Health Sciences, University of Washington, Seattle, WA

RICHARD MAYEUX, Professor and Director, Sergievsky Center, Co-Director, Taub Institute, College of Physicians and Surgeons, Columbia University, New York, NY

CHARLES POOLE, Associate Professor, Department of Epidemiology, University of North Carolina School of Public Health, Chapel Hill, NC

BEATE RITZ, Associate Professor, Department of Epidemiology and Center for Occupational and Environmental Health, School of Public Health, University of California, Los Angeles, CA

JOSEPH RODRICKS, Principal, ENVIRON Health Sciences Institute, ENVIRON International Corporation, Arlington, VA

RICHARD SCHLESINGER, Chair and Professor, Department of Biological Sciences, Dyson College of Arts and Sciences, New York, NY

JAMES TAYLOR, Head, Section of Industrial Dermatology, Department of Dermatology, Cleveland Clinic Foundation, Cleveland, OH

MARK UTELL, Professor, Departments of Medicine and Environmental Medicine, University of Rochester School of Medicine, Rochester, NY

WILLIAM VALENTINE, Associate Professor, Department of Pathology, Vanderbilt University Medical Center, Nashville, TN

JUDITH ZELIKOFF, Associate Professor, Institute of Environmental Medicine, New York University School of Medicine, Tuxedo, NY

STAFF

CAROLYN FULCO, Senior Program Officer
ABIGAIL MITCHELL, Senior Program Officer
MARY PAXTON, Senior Program Officer
MICHELLE CATLIN, Senior Program Officer
CARRIE SZLYK, Program Officer (*until December 2003*)
MICHAEL SCHNEIDER, Senior Program Associate
JUDITH URBANCZYK, Senior Program Associate
HOPE HARE, Administrative Assistant
DEEPALI PATEL, Research Associate
PETER JAMES, Research Assitant
DAMIKA WEBB, Senior Program Assistant
ROSE MARIE MARTINEZ, Director, Board on Health Promotion and Disease Prevention

CONSULTANTS

MIRIAM DAVIS, Independent Medical Writer, Silver Spring, MD
MARK GOLDBERG, McGill University, Montreal, QC
KATHERINE HOGGATT, University of California, Los Angeles, CA
JOAN DENCKLA, Harvard Medical School, Boston, MA
KIT SHAN LEE, University of British Columbia, Vancouver, BC

EDITOR

NORMAN GROSSBLATT, NRC Senior Editor

REVIEWERS

This report has been reviewed in draft form by individuals chosen for their diverse perspectives and technical expertise, in accordance with procedures approved by the National Research Council's Report Review Committee. The purpose of this independent review is to provide candid and critical comments that will assist the institution in making its published report as sound as possible and to ensure that the report meets institutional standards for objectivity, evidence, and responsiveness to the study charge. The review comments and draft manuscript remain confidential to protect the integrity of the deliberative process. We wish to thank the following individuals for their review of this report:

JOHN R. BALMES, San Francisco General Hospital, University of California, San Francisco, CA
ANNECLAIRE J. DE ROOS, Fred Hutchinson Cancer Research Center, University of Washington, Seattle, WA
ARTHUR L. FRANK, School of Public Health, Drexel University, Philadelphia, PA
PATRICK KINNEY, Mailman School of Public Health, Columbia University, New York, NY
HOWARD KIPEN, Environmental and Occupational Health Sciences Institute, Department of Environmental and Community Medicine, Rutgers, Piscataway, NJ
JANE Q. KOENIG, Department of Environmental and Occupational Health Sciences, University of Washington, Seattle, WA
FRANCINE LADEN, Channing Laboratory, Brigham and Women's Hospital and Harvard Medical School, Boston, MA
THOMAS MACK, Norris Comprehensive Cancer Center, University of Southern California, Los Angeles, CA
JONATHAN PATZ, Global Environmental Health Center for Sustainability and the Global Environment (SAGE), Nelson Institute for Environmental Studies and Department of Population Health Sciences, University of Wisconsin, Madison, WI
SAMUEL POTOLICCHIO, Department of Neurology, George Washington University Medical Center, Washington, DC
PEGGY REYNOLDS, Environmental Health Investigations Branch, California Department of Health Services, Oakland, CA
JONATHAN M. SAMET, Bloomberg School of Public Health, Johns Hopkins University, Baltimore, MD

Although the reviewers listed above have provided many constructive comments and suggestions, they were not asked to endorse the conclusions or recommendations nor did they see the final draft of the report before its release. The review of this report was overseen by **DAVID J. TOLLERUD**, School of Public Health University of Louisville, KY, and **M. DONALD WHORTON,** WorkCare, Inc., Alameda, CA, who were appointed by the Report Review Committee. They were responsible for making certain that an independent examination of this report was carried out in accordance with institutional procedures and that all review comments were carefully considered. Responsibility for the final content of this report rests entirely with the authoring committee and the institution.

PREFACE

As this report goes to press and our country is engaged in a war in Iraq, it is important to recall the 1990-1991 Gulf War. Engaging around 700,000 US military personnel, the Gulf War was of brief duration and entailed very few casualties among US troops. Yet, as they say, "war is hell", and our troops were exposed to numerous traumatic events and a multitude of hazardous substances. Not long after the war ended, many of its veterans reported a variety of chronic symptoms. Numerous studies were conducted, most of which corroborated reports of higher rates of signs and symptoms among these veterans. Some of the signs and symptoms have clearly been associated with identifiable medical diagnoses such as post-traumatic stress disorder and depression; others are outside current medical diagnostic classifications.

Veterans have been deeply concerned about whether exposures in the gulf were associated with chronic health problems after the end of the war. In response to their concerns, the Department of Veterans Affairs (VA) and Congress secured the assistance of the Institute of Medicine (IOM) in evaluating the scientific literature regarding exposures that may have occurred in the Gulf War. In a sense, this approach followed a model developed for the Vietnam War, after which there was concern about the possible health effects of exposure to dioxins in Agent Orange. In that case, the work of IOM has played a key role in informing VA decisions regarding compensation for dioxin-related chronic health effects. Following that model, Congress enacted legislation that specifically directed IOM to evaluate the effects of 33 agents; this report covers a small number of the agents: hydrazines, red fuming nitric acid, hydrogen sulfide, oil-fire byproducts, and diesel-heater fumes. In addition, VA requested that we assess potential exposures to fuels that were used in the Gulf War (gasoline, jet fuel, diesel fuel, and kerosene) and their combustion products.

Although we had a relatively small number of substances to review, the scientific literature on air pollutants from fuel combustion, as well as from exposure to fuels, is extensive. IOM appointed a committee with knowledge in the toxicology and epidemiology of fuels and combustion products; it included experts in combustion chemistry, rocket propellants, immunology, pulmonology, cancer, neurosciences, dermatology, and reproductive and developmental toxicology. The committee did not limit itself to studies of Gulf War veterans but rather reviewed all relevant literature with regard to chronic medical effects of exposure. Although the committee focused on epidemiologic studies, which are likely to identify associations between specific exposures and diagnoses in people, it also placed weight on toxicologic studies and on clinical case series that were informative about specific exposure-disease relationships. Along the lines of earlier Gulf War reports, the committee has framed its conclusions in categories of strength of association. Despite the extensive challenge of reviewing the literature and the diversity of expertise and views among committee members, the committee was able to reach consensus on all conclusions. For that, I am most grateful.

The committee identified several associations between exposures to rocket propellants and combustion products and disease. However, there is some concern among our members about the direction that the process has taken. Many of the substances to which there was potential exposure in the gulf are unique to war service (for example, nerve agents, mustard agents, and rocket propellants), but others are not and may be at least as likely to occur in noncombat military service or in civilian life as in war (for example, fuels, air pollutants, and the solvents and pesticides reviewed in *Gulf War and Health, Volume 2: Insecticides and Solvents*). Therefore, as the process has evolved from an examination of exposures unique to wartime to exposures that are ubiquitous and may be even greater in civilian life, what are VA and Congress to do with the results of this study? A second troubling issue is the lack of exposure information for individual veterans; given that many risks are clearly exposure-related, it is difficult to use the results of our review to assess whether veterans' illnesses are due to such exposures. Third, it is important to interpret the results of our review in a larger context of public health and prevention; for example, the committee found some evidence of an association between hydrazine exposure and lung cancer, but there obviously are much larger and better-established associations between lung cancer and other exposures, such as smoking and exposure to radon and asbestos. Given those circumstances, this report cannot answer the question of whether service in the gulf was associated with such exposures and whether specific health outcomes are due to the exposures. Despite those limitations, the committee hopes that its report will be helpful to all who may have been exposed to the substances in question and to those who are considering further research in the subject.

I am deeply appreciative of the expert work of our committee members, and it has been a privilege and a pleasure to work with the IOM staff. Without them, this report would not have been possible.

Lynn Goldman, MD, MPH, *Chair*

CONTENTS

Boxes, Tables, and Figures

EXECUTIVE SUMMARY

The 1991 Persian Gulf War was considered a brief and successful military operation with few injuries and deaths. The returning veterans, however, soon began reporting numerous health problems that they believed to be associated with their service in the gulf. Many Gulf War veterans returned to normal activities, but a large number have had a wide array of unexplained illnesses.

In response to the growing concerns of ill Gulf War veterans, Congress passed two laws in 1998: PL 105-277, the Persian Gulf War Veterans Act, and PL 105-368, the Veterans Programs Enhancement Act. Those laws directed the secretary of veterans affairs to enter into a contract with the National Academy of Sciences (NAS) to review and evaluate the scientific and medical literature regarding associations between illness and exposure to toxic agents, to environmental or wartime hazards, or to preventive medicines or vaccines associated with Gulf War service and to consider the NAS conclusions when making decisions about compensation. The study was assigned to the Institute of Medicine (IOM).

The Persian Gulf War legislation directs IOM to study a wide array of biologic, chemical, and physical agents. Given the large number of agents to study, IOM divided the task into several reviews. It has completed two reviews — *Gulf War and Health, Volume 1: Depleted Uranium, Pyridostigmine Bromide, Sarin, and Vaccines* and *Gulf War and Health, Volume 2: Insecticides and Solvents* — and has recently conducted an update of the sarin review in *Gulf War and Health: Updated Literature Review of Sarin.* The current volume examines the health effects of hydrazines, red fuming nitric acid, hydrogen sulfide, oil-fire byproducts, diesel-heater fumes, and fuels (for example, jet fuel and gasoline).

CHARGE TO THE COMMITTEE

In accordance with PL 105-368 and PL 105-277, IOM appointed the Committee on Gulf War and Health, Literature Review of Selected Environmental Particulates, Pollutants, and Synthetic Chemical Compounds and asked it to determine the following to the extent that available scientific data permit meaningful conclusions:

(A) whether a statistical association exists between exposure to the agent, hazard, or medicine or vaccine and the illness, taking into account the strength of the

scientific evidence and the appropriateness of the scientific methods used to detect the association,
(B) the increased risk of the illness among human or animal populations exposed to the agent, hazard, or medicine or vaccine,
(C) whether a plausible biologic mechanism or other evidence of a causal relationship exists between exposure to the agent, hazard, or medicine or vaccine and the illness.

It should be noted that the charge to IOM was not to determine whether a unique Gulf War syndrome exists or to make judgments about whether veterans were exposed to the putative agents. Nor was the charge to focus on broader issues, such as the potential costs of compensation for veterans or policy regarding compensation; such decisions are the responsibility of the secretary of veterans affairs.

Evidence of Statistical Association

The committee reviewed the available scientific evidence in the peer-reviewed literature to draw conclusions about associations between the agents of interest and adverse health effects. The committee placed its conclusions in categories that reflect the strength of the evidence of an association (described below). In an effort to determine whether a statistical association between a putative agent and a health outcome exists, the committee adapted categories of association used by the International Agency for Research on Cancer in evaluating evidence of the carcinogenicity of various agents and categories used by numerous other IOM committees.

Determining Increased Risk in Gulf War Veterans

The second part of the committee's charge, as noted in the legislation, is to determine, to the extent permitted by available scientific data, the increased risk of illness among people exposed to the putative agents during service in the Persian Gulf. Generally, to accomplish that task, the committee would have reviewed studies of Gulf War veterans. However, many of the Gulf War veteran studies were hampered by poor measures of exposure to the putative agents, used questionnaires to identify illnesses and exposure to the agents of concern, or did not include outcomes measured with clinical examinations or laboratory tests. The committee therefore based its conclusions primarily on evidence from studies of people exposed to the putative agents in occupational or clinical settings rather than evidence from studies of Persian Gulf veterans. The committee found the evidence from occupational studies adequate for drawing conclusions about associations between the putative agents and health outcomes, but the lack of adequate data on the veterans themselves complicated its consideration of the second part of the charge: determination of increased risk in Gulf War veterans.

To estimate the magnitude of risk of a particular health outcome among Gulf War veterans, the committee would need to compare the rates of disease or other health effects in veterans exposed to the putative agents with the rates in those who were not exposed. That would require information about the specific agents to which individual veterans were exposed and about their doses. However, there is a paucity of data regarding the agents and doses to which individual Gulf War veterans were exposed. Furthermore, to answer questions about increased risk of illnesses in Gulf War veterans, it would be important to know the degree to which any other differences between exposed and nonexposed veterans could influence the rates of disease or other health outcomes; such information on the Gulf War veteran population is lacking.

Because of the lack of various kinds of data on veterans, the committee could not extrapolate from the exposures in the studies that it reviewed to the exposures of Gulf War veterans. Therefore, it could not determine the likelihood of increased risk of adverse health outcomes among Gulf War veterans due to exposure to the agents examined in this report.

Existence of a Plausible Biologic Mechanism or Other Evidence of a Causal Relationship

Toxicologic data form the basis of the committee's response to the third part of its charge: to determine whether there is a plausible biologic mechanism or other evidence of a causal relationship between exposure to a particular agent and a health effect. Although toxicologic studies played a small role in determining the likelihood that an exposure to a specific agent might cause a long-term health outcome, the committee used evidence from toxicologic studies to assess biologic plausibility in support of epidemiologic data.

COMMITTEE'S APPROACH TO ITS CHARGE

Identification and Evaluation of the Literature

The committee began its evaluation by presuming neither the existence nor the absence of associations. It has sought to characterize and weigh the strengths and limitations of the available evidence. The committee's task was not to judge individual cases of particular diseases or conditions or to address questions of causation. Nor did the committee concern itself with policy issues, such as potential costs of compensation, policy regarding compensation, or any broader policy implications of its findings. Additionally, the committee reviewed epidemiologic studies of fuels and combustion products rather than the numerous components of those agents.

Extensive searches of the epidemiologic literature were conducted on the agents identified for study, and over 33,000 potentially relevant references were retrieved. After an assessment of the titles and abstracts of the initial searches, the committee focused on some 800 potentially relevant epidemiologic studies for review and evaluation.

Because only a few studies were related directly to veterans' exposures, the committee reviewed primarily occupational studies of populations that had been exposed to the agents of interest. Those studies often included people whose exposures had been over a lifetime (such as to air pollution in their communities) or included workers employed in a particular industry over many years. In contrast, the exposures of veterans in the Persian Gulf were of relatively short duration with varying intensity. Therefore, the exposures experienced during the Gulf War might only approximate the exposures described in the occupational and environmental literature reviewed in this report. The conclusions of statistical associations based on occupational studies are meant to serve as a guide to potential health effects associated with specific agents.

The committee adopted a policy of using only peer-reviewed published literature as the basis of its conclusions. Publications that were not peer-reviewed had no evidentiary value for the committee; that is, they were not used as evidence for arriving at conclusions about the degree of association between exposure to a particular agent and adverse health effects. The process of peer review by fellow professionals ensures high standards of quality but does not guarantee the validity of a study or the ability to generalize its results. Accordingly, committee members read each study critically and considered its relevance and quality. The committee did not collect original data, nor did it perform any secondary data analysis.

It should be noted that our available scientific tools—toxicology and epidemiology—are inadequate to illuminate clearly the human health effects of individual components of complex mixtures of the type experienced by Gulf War veterans. In many cases, the committee found "inadequate/insufficient evidence of an association" between the exposure of concern and a health outcome; that may have been due to a lack of clear evidence because of the inadequacy of those tools rather than to the absence of effects.

Inclusion Criteria

The committee's next step, after securing the full text of some 800 epidemiologic studies, was to determine which studies would be included in the review as primary or support studies. Therefore, the committee developed inclusion criteria. For a study to be included in the committee's review it had to meet specified criteria, for example, methodologic rigor, identification of class or agent, specificity of health outcome, an exposure assessment, and in some cases, an exposure-free interval. For relevance to the Gulf War veterans, the committee focused on long-term health outcomes that persist after exposure ceases.

Considerations in Assessing the Strength of the Evidence

The committee's process of reaching conclusions about the various agents and their potential for adverse health outcomes was collective and interactive. Once a study was included in the review because it met the committee's criteria, there were several considerations in assessing the strength of an association. They are patterned after those introduced by Hill in 1971 and include strength of the evidence for an association, dose-response relationship, temporal relationship, consistency of association, specificity of association, and biologic plausibility. The committee also considered whether alternative explanations or errors—such as bias, confounding, and chance[1]—might account for the finding of an association.

The committee's final judgment, therefore, is based on a balance between the strength of support of an association and the degree of exclusion of alternatives. The evaluation of evidence to reach conclusions about statistical associations goes beyond quantitative procedures; several stages during the review required thoughtful consideration and judgment and could not always be accomplished by adherence to a prescribed formula.

The approach described here evolved throughout the process of review and was determined in important respects by the nature of the evidence, exposures, and health outcomes being examined. Both quantitative and qualitative aspects of the process were important to the overall review. Ultimately, the conclusions expressed in this report are based on the committee's collective judgment.

CATEGORIES OF ASSOCIATION

The committee classified the evidence of an association between exposure to a specific agent and a specific health outcome into five categories. The categories have been developed by

[1]Chance refers to sampling variability.

previous IOM committees and have been used to evaluate vaccine safety, herbicides used in Vietnam, and indoor pollutants related to asthma.

Sufficient Evidence of a Causal Association

Evidence is sufficient to conclude that there is a causal association between exposure to a specific agent and a specific health outcome in humans. The evidence is supported by experimental data and fulfills the guidelines for sufficient evidence of an association (below). The evidence must be biologically plausible and satisfy several of the guidelines used to assess causality, such as strength of association, dose–response relationship, consistency of association, and temporal relationship.

Sufficient Evidence of an Association

Evidence is sufficient to conclude that there is an association. That is, a consistent association has been observed between exposure to a specific agent and a specific health outcome in human studies in which chance and bias, including confounding, could be ruled out with reasonable confidence. For example, several high-quality[2] studies report consistent associations, and the studies are sufficiently free of bias, including adequate control for confounding.

Limited/Suggestive Evidence of an Association

Evidence is suggestive of an association between exposure to a specific agent and a specific health outcome, but the body of evidence is limited by the inability to rule out chance and bias, including confounding, with confidence. For example, at least one high-quality study reports an association that is sufficiently free of bias, including adequate control for confounding, and other corroborating studies provide support for the association but are not sufficiently free of bias, including confounding. Alternatively, several studies of lower quality show consistent associations, and the results are probably not[3] due to bias, including confounding.

Inadequate/Insufficient Evidence to Determine Whether an Association Exists

Evidence is of insufficient quantity, quality, or consistency to permit a conclusion regarding the existence of an association between exposure to a specific agent and a specific health outcome in humans.

---

[2]Factors used to characterize high-quality studies include the statistical stability of the association, whether a dose-response or other trend was demonstrated, whether the association was among numerous comparisons that were made, and the quality of the assessments of exposure and outcome. Specifically, the quality of exposure assessment refers to specificity and sensitivity in relation to the association of interest. Biologic monitoring data, such as markers of exposure, are theoretically the most preferable but are almost never obtainable in the context of a nonpersistent chemical. Other kinds of efforts can obtain sensitive measures of exposure, such as use of interview techniques that minimize recall bias, an assessment of occupational history by a panel of experts, and estimating exposure intensity independent of health outcome.

[3]Factors used to make this judgment include the data on the relationship between potential confounders and related health end points in a given study, information on subject selection, and classification of exposure.

Limited/Suggestive Evidence of No Association

Evidence is consistent in not showing an association between exposure to a specific agent and a specific health outcome after exposure of any magnitude. A conclusion of no association is inevitably limited to the conditions, magnitudes of exposure, and length of observation in the available studies. The possibility of a very small increase in risk after exposure cannot be excluded.

The committee endeavored to express its judgment as clearly and precisely as the available data allowed, and it used the established categories of association from previous IOM studies because they have gained wide acceptance over more than a decade by Congress, government agencies, researchers, and veterans groups. The five categories describe different degrees of association and sound a recurring theme: the validity of an association is likely to vary with the extent to which the authors reduced common sources of error—chance variation, bias, and confounding—in drawing inferences. Accordingly, the criteria for each category express a degree of confidence based on the extent to which sources of error were reduced.

HUMAN HEALTH OUTCOMES

The committee reviewed numerous epidemiologic studies to arrive at conclusions about association. The committee weighed the strengths and limitations of all the epidemiologic studies and reached its conclusions by interpreting the data in the entire body of reviewed literature. It assigned each health outcome being considered to one of the five categories of association according to the criteria set forth above. The health outcomes that were indicated by the epidemiologic studies were numerous and include cancer, respiratory, cardiovascular, reproductive, and neurologic outcomes. In many cases, the health outcomes described might also result from genetics or lifestyle factors; for example, according to the American Cancer Society, smoking is believed to be responsible for about 80% of lung-cancer cases.

The committee's findings about the strength of the associations between the putative agents and the health outcomes are summarized in Table ES-1.

SUMMARY OF CONCLUSIONS

Although Table ES-1 provides a summary of all the committee's conclusions, the committee wishes to note that the starting point for any health outcome before study is, of course, the category of inadequate or insufficient evidence of an association. Of all the long-term health outcomes on which any evidence was culled from the epidemiologic literature, none was found to be associated in even a limited or suggestive fashion with the uncombusted fuels that veterans may have been exposed to during the Gulf War (with the exception of benzene, a component of fuels, which was reviewed by a previous IOM committee and not reassessed in this report).

The strongest finding was that there is sufficient evidence of an association between combustion products and lung cancer. The committee also found limited or suggestive evidence of an association between combustion-product exposure and cancers at several other sites (oral, nasal, laryngeal, and bladder), incident asthma, and two reproductive outcomes after exposure during pregnancy: preterm birth and low birthweight or intrauterine growth retardation. For the propellant components of Scuds and other missiles used, only hydrazines were found to have a suggestive association with lung cancer.

Finally, it should be repeated that the committee was charged with reviewing the scientific data, not with making recommendations regarding the Department of Veterans Affairs policy; therefore, conclusions are not intended to imply or suggest policy decisions. Furthermore, the conclusions are related to associations between exposure to the agents under study and health outcomes in human populations, not to the likelihood that any one person's health problem is associated with or caused by exposure to the agents.

TABLE ES.1 Summary of Findings Regarding the Association Between Exposure to Fuels, Combustion Products, Hydrazines, and Nitric Acid and Specific Health Outcomes

Sufficient Evidence of a Causal Relationship

Evidence is sufficient to conclude that there is a causal association between exposure to a specific agent and a specific health outcome in humans. The evidence is supported by experimental data and fulfills the guidelines for sufficient evidence of an association (below). The evidence must be biologically plausible and satisfy several of the guidelines used to assess causality, such as: strength of association, dose–response relationship, consistency of association, and a temporal relationship.

- No conclusions

Sufficient Evidence of an Association

Evidence is sufficient to conclude that there is a positive association. That is, a consistent positive association has been observed between exposure to a specific agent and a specific health outcome in human studies in which chance and bias, including confounding, could be ruled out with reasonable confidence. For example, several high-quality studies report consistent positive associations, and the studies are sufficiently free of bias, including adequate control for confounding.

- Combustion products and lung cancer

Limited/Suggestive Evidence of an Association

Evidence is suggestive of an association between exposure to a specific agent and a specific health outcome, but the body of evidence is limited by the inability to rule out chance and bias, including confounding, with confidence. For example, at least one high-quality study reports a positive association that is sufficiently free of bias, including adequate control for confounding. Other corroborating studies provide support for the association, but they were not sufficiently free of bias, including confounding. Alternatively, several studies of lower quality show consistent positive associations, and the results are probably not due to bias, including confounding.

Cancers

- Combustion products and
    - Cancers of the nasal cavity and nasopharynx
    - Cancers of the oral cavity and oropharynx
    - Laryngeal cancer
    - Bladder cancer

- Hydrazines and lung cancer

Reproductive Effects

- Combustion products and
    - Low birthweight/intrauterine growth retardation and exposure during pregnancy
    - Preterm birth and exposure during pregnancy

Respiratory Effects

- Combustion products and incident asthma

Inadequate/Insufficient Evidence

Evidence is of insufficient quantity, quality, or consistency to permit a conclusion regarding the existence of an association between exposure to a specific agent and a specific health outcome in humans.

Cancers

- Fuels and
    - Cancers of the oral cavity and oropharynx
    - Cancers of the nasal cavity and nasopharynx
    - Esophageal cancer
    - Stomach cancer
    - Colon cancer
    - Rectal cancer
    - Hepatic cancer
    - Pancreatic cancer
    - Laryngeal cancer
    - Lung cancer
    - Melanoma
    - Nonmelanoma skin cancer
    - Female breast cancer
    - Male breast cancer
    - Female genital cancers (cervical, endometrial, uterine, and ovarian cancers)
    - Prostatic cancer
    - Testicular cancer
    - Nervous system cancers
    - Kidney cancer
    - Bladder cancer
    - Hodgkin's disease
    - Non-Hodgkin's lymphoma
    - Multiple myeloma
    - Myelodysplastic syndromes
- Combustion products and
    - Esophageal cancer
    - Stomach cancer
    - Colon cancer

    - Rectal cancer
    - Hepatic cancer
    - Pancreatic cancer
    - Melanoma
    - Female breast cancer
    - Male breast cancer
    - Female genital cancers (cervical, endometrial, uterine, and ovarian cancers)
    - Prostatic cancer
    - Testicular cancer
    - Nervous system cancers
    - Ocular melanoma
    - Kidney cancer
    - Non-Hodgkin's lymphoma
    - Hodgkin's disease
    - Multiple myeloma
    - Leukemia
    - Myelodysplastic syndromes
- Hydrazines and
    - Hematopoietic and lymphopoietic cancers
    - Digestive tract cancers
    - Pancreatic cancer
    - Bladder cancer
    - Kidney cancer
- Nitric acid and:
    - Stomach cancer
    - Melanoma
    - Lymphopoietic cancers
    - Pancreatic cancer
    - Laryngeal cancer
    - Lung cancer
    - Bladder cancer
    - Multiple myeloma

Reproductive Effects

- Fuels and adverse reproductive or developmental outcomes (including infertility, spontaneous abortion, childhood leukemia, CNS tumors, neuroblastoma, and Prader-Willi syndrome)
- Combustion products and
    - Preterm births and exposure during any specific time period during pregnancy (for example, the first trimester)
    - Low birth weight and intrauterine growth retardation and exposure before gestation or during any specific period during pregnancy (for example, the first trimester)
    - Specific birth defects, including cardiac effects, and exposure before conception (maternal and paternal) or during early pregnancy (maternal)

- All childhood cancers identified, including acute lymphocytic leukemia, leukemia, neuroblastoma, and brain cancer

Neurologic Effects

- Fuels and
  - Peripheral neuropathy
  - Neurobehavioral effects
  - Multiple Chemical Sensitivity symptoms
- Combustion products and
  - Neurobehavioral effects
  - Posttraumatic stress disorder
  - Nervous system subgroupings (or individual nervous system diseases)
  - Multiple Chemical Sensitivity symptoms

Respiratory Effects

- Fuels and
  - Nonmalignant respiratory disease
  - Chronic bronchitis
  - Asthma
  - Emphysema

- Combustion products and:
  - Chronic bronchitis (less than 1 year of exposure)
  - Emphysema
  - Chronic obstructive pulmonary disease
- Hydrazines and emphysema

Cardiovascular Effects:

- Combustion products and ischemic heart disease or myocardial infarction (less than 2 years of exposure)
- Hydrazines and ischemic heart disease or myocardial infarction
- Nitric acid and cardiovascular diseases

Dermal Effects:

- Fuels and dermatitis—irritant and allergic
- Combustion products and dermatitis—irritant and allergic

Other Health Effects:

- Fuels and sarcoidosis
- Combustion products and sarcoidosis
- Hydrazines and hepatic disease

Limited/Suggestive Evidence of No Association

Evidence is consistent in not showing a positive association between exposure to a specific agent and a specific health outcome after exposure of any magnitude. A conclusion of no association is inevitably limited to the conditions, magnitudes of exposure, and length of observation in the available studies. The possibility of a very small increase in risk after exposure studied cannot be excluded.

- No conclusions

1

INTRODUCTION

The 1991 Persian Gulf War was considered a brief and successful military operation with few injuries and deaths among coalition forces. The returning veterans, however, soon began reporting numerous health problems that they believed to be associated with their service in the gulf. Many Gulf War veterans returned to normal activities, but a large number have had a wide array of unexplained illnesses.

In response to the growing concerns of ill Gulf War veterans, Congress passed two laws in 1998: PL 105-277, the Persian Gulf War Veterans Act, and PL 105-368, the Veterans Programs Enhancement Act. Those laws directed the secretary of veterans affairs to enter into a contract with the National Academy of Sciences (NAS) to review and evaluate the scientific and medical literature regarding associations between illness and exposure to toxic agents, environmental or wartime hazards, or preventive medicines or vaccines associated with Gulf War service and to consider the NAS conclusions when making decisions about compensation. The study was assigned to the Institute of Medicine (IOM).

The Persian Gulf War legislation directs IOM to study a wide array of diverse biologic, chemical, and physical agents (Box 1.1). Exposures to most of the Gulf War agents have been extensively studied and characterized, primarily in occupational settings (for example, exposure to pesticides, solvents, and fuels) but others have not been as well studied and characterized in human populations (for example, exposure to nerve agents and vaccines).

Given the large number of agents to study, IOM divided the task into several reviews. It has completed two reviews: *Gulf War and Health, Volume 1: Depleted Uranium, Pyridostigmine Bromide, Sarin, Vaccines* (IOM 2000) and *Gulf War and Health, Volume 2: Insecticides and Solvents* (IOM 2003). The conclusions of the first two reports are presented in Appendix A. The current volume examines the health effects of fuels, combustion products, hydrazines, and nitric acid. Those broad categories include the agents listed in the legislation (for example, hydrogen sulfide, oil-fire byproducts, and diesel-heater fumes).

BOX 1.1
Agents Specified in PL 105-368 and PL 105-277

(A) The following organophosphorous pesticides:
- (i) Chlorpyrifos.
- (ii) Diazinon.
- (iii) Dichlorvos.
- (iv) Malathion.

(B) The following carbamate pesticides:
- (i) Proxpur.
- (ii) Carbaryl.
- (iii) Methomyl.

(C) The carbamate pyridostigmine bromide used as nerve agent prophylaxis.

(D) The following chlorinated hydrocarbons and other pesticides and repellents:
- (i) Lindane.
- (ii) Pyrethrins.
- (iii) Permethrins.
- (iv) Rodenticides (bait).
- (v) Repellent (DEET).

(E) The following low-level nerve agents and precursor compounds at exposure levels below those which produce immediately apparent incapacitating symptoms:
- (i) Sarin.
- (ii) Tabun.

(F) The following synthetic chemical compounds:
- (i) Mustard agents at levels below those which cause immediate blistering.
- (ii) Volatile organic compounds.
- (iii) Hydrazine.
- (iv) Red fuming nitric acid.
- (v) Solvents.

(G) The following sources of radiation:
- (i) Depleted uranium.
- (ii) Microwave radiation.
- (iii) Radio frequency radiation.

(H) The following environmental particulates and pollutants:
- (i) Hydrogen sulfide.
- (ii) Oil fire byproducts.
- (iii) Diesel heater fumes.
- (iv) Sand micro-particles.

(I) Diseases endemic to the region (including the following):
- (i) Leishmaniasis.
- (ii) Sandfly fever.
- (iii) Pathogenic escherichia coli.
- (iv) Shigellosis.

(J) Time compressed administration of multiple live, ''attenuated,'' and toxoid vaccines.

SCOPE OF THIS VOLUME

After the 1991 Gulf War, deployed veterans began to report more symptoms than their nondeployed counterparts according to numerous population-based studies from the United States (Iowa Persian Gulf Study Group 1997; Kang et al. 2000), United Kingdom (Cherry et al.

2001; Unwin et al. 1999), Canada (Goss Gilroy Inc. 1998), and Denmark (Suadicani et al. 1999). Among the most common symptoms were fatigue, rash, headache, pain, and memory complaints. Symptoms often grouped together into clusters, which were characterized as "unexplained illnesses" because they did not fit any established medical diagnoses. Some 20-25% of deployed veterans reported symptom clusters—a rate 2 or 3 times that in nondeployed military personnel. The symptom clusters were associated with disability and poorer quality of life. But the deployed veterans did not appear to have higher rates of hospitalization or mortality, than veterans not deployed to the Persian Gulf.

The search for causes of veterans' symptoms has produced a large body of published studies. Exposures to numerous agents during the Gulf War (see Box 1.1) have been analyzed in relation to veterans' symptoms. This volume, however, will examine health outcomes only as related to exposure to fuels, combustion products, hydrazines, and nitric acid. The various ways that the veterans might have been exposed to those agents are discussed briefly below and described in more detail in Chapters 3 and 9.

During the 1991 Persian Gulf War, the Iraqis used Scud missiles that contained inhibited red fuming nitric acid (IRFNA), a highly corrosive oxidizing agent in liquid rocket fuel. It is believed that veterans might have been exposed to IRFNA when they disarmed or disposed of weapons or were downwind of the breakup, impact, or interception of a Scud. Hydrazine was probably not used in the Scuds, but it remains an agent of interest (Chapter 9).

The most visually dramatic environmental event of the Gulf War was the smoke from more than 600 oil-well fires. Veterans were probably exposed through air pollution as smoke plumes rose and combined to form giant plumes that could be seen for hundreds of kilometers. There were other potential sources of exposure to petroleum-based products, such as gasoline, kerosene, and diesel fuels used in unvented tent heaters, cooking stoves, and portable generators. Petroleum products, including diesel fuels, were used to suppress sand and dust, and petroleum fuels were used for burning waste and trash.

In light of those conditions, the committee used its collective judgment in choosing studies and occupations that it believed were most representative of the environmental exposures experienced by veterans in the Persian Gulf. The committee reviewed hundreds of studies to arrive at its conclusions about association between exposures and specific health outcomes. The committee reviewed epidemiologic studies of fuels and combustion products rather than the numerous components of those agents. Its review included all relevant experimental and epidemiologic studies. As noted above, because only a few studies were related directly to veterans' exposures, the committee reviewed occupational, environmental, and clinical studies of populations that had been exposed to the agents of interest. Those studies often included people whose exposure was over a lifetime (such as in community air pollution studies) or included workers employed in a particular industry over many years. In contrast, the exposures experienced by veterans in the Persian Gulf were relatively short although the intensity might vary from occupational exposures. Therefore, the exposures experienced in the gulf might only approximate exposures described in the occupational literature used in this report.

CHARGE TO THE COMMITTEE

In accordance with PL 105-368 and PL 105-277, IOM appointed the Committee on Gulf War and Health: Literature Review of Selected Environmental Particulates, Pollutants, and Synthetic Chemical Compounds, which was asked to assess the following for associations between illness and each agent, hazard, or medicine or vaccine to the extent that available scientific data permit meaningful determinations:

(A) whether a statistical association exists between exposure to the agent, hazard, or medicine or vaccine and the illness, taking into account the strength of the scientific evidence and the appropriateness of the scientific methodology used to detect the association;

(B) the increased risk of the illness among human or animal populations exposed to the agent, hazard, or medicine or vaccine; and

(C) whether a plausible biological mechanism or other evidence of a causal relationship exists between exposure to the agent, hazard, or medicine or vaccine and the illness.

The legislation did not provide the IOM committee with a list of illnesses suspected to be associated with exposure to the numerous agents in the Persian Gulf. The IOM staff and committee members developed such a list on the basis of the diseases and conditions that had been mentioned in the scientific literature that came to their attention through extensive literature searches, as described in Chapter 2.

It should be noted that the charge to IOM was not to determine whether a unique Gulf War syndrome exists or to make judgments regarding whether veterans were exposed to the putative agents. Nor was the charge to focus on broader issues, such as the potential costs of compensation for veterans or policy regarding such compensation; such decisions are the responsibility of the secretary of veterans affairs.

COMMITTEE'S APPROACH TO ITS CHARGE

Specific details of how the committee approached its charge and the methods it used in reaching conclusions are discussed in Chapter 2. However, a brief overview is presented here.

Evidence of Statistical Association

The committee reviewed the available scientific evidence in the peer-reviewed literature to draw conclusions about associations between the agents of interest and adverse health effects. The committee placed its conclusions in categories that reflect the strength of the evidence of an association. In an effort to determine whether a statistical association between the putative agent and a health outcome exists, the committee adapted categories of association used by the International Agency for Research on Cancer in evaluating evidence of the carcinogenicity of various agents and categories used by numerous other IOM committees. The categories and the criteria for assigning a particular health outcome to a category are described in Chapter 2. It should be noted that the categories described are related to associations between exposure to agents and health outcomes in human populations, primarily from occupational studies, not to the likelihood that any individual's illnesses are associated with a given agent.

Determining Increased Risk in Gulf War Veterans

The second part of the committee's charge is to determine, to the extent permitted by available scientific data, the increased risk of illness among people exposed to the putative agents during service in the Persian Gulf. Generally, to accomplish that task, the committee would have reviewed studies of Gulf War veterans. However, many of the Gulf War veteran studies were hampered by poor measures of exposure to the putative agents, used questionnaires to identify illnesses and exposure to the agents of concern, or did not include outcomes measured with actual clinical examinations or laboratory tests. The committee therefore based its conclusions primarily on evidence from studies of people exposed to the putative agents in occupational or clinical settings rather than from studies of Persian Gulf veterans. The committee found the evidence from occupational studies sufficient for drawing conclusions about associations between the putative agents and health outcomes, but the lack of adequate data on the veterans themselves complicated its consideration of the second part of the charge determination of increased risk in Gulf War veterans.

To estimate the magnitude of risk of a particular health outcome among Gulf War veterans, the committee would need to compare the rates of health effects or disease in veterans exposed to the putative agents with the rates in those who were not exposed. That would require information about the specific agents to which individual veterans were exposed and about their doses. However, there is a paucity of data regarding the agents and doses to which individual Gulf War veterans were exposed. Furthermore, to answer questions about increased risk of illnesses in Gulf War veterans, it would be important to know the degree to which any other differences between exposed and nonexposed veterans could influence the rates of health outcomes or diseases; such information in the Gulf War veteran population is lacking. Because of the lack of various kinds of data on veterans, the committee could not extrapolate from the exposures in the studies that it reviewed to the exposures of Gulf War veterans. Therefore, it could not determine the likelihood of increased risk of adverse health outcomes among Gulf War veterans due to exposure to the agents examined in this report.

Existence of a Plausible Biologic Mechanism or Other Evidence of a Causal Relationship

Toxicologic data form the basis of the committee's response to the third part of its charge—to determine whether there is a plausible biologic mechanism or other evidence of a causal relationship between exposure to a particular agent and a health effect. That information is summarized in general terms in Chapter 3. Specific toxicologic findings related to each health outcome are also given in the chapters that review the epidemiologic literature (Chapters 4-9).

ORGANIZATION OF THE REPORT

Chapter 2 discusses the considerations that guided the committee's review and evaluation of the scientific evidence and the criteria that it established to draw conclusions of association. Chapter 3 provides background information on fuels and combustion products, discusses how the veterans might have been exposed to those agents, and provides an overview of their toxicology. In Chapters 4 through 8 the committee presents its review of epidemiologic studies that identify health outcomes related to exposure to the putative agents and provide conclusions about those associations. Specifically, Chapter 4 discusses cancer; Chapter 5 examines respiratory outcomes; Chapter 6 presents the committee's findings with respect to cardiovascular outcomes; Chapter 7 reviews reproductive and developmental outcomes, including childhood cancers; and Chapter 8 presents remaining health outcomes, such as neurologic and dermatologic findings. Finally, Chapter 9 is organized differently from the previous five chapters in that all the health outcomes related to exposure to missile propellants—hydrazines and red fuming nitric acid—are presented.

Additionally, Chapter 9 discusses how veterans might have been exposed to those propellants and presents an overview of the their toxicology.

Appendix A provides the conclusions from the first two Gulf War reports. Appendix B provides details of the committee's search strategy of the peer-reviewed medical and scientific literature. The types of studies reviewed by the committee and comments about the nature of the Gulf War studies are discussed in Appendix C. Descriptive tables of the cohort and case-control studies included in the cancer chapter may be found in Appendix D.

REFERENCES

Cherry N, Creed F, Silman A, Dunn G, Baxter D, Smedley J, Taylor S, Macfarlane GJ. 2001. Health and exposures of United Kingdom Gulf War veterans. Part I: The pattern and extent of ill health. *Occupational and Environmental Medicine* 58(5):291-298.

Goss Gilroy Inc. 1998. *Health Study of Canadian Forces Personnel Involved in the 1991 Conflict in the Persian Gulf.* Ottawa, Canada: Goss Gilroy Inc., Department of National Defence.

IOM (Institute of Medicine). 2000. *Gulf War and Health, Volume 1: Depleted Uranium, Sarin, Pyridostigmine Bromide, Vaccines.* Washington, DC: National Academy Press.

IOM. 2003. *Gulf War and Health, Volume 2: Insecticides and Solvents.* Washington, DC: The National Academies Press.

Iowa Persian Gulf Study Group. 1997. Self-reported illness and health status among Gulf War veterans. A population-based study. The Iowa Persian Gulf Study Group. *Journal of the American Medical Association* 277(3):238-245.

Kang HK, Mahan CM, Lee KY, Magee CA, Murphy FM. 2000. Illnesses among United States veterans of the Gulf War: A population-based survey of 30,000 veterans. *Journal of Occupational and Environmental Medicine* 42(5):491-501.

Suadicani P, Ishoy T, Guldager B, Appleyard M, Gyntelberg F. 1999. Determinants of long-term neuropsychological symptoms: The Danish Gulf War Study. *Danish Medical Bulletin* 46(5):423-427.

Unwin C, Blatchley N, Coker W, Ferry S, Hotopf M, Hull L, Ismail K, Palmer I, David A, Wessely S. 1999. Health of UK servicemen who served in Persian Gulf War. *Lancet* 353:169-178.

2

CONSIDERATIONS IN IDENTIFYING AND EVALUATING THE LITERATURE

This chapter presents the committee's approach to identifying the literature for review and its considerations in evaluating the strength of evidence presented in that literature. It provides information about the types of literature the committee identified how the committee assessed the strength of the evidence, and the categories of association that the committee used to summarize its findings. The committee's approach was similar to that used in *Gulf War and Health, Volume 1: Depleted Uranium, Pyridostigmine Bromide, Sarin, and Vaccines* and *Gulf War and Health, Volume 2: Insecticides and Solvents* (IOM 2000b, 2003a). For each agent under consideration, the committee determined, to the extent that available published scientific data permitted, the strength of the evidence of associations between exposure to the agent and adverse health outcomes. The committee reviewed available epidemiologic studies of Gulf War veterans and epidemiologic studies of other populations known to have been exposed to the agents of concern.

As discussed in Chapter 1, the committee was charged with summarizing the strength of the scientific evidence regarding exposure to the putative agents and illnesses suspected to be associated with them. The legislation (PL 105-277 and PL 105-368) that directs the committee's work did not provide a specific list of diseases or illnesses for study; the diseases and illnesses discussed in the report were those dealt with in the scientific and medical literature reviewed. As the searches were conducted on the agents of concern, the studies found identified the health outcomes for review.

The committee began its evaluation by presuming neither the existence nor the absence of associations. It has sought to characterize and weigh the strengths and limitations of the available evidence. The committee's task was not to judge individual cases of particular diseases or conditions or to address questions of causation. Nor did the committee concern itself with policy issues, such as potential cost of compensation, policy regarding compensation, or any broader policy implications of its findings.

IDENTIFICATION OF THE LITERATURE

The committee's first step was to identify the literature it would review. It began its work by overseeing extensive searches of the peer-reviewed medical and scientific literature (Appendix B). It identified epidemiologic studies of persistent health outcomes associated with exposure to hydrazines, red fuming nitric acid, hydrogen sulfide, oil-fire byproducts, and diesel-heater fumes, as directed by PL 105-277 and PL 105-368. At the request of the Department of Veterans Affairs, the committee also identified epidemiologic studies on persistent health outcomes associated with exposure to fuels (for example, jet fuel and gasoline) used during the Gulf War.

The searches retrieved over 33,000 potentially relevant references. All searches were completed early in 2004; relevant studies published later will be reviewed by future IOM committees. After an assessment of the titles and abstracts in the results of the initial searches, the committee focused on some 800 potentially relevant epidemiologic studies for review and evaluation. The committee reviewed epidemiologic studies of fuels and combustion products rather than the numerous components of those agents. Those studies were assessed for evidence of associations between the agents of interest and persistent health outcomes in humans. The committee used its collective judgment in selecting studies thought to reflect the types of exposures that Gulf War veterans might have experienced. Although Gulf War veterans were exposed to multiple complex mixtures, epidemiologic studies are not typically designed to address such types of exposures.

Because only a few studies were related directly to veterans' exposures, the committee reviewed primarily occupational studies of populations that had been exposed to the agents of interest. Those studies often included people whose exposures had been over a lifetime (such as exposure to air pollution in their communities) or workers employed in particular industries over many years. In contrast, the exposures of veterans in the Persian Gulf were of relatively short duration with varying degrees of intensity. Therefore, the exposures experienced during the Gulf War might only approximate the exposures described in the occupational literature reviewed in this report. The conclusions as to statistical associations based on occupational and other types of studies are meant to serve as a guide to potential health effects associated with specific agents.

The committee adopted a policy of using only peer-reviewed published literature as the basis of its conclusions. Publications that were not peer-reviewed had no evidentiary value for the committee; that is, they were not used as evidence for arriving at conclusions about the degree of association between exposure to a particular agent and adverse health effects. The process of peer review by fellow professionals, which is one of the hallmarks of modern science, ensures high standards of quality but does not guarantee the validity of a study or the ability to generalize results. Accordingly, committee members read each study critically and considered its relevance and quality. In some instances, non-peer-reviewed publications provided background information for the committee and raised issues that required further literature searches. The committee did not collect original data, nor did it perform any secondary data analysis.

With that orientation to the committee's task, the following sections provide a brief discussion of the value of epidemiologic studies, the committee's inclusion criteria for review of those studies, considerations in evaluating the evidence or data provided by the studies, and the categories of association that are used to draw conclusions about the strength of the evidence presented in the studies.

EPIDEMIOLOGIC STUDIES

Epidemiology deals with the study of the determinants, frequency, and distribution of disease in human populations. A focus on populations distinguishes epidemiology from medical disciplines that focus on the individual. Epidemiologic studies examine the relationship between exposures to agents of interest in a studied population and the development of health outcomes, so they can be used to generate hypotheses for study or to test hypotheses posed by investigators.

Epidemiologic studies can establish statistical associations between exposure to specific agents and health effects, and associations are generally estimated by using relative risks or odds ratios. To conclude that an association exists, it is necessary for exposure to an agent to be followed by the health outcome more frequently than it would be expected to by chance alone. Furthermore, it is almost always necessary to find that the effect occurs consistently in several studies. Epidemiologists seldom consider a single study sufficient to establish an association; rather, it is desirable to replicate the findings in other studies to draw conclusions about the association. Results of separate studies are sometimes conflicting. It is sometimes possible to attribute discordant study results to such characteristics as soundness of study design, quality of execution, and the influence of different forms of bias. Studies that result in a statistically precise measure of association suggest that the observed result was unlikely to be due to chance. When the measure of association does not show a statistically precise effect, it is important to consider the size of the sample and whether the study had the power to detect an effect of a given size.

Epidemiologic study designs differ in their ability to provide valid estimates of an association (Ellwood 1998). Randomized controlled trials on comparable populations yield the most robust type of evidence; cohort or case-control studies are more susceptible to bias. Cross-sectional studies generally provide a lower level of evidence than cohort and case-control studies (Appendix C). Determining whether a given statistical association rises to the level of causation requires inference (Hill 1965). As discussed by the International Agency for Research on Cancer in the preamble of its monographs evaluating cancer risks (for example, IARC 2004), a strong association in an epidemiologic study is demonstrated by the observed association in a number of different studies, an increased risk of disease with increasing exposure or a decline in risk after cessation of exposure, and specificity of an effect. Those characteristics all strengthen the likelihood that an association seen in an epidemiologic study is a causal effect. Inferences from epidemiologic studies, however, are often limited to population or ecologic associations because of a lack of individual exposure information. Exposures might not be controlled in epidemiologic studies, and in some cases there is large uncertainty in the assessment of exposure. To assess explanations other than causality, one must bring together evidence from different studies and apply well-established criteria, which have been refined over more than a century (Evans 1976; Hill 1965; Susser 1973, 1977, 1988, 1991; Wegman et al. 1997). For a recent discussion of those criteria, a discussion is offered in the 2004 report of the US Surgeon General (Office of the Surgeon General-HHS 2004). The strengths and limitations of the various epidemiologic designs, the issues to be considered in assessing epidemiologic studies, and the outcomes measured in the studies are discussed in Appendix C.

By examining numerous epidemiologic studies, the committee addressed the question, "Does the available evidence support a causal relationship or an association between exposure to a specific agent and a health outcome?" An association between a specific agent and a specific health outcome does not mean that exposure to the agent invariably results in the health outcome or that all cases of the outcome result from exposure. Such complete correspondence between agent and disease is the exception in large populations (IOM 1994b). The committee evaluated the data and based its conclusions on the strength and coherence of the data in the selected epidemiologic studies that met its inclusion criteria.

INCLUSION CRITERIA

The committee's next step, after securing the full text of about 800 epidemiologic studies, was to determine which studies would be included in the review as primary or support studies. For a study to be included in the committee's review, it had to meet these criteria: methodologic rigor, identification of class or agent, specificity of health outcome, an exposure assessment, and in some cases an exposure-free interval. Studies that met the committee's criteria are referred to as *primary* studies. For relevance to the Gulf War veterans, the committee focused on long-term health outcomes that persist after exposure ceases.

Methodologic Rigor

The study had to be a published in a peer-reviewed journal, had to include details of its methodology, had to include a control or reference group, had to have the statistical power to detect effects, and had to include reasonable adjustment for confounders. Case studies and case series were generally excluded from the committee's consideration (see Appendix C).

Identification of Class or Agent

The study had to identify fuels, combustion products, or propellants as specified in the legislation. Because it is more difficult to draw conclusions on specific agents in studies of multiple chemical exposures, studies of this type were not considered *primary*. If agents were not specifically identified, the study would have been included if it was of an occupation that involved a fuel or combustion product exposure similar to veterans' presumed exposures in the Persian Gulf.

Specificity of Outcome

The study had to specify a distinct outcome rather than a nonspecific group of health outcomes. Studies of broad disease categories (for example, diseases of the nervous system) were not considered as *primary* studies. Lack of specificity occurs primarily in mortality studies that examine all-cause mortality (such as deaths from all nervous system diseases) as opposed to cause-specific mortality (such as from Parkinson's disease). All-cause mortality studies were excluded unless they analyzed specific health outcomes.

Exposure Assessment and Exposure-free Interval for Reversible Effects

The committee preferred studies that had an independent assessment of exposure rather than self-reported exposure. For example, studies that used assessment by an industrial hygienist or with a job-exposure matrix (JEM) were weighted more heavily by the committee.

To be relevant to Gulf War veterans, a study had to examine long-term rather than short-term outcomes. For some outcomes (for example, dermatologic, neurologic, and respiratory), long-term effects can be determined only after an exposure-free interval of weeks to months before evaluation of study subjects. The committee required an exposure-free interval specifically for effects that might be reversible (such as headache, light-headedness, poor coordination, rash, or cough) but not for irreversible effects (such as cancer).

The committee gave less weight to ecologic or toxicologic studies. Toxicologic studies had a small role in the committee's assessment of association between the putative agents and health outcomes. Like previous committees, this one used evidence from toxicologic studies to assess biologic plausibility in support of epidemiologic data rather than as part of the weight of evidence to determine the likelihood that an exposure to a specific agent causes a long-term outcome. That is because toxicologic studies can inform about disease processes (for example, cancer) but are less informative about specific diseases (for example, esophageal cancer).

Support Studies

Studies that the committee might exclude or consider as *support* (that is, they carry less weight than primary studies) are studies of self-reported exposure, multiple exposure, or exposure to specific agents that cannot be assessed; studies whose outcomes are considered "subclinical" (that is, of altered functioning consistent with later development of a diagnosis but without clear predictive validity); studies with a lack of specificity of outcomes (for example, those with a broad range of International Classification of Disease (ICD) codes that refer to all diseases of the respiratory or nervous system); and studies without an exposure-free interval for reversible effects.

CONSIDERATIONS IN ASSESSING THE STRENGTH OF EVIDENCE

The committee's process of reaching conclusions about the various agents and their potential for adverse health outcomes was collective and interactive. Once a study was included in this review because it met the committee's criteria, there were several considerations in assessing the strength of associations. They were patterned after those introduced by Hill (1971) and include strength of the evidence of an association, presence of a dose-response relationship, presence of a temporal relationship, consistency of the association; specificity of the association; and biologic plausibility.

Strength of Evidence of an Association

The strength of an association is usually expressed as the magnitude of the measure of effect, for example, relative risk or odds ratio. Generally, the higher the relative risk, the greater the likelihood that the exposure-disease association is causal and the lower the likelihood that it is due to undetected error, bias, or confounding (discussed below). Measures of statistical significance, such as p values, are not indicators of the strength of an association. Small increases in relative risks that are consistent among studies, however, might be evidence of an association, and some forms of extreme bias or confounding can produce a high relative risk. The statistical power of a study was important for it had to be able to detect effects of a certain magnitude, especially important for negative results.

Thus, studies were evaluated for their rigor and analyses. Greater weight was given to studies that were conducted in a manner that reduced sources of error, bias, and confounding. More weight was given to studies in which there was independent assessment of exposure, either based on knowledge of a specific industry; if specific exposures were associated with an occupational title or industry, such as when a JEM was used to categorize exposure; or if an assessment was made by an industrial hygienist. Studies that had self-reported exposures were considered, at best, support studies.

Dose-Response Relationship

The existence of a dose-response relationship—that is, an increased strength of association with increasing intensity or duration of exposure or other appropriate relation—strengthens an inference that an association is real. However, the lack of an apparent dose-response relationship does not rule out an association, as in the case of a threshold exposure beyond which the relative risk of disease remains constant and high. If the *relative* degree of exposure among several studies can be determined, indirect evidence of a dose-response relationship may exist. For example, if studies of presumably low-exposure cohorts show only mild increases in risk whereas studies of presumably high-exposure cohorts show larger increases in risk, the pattern would be consistent with a dose-response relationship.

Temporal Relationship

If an observed association is real, exposure must precede the onset of disease by at least the duration of disease induction. The committee considered whether a disease occurred within a period after exposure to the putative agent that was consistent with current understanding of the natural history of the disease. The committee interpreted the lack of an appropriate time sequence as evidence against association but recognized that insufficient knowledge about the natural history and pathogenesis of many of the diseases under review limited the utility of this consideration.

Consistency of Association

A consistent association requires that the association be found regularly in a variety of studies, for example, in more than one study population and with different study methods. However, consistency alone is not sufficient evidence of an association. The committee considered findings that were consistent in direction among different categories of studies to be supportive of an association. It did not require exactly the same magnitude of association in different populations to conclude that there was a consistent association. A consistent association could occur when the results of most studies were positive and the differences in measured effects were within the range expected on the basis of sampling error, selection bias, misclassification, confounding, and differences in dose.

Thus, for a health outcome to be considered associated with an agent there had to be corroboration, that is, replication of findings among studies and populations and under relevant conditions. The degree to which an effect could be consistently reproduced gave the committee confidence that they were observing a true effect.

Specificity of Association

Specificity of association is the degree to which exposure to a given agent predicts the frequency or magnitude of a particular outcome. A positive finding seems more strongly supported when the association between the exposure and the health outcome is specific to both than when the association is nonspecific to the exposure or the health outcome. The committee recognized, however, that perfect specificity could not be expected, given the multifactorial etiology of many of the diseases under examination. The committee also recognized the possibility that many of the agents under study were associated with a broad array of diseases.

The committee members did, however, require that specific outcomes be identified. Studies that provided general outcomes (for example, diseases of the nervous system) or outcomes identified by broad ranges of ICD codes (for example, codes referring to all diseases of the respiratory system) were considered, at best, supportive of an outcome.

Biologic Plausibility

Biologic plausibility reflects knowledge of the biologic mechanism by which an agent can lead to a health outcome. That knowledge comes through mechanism-of-action or other studies in pharmacology, toxicology, microbiology, physiology, and other fields—typically in studies of animals. Biologic plausibility is often difficult to establish or may not be known when an association is first documented. The committee considered such factors as evidence from animal and human studies that exposure to an agent is associated with diseases known to have biologic mechanisms similar to that of the disease in question, evidence that some outcomes are commonly associated with occupational or environmental exposures, and knowledge of routes of exposure, storage in the body, and excretion that suggest that a disease is more likely to occur in some organs than in others. Biologic plausibility was required by the committee only in drawing a conclusion of "sufficient evidence of a causal association" (see below); for the other categories of association, it is not necessary to demonstrate a biologically plausible mechanism. The extent to which all the data are consistent and subject to a biologically plausible mechanism influences the weight attached to the results of a study, as does an indication that the mechanism is similar in the animal(s) under study and humans.

Additional Considerations

The committee carefully considered whether alternative explanations or errors—such as bias and chance—might account for the finding of an association.

Bias

Bias refers to systematic or nonrandom error. Bias causes an observed value to deviate from the true value. It can weaken an association or generate a spurious association. Because all studies are susceptible to bias, a goal is to minimize bias or to adjust the observed value of an association by using special methods to correct for bias. Three kinds of bias may compromise the results of an investigation: selection bias, information bias, and confounding.

- *Selection bias* occurs when the participants in a study are not representative of the general population. The study participants differ from nonparticipants in characteristics that cannot be observed, that is, the groups differ in measured or unmeasured baseline characteristics because of how participants were selected or assigned.
- *Information bias* results from the manner in which data are collected and can result in measurement errors, imprecise measurement, and misdiagnosis. Those types of errors may be uniform in an entire study population or may affect some parts of the population more than others. Bias may result from misclassification of study subjects with respect to the outcome

variable. Other common sources of information bias are the inability of study subjects to recall accurately the circumstances of their exposure (recall bias) and the likelihood that one group more frequently reports what it remembers than another group (reporting bias). Information bias is especially harmful in interpreting study results when it affects one comparison group more than another.

- *Confounding* occurs when a variable or characteristic otherwise known to be predictive of the outcome can account for part or all of an apparent association. A confounding variable is an uncontrolled variable that influences the outcome of a study to an unknown extent, making precise evaluation of the effects of the independent variable impossible. Carefully applied statistical adjustments can often control for or reduce the influence of a confounder.

Chance

Chance is a type of error that can lead to an apparent association between an exposure to an agent and a health effect when none is present. An apparent effect of an agent on a health outcome may be the result of random variation due to sampling in assembly of the study population rather than the result of exposure to the agent under study. Standard methods that use confidence intervals, for example, allow one to assess the role of chance variation due to sampling.

Thus, the committee's final judgment is based on a balance between the strength of support of an association and the degree of exclusion of alternatives. The evaluation of evidence to reach conclusions about statistical associations goes beyond quantitative procedures, and several stages during the review required thoughtful consideration and judgment and could not always be accomplished by adherence to a prescribed formula.

The approach described here evolved throughout the process of review and was determined in important respects by the nature of the evidence, exposures, and health outcomes being examined. Both quantitative and qualitative aspects of the process were important to the overall review. Ultimately, the conclusions expressed in this report about causation are based on the committee's collective judgment.

CATEGORIES OF ASSOCIATION

The committee classified the evidence of an association between exposure to a specific agent and a specific health outcome in five categories. The categories have been developed by previous IOM committees and also have been used to evaluate vaccine safety (IOM 1991 1994a), herbicides used in Vietnam (IOM 1994b, 1996, 1999, 2001, 2003b), and indoor pollutants related to asthma (IOM 2000a).

Sufficient Evidence of a Causal Association

Evidence is sufficient to conclude that there is a causal association between exposure to a specific agent and a specific health outcome in humans. The evidence is supported by experimental data and fulfills the guidelines for sufficient evidence of an association (below). The evidence must be biologically plausible and satisfy several of the guidelines used to assess causality, such as strength of association, dose-response relationship, consistency of association, and temporal relationship.

Sufficient Evidence of an Association

Evidence is sufficient to conclude that there is an association. That is, a consistent association has been observed between exposure to a specific agent and a specific health outcome in human studies in which chance and bias, including confounding, could be ruled out with reasonable confidence. For example, several high-quality[1] studies report consistent positive associations, and the studies are sufficiently free of bias, and have adequate control for confounding.

Limited/Suggestive Evidence of an Association

Evidence is suggestive of an association between exposure to a specific agent and a specific health outcome, but the body of evidence is limited by the inability to rule out chance and bias, including confounding, with confidence. For example, at least one high-quality study reports a positive association that is sufficiently free of bias, and has adequate control for confounding. Other corroborating studies provide support for the association, but they were not sufficiently free of bias, including confounding. Alternatively, several studies of lower quality show consistent positive associations, and the results are probably not[2] due to bias, including confounding.

Inadequate/Insufficient Evidence to Determine Whether an Association Exists

Evidence is of insufficient quantity, quality, or consistency to permit a conclusion regarding the existence of an association between exposure to a specific agent and a specific health outcome in humans.

Limited/Suggestive Evidence of No Association

Evidence is consistent in not showing a positive association between exposure to a specific agent and a specific health outcome after exposure of any magnitude. A conclusion of no association is inevitably limited to the conditions, magnitudes of exposure, and length of observation in the available studies. The possibility of a very small increase in risk after the exposure studied cannot be excluded.

The committee endeavored to express its judgment as clearly and precisely as the available data allowed, and it used the established categories of association from previous IOM studies because they have gained wide acceptance over more than a decade by Congress, government agencies, researchers, and veterans groups. The five categories describe different levels of association and sound a recurring theme: the validity of an association is likely to vary

---

[1]Factors used to characterize high-quality studies include the statistical stability of the association, whether a dose–response or other trend was demonstrated, whether the association was among numerous comparisons that were made, and the quality of the assessments of exposure and outcome. Quality of exposure assessment refers to specificity and sensitivity in relation to the association of interest. Biologic monitoring data are theoretically the most preferable—such as markers of exposure—but are almost never obtainable in the context of a nonpersistent chemical. Other kinds of efforts can obtain sensitive measures of exposure, such as use of interview techniques that minimize recall bias, an assessment of occupational history by a panel of experts, and estimating exposure intensity independently of health outcome.

[2]Factors used to make this judgment include the data on the relationship between potential confounders and related health end points in a given study, information on subject selection, and classification of exposure.

with the extent to which the authors reduced common sources of error—chance variation and bias, including confounding—in drawing inferences. Accordingly, the criteria for each category express a degree of confidence based on the extent to which sources of error were reduced.

REFERENCES

Ellwood JM. 1998. *Critical Appraisal of Epidemiological Studies and Clinical Trials.* 2nd Edition. Oxford: Oxford University Press.

Evans A. 1976. Causation and disease: The Henle-Koch postulates revisited. *Yale Journal of Biology and Medicine* 49(2):175-195.

Hill A. 1965. The environment and disease: Association or causation? *Proceedings of the Royal Society of Medicine* 58:295-300.

Hill A. 1971. *Principles of Medical Statistics*. New York: Oxford University Press.

IARC (International Agency for Research Cancer). 2004. *Tobacco Smoke and Involuntary Smoking. IARC Monographs on the Evaluation of Carcinogenic Risks to Humans.* 83. Lyon, France: International Agency for Research on Cancer.

IOM (Institute of Medicine). 1991. *Adverse Effects of Pertussis and Rubella Vaccines*. Washington, DC: National Academy Press.

IOM. 1994a. *Adverse Events Associated with Childhood Vaccines: Evidence Bearing on Causality.* Washington, DC: National Academy Press.

IOM. 1994b. *Veterans and Agent Orange: Health Effects of Herbicides Used in Vietnam.* Washington, DC: National Academy Press.

IOM. 1996. *Veterans and Agent Orange: Update 1996.* Washington, DC: National Academy Press.

IOM. 1999. *Veterans and Agent Orange: Update 1998.* Washington, DC: National Academy Press.

IOM. 2000a. *Clearing the Air: Asthma and Indoor Air Exposures.* Washington, DC: National Academy Press.

IOM. 2000b. *Gulf War and Health, Volume 1: Depleted Uranium, Sarin, Pyridostigmine Bromide, Vaccines.* Washington, DC: National Academy Press.

IOM. 2001. *Veterans and Agent Orange: Update 2000.* Washington, DC: National Academy Press.

IOM. 2003a. *Gulf War and Health, Volume 2: Insecticides and Solvents.* Washington, DC: The National Academies Press.

IOM. 2003b. *Veterans and Agent Orange: Update 2002.* Washington, DC: The National Academies Press.

Office of the Surgeon General-HHS. 2004. *The Health Consequences of Smoking: A Report of the Surgeon General.* [Online]. Available: http://www.surgeongeneral.gov/library/smokingconsequences [accessed October 26, 2004].

Susser M. 1973. *Causal Thinking in the Health Sciences: Concepts and Strategies of Epidemiology.* New York: Oxford University Press.

Susser M. 1977. Judgment and causal inference: Criteria in epidemiologic studies. *American Journal of Epidemiology* 105(1):1-15.

Susser M. 1988. Falsification, verification, and causal inference in epidemiology: Reconsideration in the light of Sir Karl Popper's philosophy. In: Rothman KJ, ed. *Causal Inference*. Chestnut Hill, MA: Epidemiology Resources. Pp. 33-58.

Susser M. 1991. What is a cause and how do we know one? A grammar for pragmatic epidemiology. *American Journal of Epidemiology* 133(7):635-648.

Wegman DH, Woods NF, Bailar JC. 1997. Invited commentary: How would we know a Gulf War syndrome if we saw one? *American Journal of Epidemiology* 146(9):704-711.

3

UNCOMBUSTED FUELS AND COMBUSTION PRODUCTS: BACKGROUND INFORMATION

In addition to the partially combusted crude oil associated with the well-publicized oil-well fires, several petroleum-derived fuels were present in the Persian Gulf region during Operation Desert Shield and Operation Desert Storm, including gasoline, kerosene, diesel, and jet-propulsion fuels JP-4, JP-5, and JP-8. Those fuels were used by the military to power aircraft, ground vehicles, tent heaters, and cooking stoves. They were also used for less conventional purposes, such as suppressing sand, cleaning equipment, and burning trash. Military personnel serving in the Gulf War theater of operations could have been exposed to the uncombusted fuels, the combustion products from the burning of those fuels, or a combination of uncombusted and combusted materials.

This chapter provides background information on fuels and their combustion products separately. Information on the individual components of combustion products are discussed when it is available and relevant. The main exposure routes of concern are inhalation and dermal; ingestion of fuels by Gulf War personnel is of much less concern. As noted in Chapter 2, the committee used data from animal and in vitro studies mainly as background information and to provide support, when possible, for its conclusions. They were also used in deciding whether there is a causal relationship between exposure and disease. Most of the compounds discussed here are common pollutants on which there is a large volume of literature, including numerous reviews. In light of the committee's use of the data, this chapter provides an overview of the compounds and their toxicology. The reader is referred to reviews for more details; primary toxicology studies are discussed only as warranted.

UNCOMBUSTED FUELS

Petroleum-derived fuels are complex mixtures that contain hundreds of aliphatic and aromatic hydrocarbon compounds; most also contain performance-enhancing additives. The composition of a particular fuel varies from batch to batch, depending on such factors as the source of the crude oil from which it is derived, the refining process used in its production, and the product specifications. The toxicity of some components of the fuels (for example, benzene, toluene, and xylenes) has been well characterized, but the toxicity of many, particularly the longer-chained carbon compounds, has not been extensively studied.

This section provides an overview of toxicologic information on gasoline, kerosene, diesel, JP-4, JP-5, and JP-8. It begins with summaries of physical and chemical properties of the various fuels and a compendium of exposure limits recommended by national and international government bodies and other organizations. That information is followed by a description of the toxicokinetics of the fuels and a summary of experimental studies conducted in humans and animals, focusing on studies that yielded information on chronic adverse health effects, on genetic susceptibility, or on interactions between fuels and other substances.

The fuels discussed here have been the subjects of comprehensive reviews by the Agency for Toxic Substances and Disease Registry (ATSDR 1995a, 1995b, 1995c, 1998, 1999b), the International Agency for Research on Cancer (IARC 1989), the National Research Council (NRC 1996b, 2003), and Ritchie et al. (2003). The reader is referred to those sources for more detailed reviews of the toxicologic data on those fuels.

Several components of hydrocarbon fuels—benzene, toluene, xylenes, and naphtha—were reviewed in *Gulf War and Health, Volume 2: Insecticides and Solvents* (IOM 2003) and will not be addressed individually here. The Committee on Gulf War and Health: Literature Review of Insecticides and Solvents found sufficient evidence of a causal relationship between benzene and both acute leukemia and aplastic anemia. The reader is referred to that volume for more information on adverse health effects associated with exposures to benzene, toluene, xylenes, and naphtha.

Physical and Chemical Properties

Some of the physical and chemical properties of gasoline, kerosene, diesel, JP-4, JP-5, and JP-8 are presented in Table 3.1. They are arranged in order of increasing carbon number, that is, according to composition of relatively longer hydrocarbon chains or heavier cut of distillates. Naphthas, middle distillates used in mixing gasoline and composed primarily of C_5-C_{13} aliphatic hydrocarbons, would fall between gasoline and JP-4. Kerosene, JP-5, and JP-8 are very similar in composition, differing primarily in the additive packages that characterize them; hence they share several synonyms.

Exposure Limits

Limits of occupational exposures to several fuels have been recommended by such organizations as the American Conference of Governmental Industrial Hygienists (ACGIH), ATSDR, IARC, the National Institute for Occupational Safety and Health (NIOSH), and the Occupational Safety and Health Administration (OSHA). Those values, as summarized in Table 3.2, give a sense of what fuel exposures are currently considered safe.

TABLE 3.1 Chemical Identity and Some Physical and Chemical Properties of Selected Fuels

Properties	Gasoline	JP-4	JP-5	JP-8	Kerosene	Diesel
Synonyms	Motor fuel, motor spirit, natural gasoline, petrol, mogas	MIL-T-5624-L-Amd. 1 wide cut (registered trade name)	NATO F-44, AVCAT, MIL-T5624M	NATO F-34, AVTUR, MIL-T-83133B	Fuel oil no. 1, Deobase, kerosene, K-1, JP-1	Auto diesel, automotive diesel oil, diesel fuel oil, diesel oil, fuel oil no. 1-D, fuel oil no. 2, fuel oil no. 2-D, fuel oil no. 4, gas oil
			aviation kerosene, kerosene, fuel oil no. 1, jet kerosene, turbo fuel A, straight run kerosene, distillate fuel oils light			
CAS registry no.	8006-61-9	50815-00-4	8008-20-6 (kerosene) 70892-10-3 (fuel oil no. 1)	8008-20-6 (kerosene) 70892-10-3 (fuel oil no. 1)	8008-20-6	68334-30-5 (general diesel fuel)
Average molecular weight	108	No data found	No data found	No data found	No data found	No data found
Range of carbon numbers	C_4-C_{13}	C_4-C_{16}	C_9-C_{17}	C_9-C_{17}	C_{10}-C_{16}	C_{10}-C_{19}
Approximate composition						
-Alkanes	54.3 (wt. %)	75-78 (wt. %)	84 (vol. %)	71-78 (vol. %)	78-96 (vol. %)	64-85 (vol. %)
-Alkenes	1.8	4-7	0.5	0.5-5	0-5	1-10
-Aromatics	30.5	14-15	16	12-22	4-25	5-30
Additives	Octane enhancers, antioxidants, metal deactivators, ignition controllers, icing inhibitors, detergents/ dispersants, corrosion inhibitors	Icing inhibitors, antioxidants, corrosion inhibitors, metal deactivators, anti-static agents	Icing inhibitors, antioxidants, corrosion inhibitors, anti-static agents, lubrication improvers, biocides, thermal stability improvers	Icing inhibitors, static inhibitors, corrosion inhibitors, antioxidants, metal deactivators	No data found	Ignition improvers/centane enhancers, smoke suppressors/combustion enhancers, detergents, flow improvers, cloud-point depressors, wax anti-settlers, static inhibitors, corrosion inhibitors, antioxidants, anti-foam agents, dehazers, biocides, lubricants, odor maskers
Physical state	Liquid	Liquid	Liquid	Liquid	Liquid	Liquid
Color	Colorless to pale brown	Colorless to straw colored	Clear	Clear	Colorless to brown	Colorless to brown
Odor	Gasoline-like	Like gasoline and/or	Kerosene-like	Kerosene-like	Kerosene-like	Kerosene-like

Properties	Gasoline	JP-4	JP-5	JP-8	Kerosene	Diesel
		kerosene				
Melting point	−90.5–−95.4°C	−46°C	−46°C	−52°C	−45.6°C	−48-18°C
Boiling point	39-204°C	45-300°C	150-290°C	175-300°C	175-325°C	101-588°C
Density	0.7-0.8 g/ml (temperature not specified)	0.75-0.80 g/ml (at 15°C)	0.79-0.85 g/ml (at 15°C)	0.79-0.85 g/ml (at 15°C)	0.80 g/ml (at 20°C)	0.87-1.0 g/ml (at 20°C)
Solubility						
-Water	Insoluble (at 20°C)	57 mg/L (at 20°C)	≈5 mg/L (at 20°C)	≈5 mg/L (at 20°C)	≈5 mg/L at 20°C)	≈5 mg/L (at 20°C)
-Organic solvents	Absolute alcohol, ether, chloroform, benzene	Generally miscible with organic solvents	Miscible with other petroleum solvents	Miscible with other petroleum solvents	Miscible with other petroleum solvents	No data found
Flashpoint	−46°C	−23-1°C	60°C	38°C	38°C	38-58°C

NOTES: CAS=Chemical Abstracts Services; JP-4=jet-propulsion fuel 4; JP-5=jet-propulsion fuel 5; JP-8=jet-propulsion fuel 8.
When several data points were found for a property of a given fuel, they are presented as a range.
SOURCES: ATSDR (1995a, 1995b, 1995c, 1998, 1999b), Budavari et al. (1989), HSDB (2003a, 2003b), NRC (1996b, 2003), WHO (1996).

TABLE 3.2 Recommended Exposure Limits for Fuels

Organization	Fuel Type	Type of Exposure Limit	Recommended Exposure Value	Reference
Occupational Exposure Limits				
ACGIH	Gasoline	TLV STEL	300 ppm = 890 mg/m^3, A3 (adopted 1996) 500 ppm = 1,480 mg/m^3	ACGIH 2003
	Diesel (as a total hydrocarbons)	TLV	100 mg/m^3, A3, Skin (adopted 2001)	ACGIH 2003
	Kerosene (8088-20-6) (as a total hydrocarbon vapor)	TLV	200 mg/m^3, A3, Skin (proposed 2002)	ACGIH 2003
	Jet fuels (94114-58-6) (as a total hydrocarbon vapor)	TLV	200 mg/m^3, A3, Skin (proposed 2002)	ACGIH 2003
AFOSH	Petroleum distillates (naphtha)	PEL STEL	400 ppm 500 ppm	Air Force 1989
	JP-5	PEL STEL	350 mg/m^3 (interim) 1,000 mg/m^3 (interim)	Ritchie et al. 2003
NIOSH	Gasoline	—	Carcinogen: lowest possible concentration	NIOSH 1998
	Kerosene	REL	100 mg/m^3	NIOSH 1997
	Petroleum distillates (naphtha)	REL Ceiling (15-min) IDLH	85 ppm = 350 mg/m^3 438 ppm = 1,800 mg/m^3 10,000 ppm	NIOSH 1997 NIOSH 1997
OSHA	Gasoline (in workroom air)	PEL STEL	300 ppm = 900 mg/m^3 550 ppm = 1,500 mg/m^3	OSHA 1989 (29 CFR 1910.1000)
	Petroleum distillates (naphtha)	PEL	500 ppm = 2,000 mg/m^3	OSHA 1997 (29 CFR 1910.1000)
Exposure Limits for the General Population				
ATSDR	Gasoline (automotive)	MRL	None developed because of data gaps	ATSDR 1995a
	Diesel (fuel oil no. 2)	MRL	0.02 mg/m^3 (acute inhalation exposure)	ATSDR 1995b

Organization	Fuel Type	Type of Exposure Limit	Recommended Exposure Value	Reference
	Kerosene (fuel oil no. 1)	MRL	0.01 mg/m^3 (intermediate-duration inhalation exposure)	ATSDR 1995b
	JP-4	MRL	9 mg/m^3 (intermediate-duration inhalation exposure)	ATSDR 1995c
	JP-5/JP-8	MRL	3 mg/m^3 (intermediate-duration inhalation exposure)	ATSDR 1998
IARC	Gasoline	Evaluation of carcinogenicity	Possibly carcinogenic to humans (group 2B)	IARC 1989
	Distillate (light) diesel		Not classifiable as to its carcinogenicity to humans (group 3)	
	Jet fuel		Not classifiable as to its carcinogenicity to humans (group 3)	

NOTES: ACGIH=American Conference of Governmental Industrial Hygienists; TWA=Time-Weighted Average; TLV=Threshold Limit Value (TWA for 8-hr workday during 40-hr workweek); A3=Confirmed Animal Carcinogen with Unknown Relevance to Humans; Skin=potentially large contribution to exposure by dermal route; STEL=Short-Term Exposure Limit (15-min TWA); Ceiling=value never to be exceeded; AFOSH=Air Force Office of Safety and Health; ATSDR =Agency for Toxic Substances and Disease Registry; MRL=minimal risk level; JP-4, 5, or 8=jet-propulsion fuel 4, 5, or 8; IARC=International Agency for Research on Cancer; NIOSH=National Institute for Occupational Safety and Health; REL=Recommended Exposure Limit (TWA for 10-hr workday during 40-hr workweek); IDHL=Immediately Dangerous to Life or Health; OSHA=Occupational Safety and Health Administration; PEL=Permissible Exposure Limit (TWA for 8-hr workday during 40-hour workweek).

Toxicokinetics

Given that gasoline, kerosene, diesel, JP-4, JP-5, and JP-8 are composed of hundreds of hydrocarbon compounds, it is impractical to describe here the toxicokinetics of each component. Because fuels contain many different components, they will exhibit a wide range of variability regarding absorption, metabolism, and excretion. General aspects of the toxicokinetics of JP-8 were presented in the recent National Research Council report *Toxicologic Assessment of Jet-Propulsion Fuel 8* (NRC 2003). The principles are applicable to gasoline, kerosene, diesel, JP-4, and JP-5, and they are repeated here. The major determinants of hydrocarbon toxicokinetics after systemic uptake are disposition-related physiologic properties of the organism—such as alveolar ventilation, cardiac output and blood flow to the organs, and organ volume—and partition coefficients of the fuel components. Hydrocarbons with high blood:air partition coefficients are absorbed to a greater extent than compounds with poor blood solubility. Given that most hydrocarbons have fairly high fat:air and fat:blood partition coefficients, it is not surprising that fat or adipose tissue is a major storage depot for many of the fuel components. For hydrocarbons with high fat:blood partition coefficients, metabolic clearance after cessation of exposure is especially important. Hydrocarbons and their metabolites accumulate in lipid-rich tissues, so the absence of hydrocarbons and their metabolites in exhaled air, blood, or urine does not necessarily mean the absence of systemic exposure. Cytochrome P450 enzymes metabolize most hydrocarbons by such reactions as aliphatic hydroxylation, aromatic hydroxylation, and epoxidation. Alcohol and aldehyde dehydrogenases play an important role in metabolizing alcohols into their corresponding keto acids. Phase II reactions—including conjugation with glutathione, glucuronic acid, sulfate, and glycine—are important in formation of water-soluble metabolites.

Data on absorption, distribution, metabolism, and elimination of gasoline, kerosene, diesel, JP-4, JP-5, and JP-8 are sparse. The components of each of these fuels are processed primarily according to their own physicochemical properties. When Tsujino et al. (2002) applied 1ml of kerosene dermally to the abdomen of rats for 1, 3, or 6 hr, it was absorbed and distributed via blood circulation, but the aromatic compound trimethylbenzene was absorbed by the skin to a greater degree than the aliphatic hydrocarbons. Kimura et al. (1988) had similar results with inhaled gasoline and kerosene. Local and systemic effects observed after exposure to those fuels indicated that they are absorbed by the respiratory tract, the gastrointestinal tract, and the skin. Toxicokinetic information on several fuel components is available (in particular, benzene, toluene, and xylenes); but their interactions with each other and with other hydrocarbon components may affect their toxicokinetic properties (ATSDR 1989, 1990, 1991, 1995e; NRC 1996a).

Experimental Studies

Controlled studies of the toxicity of gasoline, kerosene, diesel, JP-4, JP-5, and JP-8 in humans and laboratory animals are summarized here, with emphasis on studies that addressed whether effects persist after cessation of exposure. Epidemiologic studies of the adverse health effects of the fuels will be discussed in later chapters.

Cancer

MacFarland et al. (1984) exposed Fischer 344 rats and B6C3F1 mice to unleaded gasoline vapors by inhalation at up to about 2,000 ppm for 2 years. There was an increased incidence of hepatocellular adenomas and carcinomas in the exposed female mice but not in the exposed males. There was an increased incidence of renal adenomas and carcinomas in the exposed male rats, but not in the exposed females; these kidney tumors were probably related to a male-rat-specific nephropathy (see discussion of renal effects later in this section) that is not considered relevant to humans (ATSDR 1995a). Gasoline contains 2-3% benzene, a known human carcinogen that has been shown to cause an increased incidence of leukemia in occupationally exposed workers (ATSDR 1991; IARC 1989). No studies that assessed cancer in laboratory animals from dermal or oral exposure to gasoline were found.

Middle-distillate fuels (MDFs)—which include kerosene, diesel, JP-5, and JP-8—have been shown to cause skin tumors in mice (reviewed in IARC 1989; and also reviewed in Nessel 1999). MDFs have low or no mutagenic activity and no tumor-initiating activity. They are, however, active skin-tumor promoters, requiring chronic dermal irritation and skin injury. That profile indicates that dermal carcinogenesis associated with MDFs is the result of a nongenotoxic process (Nessel 1999). No carcinogenicity studies that assessed cancer in laboratory animals from inhalation or oral exposure to MDFs were found.

Genotoxicity

Several in vivo and in vitro assays have shown gasoline, kerosene, diesel, JP-5, and JP-8 not to be highly genotoxic (reviewed in ATSDR 1995a, 1995b, 1995c, 1998; NRC 2003). They are not mutagenic in multiple strains of *Salmonella typhinurium* with and without activation (Brusick and Matheson 1978a, 1978b; Conaway et al. 1984; Deininger et al. 1991; McKee et al. 1994, 1989; Nessel 1999). Mixed results have been reported concerning mutagenicity from the in vitro mouse lymphoma assay and from in vitro and in vivo assays of induction of sister-chromatid exchanges (API 1988a, 1988b).

Neurologic Effects

Several studies assessed nervous system effects after cessation of exposure of laboratory animals to hydrocarbon fuels. The relevance to humans of neurobehavioral effects observed in animals, however, is not well understood.

Kainz and White (1983) exposed CD-1 mice to diesel-fuel vapors at up to 204 mg/m^3 for 8 hr/day for 5 days and followed the exposure with a 24-hr no-exposure period. They found that motor coordination, as measured by a rotarod test, was progressively decreased in the mice given the highest dose, but showed signs of recovery after 24 hr. Inconclusive results were reported for the hot-plate test, and no effects were observed when the mice were given the inclined-plane test or the corneal-reflex test.

A series of light naphtha distillates, which are used in mixing gasoline, were tested in Sprague-Dawley rats according to a common protocol: exposure at up to 7,500 ppm for 6 hr/day 5 days/week for 13 weeks followed by motor-activity evaluation, a functional observational battery, and a neuropathology examination after a 4-week no-exposure period. Significantly higher motor activity was observed in the males given high doses of light catalytic reformed naphtha, but no other nervous system effects were observed among rats exposed to that agent

(Schreiner et al. 2000), to light alkylate naphtha (Schreiner et al. 1998), or to light catalytic cracked naphtha (Lapin et al. 2001).

Nordholm et al. (1999) exposed Sprague-Dawley rats by inhalation to JP-4 vapors at 2,000 mg/m^3 for 6 hr/day for 14 days and followed the exposure with no-exposure periods of 14 or 60 days. Similarly, Sprague-Dawley rats were exposed by inhalation to JP-8 or JP-5 vapors at up to 1,000 or 1,200 mg/m^3, respectively, for 6 hr/day 5 days/week for 6 weeks, and the exposure was followed by a 65-day no-exposure period (Ritchie et al. 2001; Rossi et al. 2001). Subtle but apparently persistent changes in neurophysiologic and psychologic capacity detectable only with appropriate test batteries were observed, but no dose–response relationships were demonstrated.

Koschier (1999) reported that rats dermally exposed to hydrodesulfurized kerosene at up to 495 mg/kg for 5 days/week for 13 weeks followed by a 4-week no-exposure period did not show any adverse neurobehavioral or histologic effects compared with the control group.

Although this study was not an experimental investigation, former "gasoline-sniffers" (after at least a 6-month hiatus) showed higher rates of abnormal tandem gait, bilateral palmomental reflexes, and cognitive deficits in visual recognition memory and pattern-location paired associate learning than a control group (Goodheart and Dunne 1994). The magnitude of neurologic and cognitive effects correlated with duration of gasoline-sniffing and with blood lead concentrations, so the outcomes might not have been attributable entirely to the petrochemical components of the gasoline.

Respiratory Effects

Various respiratory effects (such as increased pulmonary resistance, interstitial edema, and damage to bronchiolar epithelium) have been observed in some subchronic and chronic animal studies immediately following exposure to hydrocarbon fuels but other studies did not find such effects (as reviewed in ATSDR 1995a, 1995b, 1995c, 1998; NRC 2003). It is not known whether the observed respiratory effects would have persisted or reversed themselves after a no-exposure period.

A single large study of persistence of respiratory effects after a no-exposure period in laboratory animals exposed to a hydrocarbon fuel was found. Bruner et al. (1993) exposed mice and rats of both sexes to JP-4 vapors at 1,000 or 5,000 mg/m^3 for 12 months. Immediately after the 12-month exposure period, the low-dose female mice showed mild pulmonary inflammation and the low-dose males of both species showed hyperplasia of the nasolacrimal duct epithelium. No effects were present in either species 12 months after exposure.

Hepatic Effects

A number of studies have assessed the potential of subchronic or chronic exposure to hydrocarbon fuels to cause hepatic effects in laboratory animals immediately after exposure (as reviewed in ATSDR 1995a, 1995b, 1995c, 1998; NRC 2003).

Several studies of subchronic or chronic exposure of mice to unleaded gasoline vapors at about 2,000 ppm showed hepatic effects, such as hypertrophy, increased cytochrome P450 content, and tumor-related necrosis and hemorrhage. Other studies of subchronic or chronic exposure at similar concentrations did not find any adverse hepatic effects in rats and monkeys (ATSDR 1995a).

Increased liver weight has been associated with subchronic exposure of mice, rats, dogs, and monkeys to JP-4 vapors at up to 5,000 mg/m^3 (MacNaughton and Uddin 1984). Reversible hepatocellular fatty changes in mice, but not in rats and dogs, have been associated with subchronic exposure to JP-4 vapors at up to 1,000 mg/m^3 (MacEwen and Vernot 1984).

Inconsistent results have been reported in inhalation-, oral-, and dermal-exposure studies of hepatic effects caused by kerosene, JP-5, and JP-8 (which are similar in composition). Several subchronic inhalation studies found hepatic effects: increased glycolysis in rats (Starek and Vojtisek 1986); increased hepatic basophilic foci in male rats but not in female rats or in mice (Mattie et al. 1991); and reversible diffuse mild swelling of hepatocytes, decreased serum glutamic pyruvic transaminase, mild hepatic hyperplasia, increased hepatocyte vacuolization, fatty changes in hepatocytes, and increased liver adenomas in rats, mice, and dogs and increased liver weight only in dogs (Keller et al. 1984). Other studies with similar exposure conditions did not report any hepatic effects (Bogo et al. 1983; Carpenter et al. 1976; Parton 1994).

Two studies assessed the persistence of hepatic effects after a no-exposure period in laboratory animals exposed to a hydrocarbon fuel. Dennis (1982) found no hepatic lesions 14 days after applying JP-4 at 2,000 mg/kg to the skin of rabbits. (Bruner et al. 1993) observed no liver toxicity in rats exposed to JP-4 vapors at 1,000 or 5,000 mg/m^3 for 6 hr/day 5 days/week for 12 months. However, after a 12-month no-exposure period, non-dose-related decreases were found in the liver weights of the male, but not female, rats. Of mice exposed at the same concentrations and for the same duration, only high-dose females had an increase in lymphocytic inflammatory infiltrates in the liver at the end of the exposure period, but that effect was no longer found at the end of the 12-month no-exposure period (Bruner et al. 1993).

Cardiovascular Effects

Because hydrocarbons historically have been used as anesthetics and abused as narcotics, inhalation of hydrocarbons is well known to have acute effects on the cardiovascular system (NRC 1996b). They can induce potentially fatal cardiac arrhythmias, but for arrhythmias to occur epinephrine must be released simultaneously with inhalation (Garb and Chenoweth 1948). Chronic effects of hydrocarbon fuels on the cardiovascular system have not been well studied.

Gastrointestinal Effects

Gastrointestinal effects have been observed in laboratory animals after oral exposure to gasoline (gastric erythema, erosion of the gastric mucosa, and ulceration of the epithelium) and kerosene (gastritis and hyperplasia) and after inhalation exposure to JP-4 (emesis) (reviewed in ATSDR 1995a, 1995b, 1995c, 1995e, 1998).

Immunologic Effects

MDFs have been shown to be weak to moderate skin sensitizers in laboratory animals (Cowan and Jenkins 1981; Kanikkannan et al. 2000; Kimber and Weisenberger 1989; Kinkead et al. 1992a, 1992b; Schultz et al. 1981).

Dermal exposure of mice to several MDFs (kerosene, JP-5, and JP-8) has been found to cause a variety of local and systemic immune effects, such as decreases in relative weights of lymph nodes and thymus, in thymocyte counts, in bone marrow nucleated cell counts, in thymic cortical lymphocytes, and in cellularity of thymic lobules, and in suppression of contact and delayed hypersensitivity responses (Ullrich 1999; Upreti et al. 1989).

Immune-system effects have also been observed in rats exposed to diesel fuel aerosol and JP-8 aerosol by inhalation (Dalbey et al. 1987; Harris et al. 1997b, 1997a, 2000), but no immune-system effects were found in rats exposed to JP-8 vapor by inhalation or in rats or monkeys exposed to gasoline by inhalation (Kuna and Ulrich 1984; Mattie et al. 1991). JP-8 aerosols are believed to be more immunotoxic than JP-8 vapors (NRC 2003).

Oral exposure of rats and mice to kerosene or JP-8 caused immune-system effects, such as decreases in white-cell count, in relative spleen weight, in thymic weight, and in antibody plaque-forming cell response to sheep red cells (Dudley et al. 2001; Mattie et al. 1995; Parker et al. 1981). Keil et al. (2003) found that in utero exposure of mice to JP-8 at 1,000 or 2,000 mg/kg by gavage on gestation days 6-15 impaired the immune function of the offspring later in life.

Renal Effects

Some hydrocarbon fuels have been shown to induce hydraline droplet nephropathy syndrome in male rats (but not in female rats or in males and females of any other species) exposed subchronically or chronically by inhalation or ingestion (reviewed in ATSDR 1995a, 1995b, 1995c, 1998; Bruner et al. 1993; Cowan and Jenkins 1981; Keller et al. 1984; Mattie et al. 1991, 1995; NRC 2003; Parker et al. 1981; Parton 1994). The components of hydrocarbon fuels determined to be largely responsible for the syndrome in the male rat are the branched alkane compounds with six or more carbons (ATSDR 1995a). Hydraline droplet nephropathy syndrome is sex- and species-specific and is not considered to be relevant to humans (Alden 1986; Flamm and Lehman-McKeeman 1991).

Reproductive and Developmental Effects

No developmental effects were observed in the fetuses of rats exposed to unleaded gasoline vapors at 1,600 ppm during gestation (Litton Bionetics 1978). Unleaded-gasoline vapors did not cause developmental defects (malformations, total variations, resorptions, low fetal body weight, or low offspring viability) in the offspring of rats exposed at up to 23,900 mg/m^3 (9,000 ppm) for 6 hr/day on gestation days 6-19 (Roberts et al. 2001). Exposure to unleaded-gasoline vapors at about 2,000 ppm for 2 years did not lead to histologic changes in the reproductive systems of rats or mice (MacFarland et al. 1984). No reproductive effects were found in a two-generation reproduction-toxicity test in which male and female rats were exposed to vapors of gasoline (presumably unleaded) at up to 20,000 mg/m^3 (McKee et al. 2000).

Inhalation exposure of pregnant rats to petroleum naphtha at 100 or 400 ppm on days 6-15 of gestation did not produce teratogenic effects (Beliles and Mecler 1982). A similar protocol to test for reproductive and developmental effects was used with three types of light naphtha distillates: alkylated (Bui et al. 1998), catalytic cracked (Schreiner et al. 1999), and catalytic reformed (Schreiner et al. 2000). The results were uniformly negative for all three test agents when male and female rats were exposed at up to 25,000 mg/m^3, at 7,500 ppm, and at 7,500 ppm, respectively, daily from 2 weeks before mating through delivery.

No studies of the reproductive- or developmental-toxicity potential of JP-4 were found, but kerosene-related fuels have been tested for reproductive and developmental effects of dermal, oral, and inhalation exposure.

No reproductive or developmental effects were observed when male and female rats were dermally exposed to hydrodesulfurized kerosene at up to 494 mg/kg per day for 7-8 weeks from before mating through gestation (Schreiner et al. 1997). No histologic changes were observed in the reproductive systems of mice dermally exposed to JP-5 at up to 8,000 mg/kg 5 times per week for 13 weeks (NTP/NIH 1998).

No reproductive effects were observed in male and female rats exposed to JP-8 by gavage at up to 1,500 (females) or 3,000 (males) mg/kg per day before and during mating and, in the case of the females, during gestation and lactation (Mattie et al. 2000, 1995). Maternal gestational weight gain and fetal body weights were reduced in rats exposed to JP-8 by gavage at 1,500 or 2,000 mg/kg per day on days 6-15 of pregnancy; the types of fetal abnormalities did not differ significantly between treated and nonexposed rats, and there was a progressive increase in the overall incidence of abnormalities with increasing dose from 500 to 1,500 mg/kg per day, but not 2,000 mg/kg per day (Cooper and Mattie 1996).

Inhalation of jet fuel A (a kerosene-like fuel) at 100 or 400 ppm on days 6-15 of gestation did not produce teratogenic effects in rats (Beliles and Mecler 1982). Similarly, exposing rats to fuel oil at concentrations of 100 or 400 ppm on gestation days 6-15 did not produce teratogenic responses (Beliles and Mecler 1982). Lock et al. (1984) also found that intermediate-duration exposure of rats to diesel-fuel aerosols did not lead to reproductive or developmental effects.

Dermal Effects

Several hydrocarbon fuels have been shown to be skin irritants. Gasoline caused dermal irritation when applied to the skin of rabbits (ATSDR 1995a). Case studies of individuals immersed in gasoline for several hours described chemical burns on the exposed skin (ATSDR 1995a). Case studies also report that dermal exposure to kerosene causes a variety of dermal effects (ATSDR 1995b). Dermal irritation was observed in laboratory animals exposed to JP-4, JP-5, and JP-8 (ATSDR 1995c, 1998).

COMBUSTION PRODUCTS

Combustion of fuels results in the formation of complex mixtures of gases and particles. The specific profile of combustion products is a function of what was burned and under what conditions the burning occurred. The primary constituents that characterize smoke from fires, exhaust from burning fuels, and products of other combustion sources are also those which characterize air pollution in general. The potential toxicity of combustion products varies with their composition, including particle size. The various components have differing toxicities, so the overall toxicity of the complex mixture will depend on the relative amounts of the individual components. Although great strides have been made in the learning about health effects of combustion products, how the relative amounts of components of the products correlate with potential health effects and how they interact with each other are not entirely understood (NRC 2004).

The gases in combustion products can include sulfur dioxide (SO_2), ozone (O_3), nitrogen oxide (NO), nitrogen dioxide (NO_2), carbon monoxide (CO), carbon dioxide (CO_2), hydrogen sulfide (H_2S), and volatile organic compounds (VOCs) (the oxides of nitrogen as a group are referred to as NO_x and the oxides of sulfur as SO_x). VOCs were reviewed by the second Institute of Medicine Gulf War committee in conjunction with its review of solvents and are not reviewed here.

The chemical composition and physical composition of particles in general vary widely. They may include elemental and organic carbon, sulfates, nitrates, pollen, microbial contaminants, and metals. Photochemical reactions of fine particles with SO_2 and NO_2 in the atmosphere form strong acids, such as sulfuric acid, nitric acid, hydrochloric acid, and acid aerosols. Polycyclic aromatic hydrocarbons (PAHs) are formed by incomplete combustion, including combustion of fossil fuels, and can be adsorbed on particulate matter (PM). A number of other hazardous pollutants (such as toxic metals) can be associated with combustion. The committee does not review the health effects of individual hazardous chemicals that might be adsorbed onto PM. The bioavailability and toxicity of such a chemical is affected by being adsorbed on the particle, so toxicity of the chemical alone cannot be directly extrapolated to its toxicity when adsorbed on the particle. In addition, the amounts of hazardous compounds adsorbed on PM are generally lower than the amounts that would be used in animal studies to assess the effects of the compounds themselves. Therefore, the committee focuses on studies of the toxicity of PM, not studies of the individual compounds that might be adsorbed on or incorporated into the PM.

Potential Exposures in the Gulf War

Gulf War veterans were involved in a number of situations with potential for considerable exposure to airborne products of combustion of petroleum or derivatives.

At the end of the Gulf War, over 600 Kuwaiti oil wells were ignited by retreating Iraqi troops. Large plumes of smoke rose from the fires. Occasionally, the smoke remained near the ground and enveloped US military personnel. No systematic monitoring occurred in the initial deployment in 1990 until May 1991, when several independent teams from multiple US and international agencies (including the US Army Environmental Health Agency and the US Environmental Protection Agency, EPA) went into Kuwait to monitor the ambient air contamination due to oil-well fire emissions (Spektor 1998). Smoke sampling was performed to improve understanding of the nature of the plumes generated by the burning oil wells. Most of the oil fires were still burning when measurements began.

Individual fires created distinct smoke plumes over short distances, but over longer distances the plumes merged into one "supercomposite" plume south of Kuwait City measuring about 40 km wide. At the base of the plume, oil falling in droplet form or emitted from uncapped wells collected in pools on the desert; the pools sometimes were on fire as well (Hobbs and Raadke 1992). The smoke plumes from individual fires varied in color and density. Black smoke plumes resulted from single well fires and had relatively high concentrations of carbon; they made up 60-65% of the fires. The densest black plumes were from the burning pools of oil. White smoke plumes, accounting for 25-30% of the fires, contained almost no carbon but had a higher concentration of inorganic salts, which is consistent with reports of the presence of brine solutions in the oil fields (Cofer et al. 1992; Spektor 1998).

The available monitoring data indicate that levels of nitrogen oxides, carbon monoxide, sulfur dioxide, hydrogen sulfide, other pollutant gases, and PAHs did not exceed those in the air of a typical US industrial city. Within the samples, PAH concentrations were low (PAC 1996). High concentrations of PM (sand and soot) were often observed at multiple monitoring sites; an estimated 20,000 tons of soot, or fine-particle mass, was generated by the fires (Thomas et al. 2000) and made up about 23% of the PM in the Persian Gulf, often at concentrations twice those considered safe (Rostker 2000).

In addition to air monitoring, potential exposures of troops to smoke and combustion products from the oil-well fires were modeled (Draxler et al. 1994). Daily and seasonal normalized air concentrations due to emissions from the oil-well fires were computed using a modified Lagrangian transport, dispersion, and deposition model for the period of February through October 1991. The highest normalized concentrations were located near the coast between Kuwait and Qatar. Peak values moved farther west and inland with each season (that is, the smoke and combustion products moved from over the Gulf in the spring to the west over the Saudi Peninsula by autumn).

In addition to exposure to smoke from oil-well fires, military personnel might have had exposures to combustion products because they were close to military vehicles, aircraft, and heaters in poorly ventilated tents.

Physical and Chemical Properties

As discussed above, combustion products are complex mixtures of substances. The physical and chemical properties of the major components of combustion products are discussed below.

Gases

Hydrogen Sulfide

As described by the (ATSDR 1999a), H_2S is a colorless, flammable gas under normal conditions. H_2S—also known as hydrosulfuric acid, stink damp, and sewer gas—has an odor similar to that of rotten eggs. It is a naturally occurring compound found in crude petroleum, natural gas, volcanic gases, and hot springs. It can also be made by people, and it can be found in human and animal waste, sewage-treatment facilities, sediments of fish aquaculture, and livestock barns or manure areas. Petroleum refineries, natural-gas plants, petrochemical plants, coke-oven plants, kraft-paper mills, food-processing plants, and tanneries are other sources of H_2S (ATSDR 1999a).

Sulfur Oxides

SO_x easily dissolve in water. Sulfur is found in raw materials, including crude oil, coal, and ore that contains common metals, such as aluminum, copper, zinc, lead, and iron. When fuel that contains sulfur is burned, SO_x is formed. SO_x can also form when gasoline is extracted from oil, or metals are extracted from ore.

SO_2 dissolves in water vapor to form sulfuric acid, and it interacts with other gases and particles in the air to form sulfates and other products. Sources of SO_2 include electric utilities, petroleum refineries, cement manufacturing, and metal-processing facilities. Locomotives, large ships, and some nonroad diesel equipment burn high-sulfur fuel and release SO_2 into the air (EPA 2003b).

Nitrogen Oxides

From the human-exposure perspective, NO_2 is the most important and common nitrogen oxide. NO_2 is a reddish brown, water-soluble, moderately oxidizing gas. The primary atmospheric reaction for NO_2 production is the rapid oxidation of NO by oxidants, such as O_3. Major sources of NO_2 include the combustion of fossil fuels from stationary sources for heating and power generation and in motor-vehicle internal-combustion engines. As in the case of many other outdoor pollutants, concentrations of NO_2 can vary with the time of day, the season, meteorologic conditions, and human activities (Gong 1992). Unvented combustion appliances, such as gas stoves and gas-fired water heaters, are major sources of indoor NO_2.

Carbon Monoxide and Carbon Dioxide

The fourth-most abundant gas in the earth's atmosphere, CO_2 is a colorless, odorless, and faintly acid-tasting gas at room temperature. It is transformed into sugars and other forms of energy by plants during photosynthesis, and it is exhaled by animals as a waste product of cellular respiration and released into the air during the burning of carbon-containing fossil fuels (oil, coal, and natural gas).

CO, also a colorless and odorless gas, is highly toxic to humans. It is formed as a result of the incomplete combustion of carbon-containing compounds. Heaters, oil- and wood-burning furnaces, and nonelectric stoves and ranges used in confined or poorly ventilated spaces can rapidly accumulate CO to dangerous concentrations.

Ozone

Ground level O_3 is a highly reactive and oxidative gas that is formed by photochemical reactions of sunlight, NO_2, and hydrocarbon vapors. Ozone concentration peaks in the late morning or afternoon and declines in the evening because of its reactions with nitric acid and terrestrial surfaces. Because hydrocarbon vapors and NO_2 persist in the atmosphere, O_3 can form far downwind of the sources; O_3 concentrations can be higher in suburbs and rural areas than in urban areas (Lippman 1992).

Particulate Matter

Airborne PM consists of a complex mixture of organic and inorganic solids and gas-liquids (aerosols) with heterogeneous physicochemical composition, size, and biologic activity (Gong 1992). PM is made up of particles of extremely diverse sizes. Particles of 3-50 nm in aerodynamic diameter are most prevalent in urban air adjacent to roadways as a result of vehicle emissions, but particles can be 100 nm or larger. The size of the PM dictates how deeply into the lungs the particles will penetrate, which is related to their potential for toxicity.

PM generated by combustion generally consists of different chemical species. PM can have adsorbed PAHs, aldehydes, sulfuric acid, and toxic metals. Even individual particles in an aerosol typically will have a complex chemical composition. The effects of a particular component of an aerosol may depend on its physical state, that is, whether it is part of a particle core or adsorbed onto the particle surface.

Toxicokinetics

Gases

Water solubility is the main determinant of how deeply into the lungs a gas penetrates. In general, highly soluble gases, such as SO_2, do not penetrate farther than the nose. Insoluble gases, such as O_3 and NO_2, penetrate deeply into the lungs and are more toxic. Highly insoluble gases, such as CO and H_2S, pass through the respiratory tract and are taken up into the bloodstream and distributed throughout the body.

Breathing rate, blood flow, and route of exposure (oral vs nasal) to the lungs also affect the bioavailability of gases. Increased airflow can increase the penetration of some gases (such as SO_2) into the lungs. Therefore, a person who is exercising will have increased bioavailability of such gases. Increased blood flow to the lungs, as occurs during exercise, also increases the bioavailability of gases that are taken up into the bloodstream.

Particulate Matter

In general, large particles (over 10 μm) will not remain suspended in the air and will not enter the air passages and therefore are not bioavailable. As particles become smaller they are deposited farther down the respiratory tract and particles smaller than 2.5μm are deposited deep in the lung.

Other hazardous pollutants, such as toxic metals, can be adsorbed onto the surface of particles, and this leads to exposure to them. The reactivity and solubility of the components of the PM also affect their bioavailability. More-reactive and more-soluble compounds interact with the lungs and are deposited more proximally than less-reactive and less-soluble compounds, which can be deposited deeper in the lungs. PAHs, which also can be present on PM, can be absorbed in humans and animals. PAHs are widely distributed in animals (there are no comparable data on humans). Metabolism occurs via many pathways. The metabolites include epoxide intermediates, dihydrodiols, phenols, and quinines. The epoxide intermediates are electrophilic and are thought to mediate the genotoxicity of PAHs. In animals, the feces are the major route of excretion after inhalation.

Toxicity Studies

Toxicity studies have been conducted on combustion product mixtures and on the individual components of combustion products. This section discusses studies of mixtures of smoke or exhaust and then the health effects seen in relevant studies after exposures to some of the individual components of combustion products. The focus is on inhalation studies because the committee considered inhalation to be the route of exposure most relevant to potential exposures in the Gulf War. A brief discussion of the potential effects of PM after dermal exposure is included.

Experimental studies of the effects of combustion products after inhalation have been conducted in air chambers and with intratracheal instillation. The method of exposure should be taken into account in interpreting and extrapolating their results. It should also be noted that the committee has focused on the initiation or induction of disease and not on the exacerbation of disease states. This section therefore focuses on effects on normal, not compromised, animals.

Mixtures of Combustion Products

Two studies investigated the effects specifically of smoke from the Kuwaiti oil-well fires. Moeller et al. (1994) studied feral cats exposed to the smoke. Cats were collected from Kuwait about 8 months after the fires began. Twelve of the animals were from Kuwait City, which was relatively smoke-free and 14 were from Ahmadi, in which there was high smoke exposure. Histopathologic tests were conducted on all major organs (for example, lung, liver, and kidney), and lung, liver, kidney, urine, and blood samples were tested for the presence of various toxicants. The authors concluded that exposure to the smoke had little or no long-term effects on the animals.

Brain et al. (1998) compared the effects of intratracheal instillation of the particles from the oil fires (smaller than 3.5 μm) at 0.15, 0.75, and 3.75 mg/100 g of body weight with those of particles collected in St. Louis, Missouri, on pulmonary inflammation in hamsters. Twenty-four hours after instillation, the hamsters exposed to the oil-fire particles had effects qualitatively similar to those in hamsters exposed to the particles from St. Louis. But they had higher concentrations of macrophages and neutrophils and lower myeloperoxidase and lactate dehydrogenase activity in their bronchoalveolar lavage than the animals exposed to the St. Louis particles. Albumin and ss-N-acetylglucosaminidase activities were comparable. Most of the measures had returned to control values by 7 days after instillation. The authors concluded that the responses in hamsters to particles from the oil fires were similar to those from typical urban summer pollution in St. Louis.

A number of acute-exposure toxicity studies have been conducted in laboratory animals, of which several are described here. A single exposure of sheep to wood smoke via inhalation resulted in dose-dependent injury to the tracheobronchial epithelium and lung parenchyma, but total antioxidant potential was not affected (Park et al. 2004). Ho and Kou (2002) studied the mechanism of wood-smoke-induced increases in nasal-airway resistance and airway reactivity in anesthetized rats. Reflex cholinergic and tachykininergic and possibly augmented nasal swelling appeared to be involved. The effects of subchronic exposure of brown Norway rats to relatively low concentrations of wood smoke—fine particles (smaller than 1 μm) at 1 or 10 mg/m^3—5 days/week for 4 or 12 weeks in whole-body chambers were investigated by Tesfaigzi et al. (2002). Mild respiratory effects were seen. At the high concentration, pulmonary function and pulmonary resistance were somewhat affected. Mild chronic inflammation and squamous metaplasia were observed in the larynx of exposed groups. Alveolar macrophage hyperplasia severity was increased and pigmentation was increased with dose, and the alveolar septa were slightly thickened.

Because epidemiologic data indicate a possible association between exposure to smoke and respiratory cancer, toxicologic studies have been conducted to further investigate the association. Studies have indicated that smoke from cooking with biofuels was associated with increased micronuclei and chromosomal aberrations in Indian women; the extent of the effects depended on the cooking fuel (Musthapa et al. 2004). Lohani et al. (2000) investigated the genotoxicity of kerosene soot in vitro in Syrian hamster embryo fibroblasts. The significant increase in induced micronuclei seen after treatment with soot (0.5-1.0 $\mu g/cm^2$ for 66 hr) indicated that kerosene soot can be genotoxic in vitro. Subcutaneous injection of extracts of soot from cooking fires into mice led to skin cancer (Liang et al. 1984), and dermal application of soot extracts from smoky-coal but not wood combustion could act as a complete carcinogen in mice (Mumford et al. 1990). Exposing rats and mice to coal and wood smoke by natural inhalation (placing the animals in rooms with cooking similar to what would occur in homes in some areas of China) resulted in a statistical increase in number of lung cancers (Liang et al. 1988). The larger increase was seen after exposure to coal smoke.

A great deal of research has also been conducted into the possible health effects of diesel exhaust, which is relevant not only because diesel fuel was burned in the Gulf War but because diesel exhaust contains many of the same components as other combustion products, such as smoke from oil-well fires. The potential health effects and experimental data on diesel exhaust have been reviewed and summarized by EPA (2002). Chronic exposure of animals to concentrations of diesel exhaust that are not acutely toxic have demonstrated respiratory effects (histopathologic and immunologic) in several animal species. Diesel exhaust has also been shown to be carcinogenic in a number of laboratory animals. Diesel exhaust given by inhalation at levels sufficient to induce particle overload has been shown to be carcinogenic in rats, but not in other rodent species (Nikula 2000). There is evidence that diesel exhaust, or some fraction of diesel exhaust, is mutagenic. What fraction might mediate effects is not well established (EPA 2002).

Gases

Hydrogen Sulfide

Histologic and biochemical changes have been seen in the respiratory system after acute toxic exposures to H_2S (for review, see ATSDR 1999a). The effects of lower concentrations of intermediate or chronic exposure are not as clear.

The Chemical Industry Institute of Toxicology (CIIT 1983a, 1983b, 1983c) exposed Fisher-344 rats, Sprague Dawley rats, and B6C3F mice to H_2S at a time-weighted average concentration of 10.1, 30.5, or 80 ppm for 6 hr/day 5 days/week for 90 days. No treatment-related effects on the cardiovascular system, the gastrointestinal system, immune function, the renal system, the hepatic system, bone marrow or bones, or the hematologic system were seen. Body weight was decreased by 10% in female Sprague Dawley rats in the 80-ppm dose group, and inflammation of the nasal mucosa was seen in mice at that dose. CIIT also looked at behavior and neuropathology end points and reproductive effects; no effects on any of those end points were seen.

Curtis et al. (1975) exposed pigs to H_2S at 8.5 ppm for 24 hr/day for 17 days; no effects on the gastrointestinal system were observed.

Hayden et al. (1990) saw an increase in parturition time and difficulty in delivery in 6 of 17 rats exposed to H_2S at 20, 50, or 75 ppm but in only one of seven control animals; no statistical analyses were performed. Although few studies have been conducted, H_2S does not appear to be genotoxic (ATSDR 1999a). No chronic bioassays have been conducted.

Researchers examined neurohistologic characteristics (Hannah and Roth 1991) and brain amino acid concentrations (Hannah et al. 1989) in rats exposed to H_2S from gestational day 5 through postpartum day 21. Some alterations in the architecture and growth characteristics of Purkinje cell dendritic fields were seen after exposure to H_2S at 20 ppm (Hannah and Roth 1991) and a decrease in brain amino acid concentrations at 75 but not 50 ppm (Hannah et al. 1989). Data from Skrajny et al. (1992) have also demonstrated altered neurotransmitter concentrations after exposure to H_2S. A decrease in norepinephrine concentrations and an increase in serotonin concentrations were seen after exposure of rats to H_2S at 20 ppm for 7 hr/day from gestational day 5 to postpartum day 21.

Taken together, the data on H_2S do not demonstrate any consistent effects at concentrations that are below those which are acutely toxic.

Sulfur Dioxide

SO_2 is a highly soluble irritating gas that is quickly absorbed in the nose and upper airway and does not reach the lower parts of the respiratory system under resting conditions (ATSDR 1998). Lower parts of the respiratory system can become targets during exercise. Immediate responses have been seen after exposure to SO_2 in many controlled human experiments at 5 ppm and above (Costa 2001). Asthmatics appear to be more sensitive to the effects of SO_2.

SO_2 has been demonstrated to decrease mucociliary clearance. Prolonged exposure of donkeys to SO_2 at 102 $\mu g/m^3$ for 1 hr/day 5 days/week for 6 months (Schlesinger et al. 1979) and rabbits at 250 $\mu g/m^3$ for 1 hr/day 5 days/week for 4, 8, or 12 months (Gearhart and Schlesinger 1989) caused persistent decreases in mucociliary clearance. Observed effects might have been mediated by a change in the mucus pH, composition, or consistency. Inhalation of SO_2 might also have altered mucus production by increasing the number of mucus-secreting cells.

Pulmonary changes due to SO_2 have been seen in exposed animals. Mild lesions in the lungs were seen in hamsters exposed to SO_2 at 650 ppm for 4 hr/day 5 days/week for 19-74 weeks (Goldring et al. 1970). Lung function was affected in rabbits exposed at 70-300 ppm for 6 weeks (Miyata et al. 1990) and guinea pigs exposed at 10 ppm for 1 hr/day for 30 days (Haider 1985). SO_2-induced lung biochemical and histologic changes in laboratory animals were also seen by Krasnowska et al. (1998) (30-40 ppm for 1 hr/day 5 days/week for 12 weeks), Lamb and Reid (1968) (400 ppm for 3 hr/day 5 days/week for up to 42 days), and Basbaum et al. (1990) (400 ppm for 3 hr/day 5 days/week for up to 3 weeks).

In chronic studies, no respiratory, cardiovascular, hematologic, hepatic, or renal effects were seen after SO_2 exposure of monkeys at 5.1 ppm for 23.3 hr/day 7 days/week for 78 weeks (Alarie et al. 1975) or guinea pigs at 5.72 ppm for 22 h/day 7 days/week for 52 weeks (Alarie et al. 1972). Oxidative effects (lipid peroxidation), however, were seen in the hearts of guinea pigs exposed at 10 ppm 1 hr/day for 30 days (Haider 1985).

Riedel et al. (1992) examined the effects of SO_2 at 5 ppm for 8 hr/day for 5 days on immune function in guinea pigs. They found an increase in sensitization to ovalbumin but no other consistent immune effects.

Reproductive effects were not seen in mice or rabbits exposed in utero to SO_2 (Murray et al. 1979; Petruzzi et al. 1996). No developmental effects were seen in mice exposed at up to 250 ppm from gestational day 7 through 17 (Singh 1982), but some neurodevelopmental effects were seen in mice exposed at 32 or 65 ppm from gestational day 7 through 18 (Singh 1989); effects on skeletal development were seen in mice at 25 ppm for 7 hr/day from gestational day 6 through 15 and rabbits at 70 ppm for 7 hr/day from gestational day 6 through 18 (Murray et al. 1979).

Peacock and Spence (1967) found some evidence of carcinogenicity of SO_2. Possible lung carcinomas and lung adenomas were seen in mice exposed to SO_2 at 50 ppm for 5 min/day 5 days/week for 2 years. However, only a single dose was tested, and further studies are needed to establish whether SO_2 is carcinogenic in animals. Any malignant effects could be caused by chronic irritation of respiratory epithelium. In addition, data indicate that SO_2 can be genotoxic (ATSDR 1998).

Nitrogen Oxides

Numerous laboratory-animal studies have been conducted on the toxicity of NO_x; most focused on NO_2. The toxicology of NO_2 has been reviewed by the World Health Organization (WHO 1997), Environmental Protection Agency (EPA 1993), and the National Research Council (NRC 1985, 2002).

The primary target of NO_2 is the lungs, although it can produce changes in the blood and other organs as well (EPA 1993). Acute high-dose exposure to NO_2 can lead to hypoxia. NO_2 reaches the lungs and rapidly diffuses to the blood, where it reacts with hemoglobin (Costa 2001). That reaction, however, is typically not seen with exposures at concentrations below 10 ppm. At lower concentrations, the main concerns about NO_2 are effects on the lungs (for example, edema, congestion, and damaged cilia) and on the host defense system in the lungs (NRC 2002; WHO 1997). The observed effects are usually reversible, although a great degree of inflammation can lead to permanent lung damage or death.

Effects on the immune system and lungs are also the primary concern when laboratory animals are repeatedly exposed to NO_2. For example, impaired resistance to *Streptococcus* sp. infections, defined as decreased survival and survival time, has been observed in mice after exposure at 0.5 ppm for 3 hr/day for 3 months (Ehrlich et al. 1979). The persistence of the effects, however, is not known. Furthermore, some data indicate that continuous exposure of mice to NO_2 at 0.5 ppm has effects, but that intermittent exposure does not (Ehrlich and Henry 1968). Immune suppression has also been observed in mice after exposure at above 5 ppm (Rose et al. 1988; Rose et al. 1989). Structural changes occurred in lungs of rats exposed to NO_2 at as low as 0.5 ppm for up to 19 months (Hayashi et al. 1987). Studies in rabbits, rats, and beagles showed that chronic exposure to NO_2 at 8, 15, and 0.64 ppm, respectively, led to emphysema of the type found in human lungs (WHO 1997).

Standard carcinogenicity bioassays of NO_2 have not been conducted. Evidence from other types of studies (acute-, subchronic-, and chronic-exposure studies) in laboratory animals did not show that NO_2 can cause tumors on its own (for review, see WHO 1997). Results of studies of the cocarcinogenic potential of NO_2 are equivocal. Overall, the effects on the potential carcinogenicity of NO_2 are inconsistent, and this requires further investigation.

Ozone

O_3 is a highly reactive oxidant that does not appear to penetrate the liquid linings of the lung (Costa 2001; EPA 1996). It can disrupt the barrier function of the lung and lead to increased permeability by other compounds and produce inflammation. Inflammation could then lead to further lung damage and a thickening of the air-blood barrier. In a number of laboratory animals, O_3 has consistently been shown to affect the ciliated epithelial cells of the airways, type 1 epithelial cells of the gas-air exchange region, and ciliated cells in the nasal region. Those effects result in a change in the cellular composition of the lung and can lead to a thickening of the air-blood barrier and decreases in mucociliary clearance.

With chronic exposure, there is an initial inflammatory response that peaks in the first few days of exposure. Epithelial hyperplasia then occurs but returns to normal on cessation of exposure. Fibrotic tissue changes occur gradually and can persist or even increase after cessation of exposure (Last et al. 1984). From studies in monkeys, it appears that intermittent exposures (for example, once a month) might have a greater effect than daily or continuous exposures at the same concentration (Reiser et al. 1987).

Pulmonary function changes are seen after acute exposures. The effects of long-term exposure on pulmonary function are not consistent and appear to be reversible on cessation of exposure (Chang et al. 1992; Costa et al. 1995; NTP 1994). Airway responsiveness was affected in animals sensitized to the allergen ovalbumin, but O_3 alone at 0.3 ppm for 4 hr/day 4 days/week for 24 weeks had no effect (Schlesinger et al. 2002).

A great deal of research has investigated the effects of O_3 on the immune system; animal studies support data from humans indicating that dose and duration are important in determining the effect. Early studies by Coffin and Blommer (1967) showed an increase in infectivity after O_3 exposure. Gilmour et al. (1993) demonstrated that the increased infectivity might be due to altered phagocytosis. Osebold et al. (1980) demonstrated an increased immune response in animals sensitized with ovalbumin after O_3 exposure. O_3 has also been shown to affect macrophage functions (Cohen et al. 1996, 2001; Zelikoff et al. 1991), and cytokines (Cohen et al. 2001).

Chronic bioassays have indicated that O_3 has some potential for carcinogenicity, but the results appear to depend on species and sex. In animals exposed at 0.12, 0.5, and 1.0 ppm of ozone for 6 hr/day 5 days/week or at 0.12 ppm for 2 years, the National Toxicology Program (NTP 1994) concluded that there is no evidence of carcinogenicity in rats. In male mice with the same treatments, increases in adenomas and carcinomas were observed in the lungs, but no concentration-dependent response was observed. In addition, in a lifetime exposure study, O_3 at

0.5 ppm or 1.0 ppm for 125 weeks did not have tumor-promoting activity in mice treated with tobacco carcinogen (NTP 1994).

O_3 can have other systemic effects. Because it does not pass the air-blood barrier, however, many of them are thought to be secondary to lung injury or due to reaction products of O_3. Oxidative intermediates can be formed from the reaction of O_3 with other compounds, and the intermediates could mediate some of the effects of O_3.

Carbon Monoxide and Carbon Dioxide

CO and CO_2 can both be toxic if the concentrations are high enough. Both can lead to death due to asphyxiation, although the underlying cause of the asphyxiation differs. The effects of both compounds at concentrations that do not cause overt symptoms, however, are not well studied.

The effects of chronic, low exposures to CO are thought to be mediated by effects of CO on oxygen-carrying capacity of the blood. Developmental effects have been seen after acute poisonings with CO in animals; the developing auditory system appears sensitive (Lopez et al. 2003; Stockard-Sullivan et al. 2003). Effects on the cardiovascular system have also been seen at concentrations that are below acutely toxic concentrations (Dubuis et al. 2002; Melin et al. 2002).

Particulate Matter

As discussed previously, the size of particles has a great effect on their toxicity. Concern typically begins with the PM that is 10 μm or less; the main concerns are associated with fine (less than 2.5 μm) and ultrafine (less than 0.1 μm) particles. Size not only affects particle deposition but also can affect the surface area and later the amount of hazardous materials adsorbed on particles. The effects of the PM found in diesel exhaust have been studied intensively. Unless results are directly related to the PM in diesel exhaust, those studies are discussed above under "Mixtures of Combustion Products". The potential health effects of PM and research priorities have recently been reviewed (EPA 2003a; NRC 2004).

One of the main concerns after exposure to PM is effects on the respiratory system. Chronic, noncancer respiratory effects seen in animals are in the lungs; dose-dependent inflammation and histopathologic changes have been seen in the lungs of rats, mice, hamsters, and monkeys (EPA 2003a). The immune response appears to be affected by both fine and ultrafine particles (Zelikoff et al. 2003). Exposure of laboratory animals to residual oil fly ash (a product of the combustion of oil and residual fuel oil that contains transition metals) can lead to inflammatory lung injury (Ghio et al. 2002).

Cardiovascular effects have also been seen after animals have been exposed to PM. Changes in heart rate have been observed, but they were not accompanied by respiratory changes (EPA 2003a). It is thought that PM has its effects on the cardiovascular system through the uptake of particles into the circulation and the release of soluble substances into circulation or through effects on the autonomic control of the heart and the circulatory system. It is not known, however, whether this effect persists or is transient. The mechanism by which particulate matter increases cardiovascular effects is not known, but recent research suggests that when mediators enter the circulation, the bone marrow is stimulated and causes the release of white blood cell precursors into the bloodstream (Goto et al. 2004; Tan et al. 2000). That response may lead to increased cardiorespiratory morbidity and mortality.

Other systemic effects have also been seen. Those effects, such as hemodynamic effects, increased the risk of heart attack and stroke and effects on hematopoiesis are thought to be secondary to the lung injury seen (EPA 2003a).

One component of PM that might provide some biologic plausibility for its toxic effects is PAHs. As discussed earlier, reactive epoxide intermediates can form in the metabolism of PAHs; the intermediates are genotoxic and could lead to carcinogenicity. Schulte et al. (1994) saw an increase in all lung tumors and a dose-dependent increase in malignant tumors in mice exposed to PAH-enriched exhaust containing benzo[a]pyrene at 0.05 or 0.09 mg/m^3. Tumors of the nasal cavity, pharynx, larynx, and trachea were seen in a dose-dependent manner in hamsters exposed to benzo[a]pyrene at 9.5 or 46.5 mg/m^3 for 109 weeks, but no lung tumors were seen in those animals (Thyssen et al. 1981). No effects were seen in the lungs, nose, and kidneys of Fischer rats exposed by nose to an aerosol of benzo[a]pyrene at 7.7 mg/m^3 for 2 hr/day 5 days/week for 4 weeks (Wolff et al. 1989).

Skin disorders have been seen in animals after dermal exposure to PAHs. In an early study, suppression of sebaceous glands was seen in Swiss mice treated with benzo[a]pyrene, benz[a]anthracene, and dibenz[a,h]anthracene, but no controls were used (Bock and Mund 1958). Increased cell proliferation and inflammation were seen after exposure to a single treatment of 16, 32, or 64 μg once a week for 29 weeks (Albert et al. 1991). There is also evidence that PAHs are photosensitizers in mice, but that effect appears to be reversible (Forbes et al. 1976) and there is evidence of skin carcinogenicity in animals treated dermally with PAHs; a number of studies showed that intermediate exposure to PAHs produces skin tumors (ATSDR 1995d).

INDIVIDUAL SUSCEPTIBILITY

Because of variations in genetic makeup, a genetically susceptible person will exhibit responses to a hydrocarbon fuel or to combustion products different from those of most persons exposed to an identical dose.

Little has been documented about specific differences in genetic susceptibility to hydrocarbon fuels and their components, but exploration of the human genome promises advances in the near future. Some information suggests that people with an erythrocyte glucose-6-phosphate dehydrogenase deficiency may have increased susceptibility to the hemolytic effects of naphthalene (ATSDR 1999b). People with aryl hydrocarbon hydroxylase that is particularly susceptible to induction and people with genetic diseases associated with DNA-repair deficiencies (such as Down syndrome and familial retinoblastoma) may be particularly susceptible to the carcinogenic effects of PAHs (ATSDR 1999b).

Little is known also about specific differences in genetic susceptibility with respect to combustion products. Some components of combustion products are metabolized to active metabolites, which are later detoxified. Differences in the activity of the enzymes involved in those toxification and detoxification pathways can alter a person's susceptibility to combustion-product components. For example, increased formation of the epoxide intermediates by increased activity of p450 enzymes that activate PAHs would increase a person's susceptibility to PAHs, whereas increased activity of epoxide hydrolase, which detoxifies epoxide metabolites, would protect against the toxicity of PAHs (Klaassen 2001). In addition to altered susceptibility resulting from enzyme activity, whether genetic or by induction of enzymes by coexposure to other compounds, people could have altered susceptibility to combustion products because of illness. An example is asthma-related increased susceptibility to many of the effects of combustion products.

INTERACTIONS

Because hydrocarbon fuels and their combustion products contain hundreds of components, it is probably not possible to identify all the possible interactions between a fuel and other substances, between components of a fuel, between combustion products and other substances, or between components of combustion products. Additive, synergistic, or antagonistic effects might occur; however, data on such effects are sparse. For example, primarily as a consequence of modifications in enzyme induction, the toxicity of benzene, a component of hydrocarbon fuels, can be altered by alcohol, drugs, industrial chemicals, radiation, metals, halogenated hydrocarbons, and pesticides (ATSDR 1995a).

Several recent studies have evaluated interactions between a hydrocarbon fuel and other substances. Peden-Adam et al. (2001) assessed immunotoxic effects of concurrent exposure of mice to pyridostigmine bromide (an anti-nerve-gas agent), *N,N*-diethyl-*m*-toluamide (DEET, an insect repellent), and JP-8. The findings of their study indicate that combined exposure to those three materials does not significantly alter many immunologic end points (body, spleen, and thymus mass; spleen and thymus cellularity; peripheral white-cell populations; lymphocyte proliferation; macrophage nitrite production; and natural killer-cell and cytotoxic T-lymphocyte activity) but does selectively target functional end points, such as delayed-type hypersensitivity responses.

Baynes et al. (2001) studied the influence of three JP-8 performance additives on dermal disposition of two fuel components: naphthalene and dodecane. Jet-A, which has the same hydrocarbon composition as JP-8 but without the performance additives, was mixed with up to three performance additives, and disposition was assayed by using isolated perfused porcine skin flaps. The data show that various combinations of the three performance additives can potentially alter the dermal disposition of the fuel components and that products of two-factor interactions were not predictable from single-factor exposures. Riviere et al. (2002) also used the isolated perfused porcine skin-flap model to evaluate potential interactions among various combinations of low sulfur mustard, JP-8, DEET, and permethrin exposures. Data from the study suggest that JP-8 exposure may modulate transdermal flux of permethrin.

There has also been research on the components of combustion products that indicated that the presence of one component affects the toxicity of other components. For example, there is evidence of antagonistic effects between O_3 and SO_2 that depend on the end point (Schlesinger and Graham 1992), and, as discussed previously, components adsorbed on PM behave differently from those not adsorbed on PM.

REFERENCES

ACGIH (American Conference of Industrial Hygienists). 2003. 2003 TLVs and BEIs: Threshold Limit Values for Chemical Substances and Physical Agents. Biological Exposure Indices. Cincinnati, OH: American Conference of Governmental Industrial Hygienists.

Air Force. 1989. *The Installation Restoration Program Toxicology Guide. Volume 4*. Oak Ridge, TN: Biomedical and Environmental Information Analysis; as cited in ATSDR 1998.

Alarie Y, Ulrich CE, Busey WM, Krumm AA, MacFarland HN. 1972. Long-term continuous exposure to sulfur dioxide in cynomolgus monkeys. *Archives of Environmental Health* 24(2):115-128.

Alarie YC, Krumm AA, Busey WM, Urich CE, Kantz RJ. 1975. Long-term exposure to sulfur dioxide, sulfuric acid mist, fly ash, and their mixtures. Results of studies in monkeys and guinea pigs. *Archives of Environmental Health* 30(5):254-262.

Albert RE, Miller ML, Cody T, Andringa A, Shukla R, Baxter CS. 1991. Benzo[a]pyrene-induced skin damage and tumor promotion in the mouse. *Carcinogenesis* 12(7):1273-1280.

Alden CL. 1986. A review of unique male rat hydrocarbon nephropathy. *Toxicologic Pathology* 14(1):109-111.

API (American Petroleum Institute). 1988a. In Vivo Sister Chromatid Exchange (SCE) Assay with API 81-07: Hydrodesulferized Kerosene. API Med. Res.Publ. 36-30043. Washington, DC: American Petroleum Institute, Health and Environmental Science Department; as cited in Skisak et al. 1995.

API. 1988b. Sister Chromatid Exchange (SCE) Assay in Chinese Hamster Ovary (CHO) Cell with API 81-07: Hydrodesulferized Kerosene. API Med. Res.Publ. 35-32482. Washington, DC: American Petroleum Institute, Health and Environmental Science Department; as cited in Skisak et al. 1995.

ATSDR (Agency for Toxic Substances and Disease Registry). 1989. *Toxicological Profile for Toluene.* Atlanta, GA: US Department of Health and Human Services, Public Health Service, ATSDR.

ATSDR. 1990. *Toxicological Profiles for 1,3-Butsdiene, 1,2-Dibromoethane, Ethylbenzene and Xylene.* Atlanta, GA: US Department of Health and Human Services, Public Health Service, ATSDR.

ATSDR. 1991. *Toxicological Profiles for Benzene and Lead.* Atlanta, GA: US Department of Health and Human Services, Public Health Service, ATSDR.

ATSDR. 1995a. *Toxicological Profile for Automotive Gasoline* . Atlanta, GA: US Department of Health and Human Services, Public Health Service, ATSDR.

ATSDR. 1995b. *Toxicological Profile for Fuel Oils.* Atlanta, GA: US Department of Health and Human Services, Public Health Service, ATSDR.

ATSDR. 1995c. *Toxicological Profile for Jet Fuels (JP4 and JP7).* Atlanta, GA: US Department of Health and Human Services, Public Health Service, ATSDR.

ATSDR. 1995d. *Toxicological Profile for Polycyclic Aromatic Hydrocarbons (PAHs) (Update).* Atlanta, GA: US Department of Health and Human Services, Public Health Service, ATSDR.

ATSDR. 1995e. *Toxicological Profile for Xylenes (Update).* Atlanta, GA: US Department of Health and Human Services, Public Health Service, ATSDR.

ATSDR. 1998. *Toxicological Profile for Jet Fuels (JP-5 and JP-8).* Atlanta, GA: US Department of Health and Human Services, Public Health Service, ATSDR.

ATSDR. 1999a. *Toxicological Profile for Hydrogen Sulfide.* Atlanta, GA: US Department of Health and Human Services, Public Health Service, ATSDR.

ATSDR. 1999b. *Toxicological Profile for Total Petroleum Hydrocarbons (TPH).* Atlanta, GA: US Department of Health and Human Services, Public Health Service, ATSDR.

Basbaum C, Gallup M, Gum J, Kim Y, Jany B. 1990. Modification of mucin gene expression in the airways of rats exposed to sulfur dioxide. *Biorheology* 27(3-4):485-489.

Baynes RE, Brooks JD, Budsaba K, Smith CE, Riviere JE. 2001. Mixture effects of JP-8 additives on the dermal disposition of jet fuel components. *Toxicology and Applied Pharmacology* 175(3):269-281.

Beliles RP, Mecler FJ. 1982. Inhalation teratology of jet fuel A, fuel oil and petroleum naphtha in rats. In: MacFarland H, Holdsworth C, MacGregor JA, Call R, Kane M, eds. *Proceedings of the Symposium: The Toxicology of Petroleum Hydrocarbons.* Washington, DC: American Petroleum Institute. Pp. 233-238.

Bock FG, Mund R. 1958. A survey of compounds for activity in the suppression of mouse sebaceous glands. *Cancer Research* 18(8 Part 1):887-892.

Bogo B, Young RW, Hill TA, Feser CL, Nold J, Parker GA, Cartledge. R.M. 1983. The Toxicity of Petroleum and Shale JP5. AFRRI SR83-26. Bethesda, MD: Armed Forces Radiobiology Research Institute. Pp. 46-66.

Brain JD, Long NC, Wolfthal SF, Dumyahn T, Dockery DW. 1998. Pulmonary toxicity in hamsters of smoke particles from Kuwaiti oil fires. *Environmental Health Perspectives* 106(3):141-146.

Bruner RH, Kinkead ER, O'Neill TP, Flemming CD, Mattie DR, Russell CA, Wall HG. 1993. The toxicologic and oncogenic potential of JP-4 jet fuel vapors in rats and mice: 12-month intermittent inhalation exposures. *Fundamental and Applied Toxicology* 20(1):97-110.

Brusick DJ, Matheson DW. 1978a. *Mutagen and Oncogen Study on JP-4. AMRL-TR-78-24.* Wright Patterson Air Force Base, OH: Aerospace Medical Research Laboratory.

Brusick DJ, Matheson DW. 1978b. *Mutagen and Oncogen Study on JP-8 AMRL-TR-78-20.* Wright Patterson Air Force Base, OH: Aerospace Medical Research Laboratory.

Budavari S, O'Neil MJ, Smith A. 1989. *The Merck Index: An Encyclopedia of Chemicals, Drugs, and Biologicals.* Rahway, NJ: Merck and Co.

Bui QQ, Burnett DM, Breglia RJ, Koschier FJ, Lapadula ES, Podhasky PI, Schreiner CA, White RD, Dalbey WE, Feuston MH. 1998. Toxicity evaluation of petroleum blending streams: Reproductive and developmental effects of a distillate from light alkylate naphtha. *Journal of Toxicology and Environmental Health. Part A.* 53(2):121-133.

Carpenter CP, Geary DL Jr, Myers RC, Nachreiner DJ, Sullivan LJ, King JM. 1976. Petroleum hydrocarbon toxicity studies. XI. Animal and human response to vapors of deodorized kerosene. *Toxicology and Applied Pharmacology* 36(3):443-456.

Chang LY, Huang Y, Stockstill BL, Graham JA, Grose EC, Menache MG, Miller FJ, Costa DL , Crapo JD. 1992. Epithelial injury and interstitial fibrosis in the proximal alveolar regions of rats chronically exposed to a simulated pattern of urban ambient ozone. *Toxicology and Applied Pharmacology* 115(2):241-252.

CIIT (Chemical Industry Institute of Toxicology). 1983a. *Ninety-day vapor inhalation toxicity study of hydrogen sulfide in B6C3F1 mice. CIIT Docket No. 42063.* Research Triangle Park, NC: Chemical Industry Institute of Toxicology.

CIIT. 1983b. *Ninety-day vapor inhalation toxicity study of hydrogen sulfide in Fischer-344 rats. CIIT Docket No. 22063.* Research Triangle Park, NC: Chemical Industry Institute of Toxicology.

CIIT. 1983c. *Ninety-day vapor inhalation toxicity study of hydrogen sulfide in Sprague-Dawley rats. CIIT Docket No. 32063.* Research Triangle Park, NC: Chemical Industry Institute of Toxicology.

Cofer WR, Stevens RK, Winstead EL. 1992. Kuwaiti oil fires: Compositions of source smoke. *Journal of Geophysical Research* 97:14521-14525.

Coffin DL, Blommer EJ. 1967. Acute toxicity of irradiated auto exhaust. Its indication by enhancement of mortality from streptococcal pneumonia. *Archives of Environmental Health* 15(1):36-38.

Cohen MD, Sisco M, Li Y, Zelikoff JT, Schlesinger RB. 2001. Ozone-induced modulation of cell-mediated immune responses in the lungs. *Toxicology and Applied Pharmacology* 171(2):71-84.

Cohen MD, Zelikoff JT, Qu Q, Schlesinger RB. 1996. Effects of ozone upon macrophage-interferon interactions. *Toxicology* 114(3):243-252.

Conaway DD, Schreiner CA, Cragg ST. 1984. Mutagencity evaluation of petroleum hydrocarbons. In: MacFarland HN, Holdsworth CE, MacGregor JA, Call RW, Lane ML, eds. *Advances in Modern Environmental Toxicology. Vol. 6, Applied Toxicology of Petroleum Haydrocarbons.* Princeton, NJ: Princeton Scientific. Pp. 89-197; as cited in IARC 1989.

Cooper JR, Mattie DR. 1996. Developmental toxicity of JP-8 jet fuel in the rat. *Journal of Applied Toxicology* 16(3):197-200.

Costa DL. 2001. Air Pollution. In: Klaassen C, ed. *Casarett and Doull's Toxicology: The Basic Science of Poisons.* 6th ed. New York: McGraw-Hill. Pp. 979-1012.

Costa DL, Tepper JS, Stevens MA, Watkinson WP, Doerfler DL, Gelzleichter TR, Last JA. 1995. Restrictive lung disease in rats exposed chronically to an urban profile of ozone. *American Journal of Respiratory and Critical Care Medicine* 151(5):1512-1518.

Cowan MJ, Jenkins LJ. 1981. U.S. Navy toxicity study of shale and petroleum JP-5 aviation fuel and diesel fuel marine. In: Guerin MR, Griest WH, Coffin DI, eds. *Health Effects Investigation of Oil Shale Development.* Ann Arbor, MI: Ann Arbor Science. Pp. 129-140.

Curtis SE, Anderson CR, Simon J, Jensen AH, Day DL, Kelley KW. 1975. Effects of aerial ammonia, hydrogen sulfide and swine-house dust on rate of gain and respiratory-tract structure in swine. *Journal of Animal Science* 41(3):735-739.

Dalbey W, Henry M, Holmberg R, Moneyhun J, Schmoyer R, Lock S. 1987. Role of exposure parameters in toxicity of aerosolized diesel fuel in the rat. *Journal of Applied Toxicology* 7(4):265-275.

Deininger G, Jungen H, Wenzel-Hartung RP. 1991. *Middle Distillates: Analytical Investigations of Mutagenicity Studies. Research Reports No. 412-1*. Hamburg, Germany: DGMK; as cited in NRC 2003.

Dennis MW. 1982. *Acute Dermal LD50 Toxicity Study E-2B, E-6-B, E-8B, E-10, E-12*. Document #88-8100360. Washington, DC: U.S. Environmental Protection Agency, Office of Toxic Substances; as cited in ATSDR 1995c.

Draxler RR, McQueen JT, Stunder BJB. 1994. An evaluation of air pollutant exposures due to the 1991 Kuwait oil fires using a Lagrangian model. *Atmospheric Environment* 28(13):2197-2210.

Dubuis E, Gautier M, Melin A, Rebocho M, Girardin C, Bonnet P, Vandier C. 2002. Chronic carbon monoxide enhanced IbTx-sensitive currents in rat resistance pulmonary artery smooth muscle cells. *American Journal of Physiology. Lung Cellular and Molecular Physiology* 283(1):L120-L129.

Dudley AC, Peden-Adams MM, EuDaly J, Pollenz RS, Keil DE. 2001. An aryl hydrocarbon receptor independent mechanism of JP-8 jet fuel immunotoxicity in Ah-responsive and Ah-nonresponsive mice. *Toxicological Sciences* 59(2):251-259.

Ehrlich R, Findlay JC, Gardner DE. 1979. Effects of repeated exposures to peak concentrations of nitrogen dioxide and ozone on resistance to streptococcal pneumonia. *Journal of Toxicology and Environmental Health* 5(4):631-642.

Ehrlich R, Henry MC. 1968. Chronic toxicity of nitrogen dioxide. I. Effect on resistance to bacterial pneumonia. *Archives of Environmental Health* 17(6):860-865.

EPA (Environmental Protection Agency). 1993. *Air Quality Criteria for Oxides of Nitrogen. EPA-600/8-91/049aF*. Research Triangle Park, NC: Environmental Criteria and Assessment Office.

EPA. 1996. *Air Quality Criteria for Ozone and Related Photochemical Oxidants. EPA-600/P-93-004aF-cF*. Research Triangle Park, NC: National Center for Environmental Assessment-RTP Office.

EPA. 2002. *Health Assessment Document for Diesel Engine Exhaust. EPA/600/8-90/057F*. Research Triangle Park, NC: National Center for Environmental Assessment.

EPA. 2003a. *Air Quality Criteria for Particulate Matter, Volume 2. EPA/600/P-99/002bD*. Research Triangle Park, NC: National Center for Environmental Assessment-RTP.

EPA. 2003b. *SO_2: What Is It? Where Does It Come From?* [Online]. Available: http://www.epa.gov/air/urbanair/so2/what1.html [accessed February 2004].

Flamm WG, Lehman-McKeeman LD. 1991. The human relevance of the renal tumor-inducing potential of d-limonene in male rats: Implications for risk assessment. *Regulatory Toxicology and Pharmacology* 13(1):70-86.

Forbes PD, Davies RE, Urbach F. 1976. Phototoxicity and photocarcinogenesis: comparative effects of anthracene and 8-methoxypsoralen in the skin of mice. *Food and Cosmetics Toxicology* 14(4):303-306.

Garb J, Chenoweth MB. 1948. Studies on hydrocarbon-epinephrine induced ventricular fibrillation. *Journal of Pharmacology and Experimental Therapeutics* 94:12-18; as cited in NRC 1996b.

Gearhart JM, Schlesinger RB. 1989. Sulfuric acid-induced changes in the physiology and structure of the tracheobronchial airways. *Environmental Health Perspectives* 79:127-136.

Ghio AJ, Silbajoris R, Carson JL, Samet JM. 2002. Biologic effects of oil fly ash. *Environmental Health Perspectives* 110(Suppl 1):89-94.

Gilmour MI, Park P, Selgrade MK. 1993. Ozone-enhanced pulmonary infection with Streptococcus zooepidemicus in mice. The role of alveolar macrophage function and capsular virulence factors. *American Review of Respiratory Disease* 147(3):753-760.

Goldring IP, Greenburg L, Park SS, Ratner IM. 1970. Pulmonary effects of sulfur dioxide exposure in the Syrian hamster. II. Combined with emphysema. *Archives of Environmental Health* 21(1):32-37.

Gong H Jr. 1992. Health effects of air pollution. A review of clinical studies. *Clinics in Chest Medicine* 13(2):201-214.

Goodheart RS, Dunne JW. 1994. Petrol sniffer's encephalopathy. A study of 25 patients. *Medical Journal of Australia* 160(4):178-181; as cited in ATSDR 1995a.

Goto Y, Ishii H, Hogg JC, Shih CH, Yatera K, Vincent R, van Eeden SF. 2004. Particulate matter air pollution stimulates monocyte release from the bone marrow. *American Journal of Respiratory and Critical Care Medicine* 170(8):891-897.

Haider SS. 1985. Effects of exhaust pollutant sulfur dioxide on lipid metabolism of guinea pig organs. *Industrial Health* 23(2):81-87.

Hannah RS, Hayden LJ, Roth SH. 1989. Hydrogen sulfide exposure alters the amino acid content in developing rat CNS. *Neuroscience Letters* 99(3):323-327.

Hannah RS, Roth SH. 1991. Chronic exposure to low concentrations of hydrogen sulfide produces abnormal growth in developing cerebellar Purkinje cells. *Neuroscience Letters* 122(2):225-228.

Harris DT, Sakiestewa D, Robledo RF, Witten M. 1997a. Immunotoxicological effects of JP-8 jet fuel exposure. *Toxicology and Industrial Health* 13(1):43-55.

Harris DT, Sakiestewa D, Robledo RF, Witten M. 1997b. Protection from JP-8 jet fuel induced immunotoxicity by administration of aerosolized substance P. *Toxicology and Industrial Health* 13(5):571-588.

Harris DT, Sakiestewa D, Robledo RF, Young RS, Witten M. 2000. Effects of short-term JP-8 jet fuel exposure on cell-mediated immunity. *Toxicology and Industrial Health* 16(2):78-84.

Hayashi Y, Kohno T, Ohwada H. 1987. Morphological effects of nitrogen dioxide on the rat lung. *Environmental Health Perspectives* 73:135-145.

Hayden LJ, Goeden H, Roth SH. 1990. Growth and development in the rat during sub-chronic exposure to low levels of hydrogen sulfide. *Toxicology and Industrial Health* 6(3-4):389-401.

Ho CY, Kou YR. 2002. Mechanisms of wood smoke-induced increases in nasal airway resistance and reactivity in rats. *European Journal of Pharmacology* 436(1-2):127-134.

Hobbs PV, Raadke LF. 1992. Airborne studies of the smoke from Kuwait oil fires. *Science* 256:987-991.

HSDB (Hazardous Substances Data Bank). 2003a. *Gasoline*. [Online]. Available: http://toxnet.nlm.nih.gov/cgi-bin/sis/htmlgen?HSDB [accessed August 2004].

HSDB. 2003b. *Kerosene*. [Online]. Available: http://toxnet.nlm.nih.gov/cgi-bin/sis/htmlgen?HSDB [accessed August 2004].

IARC (International Agency for Research on Cancer). 1989. *Occupational Exposures in Petroleum Refining: Crude Oil and Major Petroleum Fuels. IARC Monographs on the Evaluation of Carcinogenic Risk to Humans.* 45. Lyon, France: IARC.

IOM (Institute of Medicine). 2003. *Gulf War and Health, Volume 2: Insecticides and Solvents.* Washington, DC: The National Academies Press.

Kainz R, White L. 1983. Consequences associated with the inhalation of uncombusted diesel vapor. In: MacFarland H, Holdsworth C, MacGregor J, Call R, Kane M, eds. *Proceedings of the Symposium: The Toxicology of Petroleum Hydrocarbons May, 1982 Washington, DC.* Washington DC: American Petroleum Institute. Pp. 233-243.

Kanikkannan N, Jackson T, Sudhan Shaik M, Singh M. 2000. Evaluation of skin sensitization potential of jet fuels by murine local lymph node assay. *Toxicology Letters* 116(1-2):165-170.

Keil DE, Warren DA, Jenny MJ, EuDaly JG, Smythe J, Peden-Adams MM. 2003. Immunological Function in Mice Exposed to JP-8 Jet Fuel In Utero. *Toxicological Sciences* 76(2):347-356.

Keller WC, Olson CT, Back KC, Gaworski CL. 1984. Teratogenic assessment of three methylated hydrazine derivatives in the rat. *Journal of Toxicology and Environmental Health* 13(1):125-131.

Kimber I, Weisenberger C. 1989. A murine local lymph node assay for the identification of contact allergens. Assay development and results of an initial validation study. *Archives of Toxicology* 63(4):274-282.

Kimura K, Nagata T, Hara K, Kageura M. 1988. Gasoline and kerosene components in blood—a forensic analysis. *Human Toxicology* 7(4):299-305.

Kinkead ER, Salins SA, Wolfe RE. 1992a. Acute irritation and sensitization potential of JP-9 fuel. *Journal of the American College of Toxicology* 11(6):700.

Kinkead ER, Wolfe RE, Salins SA. 1992b. Acute irritation and sensitization potential of shale-derived JP-5 jet fuel. *Journal of the American College of Toxicology* 11(6):705.

Klaassen C, ed. 2001. *Casarett and Doull's Toxicology: The Basic Science of Poison*. 6th ed. New York: McGraw-Hill.

Koschier FJ. 1999. Toxicity of middle distillates from dermal exposure. *Drug and Chemical Toxicology* 22(1):155-164.

Krasnowska M, Kwasniewski A, Rabczynski J, Fal A, Kuryszko J. 1998. Effect of heparin on the course of sulphur dioxide induced bronchitis in rats. *Archivum Immunologiae Et Therapiae Experimentalis* 46(1):17-24.

Kuna RA, Ulrich CE. 1984. Subchronic inhalation toxicity of two motor fuels. *Journal of the American College of Toxicology* 3:217-229; as cited in ATSDR 1995a.

Lamb D, Reid L. 1968. Mitotic rates, goblet cell increase and histochemical changes in mucus in rat bronchial epithelium during exposure to sulphur dioxide. *Journal of Pathology and Bacteriology* 96(1):97-111.

Lapin C, Bui Q, Breglia R, Koschier F, Podhasky P, Lapadula E, Roth R, Schreiner C, White R, Clark C, Mandella R, Hoffman G. 2001. Toxicity evaluation of petroleum blending streams: Inhalation subchronic toxicity/neurotoxicity study of a light catalytic cracked naphtha distillate in rats. *International Journal of Toxicology* 20(5):307-319.

Last JA, Reiser KM, Tyler WS, Rucker RB. 1984. Long-term consequences of exposure to ozone. I. Lung collagen content. *Toxicology and Applied Pharmacology* 72(1):111-118.

Liang CK, Quan NY, Cao SR, He XZ, Ma F. 1988. Natural inhalation exposure to coal smoke and wood smoke induces lung cancer in mice and rats. *Biomedical and Environmental Sciences* 1(1):42-50.

Liang CK, Quan NY, Ma F, Zhang Y, Wang EM, Yin XR. 1984. Carcinogenicity of extract of soot from Xuan Wei County administering subcutaneously to mice. *Environmental Science Research* 31:826-827; as cited in Liang et al. 1988.

Lippman M. 1992. Ozone. In: Rom WN, ed. *Environmental and Occupational Medicine*. 2nd ed. Boston: Little, Brown and Company. Pp. 489-502.

Litton Bionetics I. 1978 . *Teratology study in rats: Unleaded gasoline.* Kensington, MD: Litton Bionetics, Inc.; as cited in ATSDR 1995a.

Lock S, Dalbey W, Schmoyer R. 1984. *Chemical Characterization and Toxicologic evaluation of airborne mixtures: Inhalation toxicology of diesel fuel obscurant aerosol in Sprague-Dawley rats. ORNL/TM-9403.* Oak Ridge TN: Oak Ridge National Laboratory; as cited in ATSDR 1995b.

Lohani M, Dopp E, Weiss DG, Schiffmann D, Rahman Q. 2000. Kerosene soot genotoxicity: enhanced effect upon co-exposure with chrysotile asbestos in Syrian hamster embryo fibroblasts. *Toxicology Letters* 114(1-3):111-116.

Lopez I, Acuna D, Webber DS, Korsak RA, Edmond J. 2003. Mild carbon monoxide exposure diminishes selectively the integrity of the cochlea of the developing rat. *Journal of Neuroscience Research* 74(5):666-675.

MacEwen JD, Vernot EH. 1984. *Toxic Hazards Research Unit Annual Technical Report. AMRL-TR-84-001*. Wright-Paterson Air Force Base, OH: Aerospace Medical Research Laboratory.

MacFarland HN, Ulrich CE, Holdsworth CE. 1984. A chronic inhalation study with unleaded gasoline vapor. *Journal of the American College of Toxicology* 3:231-248; as cited in ATSDR 1995a and IARC 1989.

MacNaughton MG, Uddin DE. 1984. Toxicology of mixed distillate and high-energy synthetic fuels. In: Mehlman MA, Hemstreet GP III, Thorpe JJ, Weaver NK, eds. *Renal Effects of Petroleum Hydrocarbons*. Princeton, NJ: Princeton Scientific Publishers.

Mattie DR, Alden CL, Newell TK, Gaworski CL, Flemming CD. 1991. A 90-day continuous vapor inhalation toxicity study of JP-8 jet fuel followed by 20 or 21 months of recovery in fischer 344 rats and C57BL/6 mice. *Toxicologic Pathology* 19(2):77-87.

Mattie DR, Marit GB, Cooper JR, Sterner TR, Flemming CD. 2000. *Reproductive Effects of JP-8 Jet Fuel on Male and Female Sprague-Dawley Rats After Exposure by Oral Gavage. AFRL-HE-WP-TR-2000-0067.* Wright Patterson Air Force Base, OH: Aerospace Medical Research Laboratory.

Mattie DR, Marit GB, Flemming CD, Cooper JR. 1995. The effects of JP-8 jet fuel on male Sprague-Dawley rats after a 90-day exposure by oral gavage. *Toxicology and Industrial Health* 11(4):423-435.

McKee RH, Amoruso MA, Freeman JJ, Przygoda RT. 1994. Evaluation of the genetic toxicity of middle distillate fuels. *Environmental and Molecular Mutagenesis* 23(3):234-238.

McKee RH, Plutnick RT, Przygoda RT. 1989. The carcinogenic initiating and promoting properties of a lightly refined paraffinic oil. *Fundamental and Applied Toxicology* 12(4):748-756.

McKee RH, Trimmer GW, Whitman FT, Nessel CS, Mackerer CR, Hagemann R, Priston RA, Riley AJ, Cruzan G, Simpson BJ, Urbanus JH. 2000. Assessment in rats of the reproductive toxicity of gasoline from a gasoline vapor recovery unit. *Reproductive Toxicology* 14(4):337-353.

Melin A, Obert P, Rebocho M, Bonnet P. 2002. Cardiac morphology and function following long-term exposure to carbon monoxide at high altitude in rats. *Journal of Toxicology and Environmental Health. Part A* 65(23):1981-1998.

Miyata T, Ishii T, Sugiyama N, Okano Y, Nishi N, Takahama K, Ogasawara S, Oda Y, Yokoyama K, Murata Y, Kai H. 1990. Effect of N-acetylneuraminic acid on respiratory tract secretion and inflammation in the bronchitic rabbit. *Archives Internationales De Pharmacodynamie Et De Therapie* 304:277-289.

Moeller RB Jr, Kalasinsky VF, Razzaque M, Centeno JA, Dick EJ, Abdal M, Petrov II, DeWitt TW, al-Attar M, Pletcher JM. 1994. Assessment of the histopathological lesions and chemical analysis of feral cats to the smoke from the Kuwait oil fires. *Journal of Environmental Pathology, Toxicology and Oncology* 13(2):137-149.

Mumford JL, Helmes CT, Lee XM, Seidenberg J, Nesnow S. 1990. Mouse skin tumorigenicity studies of indoor coal and wood combustion emissions from homes of residents in Xuan Wei, China with high lung cancer mortality. *Carcinogenesis* 11(3):397-403.

Murray FJ, Schwetz BA, Crawford AA, Henck JW, Quast JF, Staples RE. 1979. Embryotoxicity of inhaled sulfur dioxide and carbon monoxide in mice and rabbits. *Journal of Environmental Science and Health. Part C: Environmental Health Sciences* 13(3):233-250.

Musthapa MS, Lohani M, Tiwari S, Mathur N, Prasad R, Rahman Q. 2004. Cytogenetic biomonitoring of Indian women cooking with biofuels: Micronucleus and chromosomal aberration tests in peripheral blood lymphocytes. *Environmental and Molecular Mutagenesis* 43(4):243-249.

Nessel CS. 1999. A comprehensive evaluation of the carcinogenic potential of middle distillate fuels. *Drug and Chemical Toxicology* 22(1):165-180.

Nikula KJ. 2000. Rat lung tumors induced by exposure to selected poorly soluble nonfibrous particles. *Inhalation Toxicology* 12(1-2):97-119.

NIOSH (National Institute for Occupational Safety and Health). 1997. *NIOSH Pocket Guide to Chemical Hazards*. Cincinnati, OH: US Department of Health and Human Services, Public Health Service, Centers for Disease Control and Prevention, NIOSH.

NIOSH. 1998. *International Chemical Safety Cards*. [Online]. Available: http:www.cdc.gov/niosh/ipcsneng/neng0183.html [accessed February 10, 2004].

Nordholm AF, Rossi J 3rd, Ritchie GD, McInturf S, Hulme ME, McCool C, Narayanan L, MacMahon KL, Eggers J, Leahy HF, Wolfe RE. 1999. Repeated exposure of rats to JP-4 vapor induces changes in neurobehavioral capacity and 5-HT/5-HIAA levels. *Journal of Toxicology and Environmental Health. Part A.* 56(7):471-499.

NRC (National Research Council). 1985. *Emergency Exposure Guidance Level.* Vol 4. Washington, DC: National Academy Press.

NRC. 1996a. Hydrazine. In: NRC. *Spacecraft Maximum Allowable Concentrations for Selected Airborne Contaminants*. Vol. II. Washington, DC: National Academy Press. Pp. 213-234.

NRC. 1996b. *Permissible Exposure Levels for Selected Military Fuel Vapors*. Washington, DC: National Academy Press.

NRC. 2002. *Review of Submarine Escape Action Levels for Selected Chemicals*. Washington, DC: The National Academies Press.

NRC. 2003. *Toxicologic Assessment of Jet-Propulsion Fuel 8*. Washington, DC: The National Academies Press.

NRC. 2004. *Research Priorities for Airborne Particulate Matter: IV. Continuing Research Progress.* Washington, DC: The National Academies Press.

NTP (National Toxicology Program). 1994. *Toxicology and Carcinogenesis Studies of Ozone and Ozone/NNK in F344/N Rats and B6C3F1 Mice (Inhalation Studies)*. Bethesda, MD: NTP.

NTP/NIH. 1998. *National Toxicology Program Technical Report Series No. 310: Toxicology and Carcinogenesis Studies of Marine Diesel Fuel and JP-5 Navy Fuel in B6C3F1 Mice (Dermal Studies). NIH Publication No. 86-2566*. Research Triangle Park, NC: National Toxicology Program/National Institutes of Health; as cited in ATSDR 1998.

Osebold JW, Gershwin LJ, Zee YC. 1980. Studies on the enhancement of allergic lung sensitization by inhalation of ozone and sulfuric acid aerosol. *Journal of Environmental Pathology and Toxicology* 3(5-6):221-234.

PAC (Presidential Advisory Committee on Gulf War Veterans' Illnesses). 1996. *Presidential Advisory Committee on Gulf War Veterans' Illnesses: Final Report*. Washington, DC: US Government Printing Office.

Park MS, Cancio LC, Jordan BS, Brinkley WW, Rivera VR, Dubick MA. 2004. Assessment of oxidative stress in lungs from sheep after inhalation of wood smoke. *Toxicology* 195(2-3):97-112.

Parker GA, Bogo V, Young RW. 1981. Acute toxicity of conventional versus shale-derived JP5 jet fuels: Light microscopic, hematologic, and serum chemistry studies. *Toxicology and Applied Pharmacology* 57(3):302-317.

Parton KH. 1994. *The Effects of JP-8 Jet Fuel Inhalation on Liver and Kidney Function in Male F-344 Rats*. MS Thesis. Tucson, AZ: University of Arizona.

Peacock PR, Spence JB. 1967. Incidence of lung tumours in LX mice exposed to (1) free radicals; (2) SO2. *British Journal of Cancer* 21(3):606-618.

Peden-Adam MM, Eudaly J, Eudaly E, Dudley A, Zeigler J, Lee A, Robbs J, Gilkeson G, Keil DE. 2001. Evaluation of immunotoxicity induced by single or concurrent exposure to N,N-diethyl-m-toluamide (DEET), pyridostigmine bromide (PYR), and JP-8 jet fuel. *Toxicology and Industrial Health* 17(5-10):192-209.

Petruzzi S, Dell'Omo G, Fiore M, Chiarotti F, Bignami G, Alleva E. 1996. Behavioural disturbances in adult CD-1 mice and absence of effects on their offspring upon SO2 exposure. *Archives of Toxicology* 70(11):757-766.

Reiser KM, Tyler WS, Hennessy SM, Dominguez JJ, Last JA. 1987. Long-term consequences of exposure to ozone. II. Structural alterations in lung collagen of monkeys. *Toxicology and Applied Pharmacology* 89(3):314-322.

Riedel F, Naujukat S, Ruschoff J, Petzoldt S, Rieger CH. 1992. SO2-induced enhancement of inhalative allergic sensitization: Inhibition by anti-inflammatory treatment. *International Archives of Allergy and Immunology* 98(4):386-391.

Ritchie G, Still K, Rossi J3rd, Bekkedal M, Bobb A, Arfsten D. 2003. Biological and health effects of exposure to kerosene-based jet fuels and performance additives. *Journal of Toxicology and Environmental Health B Critical Review* 6(4):357-451.

Ritchie GD, Rossi J 3rd, Nordholm AF, Still KR, Carpenter RL, Wenger GR, Wright DW. 2001. Effects of repeated exposure to JP-8 jet fuel vapor on learning of simple and difficult operant tasks by rats. *Journal of Toxicology and Environmental Health* 64(5):385-415.

Riviere JE, Monteiro-Riviere NA, Baynes RE. 2002. Gulf War related exposure factors influencing topical absorption of 14C-permethrin. *Toxicology Letters* 135(1-2):61-71.

Roberts L, White R, Bui Q, Daughtrey W, Koschier F, Rodney S, Schreiner C, Steup D, Breglia R, Rhoden R, Schroeder R, Newton P. 2001. Developmental toxicity evaluation of unleaded gasoline vapor in the rat. *Reproductive Toxicology* 15(5):487-494.

Rose RM, Fuglestad JM, Skornik WA, Hammer SM, Wolfthal SF, Beck BD, Brain JD. 1988. The pathophysiology of enhanced susceptibility to murine cytomegalovirus respiratory infection during short-term exposure to 5 ppm nitrogen dioxide. *American Review of Respiratory Disease* 137(4):912-917.

Rose RM, Pinkston P, Skornik WA. 1989. Altered susceptibility to viral respiratory infection during short-term exposure to nitrogen dioxide. *Research Report/Health Effects Institute* (24):1-24.

Rossi J 3rd, Nordholm AF, Carpenter RL, Ritchie GD, Malcomb W. 2001. Effects of repeated exposure of rats to JP-5 or JP-8 jet fuel vapor on neurobehavioral capacity and neurotransmitter levels. *Journal of Toxicology and Environmental Health. Part A.* 63(6):397-428.

Rostker, Bernard. 2000. *Environmental Exposure Report: Oil Well Fires*. [Online]. Available: http://www.gulflink.osd.mil/owf_ii/ [accessed August 6, 2004].

Schlesinger RB, Cohen MD, Gordon T, Nadziejko C, Zelikoff JT, Sisco M, Regal JF, Menache MG. 2002. Ozone differentially modulates airway responsiveness in atopic versus nonatopic guinea pigs. *Inhalation Toxicology* 14(5):431-457.

Schlesinger RB, Graham JA. 1992. Health effects of atmospheric acid aerosols: A model problem in inhalation toxicology and air pollution risk assessment. *Fundamental and Applied Toxicology* 18(1):17-24.

Schlesinger RB, Halpern M, Albert RE, Lippmann M. 1979. Effect of chronic inhalation of sulfuric acid mist upon mucociliary clearance from the lungs of donkeys. *Journal of Environmental Pathology and Toxicology* 2(6):1351-1367.

Schreiner C, Bui Q, Breglia R, Burnett D, Koschier F, Lapadula E, Podhasky P, White R. 2000. Toxicity evaluation of petroleum blending streams: Inhalation subchronic toxicity/neurotoxicity study of a light catalytic reformed naphtha distillate in rats. *Journal of Toxicology and Environmental Health. Part A* 60(7):489-512.

Schreiner C, Bui Q, Breglia R, Burnett D, Koschier F, Podhasky P, Lapadula E, White R, Schroeder RE. 1999. Toxicity evaluation of petroleum blending streams: Reproductive and developmental effects of light catalytic cracked naphtha distillate in rats. *Journal of Toxicology and Environmental Health* 58(6):365-382.

Schreiner C, Bui Q, Breglia R, Burnett D, Koschier F, Podhasky P, Lapadula L, White R , Feuston M, Krueger A, Rodriquez S. 1997. Toxicity evaluation of petroleum blending streams: Reproductive and developmental effects of hydrodesulfurized kerosine. *Journal of Toxicology and Environmental Health* 52(3):211-229.

Schreiner C, Lapadula E, Breglia R, Bui Q, Burnett D, Koschier F, Podhasky P, White R, Mandella R, Hoffman G. 1998. Toxicity evaluation of petroleum blending streams: Inhalation subchronic toxicity/neurotoxicity study of a light alkylate naphtha distillate in rats. *Journal of Toxicology and Environmental Health. Part A.* 55(4):277-296.

Schulte A, Ernst H, Peters L, Heinrich U. 1994. Induction of squamous cell carcinomas in the mouse lung after long-term inhalation of polycyclic aromatic hydrocarbon-rich exhausts. *Experimental and Toxicologic Pathology* 45(7):415-421.

Schultz TW, Witschi H, Smith LH, Haschek WM, Holland JM, Epler JL, Fry RM, Rao TK, Larimer FW, Dumont JN. 1981. *Health Effect Research in Oil Shale Development (ORNL/TM-8034)*. Oak Ridge, TN: Oak Ridge National Laboratory; as cited in NRC 2003.

Singh J. 1982. Teratological evaluation of sulfur dioxide. *Proceedings of the Institute of Environmental Sciences* (28):144-145.

Singh J. 1989. Neonatal development altered by maternal sulfur dioxide exposure. *Neurotoxicology* 10(3):523-527.

Skisak C, DiGiovanni J, Conti CJ, Slaga TJ, Sharma S, Sagartz JW, Walborg EF Jr. 1995. Induction of short-term biomarkers of tumor promotion in skin of CD-1 mice by petroleum middle distillates: Preliminary observations. *Progress in Clinical & Biological Research.* 391:439-44.

Skrajny B, Hannah RS, Roth SH. 1992. Low concentrations of hydrogen sulphide alter monoamine levels in the developing rat central nervous system. *Canadian Journal of Physiology and Pharmacology* 70(11):1515-1518.

Spektor DM. 1998. *A Review of the Scientific Literature as It Pertains to Gulf War Illnesses, Volume 6: Oil Well Fires*. Santa Monica, CA: RAND.

Starek A, Vojtisek M. 1986. Effects of kerosene hydrocarbons on tissue metabolism in rats. *Polish Journal of Pharmacology and Pharmacy* 38(5-6):461-469; as cited in ATSDR 1998.

Stockard-Sullivan JE, Korsak RA, Webber DS, Edmond J. 2003. Mild carbon monoxide exposure and auditory function in the developing rat. *Journal of Neuroscience Research* 74(5):644-654.

Tan WC, Qiu D, Liam BL, Ng TP, Lee SH, van Eeden SF, D'Yachkova Y, Hogg JC. 2000. The human bone marrow response to acute air pollution caused by forest fires. *American Journal of Respiratory and Critical Care Medicine* 161(4 Pt 1):1213-1217.

Tesfaigzi Y, Singh SP, Foster JE, Kubatko J, Barr EB, Fine PM, McDonald JD, Hahn FF, Mauderly JL. 2002. Health effects of subchronic exposure to low levels of wood smoke in rats. *Toxicological Sciences* 65(1):115-125.

Thomas R, Vigerstad T, Meagher J. 2000. *Particulate Matter Exposure During the Persian Gulf War*. Falls Church, VA: Department of Defense Office of the Special Assistant for Gulf War Illness.

Thyssen J, Althoff J, Kimmerle G, Mohr U. 1981. Inhalation studies with benzo[a]pyrene in Syrian golden hamsters. *Journal of the National Cancer Institute* 66(3):575-577.

Tsujino Y, Hieda Y, Kimura K, Eto H, Yakabe T, Takayama K, Dekio S. 2002. Distribution of kerosene components in rats following dermal exposure. *International Journal of Legal Medicine* 116(4):207-211.

Ullrich SE. 1999. Dermal application of JP-8 jet fuel induces immune suppression. *Toxicological Sciences* 52(1):61-67.

Upreti RK, Das M, Shanker R. 1989. Dermal exposure to kerosene. *Veterinary and Human Toxicology* 31(1):16-20.

WHO (World Health Organization). 1996. *Environmental Health Criteria 171. Diesel Fuel and Exhaust Emissions*. Geneva: WHO.

WHO. 1997. *Environmental Health Criteria 188. Nitrogen Oxides (2nd Edition)*. Geneva: WHO.

Wolff RK, Bond JA, Sun JD, Henderson RF, Harkema JR, Griffith WC, Mauderly JL, McClellan RO. 1989. Effects of adsorption of benzo[a]pyrene onto carbon black particles on levels of DNA adducts in lungs of rats exposed by inhalation. *Toxicology and Applied Pharmacology* 97(2):289-299.

Zelikoff JT, Chen LC, Cohen MD, Fang K, Gordon T, Li Y, Nadziejko C, Schlesinger RB. 2003. Effects of inhaled ambient particulate matter on pulmonary antimicrobial immune defense. *Inhalation Toxicology* 15(2):131-150.

Zelikoff JT, Kraemer GL, Vogel MC, Schlesinger RB. 1991. Immunomodulating effects of ozone on macrophage functions important for tumor surveillance and host defense. *Journal of Toxicology and Environmental Health* 34(4):449-467.

4

CANCER

Cancer is a group of diseases characterized by uncontrolled growth and spread of abnormal cells (ACS 2003g; WHO 2003). Cancer can affect almost any tissue of the body. Known causes include external factors (such as chemicals, radiation, and infectious agents) and internal factors (such as mutations, hormones, and immune conditions). Such factors may act together or in sequence to initiate or promote carcinogenesis (ACS 2003g). In adults, a latent period of 10 years or more may elapse between exposure or mutation and the detection of cancer.

Cancer is the second-leading cause of death in the United States, exceeded only by heart disease. Among the member states of the World Health Organization (WHO), cancer is the third-leading cause of death, after heart disease and infectious or parasitic diseases (WHO 2003). In the United States in 2000, lung cancer was the leading cause of cancer deaths among both men and women, followed by prostatic cancer in men and breast cancer in women (Jemal et al. 2003). Each year, cancer leads to 12% of deaths worldwide, equivalent to about 6 million deaths (WHO 2003). Among men, lung and stomach cancers are the most common worldwide; among women, breast and cervical cancers are the most common (WHO 2003).

This chapter summarizes the results of epidemiologic studies of cancer outcomes related to exposure to fuels and combustion products. The committee considered the findings of those investigations as a means of determining what types of cancers Gulf War veterans might be at increased risk for as a consequence of exposure to fuels in the course of using military equipment, to tent heater fumes, and to smoke from oil-well fires. Because only a dozen years have passed since the Gulf War, studies of the Gulf War veterans themselves for cancer outcomes, which are characterized by considerable latent periods, would not yet be expected to be informative. Chapter 3 presented a general introduction on fuels and combustion products and a summary of toxicologic information on them. Appendix D contains tables that describe studies of populations exposed to relevant agents; many of the studies are referred to repeatedly in this chapter because their findings are related to several cancers of the specific anatomic sites and tissues reviewed.

In this chapter, the section on each type of cancer contains pertinent findings from cohort studies and then from case-control studies, first for fuels and then for combustion products, followed by the committee's conclusions regarding the relationship between cancer of the specific type and exposure to fuels or combustion products. The tables included at the end of this chapter contain results from the primary studies on which the committee bases its conclusions.

Those tables are presented in reverse chronological order by each type of study design. The committee reviewed over 500 epidemiologic studies on cancer related to exposure to fuels and combustion products and selected studies that met its inclusion criteria for more thorough evaluation. Briefly, the studies had to appear in peer-reviewed publications, identify exposure relevant to the committee's charge, and identify a specific health outcome (for example, the study must specify a type of cancer as opposed to considering all cancers together). Chapter 2 discusses the committee's inclusion criteria in more detail.

This chapter reviews epidemiologic studies of cancer in adults, which would be pertinent to the occurrence of cancer in Gulf War veterans themselves; studies of childhood cancer are reviewed in Chapter 7, on reproductive and developmental effects, because the committee was concerned with such outcomes in the offspring of Gulf War veterans as a possible result of parental exposure. Epidemiologic studies assessing gender-specific cancers (for example, female breast cancer and prostate cancer) are included in the committee's review. Seven percent of the 697,000 US military personnel sent to the Persian Gulf were women.

For the combustion products of crude oil and petroleum-derived fuels, the epidemiologic data complement the vast amount of toxicologic information on polycyclic aromatic hydrocarbons (PAHs) (particularly benzo[a]pyrene), other combustion products, and soot. There are numerous studies of occupational cohorts heavily exposed to PAHs (for example, from coal tar and asphalt), usually in combination with other products of combusted petroleum-derived fuels (for example, exhausts from various sources and metals) and soot. The conclusions from that large, complex body of information have been addressed by several expert bodies, including the International Agency for Research on Cancer (IARC 1985), which (IARC 1984a, 1984b) have been virtually unanimous in judging that PAHs and soot are most probably human carcinogens, particularly for skin after dermal exposure.

Urban firefighter studies were not included in the committee's review. The committee agreed that urban firefighters are likely exposed to a number of compounds that are not found in combustion products produced from oil-well fires, tent heaters, and vehicles (for example, plastics, asbestos, and PCBs). It would not be possible for the committee to distinguish between health effects in urban firefighters attributable to those compounds versus combustion products as were experienced in the Gulf War. Therefore, the committee made a decision not to include urban firefighter studies in this report.

Cancer sites or types are addressed in this chapter largely according to the ninth revision of the *International Classification of Disease* (ICD-9).[1] That approach is taken in an effort to organize the multitude of site-specific evidence presented in the chapter. In many cases, the findings by various investigators do not follow the strict categorization of the ICD-9.

CANCERS OF THE ORAL CAVITY AND OROPHARYNX

The cancers reviewed in this section include those of the oral cavity, that is, the lips, the lining of the lips and cheeks, the teeth, the gums, the tongue, the floor and roof of the mouth, and the area behind the wisdom teeth) (ICD-9 140-145); and the oropharynx and hypopharynx, the parts of the throat just behind the mouth (ICD-9 146 and 148, respectively). With cancers of the

[1] ICD codes are revised and updated by WHO. Although ICD-10 codes have been published, ICD-9 codes remain the most widely recognized and used. ICD codes were established by WHO to promote international comparability in the collection, processing, classification, and presentation of mortality statistics. The codes group cancers according to their organ or tissue of origin and their histologic features.

nasopharynx (ICD-9 147) and of the nasal cavity and paranasal sinuses (ICD-9 160)—the next section is on cancers of the nasal cavity and nasopharynx—these cancers were formerly denoted "head and neck cancers". Recently, some cancer epidemiologists (for example, Berrino et al. 2003; Boffetta et al. 2003) have chosen to consider the hypopharynx with the larynx (ICD-9 161), which it is next to, when assessing risks at that site associated with occupational exposure. In discussing the epidemiologic literature on cancer of the oral, nasal, and upper respiratory tissues, the committee has decided to specify exactly which sites individual researchers were reporting on. The committee has opted to draw conclusions related to the separate tissues that would be exposed during inhalation: along the oral pathway, along the nasal pathway, and their juncture near the larynx.

As for all head and neck cancers, the most important risk factor for cancers of the oral cavity and oropharynx is tobacco use, particularly cigarette-smoking (ACS 2003b, 2003c, 2003d). Additional risk factors for this site are alcohol consumption, vitamin A deficiency, exposure to ultraviolet radiation (sunlight), and increasing age. Some genetic factors, a weakened immune system, chronic irritation, and infection with human papillomavirus also may contribute to the occurrence of oral cancers.

In 2000, there were 10.6 new cases of cancer of the oral cavity and oropharynx per 100,000 people (15.9 among men and 6.2 among women) and 2.7 deaths per 100,000 (4.1 among men and 1.6 among women) in the United States (Ries et al. 2004).

Fuels

Table 4.1 presents the most relevant findings reviewed by the committee in drawing its conclusion on the possibility of an association between exposure to fuels and cancers of the oral cavity and oropharynx.

Cohort Studies

With the assistance of industrial hygienists and others familiar with a uranium-processing facility in Fernald, Ohio, Ritz (1999) conducted a secondary exposure assessment by using available data on the exposure of 4,128 male workers to kerosene (and to cutting fluids and trichloroethylene). The potential confounding effects of smoking were assessed by examining whether smoking habits were related to chemical exposure in a subset of 20% of the workers on whom smoking information was available in recent personnel files. There was no clear pattern of smoking behavior and exposure, so differences in smoking habits among exposure groups probably did not explain study results. Compared with the US population, the risk of death from oropharyngeal cancers (ICD-8 140-149) in the entire cohort was not notably increased (standardized mortality ratio [SMR] 1.05, 95% confidence interval [CI] 0.48-1.99). Among workers exposed to kerosene, the risks of oropharyngeal cancers derived with conditional logistic regression adjusted for pay status, time of hire, and cumulative radiation dose increased with exposure, but were imprecise (low kerosene exposure relative risk [RR] 1.85, 95% CI 0.37-9.36; moderate kerosene exposure RR 2.87, 95% CI 0.43-19.2; no workers had been categorized with heavy kerosene exposure).

Lagorio et al. (1994) tracked the mortality experience of 2,308 men through 1992; the men had been managers of Italian service stations in 1980. The effort complemented a detailed assessment of exposure at service stations in which 111 attendants were monitored in 1992 (Lagorio et al. 1993). Observation of only a single death from oropharyngeal cancer (ICD-9 140-

149) (SMR 0.38, 90% CI 0.02-1.79) during the follow-up period rendered this study uninformative.

Jarvholm et al. (1997) investigated cancer morbidity in a cohort of 4,128 male Swedish workers found by reviewing personnel files of 26 different refineries, distribution companies, lubrication-oil manufacturing industries, tank-cleaning companies, and companies that handled fuel. Exposure was determined from job titles combined with a retrospective review of air monitoring of work areas and personal exposure. The cohort was linked to the Swedish cancer and mortality registers. When the full array of oropharyngeal cancers were grouped (ICD-9 140-149), only six cases were identified in the cohort, so the somewhat increased risk estimates could not be distinguished from no effect, even for the subgroup of distribution workers with long duration and latency (standardized incidence ratio [SIR] 2.5, 95% CI 0.44-7.9).

Case-Control Studies

Zheng et al. (1996) conducted a case-control study to investigate the risk of salivary gland cancer (ICD-9 142) among residents of urban Shanghai. Cases were ascertained from 1988 and 1990. A total of 44 cases and 414 controls (frequency matched by sex and age) were interviewed to determine use of specific cooking fuels. Self-reported use of kerosene was associated with the risk of salivary gland cancer in models adjusted for sex, age, and income (odds ratio [OR] 3.5, 95% CI 1.6-7.4). Similar associations were found in multivariate models that included other possible risk factors but were not adjusted for smoking, which had not been found to be associated with salivary gland cancer.

A large population-based case-control study relying on several cancer registries was conducted in New Jersey, Los Angeles, Atlanta, and Santa Clara and San Mateo Counties, California, in January 1984-April 1985 (Huebner et al. 1992). Data were obtained on 1,114 cases (762 men and 352 women) of histologically confirmed primary oral and pharyngeal cancers (ICD-9 141, 143-146, 148, 149) diagnosed in January 1984-April 1985. The results for men working in selected industries were imprecise with some suggestion of an increased risk in petroleum-industry workers (OR 1.79, 95% CI 0.75-4.25). Employment history was obtained through interviews, and exposure was determined by job category. Smoking did not have an effect on the results.

Combustion Products

Table 4.2 presents the most relevant findings reviewed by the committee in drawing its conclusion on the possibility of an association between exposure to combustion products and cancers of the oral cavity and oropharynx.

Case-Control Studies

Gustavsson et al. (1998) identified incident cancers of the oral cavity (ICD-9 141, 143-145) or of the oropharynx or hypopharynx (ICD-9 146, 148) diagnosed in Sweden in 1988-1991. A total of 545 cases in men were identified by monitoring weekly medical reports and verified with the regional cancer registry; 641 controls were matched to the cases by region and age. Each case and control was interviewed by a trained interviewer according to a standardized protocol. Work histories were reviewed by industrial hygienists blinded to case status to estimate occupational exposure to 17 agents, including PAHs in a job-exposure matrix (JEM) approach. After adjustment for region, age, alcohol consumption, and smoking, high PAH exposure was associated with both cancer at all sites (RR 1.48, 95% CI 1.09-2.01) and pharyngeal cancer (RR 1.52, 95% CI 0.94-2.45). No dose–response relationship, however, was evident in the case of PAH exposure.

Pintos et al. (1998) conducted a study in Sao Paulo, Curitiba, and Loiania, Brazil, to examine the risk of oral cancer (ICD-9 140-145) or pharyngeal cancer (ICD-9 146-149) in relation to the use of wood stoves. The researchers identified 784 incident cases of cancer of the pharynx and mouth from local hospitals and selected two controls for each case from among other hospital inpatients (patients with other cancers or mental disorders were excluded), matching them to cases on age, sex, and trimester of hospital admission. Exposure to products of wood stoves was ascertained with a single yes-no question. After adjustment for lifetime cumulative tobacco use (pack-years), alcohol consumption (kilograms of ethanol), sociodemographic variables, diet, and history of employment in specific industries, the reported use of wood stoves was associated with an increased risk of cancer of the mouth (OR 2.73, 95% CI 1.76-4.24) and pharynx (OR 3.82, 95% CI 1.96-7.42).

The Shanghai case-control study of salivary gland cancer (ICD-9 142) (Zheng et al. 1996) found self-reported use of kerosene for cooking was associated with risk of salivary gland cancer in models adjusted for sex, age, and income (OR 3.5, 95% CI 1.6-7.4). The increases in risk associated with use of coal, gas, and wood for cooking were not as precise.

Dietz et al. (1995) identified incident cancers of the oral cavity (ICD-9 141-145), oropharynx (ICD-9 146), or hypopharynx (ICD-9 148) in Heidelberg, Germany, and evaluated the effects of using fossil-fuel stoves for heating and cooking. Cases were ascertained in 1989-1992 from all patients seeking treatment at the Otorhinolaryngology Department at the University of Heidelberg within 3 years after first diagnosis. They identified 100 and 105 cases of oral cavity and pharyngeal cancer, respectively. Controls were recruited from the same medical center and general outpatient department and matched to cases on sex, age, and size of place of residence. All subjects were interviewed to ascertain risk-factor information, including alcohol consumption (grams/day), smoking (tobacco-years), and use of fossil-fuel stoves and cookers (coal, briquette, coke, peat, gas, and oil). After adjustment for tobacco and alcohol, use of fossil-fuel single stove heating units for more than 40 years vs 0-20 years was associated with pharyngeal cancer (OR 3.3, 95% CI 1.43-7.55). Fossil-fuel stove use for cooking in kitchen units also increased risk (OR 2.5, 95% CI 1.03-6.30) for more than 40 years of stove use (compared with 0-20 years). The OR for oral cavity cancer (ICD-9 141-145), adjusted for tobacco and alcohol, was 2.4 (95% CI 1.26-4.40) for more than 40 years (compared with 0-20 years) of exposure to fossil-fuel heating units. For exposure to kitchen cooking units, the OR for oral cavity cancer, adjusted for tobacco and alcohol, was 1.6 (95% CI 0.90-2.97) for more than 40 years of stove use (compared with 0-20 years).

Pukkala (1994) examined cancer incidence in Finland in 1971-1985 in 2,369 men and 809 women employed in various occupations. Occupation was ascertained by linking cancer-registry data with occupational and social-class data from the 1970 Finnish Population Census. SIRs were calculated from sex, age, site, and calendar-year-specific rates in the general Finnish population and were adjusted for social class. Risks of various cancers among men employed in transport and communications (lip cancer SIR 0.91, 95% CI 0.73-1.12; tongue cancer SIR 1.17, 95% CI 0.74-1.76; oral cavity cancer SIR 1.17, 95% CI 0.71-1.81; pharyngeal cancer SIR 0.97, 95% CI 0.66-1.39) were not found to be increased; there was a small increase in motor vehicle drivers (tongue cancer SIR 1.56, 95% CI 0.94-2.44), but the 95% CI contained the null.

In the study by Huebner et al. (1992) of fuel exposures described above, the relationship between job categories potentially involving exposure to combustion products and primary cancers of the oral cavity and pharyngeal region were also assessed. The effect estimates derived for boiler or furnace and heavy-equipment operators (OR 1.50, 95% CI 0.68-3.34), heavy-equipment operators only (OR 1.25, 95% CI 0.78-2.01), motor-vehicle operators (OR 1.01, 95% CI 0.75-1.35), railroad transport workers (OR 1.00, 95% CI 0.30-3.35), mechanics or repairers (OR 0.86, 95% CI 0.66-1.12), and firefighters (OR 0.65, 95% CI 0.23-1.85) were imprecise and suggested no increases for these jobs. Similarly, the results for men working in selected industries were imprecise; no increased risk was observed for transportation workers (OR 1.07, 95% 0.74-1.56) and trucking or warehousing workers (OR 0.86, 95% CI 0.56-1.31). Among women, point estimates exceeded 1 for oral or pharyngeal cancer in association with employment as a motor-vehicle operator, but results were imprecise because of the small numbers (OR for motor-vehicle operator 2.80, 95% CI 0.61-12.9).

Incident oral and pharyngeal cancer was assessed in Shanghai, China (Zheng et al. 1992). A total of 204 cases 20-75 years old were ascertained in 1988-1990 and matched to 414 controls on age and sex. Exposure to potential risk factors was ascertained by interview. The prevalence of men using kerosene stoves among cases was reported to be 27.0% compared with 14.1% of controls ($p \leq 0.01$), but no difference was reported for women.

Merletti et al. (1991) conducted a population-based case-control study in Turin, Italy. From July 1982 to December 1984, 103 incident male cases of oral cavity or oropharyngeal cancer were identified. The questionnaire included a detailed occupational history. That information was reviewed by industrial hygienists and physicians experienced in occupational medicine, who determined the probability and intensity of exposure to 16 agents, including PAHs. After adjustment for age, education, geographic region of birth, tobacco-smoking, and alcohol consumption, probable or definite exposure to PAHs was not associated with cancer risk (OR 0.6; study authors stated that confidence interval included 1).

Patient records were abstracted for a case-control study at the Roswell Park Memorial Institute in Buffalo, New York (Decoufle and Stanislawczyk 1977; Viadana et al. 1976). All persons referred to the Institute in 1956-1965 were asked to report their lifetime occupational history and job activities. Their risk of cancer of the buccal cavity and pharynx was compared with that of noncancer controls according to jobs they had ever held or had held for 5 years or more. Data were analyzed and stratified by age at diagnosis (with the cut point at 60 years), and the results were adjusted for smoking. Compared with the risk in clerical workers, no increased risk of cancer of the buccal cavity and pharynx was reported for bus, taxicab, and truck drivers; deliverymen and routemen; locomotive engineers and firemen; mechanics and repairmen; or mine operatives and laborers.

Conclusion

The three cohort mortality studies that assessed the relationship between cancer of the oral cavity and oropharynx and fuels (Jarvholm et al. 1997; Lagorio et al. 1994; Ritz 1999) had limited statistical power and therefore were mostly uninformative. The case-control studies failed to report any consistent relationships between occupational or other self-reported potential exposures to fuels and cancer of the oral cavity and oropharynx (Huebner et al. 1992; Zheng et al. 1996).

The committee concludes, from its assessment of the epidemiologic literature, that there is inadequate/insufficient evidence to determine whether an association exists between exposure to fuels and cancers of the oral cavity and oropharynx.

All available studies of exposure to combustion products and cancer of the oral cavity and oropharynx were of the case-control design, and all were adjusted for cigarette-smoking and other confounders. Results of several studies suggest an association between cancers of the oral cavity and oropharynx and exposure to combustion products. Pintos et al. (1998) demonstrated an association between wood-stove use and cancers of the upper aerodigestive tract, and there were supportive findings from Dietz et al. (1995) that were based on exposure from fossil-fuel stove use in Germany, from Gustavsson et al. (1998) on PAH exposure in Sweden, and from Zheng et al. (1992, 1996) on kerosene-stove use in China.

The committee concludes, from its assessment of the epidemiologic literature, that there is limited/suggestive evidence of an association between exposure to combustion products and cancers of the oral cavity and oropharynx.

CANCERS OF THE NASAL CAVITY AND NASOPHARYNX

Cancers of the nasopharynx (ICD-9 147) or of the nasal cavity and paranasal sinuses (ICD-9 160), which previously have been grouped with oral cancers as "head and neck cancers" were considered as a separate group by the committee. The tissues of the nasal cavity and nasopharynx are subject to exposures that may be somewhat different from those of the tissues of the oral cavity. Nasopharyngeal carcinoma (NPC) is the most frequent malignant tumor of the nasopharynx.

As for other cancers of the head and neck, the most important risk factor for cancers of the nasal cavity and nasopharynx is smoking (ACS 2003b, 2003c, 2003d). Others include diets high in salt-cured fish and meats and infection with the Epstein-Barr virus. Cancers of the nasal cavities and sinuses have been found to be associated with occupational exposures, such as to dusts from wood, textiles, leather, and metals; glues; formaldehyde; solvents used in furniture and shoe production; mustard gas; isopropyl alcohol; and radium.

In 2000, there were 1.4 new cases of cancers of the nasal cavity and nasopharynx per 100,000 in the US (1.9 among men and 0.9 among women) and 0.4 deaths per 100,000 (0.5 among men and 0.2 among women) (Ries et al. 2004). NPC is rare in most parts of the world, with incidences generally less than 1 per 100,000 persons per year (Muir et al. 1987). The highest incidence is observed among southern Chinese (30-50 per 100,000 person-years); it might be attributable to the consumption of salted fish and preserved foods early in life. Several studies of NPC focused on Chinese populations because of the large number of available cases.

Fuels

Table 4.3 presents the most relevant findings reviewed by the committee in drawing its conclusion on the possibility of an association between exposure to fuels and cancers of the nasal cavity and nasopharynx.

Case-Control Studies

Increased risk of nasopharyngeal cancer posed by 20 occupational exposures was assessed in a case-control study (Armstrong et al. 2000). During a 2-year period, 530 subjects with histologically confirmed NPC were identified from four hospitals in Malaysia and 282 cases underwent interviews that included occupational history and work exposure. Each case was matched by sex and age to a general population control without a history of cancer of the head, neck, or respiratory system. Exposure to motor fuel or oil, assigned according to type of job, was associated with a greater risk of NPC in a crude analysis (OR 1.79, 95% CI 1.16-2.82). However, after adjustment for smoking, passive smoke exposure, and diet, the association was largely reduced, and the CI suggested no effect (OR 1.33, 95% CI 0.81-2.20). A case-control study conducted by Teschke (1997) had only four cases, and no increased risk of sinonasal cancer was observed.

Combustion Products

Table 4.4 presents the most relevant findings reviewed by the committee in drawing its conclusion on the possibility of an association between exposure to combustion products and cancers of the nasal cavity and nasopharynx.

Case-Control Studies

A case-control study of NPC was conducted in rural Zangwu County in the middle 1980s (Zheng et al. 1994). Beginning in 1986, 88 cases of NPC were recruited with 176 controls matched on neighborhood, sex, and age. Subjects were interviewed to determine their use of wood fuels in the year before diagnosis. Use of wood fuels was associated with an increased risk of NPC in unadjusted models (OR 3.7, $p = 0.02$), models adjusted for a sociodemographic confounder score (OR 6.4, $p = 0.003$), and models adjusted for the confounder score, childhood consumption of salted fish, and consumption of herbal tea in the year before diagnosis (OR 5.4, 95% CI 1.5-19.8). There was some evidence that the risk of NPC was increased by household factors that can affect fume concentrations; specifically, the observed wood-fuel association increased in households with lower ventilation (for example, households that had no windows or no windows in the kitchen).

A hospital-based case-control study was conducted in Guangzhou City, China, in March 1983-August 1985 (Yu et al. 1990). Because Chinese living in the area have a high risk of NPC because of dietary factors, the researchers evaluated diet in detail and controlled for its influence in their analyses. There were 306 histologically confirmed incident cases of cancer of the nasal cavity and nasopharynx in subjects who were all less than 50 years old, and 306 controls were selected from the index cases' neighborhoods of residence and matched on age, sex, and neighborhood. Exposure was based on self-reporting of occupation and exposure to specific risk factors. Subjects were interviewed in a standardized fashion that included inquiries about lifetime occupational history; exposure to dust, smoke, and chemical fumes; use of specific cooking fuels; and exposure to smoke from incense or mosquito coils. When associations were found for a self-reported occupational exposure, an occupational-medicine specialist reviewed the occupational information (job title and activity in job and industry) blindly to determine exposure status independently of case status. Exposure to smoke in a job held for at least 6 months (ever vs never) was found to be associated with an increased risk of NPC (RR adjusted for dietary risk factors in childhood based on self-reported exposure ever 2.4; 1-9 years of exposure 1.6; 10 years or more of exposure 7.6). No confidence intervals were reported, but the authors stated that the results for "ever" exposed or exposed for 10 years or more had a "2-sided p value for the adjusted RR of less than 0.05". Those results were attenuated when exposure was based on the specialist's assessment (RR with 1-9 years of exposure 1.6, 95% 1.1-2.5; RR with 10 years or more of exposure 2.7, 95% CI 1.4-5.5). There was no association with domestic exposure to cooking fire, burning incense, or antimosquito coils.

Two case-control studies that collected occupational and environmental risk-factor information for NPC were conducted in Malaysia and included subjects of Chinese origin. The first was a hospital-based study (Armstrong and Armstrong 1983) of 117 histologically confirmed cases diagnosed in 1973-1980 and treated at the only radiotherapy center for NPC in Malaysia. In addition, the researchers interviewed 200 population controls (matched on neighborhood, sex, and ethnicity) to determine risk-factor information, including exposure to smoke and dust in the workplace. Exposure to both smoke and dust was associated with an increased risk of NPC among Chinese participants (RR for smoke exposure 6.0, $p = 0.006$; RR for dust exposure 4.0, $p < 0.001$). There was some evidence of an increased risk for Malays and Indians associated with smoke exposure, but the number of exposed cases was too small (four) to reach any conclusions. Smoke exposure was generated from the burning of wood, paper, grass, and oil and tar from in such occupations as rubber-tapping (wood-smoke exposure) and street-hawking. Some of the jobs seemed to involve more than one type of exposure; from the description of the analyses, the estimates do not seem to have been adjusted for multiple exposure or for risk factors other than age and sex.

The same researchers conducted a second case-control study on histologically confirmed cases of squamous-cell NPC which is described above (Armstrong et al. 2000). There were 119 prevalent cases (diagnosed before 1990) and 163 incident cases (diagnosed in 1990-1992). Exposures to inhalants were coded in a JEM approach by one of the authors blinded to case-control status. Cases and controls did not differ with respect to exposure amount or to median number of hours exposed to engine exhaust after adjustment for smoking and diet. No increased risk of NPC was associated with exposure to engine exhaust.

In addition to those largely Asian studies of wood-burning and other cooking fuels, the committee considered a large pooled reanalysis of cancers of nasal cavities and paranasal sinuses (ICD-9 160). Leclerc et al. (1997) assembled data from 12 previous studies in seven countries that included occupational-exposure information—the same set of 12 studies as reviewed in Demers et al. (1995) and in Luce et al. (2002). The dates of cancer diagnosis spanned 1968-1990. The inclusion criteria for the selected studies were histologic confirmation of cases; age, sex, and smoking information available on both cases and controls; and occupational histories of cases and controls obtained by interviews or questionnaires given to subjects or survivors (proxies). In 10 of the 12 studies, there were a total of 680 male cases of sinonasal cancer (330 squamous-cell carcinomas, 169 adenocarcinomas, 156 cases of other histologic types, and 25 cases of unknown histology) and 250 female cases of sinonasal cancer (102 squamous-cell carcinomas, 26 adenocarcinomas, 104 cases of other histologic types, and 18 cases of unknown histology). For the pooled analysis, subjects' self-reported occupational information was recoded with the one- or two-digit International Standard Classification of Occupations. The researchers state that they controlled only for study and age category because they found that "introduction of cigarette smoking into the models, in addition to age and study, had no appreciable effect" on the risk of squamous-cell carcinoma. Among men, employment as a motor-vehicle driver was associated with an increased risk of adenocarcinoma (OR adjusted for study and age 2.50, 95% CI 1.03-

6.10) but not of squamous-cell carcinoma (OR 1.13, 95% CI 0.78-1.63). Duration of exposure did not change the point estimates for squamous-cell carcinoma, and only shorter exposure duration was linked to the increased risk of adenocarcinomas (OR <10 years 3.29, no CI; OR ≥10 years 0.80, no CI given). Also among men, employment as a cook was associated with an increased risk of squamous-cell carcinoma only in the shorter-duration group (OR adjusted 1.99, 95% CI 1.04-3.83; OR <10 years 2.72; OR ≥10 years 1.25). Among women, however, employment as a cook was associated with a suggestion of a decreased risk of squamous-cell carcinoma (based on only three exposed cases; OR ever employed vs never employed 0.51, 95% CI 0.15-1.77; OR <10 years 0.27; OR ≥10 years 0.69).

A population-based case-control study of incident nasal cavity and sinus cancer was conducted in British Columbia, Canada (Teschke et al. 1997). There were 48 cases identified in 1990-1992, and 159 population controls were frequency matched to cases on sex and age. Exposure was ascertained in interviews that included occupational history and items on individual exposures. Occupation-disease associations were estimated in models adjusted for age, sex, and tobacco use. There was no association with any particular occupation.

The incidence of pharyngeal, sinonasal, and oropharyngeal or hypopharyngeal cancer was assessed in a population-based case-control study from the Washington state cancer registry (Vaughan 1989). There were 231 cases aged 20-74 years diagnosed in 1979-1983 (sinonasal cancer) or 1980-1983 (pharyngeal cancer) and 552 population controls frequency matched to cases on age and sex (also de facto matched on telephone prefix because they were recruited with random-digit dialing). Histories for all jobs held at least 6 months were taken in interviews with subjects or their proxies. People were classified into 31 industrial and 59 occupational groups, and duration of employment was calculated on the basis of the start and end dates of employment. Models for oropharyngeal, hypopharyngeal, or sinonasal cancer were adjusted for age, sex, tobacco use, and alcohol consumption. Models for NPC were adjusted for age, sex, and race. Employment as a motor vehicle operator or other transportation worker was not associated with sinonasal cancer or pharyngeal cancer.

Conclusion

Little information is available on exposure to fuels and cancers of the nasal cavity and nasopharynx. The two studies reviewed by the committee did not report convincingly positive findings (Armstrong et al. 2000; Teschke et al. 1997).

The committee concludes, from its assessment of the epidemiologic literature, that there is inadequate/insufficient evidence to determine whether an association exists between exposure to fuels and cancers of the nasal cavity and nasopharynx.

Overall, the results of studies of the relationship between combustion products and cancers of the nasal cavity and nasopharynx are inconsistent, and indirect methods were used to assess exposure. However, positive associations were reported by studies conducted in China (Yu et al. 1990; Zheng et al. 1994) between combustion products (particularly wood smoke) and cancer of the nasopharynx. Those findings are supported by the work of Leclerc et al. (1997) and Armstrong and Armstrong (1983). The committee believes that the evidence is strong enough to suggest an association between combustion products and cancers of the nasal cavity and nasopharynx.

The committee concludes, from its assessment of the epidemiologic literature, that there is limited/suggestive evidence of an association between exposure to combustion products and cancers of the nasal cavity and nasopharynx.

ESOPHAGEAL CANCER

This review focuses on esophageal cancer (ICD-9 150). Risk factors for that cancer are increasing age, sex, ethnicity, dietary habits, chronic reflux esophagitis, alcohol and tobacco use, and work exposure (ACS 2004q, 2004w).

In the United States in 2000, there were 4.7 new cases of esophageal cancer per 100,000 people (7.9 among men and 2.1 among women) and 4.4 deaths per 100,000 (7.7 among men and 1.8 among women) (Ries et al. 2004).

Fuels

Table 4.5 presents the most relevant findings reviewed by the committee in drawing its conclusion on the possibility of an association between exposure to fuels and esophageal cancer.

Cohort Studies

A cohort of 3,814 male uranium-processing workers in Ohio in 1951-1989 was used to assess the potential relationship between esophageal and stomach cancers and kerosene exposure (Ritz 1999). Kerosene exposure based on a detailed industrial hygiene assessment (light or medium exposure) was associated with an increased risk of esophageal and stomach cancers; those cancers were analyzed together. Light kerosene exposure for 2 years or more with a 15-year lag before disease onset was associated with an RR of 3.46 (95% CI 1.22-9.80); medium kerosene exposure of the same duration and lag were also associated with an increased risk of esophageal and stomach cancer (RR 7.71, 95% CI 2.04-29.1).

Mortality was assessed in a cohort of 15,032 men with 5 years or more of work in 1964-1973 at Imperial Oil Limited refinery in Canada (Hanis et al. 1979). No specific industrial-hygiene assessment was available. There was an additional 11-year update that included 34,597 workers, including those hired in 1964-1983 (Lewis et al. 2000b; Schnatter et al. 1992). In followup through 1973, potential daily exposure to petroleum was associated with a greater risk of combined esophageal and stomach cancers (RR 3.25, $p < 0.05$); the increase was greater with increasing years of employment (Hanis et al. 1979). However, the risk was not consistently observed in later followup studies of the cohort (Lewis et al. 2000b; Schnatter et al. 1992).

In a nationwide survey of gasoline-station attendants in Italy, the SMR for esophageal cancer was 2.34 (90% CI 0.80-5.35) (Lagorio et al. 1994). In small stations, where there were higher sales per employee, the risk of esophageal cancer was greater (SMR 3.42, 90% CI 1.17-7.82). Workers in small stations with higher sales of super-premium gasoline may have experienced higher exposure.

Combustion Products

Table 4.6 presents the most relevant findings reviewed by the committee in drawing its conclusion on the possibility of an association between exposure to combustion products and esophageal cancer.

Cohort Studies

Mortality and cancer incidence were determined in a retrospective cohort study conducted in Stockholm in relation to diesel exhaust and asbestos exposure in bus-garage workers (Gustavsson et al. 1990). Although the primary focus of the work was lung-cancer incidence, esophageal-cancer incidence was also included. An increase was observed in the incidence of esophageal cancer in bus-garage workers compared with a local reference population, but the CI included the null (SMR 3.27, 95% CI 0.89-8.37).

The incidence of esophageal cancer among occupational groups in Sweden as recorded in the 1960 census was evaluated (Chow et al. 1995). SIRs were not increased for "transportation and communication" as a major industrial or occupational category. Of the reported occupations that might involve exposure to exhausts, only locomotive and traffic workers showed any increase in risk (SIR 1.1; $p > 0.05$). The database did not permit adjustment for possible confounders.

Case-Control Studies

In a case-control study of 99 cases of confirmed esophageal cancer and age-matched population controls, no associations were reported between esophageal cancer and exposure to a number of combustion products, including nitrogen oxides (NO_x), gasoline emissions, carbon monoxide, PAHs from any source, and mononuclear aromatic hydrocarbons (Parent et al. 2000b). Increases in the risk of esophageal cancer were reported in association with exposures to benzo[a]pyrene, PAHs specifically derived from coal, and PAHs specifically derived from petroleum, but the CIs all included the null. Exposure information was obtained with detailed questionnaires that were analyzed by chemists and industrial hygienists.

The relationship between PAH exposure and squamous-cell carcinoma of the esophagus was determined in a case-control study conducted in Sweden (Gustavsson et al. 1998). Participants were administered a questionnaire to determine exposure information, and work histories were reviewed and coded by an occupational hygienist. Occupational exposure to PAHs was associated with an increased risk of esophageal cancer. Estimated RR attributable to low PAH exposure was 2.01 (95% CI 1.16-3.48), and the RR of high PAH exposure was 1.87 (95% CI 1.11-3.16).

Another occupational case-control study evaluated the relationship between exposure to several types of engine exhausts and combustion products and esophageal cancer (Siemiatycki et al. 1988). Increased risk of esophageal cancer was associated with exposure to wood combustion products (OR 2.3, 90% CI 1.2-4.5) on the basis of only eight cases, but no increased risk was associated with exposure to gasoline exhaust, diesel exhaust, jet-fuel exhaust, propane exhaust, or products of combustion of propane, natural gas, liquid fuel, coal, or coke.

Conclusion

Studies of an association between fuel exposure and esophageal cancer are few, and their results are inconsistent. Two of the studies (Hanis et al. 1979; Ritz 1999) analyzed esophageal and stomach cancer together, so the committee cannot determine which cancer type may have been associated with exposure. Despite the larger number of studies of combustion products and esophageal cancer, no consistent association was observed.

The committee concludes, from its assessment of the epidemiologic literature, that there is inadequate/insufficient evidence to determine whether an association exists between exposure to fuels or combustion products and esophageal cancer.

STOMACH CANCER

This review focuses on gastric cancer (commonly known as stomach cancer) (ICD-9 151). Risk factors for stomach cancers are increasing age, sex, ethnicity, family history, dietary habits, and tobacco and alcohol use (ACS 2004q, 2004w). *Heliobacter pylori* infection is also a known cause of stomach cancer.

In 2000, there were 8.0 new cases of stomach cancer per 100,000 people (11.6 among men and 5.3 among women) and 4.6 deaths per 100,000 (6.4 among men and 3.2 among women) in the United States (Ries et al. 2004).

Fuels

Table 4.7 presents the most relevant findings reviewed by the committee in drawing its conclusion on the possibility of an association between exposure to fuels and stomach cancer.

Cohort Studies

Two cohort studies assessed the risk of combined esophageal and stomach cancer posed by exposure to fuels (Hanis et al. 1979; Ritz 1999). The results are presented in the previous section on esophageal cancer. No increased risk of stomach cancer was found in a nationwide survey of gasoline-station attendants in Italy (Lagorio et al. 1994). Amoco Oil Company employees in 1970-1980 who worked in operations were at increased risk for stomach cancer, with an SMR of 2.06 (Nelson et al. 1987), but those working in administration (and presumably were not exposed to petroleum products) had an SMR of 1.80.

Case-Control Studies

A case-control study of 3,726 cases of cancer in men in 19 Montreal hospitals was conducted to determine whether there was an association exists between exposure to fuels and various cancers, including stomach cancer (Siemiatycki et al. 1987a). Exposure was assessed with an industrial-hygiene assessment of exposure based on occupational history. The authors presented 90% confidence intervals and reported borderline increased risks for participants with automotive-gasoline exposure (OR 1.5, 90% CI 1.2-1.9). The risk of stomach cancer also was increased after exposure to kerosene (OR 1.7, 90% CI 1.2-2.3).

Combustion Products

Table 4.8 presents the most relevant findings reviewed by the committee in drawing its conclusion on the possibility of an association between exposure to combustion products and stomach cancer.

Cohort Studies

Several epidemiologic studies examined rates of stomach cancer in defined populations compared with the general population. Occupational information on persons with stomach cancer as reported to the Shanghai Cancer Registry in 1980-1984 was assessed (Kneller et al. 1990). Increased SIRs were reported for fuel suppliers (p value not given), petroleum-refinery workers ($p < 0.05$), and boiler firemen ($p < 0.01$).

A similar approach was taken to evaluating the incidence of stomach cancer that was linked to occupation as reported in the 1960 Swedish census (Chow et al. 1994). There were 16,872 men diagnosed with stomach cancer in 1961-1979, but no increased risk was observed for "transportation and communication workers" as a major industrial or occupational category. Among machine and engine maintenance workers, crane operators were found to have an increased risk of stomach cancer (SIR 1.5, $p < 0.01$). The database did not permit adjustment for potential confounders.

Case-Control Studies

Wu-Williams et al. (1990b) reported on a case-control study of 137 men with stomach cancer as reported to the Los Angeles County cancer registry. Exposure was determined by interviewing participants (or in some cases, surrogates) about occupational history using a structured questionnaire. No relationship was found between exposure to "smoke/exhaust" and stomach cancer.

A case-control study in Italy examined the relationship between occupational exposures and stomach cancer (Cocco et al. 1994). Men with histologically confirmed stomach cancer were interviewed to determine their occupational history. Controls were randomly selected from community and local health-unit registers of the resident population and matched on sex and age. A relative risk of 1.0 for stomach cancer was reported for men in several job categories in which exposure to combustion products might have occurred (for example, mechanics, repairmen, and railroad workers), but the CIs included the null. A small increase in risk was reported in men occupationally exposed to NO_x (OR 1.4, 95% CI 1.0-2.1).

An occupational case-control study evaluated the relationship between exposure to several types of engine exhausts and combustion products and stomach cancer on the basis of an industrial-hygiene assessment of occupational history (Siemiatycki et al. 1988). No increased risk was associated with exposure to gasoline exhaust, diesel exhaust, jet-fuel exhaust, propane exhaust, or products of combustion of propane, natural gas, liquid fuel, coal, or coke.

A case-control study was conducted to assess the relationship between heating and cooking fuel-related exposures and stomach cancer in a coal-mining region of Pennsylvania (Weinberg et al. 1985). Cases were identified from death certificates, and followup interviews were conducted with next of kin to determine exposures. Increases in stomach-cancer risk were reported for coal cooking and heating, but the CIs included the null. No increased risks were found for gas cooking and heating. The results were not adjusted for smoking.

Occupational history was obtained by interviewing patients admitted to Roswell Park Memorial Institute in Buffalo, New York (Viadana et al. 1976). Nonneoplastic controls were selected from the same hospital and matched for age and smoking status. An association between the occupations of bus, taxicab, or truck driver and stomach cancer was reported (RR 1.6, $p > 0.05$).

Conclusion

No consistent association between fuels or combustion products and stomach cancer was observed in the studies reviewed by the committee. Two of the studies of fuel exposure (Hanis et al. 1979; Ritz 1999) analyzed esophageal and stomach cancers together, so the committee cannot determine which cancer type may have been associated with exposure. For combustion-product exposure, two studies reported an increased risk of stomach cancer; however, the method used to assess exposure was limited and there was no adjustment for confounders.

The committee concludes, from its assessment of the epidemiologic literature, that there is inadequate/insufficient evidence to determine whether an association exists between exposure to fuels or combustion products and stomach cancer.

COLON CANCER

This review focuses on cancer of the colon (ICD-9 153). Risk factors for this cancer are family history, increasing age, ethnicity, dietary habits, weight and inactivity, and tobacco and alcohol use (ACS 2004p).

In 2000, there were 38.5 new cases of colon cancer per 100,000 people (43.5 among men and 34.8 among women) and 17.6 deaths per 100,000 (21.1 among men and 15.2 among women) in the United States (Ries et al. 2004).

Fuels

Table 4.9 presents the most relevant findings reviewed by the committee in drawing its conclusion on the possibility of and association between exposure to fuels and colon cancer.

Cohort Studies

In a cohort of 3,814 uranium-processing workers, kerosene exposure was associated with a greater risk of death from large intestine cancer, but the CIs included the null (Ritz 1999). Kerosene exposure was assessed with a detailed industrial hygiene survey.

A cohort of 10,763 workers employed at an Amoco Corporation oil refinery in 1970-1980 was retrospectively studied (Nelson et al. 1985, 1987). Exposure was classified by an industrial hygienist on the basis of job type and "rough exposure categories". Increased SMRs were found for jobs associated with exposure to light aromatic hydrocarbons for all digestive tract cancers (SMR 1.39). Occasional exposure to heavy oils was also associated with increased SMRs for digestive tract cancers (SMR 1.79). No specific digestive-cancer sites were included in the analysis. On the basis of data from the National Cancer Institute, the age-adjusted incidences of gastrointestinal cancers indicate that men are much more likely to be diagnosed with colorectal cancer than esophageal and stomach cancers (Ries et al. 2003). Therefore, it is likely that the increase in digestive tract cancers in the Amoco Corporation oil-refinery workers is due to colorectal cancer.

A cohort of workers at Imperial Oil Limited in Canada was evaluated for cancer outcomes, including colorectal cancer (Hanis et al. 1979; Lewis et al. 2000b; Schnatter et al. 1993). Moderate exposure (defined as less than daily contact with petroleum or its products) and daily exposure were not associated with a greater risk of cancers of the intestines and rectum (the result of the analysis of these cancers was presented together) (Hanis et al. 1979). In a subcohort of 6,672 male marketing and distribution workers who probably were exposed to finished products (gasoline and diesel fuel), the risk of large intestinal cancer was increased (SMR 1.50, 95% CI 0.97-2.21) (Schnatter et al. 1993); employment for 30 years or more (with a 10-year latency) was associated with a greater risk of large intestine cancer than shorter employment (SMR 2.33, $p < 0.05$). In another subcohort of 25,292 Imperial Oil Limited workers, an increased risk of large intestine cancer was found, but the CIs included the null (Lewis et al. 2003).

Case-Control Studies

A population-based case-control study conducted in Sweden assessed the potential for an association between occupational exposure and colon cancer (Gerhardsson de Verdier et al. 1992). Exposure to specific substances was assessed by self-report; although an association was noted with fuels or with work in automotive repair or gasoline stations, the CI included the null (OR 1.8, 95% CI 0.6-5.2).

In a case-control study in Montreal, exposures to multiple fuels were examined with industrial-hygienist review of occupational history, and exposure intensity and probability were estimated (Siemiatycki et al. 1987a). The ORs were not increased (as judged with 90% CIs) for automotive gasoline, aviation gasoline, kerosene, jet fuel, or diesel fuel.

In a case-control study of occupational exposure and colorectal cancer that used a subset of the National Cancer Survey database and the National Occupational Hazard Survey, the probability of exposure to specific substances was assigned with a JEM based on occupational history (Spiegelman and Wegman 1985). A medium-high cumulative-exposure probability score, which summed the products of probability of exposure in each job and duration of exposure, was associated with a greater risk of colorectal cancer (OR 1.53, $p = 0.01$) and colon cancer alone (OR 1.61; $p = 0.02$) among men exposed to fuel oil. Among women exposed to fuel oil, there was no clear increase in risk of colorectal cancer (OR 1.24, $p = 0.21$).

Combustion Products

Table 4.10 presents the most relevant findings reviewed by the committee in drawing its conclusion on the possibility of and association between exposure to combustion products and colon cancer.

Case-Control Studies

(Goldberg et al. 2001) conducted a case-control study of 497 Canadian men with colon cancer and two sets of controls, one population-based and the other a cancer case-control group. Exposure was based on a review of occupational history and expert opinion. Increasing risks were related to a number of occupational exposures, among them diesel-engine emissions (adjusted OR 1.6, 95% CI 1.0-2.5 for those with "substantial" exposure, and adjusted OR 1.2, 95% CI 0.8-1.8 for those with "nonsubstantial" exposure). There was no evidence of increasing risk with duration of exposure.

In the study in Sweden, the potential association between occupational exposure to combustion products and colon cancer was assessed (Gerhardsson de Verdier et al. 1992). Small increases in risk of colon cancer were associated with exposure to combustion gases from coal, coke, wood, and soot and with railway work, but the 95% CIs included the null. Exposure to tar and asphalt did not increase the risk of colon cancer.

An occupational case-control study evaluated the relationship between exposure to several types of engine exhausts and combustion products, based on an industrial-hygiene assessment of occupational history, and colon cancer (Siemiatycki et al. 1988). Exposure to diesel exhaust led to an increased risk of colon cancer (OR 1.3, 90% CI 1.1-1.6). Exposure to jet-fuel exhaust and products of wood combustion also led to increases in colon-cancer risk, but the 90% CI included the null. No increased risk was reported in association with exposure to gasoline exhaust, propane exhaust, or products of combustion of propane, natural gas, liquid fuel, coal, or coke.

Conclusion

No consistent association was observed in the studies of fuels and colon cancer reviewed by the committee. Three of the studies analyzed colon cancer and rectal cancer together (Hanis et al. 1979; Nelson et al. 1987; Ritz 1999), so the committee could not determine whether exposure to fuels may have been associated with a specific type of cancer. Although the three studies of exposure to combustion products and colon cancer reported positive associations (Gerhardsson de Verdier et al. 1992; Goldberg et al. 2001; Siemiatycki et al. 1988), the committee believes that the evidence of an association is inadequate because of the small number of studies available.

The committee concludes, from its assessment of the epidemiologic literature, that there is inadequate/insufficient evidence to determine whether an association exists between exposure to fuels or combustion products and colon cancer.

RECTAL CANCER

This review focuses on cancers of the rectum, rectosigmoid junction, and anus (ICD-9 154). Risk factors for those cancers are family history, increasing age, ethnicity, dietary habits, weight and inactivity, and tobacco and alcohol use (ACS 2004p).

In 2000, there were 14.6 new cases of rectal cancer per 100,000 people in the US (19.0 among men and 11.1 among women), and 3.0 deaths per 100,000 (4.0 among men and 2.3 among women) (Ries et al. 2004).

Fuels

Table 4.11 presents the most relevant findings reviewed by the committee in drawing its conclusion on the possibility of an association between exposure to fuels and rectal cancer.

Cohort Studies

As described in the colon-cancer section, a cohort of 10,763 workers at an Amoco Corporation oil refinery employed in 1970-1980 was retrospectively studied (Nelson et al. 1985, 1987). No specific digestive-tract cancer sites were included in analysis. Increased SMRs were found for jobs associated with light aromatic hydrocarbon exposure and occasional exposure to heavy oils. For the reasons described above, it is likely that most of the digestive-tract cancers were colorectal cancers.

In a cohort of workers at Imperial Oil Limited in Canada, increased risk of colorectal cancer was assessed (Hanis et al. 1979; Lewis et al. 2000b; Schnatter et al. 1993). Colon and rectal cancers were analyzed together, and the results are summarized in the colon-cancer section above. No increased risk of colorectal cancer was found in the workers. In another followup study, no increased risk of cancer of the rectum and rectosigmoid junction was found in the cohort (Lewis et al. 2003). However, cancer of the rectum was increased in the marine-operating subgroup employed for 35 years or more (SMR 2.75, 95% CI 1.19-5.41) (Lewis et al. 2000b). Exposure to fuels in this subgroup most likely occurred during loading and unloading operations.

Case-Control Studies

A hospital-based case-control study conducted in Sweden assessed the potential association between occupational exposure and rectal cancer (Gerhardsson de Verdier et al. 1992). Exposure to specific substances was assessed by self-reporting, and no association was noted between fuels and rectal cancer. There was a suggestion of an increased risk in automotive-repair or gas-station workers (OR 1.5, 95% CI 0.4-5.6), but the effect estimates were imprecise.

In a case-control study in Montreal, exposure to multiple fuels was examined with an industrial-hygiene review of occupational history, and exposure intensity and probability were estimated (Siemiatycki et al. 1987a). An increased risk of rectal cancer was reported for exposure to automotive gasoline, aviation gasoline, jet fuel, diesel fuel, and heating oil, but the 90% CIs included the null. No increased risk of rectal cancer was found in association with kerosene.

In a case-control study of occupational exposure and colorectal cancer that used a subset of the National Cancer Survey database and the National Occupational Hazard Survey, a medium-high cumulative exposure probability score was associated with a greater risk of colorectal cancer (OR 1.53, $p = 0.01$) among men exposed to fuel oil (Spiegelman and Wegman 1985). Among women exposed to fuel oil, there was no clear increase in risk of colorectal cancer (OR 1.24, $p = 0.21$). There was no evidence of an exposure-response relationship.

Combustion Products

Table 4.12 presents the most relevant findings reviewed by the committee in drawing its conclusion on the possibility of an association between exposure to combustion products and rectal cancer.

Case-Control Studies

No evidence of increased rectal cancer risk posed by occupational exposure to soot, wood, and coal combustion products was reported in a population-based case-control study of 257 Canadians (Dumas et al. 2000).

In the study in Sweden, the potential association between occupational exposure to combustion products and rectal cancer was assessed (Gerhardsson de Verdier et al. 1992). Exposure was self-reported. Associations were found between rectal cancer and exposure to combustion gases from coal, coke, and wood (OR 2.1, 95% CI 1.0-4.6), soot (OR 2.7, 95% CI 1.2-5.7), and tar and asphalt (OR 1.0, 95% CI 0.3-2.8).

A case-control study conducted in Montreal did not report an increased risk of rectal or rectosigmoid cancer in people exposed to diesel exhaust, jet-fuel exhaust, propane exhaust, or products of combustion from natural gas, liquid fuel, coal, or coke (Siemiatycki et al. 1988). A JEM classification of exposure was used. There was a slight increase in rectal cancer in people exposed to gasoline exhaust (OR 1.2, 90% CI 1.0-1.5), particularly in a subgroup exposed at high concentrations for more than 10 years (OR 1.6, 90% CI 1.1-2.3).

Conclusion

Although some studies reported positive associations between fuels or combustion products and rectal cancer, the results were not consistent, and the number of studies was small. The positive studies failed to include at least one high-quality study supported by an adequate exposure assessment.

The committee concludes, from its assessment of the epidemiologic literature, that there is inadequate/insufficient evidence to determine whether an association exists between exposure to fuels or combustion products and rectal cancer.

LIVER CANCER

This review focuses on hepatic cancer (more commonly referred to as liver cancer) (ICD-9 155) (ACS 2003f). Known risk factors include infection with hepatitis B and hepatitis C viruses; cirrhosis caused by alcohol abuse, hepatitis B and hepatitis C, and excess iron in the liver (from hemochromatosis); aflatoxin; vinyl chloride; thorium dioxide; tobacco use; anabolic steroids; and arsenic.

In 2000, there were 5.3 new cases of liver cancer per 100,000 people (8.1 among men and 3.0 among women) and 4.7 deaths per 100,000 (6.8 among men and 2.9 among women) in the United States (Ries et al. 2004).

Fuels

Table 4.13 presents the most relevant findings reviewed by the committee in drawing its conclusion on the possibility of an association between exposure to fuels and hepatic cancer.

Case-Control Studies

A case-control study reported on cases of primary liver cancer that occurred in New Jersey in 1975-1980 (Stemhagen et al. 1983). A questionnaire was used to determine occupational history and other factors, such as lifetime residence, medical history, smoking habits, and alcohol consumption. Of many occupations and industries that were examined in the study, the authors report results only for agricultural occupations (the primary purpose of the study) and for occupations and industries for which the relative risks were greater than 2.0 or for which the relative risks were greater than 1.0 and the CIs did not include the null. A total of 11 occupation and industries were in the latter category, including one that is possibly relevant to the Gulf War fuel exposures—gasoline service stations (RR 2.88, 95% CI 1.20-6.88).

Combustion Products

Table 4.14 presents the most relevant findings reviewed by the committee in drawing its conclusion on the possibility of an association between exposure to combustion products and hepatic cancer.

Case-Control Study

The study by Stemhagen et al. included two occupations that are possibly relevant to the Gulf War combustion exposures—road-building (RR 2.60, 95% CI 0.83-8.19) and bus lines (RR 2.80, 95% CI 0.93-8.40) (Stemhagen et al. 1983). Employment at gasoline service stations (RR 2.88, 95% CI 1.20-6.88) probably involved exposure to a mixture of fuel and combustion products.

Conclusion

Only one relevant study that evaluated exposure to fuels or combustion products and hepatic cancer was identified (Stemhagen et al. 1983). Although associations were noted for some occupations, there were few cases with relevant exposure, and the study did not consider all pertinent risk factors.

The committee concludes, from its assessment of the epidemiologic literature, that there is inadequate/insufficient evidence to determine whether an association exists between exposure to fuels or combustion products and hepatic cancer.

PANCREATIC CANCER

This review focuses on pancreatic cancer (ICD-9 157), for which tobacco use stands out as the most import risk factor among increasing age, ethnicity, sex, dietary habits, alcohol use, family history, and some occupational exposures (ACS 2004m, 2004p, 2004q). In addition, diabetes and pancreatitis are risk factors for pancreatic cancer.

In 2000, there were 10.9 new cases of pancreatic cancer per 100,000 people (12.8 among men and 9.4 among women) and 10.6 deaths per 100,000 (12.2 among men and 9.3 among women) in the United States (Ries et al. 2004).

Fuels

Table 4.15 presents the most relevant findings reviewed by the committee in drawing its conclusion on the possibility of an association between exposure to fuels and pancreatic cancer.

Cohort Studies

In a cohort of 3,814 uranium-processing workers, the relationship between kerosene exposure and pancreatic cancer was imprecise (Ritz 1999). For example, moderate exposure to kerosene for more than 5 years with a 15-year lag yielded an RR of 2.78 (95% CI 0.51-15.2). Kerosene exposure was based on a detailed industrial-hygiene assessment.

No increased risk of pancreatic cancer was found in a cohort of petroleum-refinery workers at Imperial Oil Limited in Canada (Lewis et al. 2003, 2000b; Schnatter et al. 1993), but only a small number of cases were noted. No specific industrial-hygiene assessment was available.

Combustion Products

Table 4.16 presents the most relevant findings reviewed by the committee in drawing its conclusion on the possibility of an association between exposure to combustion products and pancreatic cancer.

Case-Control Studies

Alguacil et al. (2000) conducted a case-control study in Spain to assess the relationship between occupational exposure and pancreatic cancer. A JEM was used to determine exposures to chemicals on the basis of jobs reported in the occupational history. There were few cases of exposure to combustion products, and the relationships reported were imprecise.

A population-based case-control study in Finland examined the relationship between a number of occupational exposures and pancreatic cancer (Kauppinen et al. 1995). Exposure analysis included a JEM. No association was found with exposure to engine exhaust (OR 0.89, 95% CI 0.51-1.53). An increased risk of pancreatic cancer was reported in association with exposure to PAHs, but the CI included the null (OR 1.33, 95% CI 0.69-2.57).

The association between occupational exposure and pancreatic cancers was evaluated in a case-control study in France (Pietri et al. 1990). Overall, transportation workers did not show an increased risk of pancreatic cancer (RR 0.87, 95% CI 0.42-1.77, on the basis of 13 exposed cases).

A case-control study in Montreal reported that exposure to coal combustion products was associated with an increased risk of pancreatic cancer (OR 2.3, 90% CI 1.4-4.0) (Siemiatycki et al. 1988). A JEM classification of exposure was used. The same study did not find increased risk of pancreatic cancer associated with exposures to gasoline exhaust, diesel exhaust, jet fuel exhaust, propane exhaust, or products of combustion of propane, natural gas, liquid fuel, wood, or coke.

Conclusion

Information on the risk of pancreatic cancer posed by fuel exposure is limited. One study reported an association between kerosene exposure and pancreatic cancer (Ritz 1999), but the results were imprecise. One of the four reviewed studies of combustion-product exposure and pancreatic cancer reported a positive finding (Siemiatycki et al. 1988). It found an association between exposure to coal combustion products and increased risk of pancreatic cancer, but it did not find a link between nine other types of combustion products and pancreatic cancer.

> **The committee concludes, from its assessment of the epidemiologic literature, that there is inadequate/insufficient evidence to determine whether an association exists between exposure to fuels or combustion products and pancreatic cancer.**

LARYNGEAL CANCER

This section addresses cancer of the larynx (ICD 161). The most important risk factor for this cancer is tobacco use, particularly cigarette-smoking (ACS 2003a). Additional risk factors include alcohol consumption (which has a synergistic effect with tobacco), dietary habits, vitamin deficiency, exposure to ultraviolet (UV) radiation (sunlight), increasing age, a weak immune system, genetic factors, and some occupational exposures, such as to dusts from wood, textiles, and leather; glues; formaldehyde; solvents used in furniture and shoe production; mustard gas; isopropyl alcohol; and radium.

In 2000, there were 4.0 new cases of laryngeal cancer per 100,000 people in the US (7.2 among men and 1.4 among women), and 1.4 deaths per 100,000 (2.6 among men and 0.5 among women) (Ries et al. 2004).

Fuels

Table 4.17 presents the most relevant findings reviewed by the committee in drawing its conclusion on the possibility of an association between exposure to fuels and laryngeal cancer.

Cohort Study

Lagorio et al. (1994) tracked the mortality experience of 2,308 men who had been managers of Italian service stations in 1980-1992. Laryngeal cancer was not associated with employment at the service stations (on the basis of three cases). Managers at all stations had an OR of 1.05 (90% CI 0.29-2.72); the OR for managers at small stations was 1.53 (90% CI 0.42-3.96).

Case-Control Studies

De Stefani et al. (1998) conducted a case-control study in Montevideo, Uruguay in 1993-1995. They enrolled 112 incident, histologically confirmed laryngeal-cancer cases in males and 509 controls (from among all other cancer cases, excluding those in sites proximal to the larynx or related to tobacco or alcohol consumption). Exposure was based on self-reported occupational history and exposure, and risks were adjusted for age, smoking, alcohol consumption, residence, education, and income. Cases with self-reported exposure to gasoline who worked as gasoline fillers had increased RRs, but the CIs included the null. There is a suggestion of a dose–response relationship with increased years of exposure to gasoline.

Wortley et al. (1992) conducted a population-based case-control study in western Washington from September 1983 to February 1987 and enrolled 235 incident cases of laryngeal cancer identified from a population-based Surveillance, Epidemiology, and End Results (SEER) registry. They matched 547 population controls to cases by sex and age with random-digit dialing. Subjects were interviewed with a questionnaire that included items on job titles, description of tasks, and nature of industry for each job held 6 months or longer. Job title and industry were coded according to 1980 US census codes. Some 505 individual occupations were collapsed into 62 categories. Job titles were categorized according to duration of exposure: less than 10 years vs 10 years or longer. Furthermore, industrial hygienists created a JEM for some chemical categories, such as diesel fumes, but not for combustion-product exposure. Risks were not found to be increased in vehicle mechanics (OR 1.2, 95% CI 0.6-2.1) or for garage- and gas-station-related work (OR 0.8, 95% CI 0.4-1.8). All results were adjusted for age, education, smoking, and alcohol.

Ahrens et al. (1991) conducted a case-control study to investigate the relationship between occupational factors and laryngeal cancer. A hospital in Bremen, Germany, was the source of 55 men newly diagnosed with histologically confirmed primary laryngeal cancer and 30 more who had been diagnosed during the previous 2 years. Each case was matched to a male patient from the same hospital without a history of cancer or other smoking-related diseases by age. Standardized interviews were conducted and included occupational history with an exposure checklist and questions on smoking and drinking behavior. Broad industrial and occupational categories related to transportation showed moderately increased risks. Increased ORs were associated with self-reported exposure to diesel oil (OR 1.7, 95% CI 0.8-3.5) and gasoline (OR 2.8, 95% CI 1.0-7.7). Self-reported exposure to gasoline was most frequent in mechanics and drivers; diesel-oil exposure was most prevalent among those employed in shipping and in drivers and train operators.

Brown et al. (1988) enrolled 183 histologically confirmed incident cases of squamous-cell carcinoma of the larynx from 56 Texas hospitals in 1975-1980 and obtained 250 population controls (ascertained from death records, driver's license files, and Health Care Financing Administration [HCFA] records) that were matched to cases on age, vital status, ethnicity, and county of residence. Subjects working in petroleum refining or chemical manufacturing had an adjusted RR of 0.93 (95% CI 0.59-1.46). For subjects with self-reported exposure to diesel and gasoline fumes, they calculated an adjusted RR of 1.50 (95% CI 1.00-2.26). However, it is not apparent from the description in the article whether diesel and gasoline fumes were the uncombusted and combusted form of those agents.

Combustion Products

Table 4.18 presents the most relevant findings reviewed by the committee in drawing its conclusion on the possibility of an association between exposure to combustion products and laryngeal cancer.

Case-Control Studies

A large IARC study assessed 1,010 male cases of laryngeal or hypopharyngeal cancer and 2,176 male population controls identified and interviewed at six European centers in 1980-1983 (for example, Berrino et al. 2003; Boffetta et al. 2003). Exposure in a specific industry or job was defined as working for at least 1 year since 1945 (Boffetta et al. 2003). Results were controlled for study area, age, smoking, and alcohol consumption. Employment in the railway-transport industry was associated with an increased risk of laryngeal cancer overall (OR 1.52, 95% CI 0.97-2.39) and showed a trend with duration of employment ($p = 0.02$). Other transportation-related occupations with the potential for exhaust exposure (motor-vehicle mechanics, other mechanics, railway vehicle loaders, lorry drivers, local and long-distance lorry drivers, and other motor-vehicle drivers) were also associated with increased risks, but the CIs were wide and included the null value. PAHs were among 16 industrial agents for which duration, intensity, and likelihood of exposure were estimated with a JEM (Berrino et al. 2003). For the 695 cases 55 years old or older, the adjusted risk associated with PAH exposure was essentially unity (95% CI 0.7-1.3); for the younger 315 cases, the adjusted OR for PAH exposure for those who had been exposed 20 years or more was 1.1 (95% CI 0.5-2.4).

In a hospital-based case-control study of incident laryngeal cancer in Istanbul, Turkey, 940 cases were identified in 1979-1984, and 1,519 other patients with diagnoses not thought to share risk factors with laryngeal cancer were selected as controls (Elci et al. 2003). Cases and controls were interviewed on admission to the hospital with a questionnaire that included occupational history. After adjustment for age, smoking, and alcohol consumption, Elci et al. (2001) found that drivers had increased risks of laryngeal cancer (OR 1.7, 95% CI 1.1-2.4), but mechanics did not (OR 0.8, 95% CI 0.5-1.3). Elci et al. (2003) described the results of applying a

JEM to work histories to estimate specific exposures. The adjusted risks of laryngeal cancer were positively associated with ever having been exposed to diesel exhaust (OR 1.5, 95% CI 1.3-1.9), to gasoline exhaust (OR 1.6, 95% CI 1.3-2.0), or to PAHs (OR 1.3, 95% CI 1.1-1.6), and these associations were similar and generally positive for all the specific sites (supraglottic, glottic, and others). The risk of laryngeal cancer was similar for all three intensity and probability levels of exposure.

In the previously described case-control study of laryngeal cancer in Montevideo, Uruguay (De Stefani et al. 1998) truck drivers had an increased risk of cancer in the glottic area (OR 2.7, 95% CI 0.7-10.7) but not the supraglottic area (OR 0.6, 95% CI 0.1-2.9). When stratified by subsite, self-reported exposure to diesel or gasoline exhaust was positively associated with glottic cancer (diesel exhaust OR 1.9, 95% CI 0.6-5.8; gasoline exhaust OR 1.8, 95% CI 0.6-5.7) but not supraglottic cancer (diesel exhaust OR 0.7, 95% CI 0.2-1.9; gasoline exhaust OR 0.8, 95% CI 0.3-2.1). The authors speculated that the glottic area is potentially more affected by smaller particles, such as those found in exhaust, than the supraglottic area.

Gustavsson et al. (1998) identified incident cancers of the oral cavity (ICD-9 141, 143-145) or the oropharynx or hypopharynx (ICD-9 146, 148) diagnosed in Sweden in 1988-1991. In models adjusted for region, age, alcohol consumption, and smoking, high PAH exposures (categorized on the basis of an industrial-hygiene assessment of the participant's occupational history) were associated with laryngeal cancer (RR 1.47, 95% CI 0.96-2.24).

Pintos et al. (1998) conducted a case-control study in Sao Paulo, Curitiba, and Loiania, Brazil, that examined the risk of laryngeal cancer in relation to the use of stoves. Reported use of wood stoves was associated with an increased risk of laryngeal cancer (OR adjusted for tobacco and alcohol consumption 2.34, 95% CI 1.17-4.67). In men, the OR was 2.03 (95% CI 1.12-3.67); in women, 16.24 (95% CI 2.66-99.1). Relatively few women were included in the study.

Goldberg et al. (1997) conducted a hospital-based case-control study in France that assessed the risk of laryngeal and hypopharyngeal cancer associated with occupation. The study included 528 male cases and 305 male controls with various other types of cancer. Interviews were conducted to obtain information on occupational history, demographic characteristics, alcohol consumption, and tobacco use. After adjustment only for age, alcohol use, and smoking, an increase in laryngeal-cancer and hypopharyngeal-cancer risk was reported for transportation-equipment operators (OR 1.5, 95% CI 1.0-2.5). When education was included in the adjustments, there was still an increase in risk, but the CI included the null (OR 1.4, 95% CI 0.9-2.3). With full adjustment, small increases in laryngeal-cancer and hypopharyngeal-cancer risk were reported for motor-vehicle mechanics (OR 1.2, 95% CI 0.5-2.5) and for workers employed in railway transportation (OR 1.4, 95% CI 0.6-3.1) and road transportation (OR 1.0, 95% CI 0.4-2.1), but all the CIs included the null.

Pollan and Lopez-Abente (1995) identified 50 incident laryngeal-cancer cases in Madrid in 1982-1985 and recruited 46 population controls matched on age, sex, and residential area and 45 hospital controls (excluding patients with alcohol- or tobacco-related diseases) matched on age, sex, and admission date. Exposure was based on self-reported job history and occupational codes; the researchers collected detailed data on year of hire and termination, occupational activity, and unit. Employment as a transport driver was associated with an increased risk of laryngeal cancer, but this result was based on only eight cases (OR adjusted for age, tobacco use, and alcohol use 2.71, 95% CI 0.85-8.64) and thus imprecise.

Muscat and Wynder (1995) reported on 235 white men with primary laryngeal cancer age-matched to 205 hospital controls with a variety of non-tobacco-related diseases. Although there was an association between laryngeal cancer and self-reported exposure to diesel exhaust, an independent review and coding of occupations and industries potentially exposed to diesel exhaust found no association with diesel-exhaust-exposed jobs.

Researchers at the University of Heidelberg, Germany, conducted a hospital-based case-control study with 164 male incident laryngeal-cancer cases ascertained in February-June 1988 and November 1988-May 1989 (Dietz et al. 1995; Maier and Tisch 1997). They recruited 656 male controls from the same outpatient clinic (excluding those with evidence of cancer) matched to cases on age and residential area. Exposure was based on occupation and exposure to environmental factors such as heating or cooking with fossil-fuel stoves. After adjustment for alcohol consumption and tobacco use, heating and cooking with fossil-fuel stoves were associated with laryngeal cancer (OR for heating with fossil-fuel stoves over 40 years 2.11, 95% CI 1.43-3.12; OR for cooking with fossil fuel stoves over 20 years 1.47, 95% CI 0.92-2.33; and OR for heating with coal, briquettes, or coke 1.52, 95% CI 0.94-2.47). ORs and 95% CIs were calculated by the committee with standard methods from the observed numbers presented in the original paper.

Wortley et al. (1992) conducted a population-based case-control study in western Washington. On the basis of on occupational titles, some jobs with the potential for diesel-exhaust exposure were associated with a small increased risk of laryngeal cancer but all estimates were imprecise: motor-vehicle operator (OR ever employed 1.3, 95% CI 0.8-2.1; OR less than 10 years 1.6; OR at least 10 years 0.8); work in motor-vehicle transportation (OR ever employed 1.3, 95% CI 0.6-2.8; OR less than 10 years 1.1; OR at least 10 years 0.8); cook (OR 1.3, 95% CI 0.4-4.1); and firefighter (OR 0.5, 95% CI 0.0-2.9). All those results were adjusted for age, education, smoking, and alcohol.

In the previously described case-control study investigating the relationship between laryngeal cancer and occupational factors conducted by Ahrens et al. (1991) in Bremen, Germany, a modest increase in risk was observed in subjects employed in the transport and communication industry (OR 1.3, 95% CI 0.64-2.59) and subjects employed as transportation and store workers (OR 1.83, 95% CI 0.94-3.56). Self-reported exposure to fumes and smoke was not associated with an increase in risk (OR 0.7, 95% CI 0.3-1.4).

In the case-control study of incident squamous cell carcinoma conducted by Brown et al. (1988) in Texas, self-reporting ever having been employed in transportation or as a driver was associated with an increase in risk of laryngeal cancer, but the CIs were wide and included the null (OR transportation 1.42, 95% CI 0.86-2.36; OR driver 1.69, 95% CI 0.75-3.83).

An early case-control study by Decoufle and Stanislawczyk (1977) was the result of abstracting the records of about 14,000 white cancer patients at the Roswell Park Memorial Institute in Buffalo, New York. Occupational histories routinely constituted a section of the medical charts. Patients with laryngeal cancer were compared with noncancer controls with respect to jobs ever held or held for 5 years or more. Analyses were stratified by age at diagnosis (with the cutpoint at 60 years), and the results for this type of cancer were adjusted for smoking. Of several exhaust-associated occupations, drivers most consistently showed increased RRs of about 1.5, adjusted for smoking, but the CIs were wide.

Conclusion

Overall, the results regarding exposure to fuels and laryngeal cancer are inconsistent. Two studies reviewed by the committee reported a modest increase in the risk of laryngeal cancer associated with exposure to fuels; however, the exposures in both studies were self-reported (Ahrens et al. 1991; Brown et al. 1988). Wortley et al. (1992) used a JEM and reported an increased risk of laryngeal cancer in vehicle mechanics that was imprecise but no increase in garage and gasoline-station workers.

The committee concludes, from its assessment of the epidemiologic literature, that there is inadequate/insufficient evidence to determine whether an association exists between exposure to fuels and laryngeal cancer.

A number of studies evaluated the potential link between exposure to combustion products and laryngeal cancer. Several studies reported positive findings, including Maier and Tisch (1997) and Dietz et al. (1995) regarding exposure to the emissions of fossil-fuel stoves and Pintos et al. (1998) regarding exposure to wood-stove emissions. There was supportive evidence from Gustavsson et al. (1998) and Elci et al. (2003). Several studies reported small increases in laryngeal-cancer risk for some exposures: Boffetta et al. (2003), De Stefani et al. (1998), Goldberg et al. (1997), Muscat and Wynder (1995), Pollan and Lopez-Abente (1995), Wortley et al. (1992), Ahrens et al. (1991) and Brown et al. (1988); however, the overall results are inconsistent.

The committee concludes, from its assessment of the epidemiologic literature, that there is limited/suggestive evidence for an association between combustion products and laryngeal cancer.

LUNG CANCER

Lung cancer (ICD-9 162) is the leading cause of cancer death of both men and women (ACS 2004s); its incidence is higher in men than in women. The major risk factor for lung cancer is tobacco-smoking. Smoking is believed to be responsible for about 80% of lung-cancer cases. Other risk factors are exposure to environmental tobacco smoke, ionizing radiation (including radon gas), arsenic, PAHs (particularly benzo[a]pyrene), asbestos, chromium, and silica; tuberculosis and some forms of pneumonia that leave scars in the lungs; family history; and some aspects of diet.

Lung cancer is classified into two main types based on the appearance of the cells (ACS 2004n). Small cell lung cancer (SCLC), also called oat cell cancer, accounts for 20% of all cancers and is almost exclusively associated with smoking. It originates primarily in the bronchi or central portion of the lungs, though it can spread rapidly throughout the body. The second type of lung cancer, non-small cell lung cancer, makes up the remaining 80% and is divided into 3 subtypes: squamous cell carcinoma, 25-30% of all lung cancers; adenocarcinoma, 40%; and large-cell undifferentiated carcinoma, 10-15%. Squamous cell carcinoma is also associated with smoking and is found centrally within the lungs. Adenocarcinoma appears in the outer regions of the lungs, and large-cell undifferentiated carcinoma can be found anywhere and can metastasize quickly.

In 2000, there were 62.3 new cases of lung cancer per 100,000 people (79.8 among men and 49.8 among women) and 56.1 deaths per 100,000 (76.9 among men and 41.2 among women), in the United States (Ries et al. 2004).

Fuels

Table 4.19 presents the most relevant findings reviewed by the committee in drawing its conclusion on the possibility of an association between exposure to fuels and lung cancer.

In a hospital-based case-control study conducted in Montreal in which exposures to multiple fuels were examined with an industrial-hygiene review of occupational history, exposure to kerosene was associated with an increased risk of squamous-cell lung cancer (OR 1.4, 90% CI 1.0-1.9) and adenocarcinoma of the lung (OR 1.5, 90% CI 1.0-2.3) (Siemiatycki et al. 1987a); exposure to heating oil, an increased risk of oat-cell lung cancer (OR 1.7, 90% CI 1.0-2.7); exposure to crude oil, an increased risk of squamous-cell lung cancer (OR 2.8, 90% CI 1.0-7.6); and exposure to diesel fuel, an increased risk of nonadenocarcinoma lung cancer (OR 1.6, 90% CI 1.1-2.4) with indications of an exposure-response relationship. In multivariate analyses, those risks were also increased.

Mortality was assessed in workers at an Imperial Oil Limited refinery in Canada (Hanis et al. 1979; Lewis et al. 2000b; Schnatter et al. 1993). In followup through 1973 of a subcohort with daily exposure to petroleum products, there was an increase in lung cancer (RR 1.89) and a greater increase with increasing years of employment (Hanis et al. 1979). However, there was a greater rate of lung cancer in office workers with no occupational exposure to petroleum products. The study did not control for smoking, and it is possible that the office workers smoked at a higher rate than the refinery workers.

A retrospective cohort study assessed mortality in 7,119 workers at a petroleum refinery in Beaumont, Texas, who worked at least 1 year in 1945-1978 (Raabe et al. 1998). The refinery produced a variety of fuels, including gasoline and jet fuel, and feedstocks for the petrochemical industry. The study did not control for smoking. No association between refinery employment and lung cancer was observed except for an increased SMR in maintenance-craft workers (SMR 1.20, 95% CI 0.99-1.45). A followup of the Beaumont cohort that extended enrollment and vital-status followup to December 31, 1996, found no association between refinery employment and lung cancer (Wong et al. 2001). A nested case-control study was conducted to assess the relationship between lung cancer and employment in the Beaumont, Texas refinery (Rosamilia et al. 1999). There were 112 cases of lung-cancer death that were matched to controls (n = 490) by birth date and race. The analysis compared each job category (an indication of the likelihood of fuel exposure) and included some individual information on smoking. No increased risk of lung cancer was found in connection with any specific job category.

Combustion Products

Table 4.20 presents the most relevant findings reviewed by the committee in drawing its conclusion on the possibility of an association between exposure to combustion products and lung cancer. Figures 4.1, 4.2, and 4.3 present results of some of the studies on exhaust-exposed workers, indoor air pollution, and ambient air pollution, respectively. Results were sorted in descending order of relative risk, except for studies in which there are multiple results, which are contiguous entries.

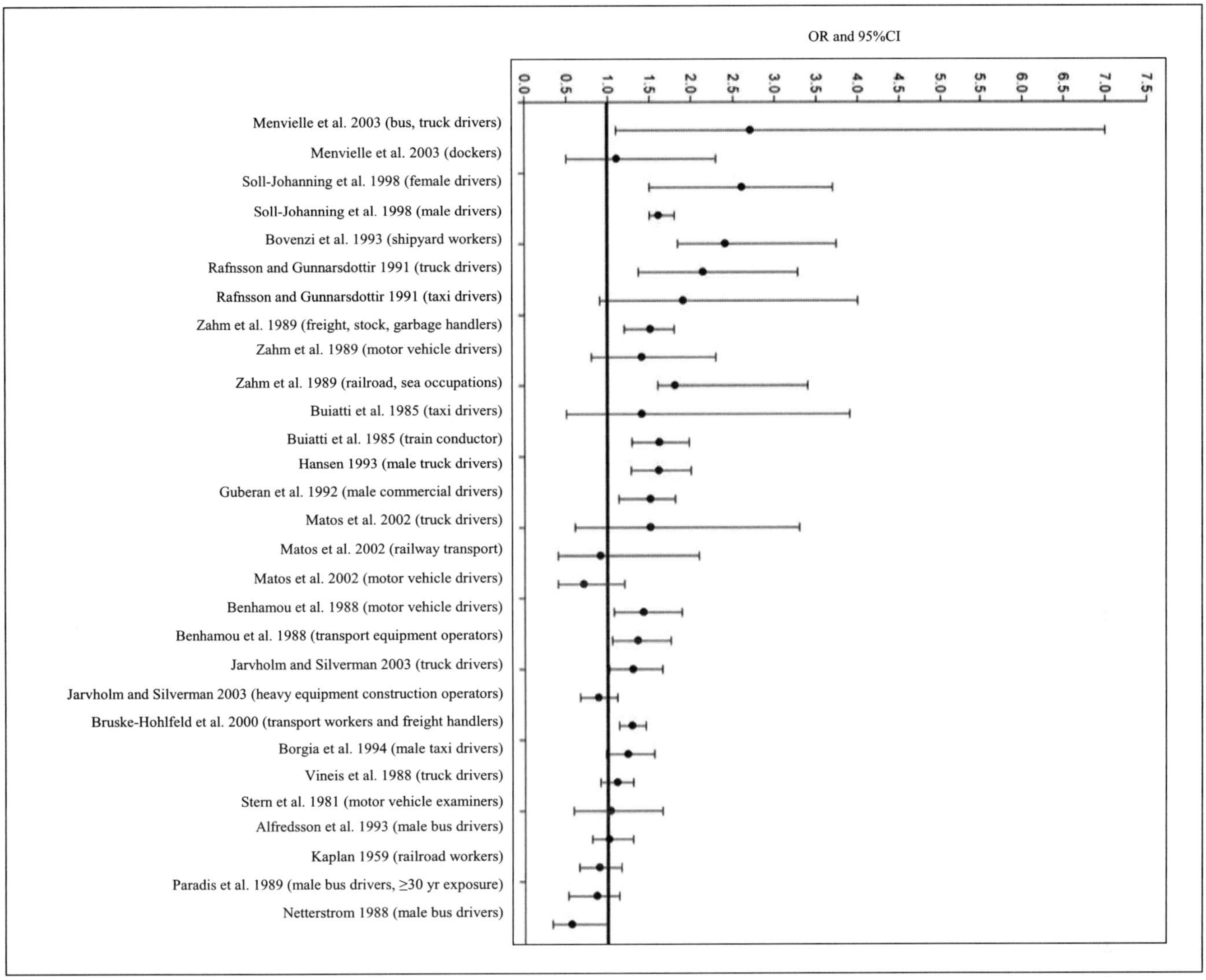

FIGURE 4.1 Lung cancer and occupations with exposure to combustion products

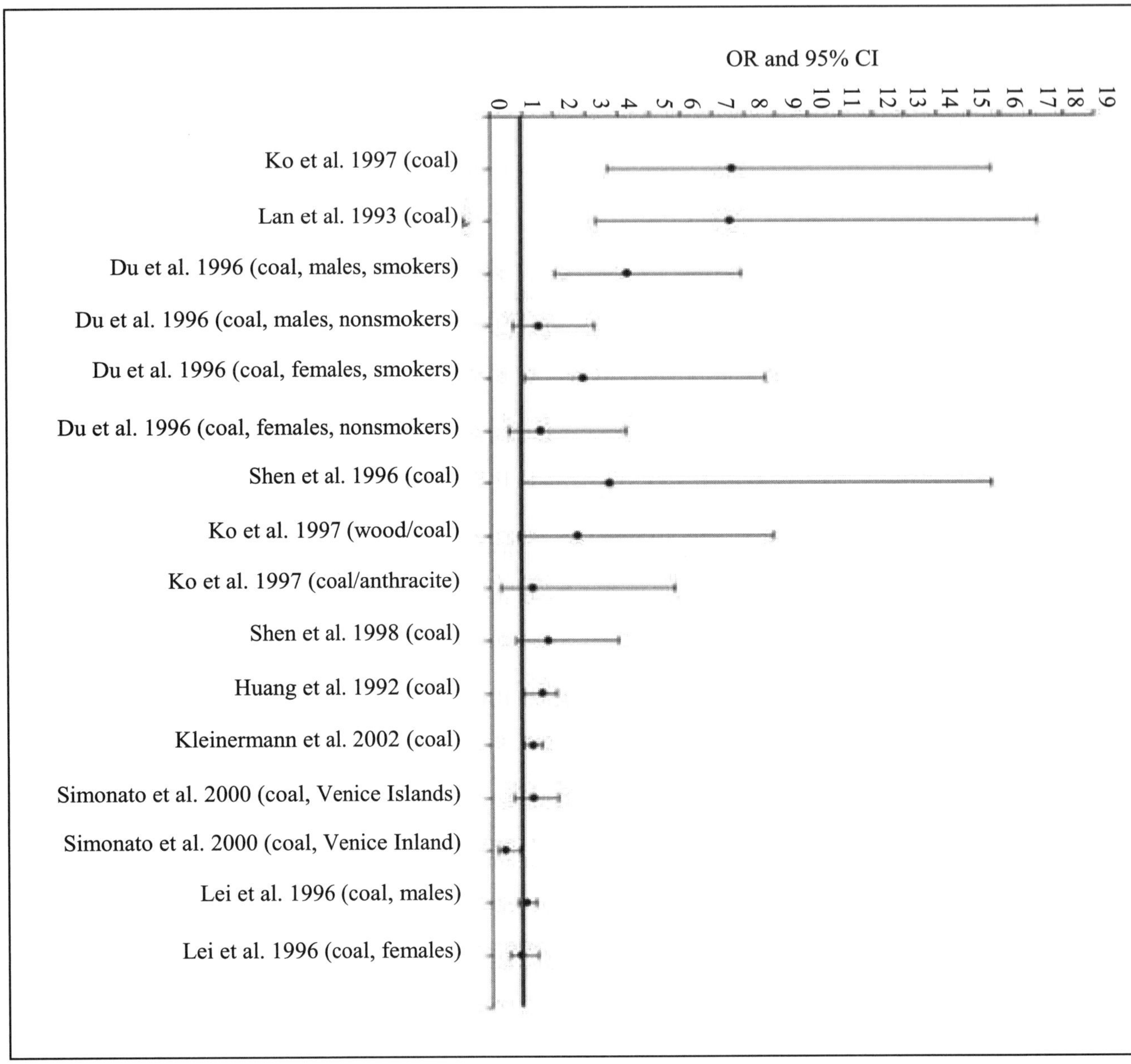

FIGURE 4.2 Lung cancer and indoor air pollution from combustion of fuels

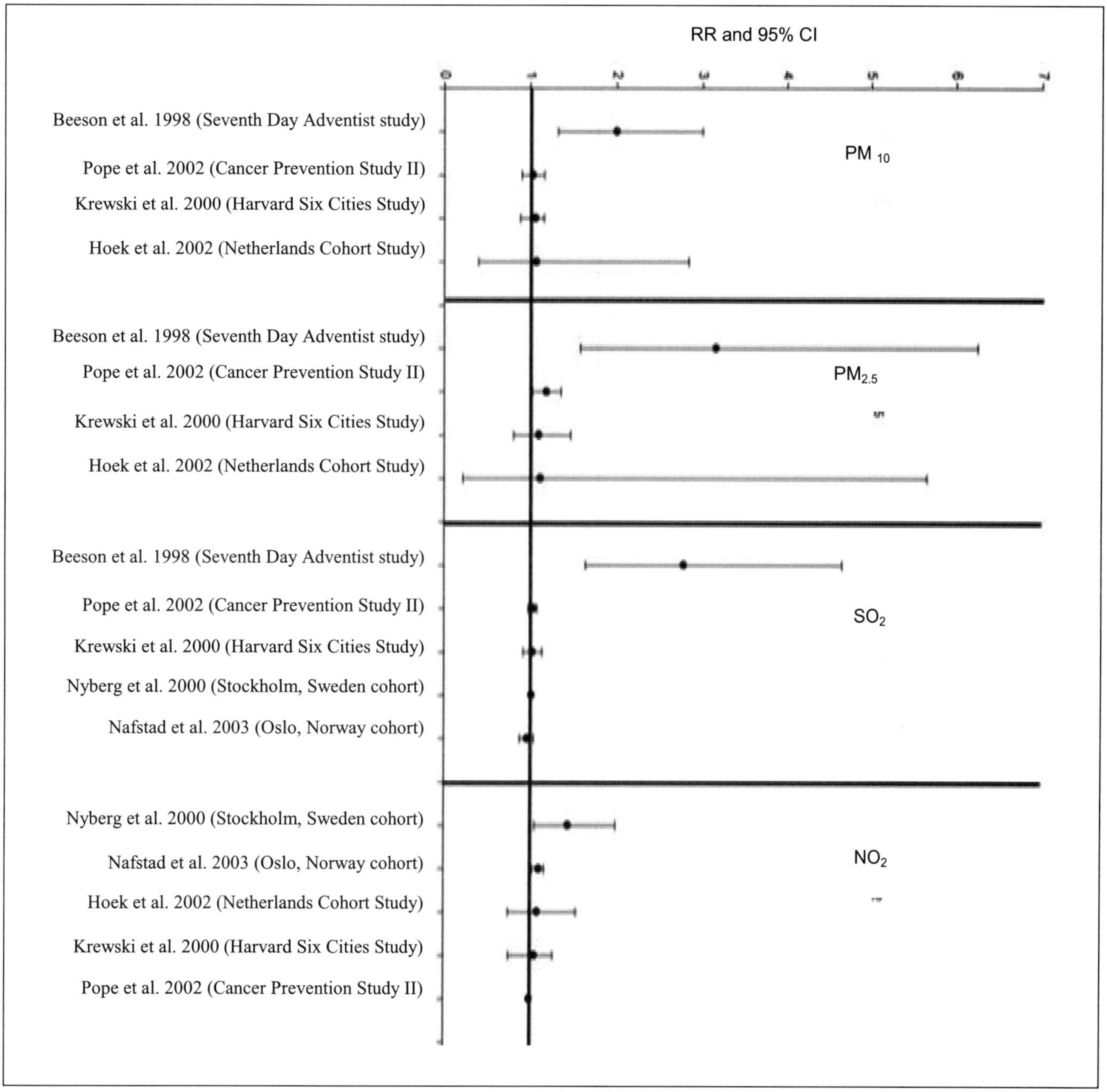

FIGURE 4.3 Lung cancer and ambient air pollution from combustion of fuels

Ambient Air-Pollution Studies

Five cohort studies have investigated the association between ambient air pollution and lung cancer: the Harvard Six Cities study (Krewski et al. 2000), the American Cancer Society (ACS) CPS-II Study (Pope et al. 1995, 2002), the California Seventh-Day Adventist Study (Abbey et al. 1999; Beeson et al. 1998), a Dutch study of diet and health (Hoek et al. 2002), and a cardiovascular cohort study in Norway (Nafstad et al. 2003). All except the Norwegian study used fixed-site air-pollution monitors to estimate exposure to ambient air pollution. In the Harvard Six Cities and ACS studies, subjects were assigned at the time of entry into the studies average annual exposure in their city of residence. In the Seventh-Day Adventist study, geostatistical interpolation of annual fixed-site monitor data was assigned to the address of each subject. In the Dutch study, a complicated exposure-assessment algorithm based on regional and local pollution and accounting for land use was used to estimate annual exposure of each subject. In the Norwegian study, dispersion models coupled with emission data were used to estimate annual sulfur dioxide (SO_2) and NO_x at each subject's residence.

Table 4.20 shows that in the Harvard Six Cities study and in the Dutch study, RRs of lung cancer were increased with exposure to fine particulate matter (PM) although the CIs included the null. In the Harvard Six Cities study, the RR associated with an increase in $PM_{2.5}$ of 18.5 $\mu g/m^3$ was 1.17 (95% CI 0.67-2.04). In the Dutch study, the RRs associated with an increase in air pollution from the 5th to the 95th percentile were 1.1 (95% CI 0.4-2.6) for black smoke (a measure of $PM_{2.5}$ and elemental carbon) and 1.3 (95% CI 0.4-3.7) for nitrogen dioxide (NO_2). In the ACS study, the RR associated with a 10 $\mu g/m^3$ increase in fine PM was 1.14 (95%CI 1.04-1.23). In the Seventh-Day Adventist Study, RRs increased with increasing exposure: with an increase in PM_{10} of 24.8 $\mu g/m^3$, men had an RR of 3.36 (95% CI 1.57-7.19), and women an RR of 1.33 (95% CI 0.60-2.96); with an increase in SO_2 of 3.72 ppb, men had an RR of 1.99 (95% CI 1.24-3.20), and women an RR of 3.01 (95% CI 1.88-4.84); and with an increase in NO_2 of 19.78 ppb, men had an RR of 1.82 (95% CI 0.93-3.57), and women an RR of 2.81 (95% CI 1.15-6.89). Finally, an association with NO_x (a marker of traffic-related combustion products) was found in the Norwegian study: for an increase in NO_x of 10 $\mu g/m^3$, the adjusted hazard ratio was 1.08 (95% CI 1.02-1.15). No associations were found with exposure to SO_2.

A number of case-control studies of the association between lung cancer and air pollution have been published. After adjusting for age, smoking, and occupation, Vena (1982) found a 26% increase in risk in persons living for at least 50 years in areas of Erie County, New York, that had high concentrations of total suspended particles (TSP). In a mortality case-control study in Krakow, Poland, an association was found among men living in areas with high concentrations of SO_2 and TSP (OR 1.46, 95% CI 1.06-1.99), but no excess risks were found among women (OR for medium or high concentrations 1.17) (Jedrychowski et al. 1990). A study in Trieste, Italy, found lung cancer to be associated with high estimated concentrations of deposited of particles (OR for over 0.298 g/m^2 per day compared with less than 0.175 g/ m^2 per day 1.4, 95% CI 1.1-1.8) (Barbone et al. 1995; Biggeri et al. 1996). Lung-cancer risk was also associated with living near an incinerator in the city (OR 2.6, 95% CI 1.3-5.1). (Alarie et al. 1972; Xu et al. 1996a) found that in northeastern China ORs in men increased with perceived smokiness in the outdoor environment (OR for "somewhat smoky" 1.5, 95% CI 1.2-2.0; OR for "smoky" 2.3, 95% CI 1.7-2.9). Similar results were found in women. In a small study among women living in Athens, Katsouyanni et al. (1991) investigated the association between lung cancer and ambient concentrations of soot. They did not find an association among nonsmoking women (smoking-adjusted, comparing highest quartile with lowest quartile OR 0.7), but found a strong association among women who smoked for long durations (30 years of smoking, comparing highest quartile with lowest quartile OR of 2.23). Nyberg et al. (2000) conducted a case-control study of lung cancer and traffic-related pollution in Stockholm, Sweden, and estimated traffic-related concentrations of NO_2 and heating-related concentrations of SO_2, using patterns of traffic density and dispersion models. After adjusting for smoking, occupation, exposure to radon, and other risk factors, they found little evidence of an association when they used exposures to NO_2 averaged over a 30-year period. A trend in risk was observed with a 20-

year lagged metric for exposure (NO_2 over 29 μg/m^3 OR 1.4, 95% CI 1.1-2.0; SO_2 over 129μg/m^3 OR 1.2, 95% CI 0.9-1.7). There was no evidence of an interaction with smoking status.

Some studies were methodologically less rigorous. Yang (1999) conducted a death-certificate case-control study in Taiwan and found an association between lung cancer and a petrochemical air-pollution index defined by the proportion of employees working in the petrochemical industry in each municipality. In a study of occupational and environmental exposures, Jockel et al. (1992) did not find an association with air pollution. Theirs was a small study, and the exposure assessments were not well described; no associations were found with estimated concentrations of SO_2. In an ecologic study in Rome, Italy, Michelozzi et al. (1998) did not find an association with distance from incinerators and oil refineries.

Occupational Exposure to Engine Exhaust

This review includes findings from occupational studies in which subjects were considered to be probably exposed to exhaust emissions from internal-combustion engines. The studies have been organized according to whether job titles were used to infer such exposures (that is, no specific estimates of exposure to exhaust-related pollutants were provided) or exposure to exhausts, diesel fumes, or PAHs was estimated with generally accepted principles of occupational epidemiology (that is, use of JEMs, detailed assessment of exposure by experts, and actual measurement of exposures). For studies that used job titles, the assumption regarding exposure was based on general industrial-hygiene information about job types, not necessarily on details of subjects' occupations. Consequently, one would expect misclassification of exposure to weaken RR estimates.

General Exposure to Exhaust

Three incidence and two mortality cohort studies of bus drivers yielded no strong indication of an association of exposure to exhaust with lung cancer (Alfredsson et al. 1993; Netterstrom 1988; Paradis et al. 1989; Soll-Johanning et al. 2003). An increased relative risk was found in a study of commercial drivers (truck, taxi, and bus drivers) in Geneva (RR 1.61, 95% CI 1.29-1.98) (Guberan et al. 1992), a study of truck drivers in Denmark (RR 1.60, 95% CI 1.28-1.98) (Hansen 1993), a study of truck drivers in Sweden (RR 1.29, 95% CI 0.99-1.65) (Jarvholm and Silverman 2003), and a study of truck drivers in Iceland (RR 2.14, 95% CI 1.37-3.18) (Rafnsson and Gunaarsdottir 1991). There was little evidence that risk increased with duration of employment in the few studies in which the risk was reported.

Almost all the case-control studies showed an increased risk of lung cancer among professional drivers (Bruske-Hohlfeld et al. 1999, 2000; Buiatti et al. 1985; Hansen et al. 1998; Hayes et al. 1989; Menvielle et al. 2003; Muscat et al. 1998; Steenland et al. 1990; Swanson et al. 1993; Zahm et al. 1989). RRs were found to increase with duration of employment in a Danish study (Hansen et al. 1998); a US study of teamster-union drivers (especially diesel- and gasoline-truck drivers) (Steenland et al. 1990); a study in Detroit, Michigan (Swanson et al. 1993); a study in New Caledonia (Menvielle et al. 2003); and a pooled analysis of three American case-control studies (Hayes et al. 1989). No clear-cut trends for professional drivers were found in a German study (Bruske-Hohlfeld et al. 1999, 2000) and in a Swedish study (Damber and Larsson 1985, 1987). Other professions that probably entail exposure to engine exhaust were found to be associated with increased risks of lung cancer, including dock work

(Jockel et al. 1998; Menvielle et al. 2003), transportation-equipment management (Menvielle et al. 2003), and shipyard work (Bovenzi et al. 1993; Hayes et al. 1989; Zahm et al. 1989).

Estimated Exposure to Compounds in Exhaust Fumes

The Dutch dietary cohort study (van Loon et al. 1997), from which exposure to ambient air pollution was estimated, was also used to estimate the incidence of occupational exposure to PAHs. Adjustment only for age showed that the RR of lung cancer increased by tertile of exposure. However, adjustment for age, smoking, and other occupational exposures led to risks that declined with increasing exposure. It is possible that the latter analysis, in which other occupational agents were included, was overmatched. An analysis adjusting for all potential confounding factors, excluding the occupational ones, was not conducted. A large census cohort study in Sweden that used a JEM to assign probability and intensity of exposure to diesel emissions on the basis of job titles collected in the 1960 and 1970 censuses showed that risks of lung cancer increased with the magnitude and probability of exposure among men but not among women (Boffetta et al. 2001). A study from the Kaiser Permanente Medical Care Program in California showed a 61% excess of lung cancer among bus-garage mechanics and showed that RRs increased by an index of cumulative diesel exhaust (Van Den Eeden and Friedman 1993).

Male firefighters in Philadelphia did not appear to be at increased risk for death from lung cancer when a surrogate index of exposure to diesel exhaust was used, although the power of the study was likely to be low because of small numbers of cases and a surrogate index of exposure (Baris et al. 2001). In a cohort of US railroad workers, younger diesel-exposed workers were found to be at higher risk, presumably because the younger workers had the greatest duration of exposure (Garshick et al. 1987, 1988; Larkin et al. 2000). Potash miners in Germany were at higher RR for death, but the 95% CIs included the null (Saverin et al. 1999). Risk was found to increase with cumulative exposure to diesel among a cohort of bus garage mechanics in Stockholm (Gustavsson et al. 1990). In the ACS CPS II study, it was reported that risk increased with duration of self-reported exposure to diesel exhaust (Boffetta et al. 1988); a limitation of this analysis is the use of self-reported exposure.

Risk estimates associated with exposure to specific components of exhaust have come out of a number of studies. Increased lung-cancer risk with cumulative exposure to diesel exhaust and to PAHs from occupational sources was found in a previously cited case-control study in Germany (Bruske-Hohlfeld et al. 2000) and in a study in Stockholm (Gustavsson et al. 2000). However, exposure to diesel exhaust from occupational sources was not found to increase the risk of lung cancer in a US hospital-based case-control study (Boffetta et al. 1990) and exposure to PAHs was not found to increase the risk in occupational studies in Buenos Aires (Matos et al. 2000), Montreal (Nadon et al. 1995), and Sweden (Emmelin et al. 1993).

Many studies have assessed the association of indoor air quality related to types of heating or cooking fuels, such as coal, with lung cancer. Studies of exposure to heating or cooking fuels included a number from China (Alarie et al. 1972; Dai et al. 1996; Du et al. 1996; He et al. 1991; Huang et al. 1992; Kleinerman et al. 2002; Lan et al. 1993; Lei et al. 1996; Liu et al. 1993; Metayer et al. 2002; Shen et al. 1996; Wu-Williams et al. 1990a, 1993; Xu et al. 1989, 1996a; Zhong et al. 1999), Hong Kong (Koo et al. 1983) and Taiwan (Chen et al. 1990; Ko et al. 1997), many of which showed such associations. Only one cohort study investigated the effects of indoor air pollution on the risk of developing lung cancer (Lan et al. 2002). That population-based interview study included more than 31,000 farmers living in Xuanwei, China, who were followed from 1976 to 1992. The analysis was based on subjects whose parents used unvented firepits and smoky coal throughout their lives. It showed that changing to stoves that had chimneys decreased the risk of lung cancer (RR < 0.6) and that the reduction occurred more than 10 years after the change.

Gulf War Veteran Study

A study assessing respiratory cancer in Gulf War Veterans was identified and reviewed by the committee (Smith et al. 2002). The study population consisted of 405,142 regular active-duty US military personnel who were in the gulf region during the Kuwaiti oil-well fires. Hospitalization records were examined from Department of Defense military treatment facilities from August 1, 1991 until hospitalization, separation from active-duty service, or July 31, 1999. Modeling was used to estimate troop exposure to oil-well fire smoke. The risk of malignant neoplasms of the respiratory and intrathoracic organs was modestly increased in the exposed group, but the CI included the null (adjusted RR 1.10, 95% CI 0.56-2.17). The relatively short observation period (8 years) is a limitation of this study for assessing cancer risk.

Conclusion

Results of studies of fuel exposure and lung-cancer risk are inconsistent. Siemiatycki et al. reported an association between kerosene and crude-oil exposure and squamous-cell lung cancer, between diesel-fuel exposure and nonadenocarcinoma, and between heating-oil exposure and oat-cell lung cancer (Siemiatycki et al. 1987a). Two cohort studies (Imperial Oil and Texas cohorts) did not find an association in workers most likely to have been exposed to fuels.

The committee concludes, from its assessment of the epidemiologic literature, that there is inadequate/insufficient evidence to determine whether an association exists between exposure to fuels and lung cancer.

There was evidence of associations between exposure to ambient air pollution, engine exhausts, and heating sources (coal) and lung cancer. Cohort and case-control studies showed consistently that risks increased with increasing ambient air pollution. There was evidence from both cohort and case-control studies that increasing exposure to engine exhausts and to its components (such as PAHs) increased the risk of lung cancer. As supporting evidence, the case-control studies of heating with coal showed increasing risks of developing lung cancer, and the risks were independent of active smoking and exposure to environmental tobacco smoke. The one cohort study showed that reduction in combustion products from smoky coal, by use of stoves that had chimneys, decreased the risk of lung cancer. Experimental evidence has shown that many compounds present in combustion products of oils in Chinese-style cooking are carcinogenic and some mutagenic. There is additional evidence that kerosene and soot are genotoxic in in vivo and in vitro models and that diesel exhaust is mutagenic. Toxicologic studies found that rats and mice exposed to coal and wood smoke had an increased incidence of lung cancer.

The committee concludes, from its assessment of the epidemiologic literature, that there is sufficient evidence of an association between exposure to combustion products and lung cancer.

MALIGNANT MELANOMA OF THE SKIN

Skin cancer is the most common type of cancer (ACS 2004u). There are two forms of skin cancer: melanoma (ICD-9 172) and nonmelanoma (basal-cell and squamous-cell carcinomas) (ICD-9 173). The major risk factor for both types of skin cancer is exposure to the sun and other sources of UV radiation. Family history, fair skin, moles, male sex, the inherited disease xeroderma pigmentosum, and immune suppression also play a role in the development of melanoma skin cancers. Melanoma is a much less common form of skin cancer than basal-cell or squamous-cell carcinoma, but is much more serious, usually being fatal if not treated in its early stages (ACS 2004u).

In 2000, malignant melanoma accounted for 17.7 new cases per 100,000 people (22.5 among men and 14.4 among women) and 2.7 deaths per 100,000 (3.8 among men and 1.8 among women) in the United States (Ries et al. 2004).

Most of the studies identified by the committee as meeting its criteria for assessing a potential association between exposure to fuels or their combustion products and skin cancer focused on melanoma. Mortality studies are likely to focus on melanoma, because it is unusual to die of other forms of skin cancer. Several studies of ocular melanoma or uveal melanoma (ICD-8 191) were identified; these are considered separately from cutaneous melanoma because they are classified as malignant neoplasms of nervous tissue. Mortality and morbidity studies of cutaneous melanoma are presented below; information gathered on malignant nonmelanoma skin cancer is summarized in the next section.

Fuels

Table 4.21 presents the most relevant findings considered by the committee in drawing its conclusion on the possibility of an association between exposure to fuels and melanoma skin cancer.

Cohort Studies

In the large Amoco cohort of oil refinery workers, Nelson et al. (1987) found the risk of skin-cancer death among white men increased (SMR 2.01, 95% CI 1.00-3.60), even though the usual "healthy-worker effect" of reduced overall mortality and cancer mortality was seen. The study combined both melanoma and nonmelanoma skin cancer in its definition of skin cancer; however, because death was the end point, virtually all the skin-cancer cases were probably melanoma. When latent period was considered, the mortality was greatest among those with less than 15 years since first exposure (SMR 5.24, $p < 0.05$). The work histories of the people in the cohort were reviewed by industrial hygienists and classified for specific exposures (Nelson et al. 1985). There were 11 skin cancers, and the excess appeared to be concentrated among the maintenance workers (SMR 3.78, $p < 0.05$). Routine exposure to refinery processes was also associated with skin-cancer mortality (SMR 2.68, $p < 0.05$). The failure to adjust for possible confounders (particularly sun exposure) reduces confidence in the finding.

Jarvholm et al. (1997) investigated the incidence of melanoma and nonmelanoma skin cancer separately in a cohort of Swedish refinery workers. A minor increase in the risk of melanoma (SIR 1.1, 90% CI 0.49-2.0) was based on seven exposed cases, who had all received their diagnoses within 20 years of their first exposure.

Mortality has been assessed periodically among workers of Imperial Oil Limited of Canada (Hanis et al. 1979; Lewis et al. 2000b; Schnatter et al. 1992). In comparison with the Canadian general population, the estimated risk of death from melanoma in 1964-1994 among men working in all sectors of the industry was somewhat increased (SMR 1.32, 95% CI 0.83-2.00). Risks had diminished from the previous followup period (1964-1983) for upstream operations and for the marketing and distribution segment (Schnatter et al. 1992). Only two additional cases were observed among marketing and distribution workers in the 11 years of followup through 1994, so SMR was reduced from 2.56 (95% CI 0.94-5.57) to 1.59 (95% CI 0.69-3.14). The occurrence of only a single new case among exploration, drilling, production, or pipeline (upstream) workers reduced the risk considerably from 6.00 (95% CI 2.19-13.06) to 2.82 (95% CI 1.13-5.81). The increased risk of melanoma among the upstream subcohort may be related to exposure to crude oil, but it also coincides with the greater potential for sun exposure of these workers, who spend a considerable amount of time outdoors.

From the Imperial Oil cohort followup through 1994, Lewis et al. (2003) defined an "inception cohort" of younger workers with exposure experience only under more recent occupational-hygiene standards; the cohort consisted of those hired in 1964-1993. In these younger men, the estimated risk of melanoma (SIR 1.25, 95% CI 0.82-1.83) was effectively equivalent to the estimated mortality among the men in the full cohort; it must be noted that the incident cases include many (if not all) of the instances of melanoma deaths in the first analysis. The contrast between mortality among the (few) older female workers and incidence among the newly hired women, however, was considerable, although the CIs overlap slightly. The women's estimated risk of melanoma (SIR 1.46, 95% CI 0.83-2.37) was similar to both findings for men. The Imperial Oil findings present a fairly coherent picture of an association of exposure to petroleum and derived fuels with melanoma, except that there is no suggestion of a dose–response relationship by duration of employment or intensity of exposure to fuel-related hydrocarbons. Additional uncertainty arises from the lack of control for possible confounders, especially exposure to sunlight.

Case-Control Studies

In an analysis of the data from the multicancer case-control study conducted in Montreal that specifically addressed association between work in various occupations and melanoma, Fritschi and Siemiatycki (1996a) found no association with any industry, occupation, or industrial-hygiene-determined substance related to petroleum. Those substances included C_1-C_4 alkanes, C_5-C_{17} alkanes, C_{18+} alkanes, and leaded gasoline with 10, 22, 18, and six exposed cases, respectively. The study has the advantages of addressing incident cases, having full exposure histories interpreted by industrial hygienists, and incorporating information on many potential confounding variables, but the researchers note the study's limited power to exclude definitively the possibility of an association with any particular exposure.

Combustion Products

Table 4.22 presents the most relevant findings considered by the committee in drawing its conclusion on the possibility of an association between exposure to combustion products and melanoma skin cancer.

Cohort Studies

Boffetta et al. (1988) analyzed the mortality experience of the prospective cohort established by the ACS in 1982 from the perspective of occupational exposure to diesel exhaust. The sample was defined as men found in followup who had been 40-79 years old at enrollment and had provided usable information on both smoking and exposure to diesel exhaust (and extensive other information gathered in the self-administered questionnaire). Although only 2 years of followup had accumulated, 7,499 deaths had occurred in the sample of 369,943 people (the above data constraints and loss to followup reduced the original sample by about 25%). When adjusted for age, smoking, and other occupational exposures, an imprecise estimate of risk of melanoma death of those exposed to diesel exhaust was increased (RR 1.67, $p > 0.05$).

Pion et al. (1995) conducted a nested case-control study on the data generated on the ACS cohort at the time of its 6-year followup. The set of 2,780 melanoma cases was made up (in unspecified proportions) of men and women of all ages who had already been so diagnosed at the time of enrollment or were newly diagnosed during the followup period. Three controls without melanoma—matched by sex, age, race, and area of residence—were drawn from the cohort for each case. Although their accuracy might still be questioned, self-reports of exposure would not be expected to be subject to recall bias in a (strictly) prospective study. Several exposures of interest to the committee were addressed (coal tar, pitch, or asphalt; diesel engine exhaust; and gasoline exhaust), but none had an OR exceeding unity. Occupations were analyzed separately by sex. The risk of melanoma was less than 1 for truck drivers (OR 0.72, 95% CI 0.40-1.30); the most marked increase for a male occupation was for (generic) firefighters (OR 2.29, 95% CI 0.85-6.16). No adjustments were made by using information on possible confounders, whose availability is one of the primary merits of the ACS prospective cohort. The commingling of cross-sectional and prospective designs in this analysis raises the possibility that exposure occurred after the cancer event for the subset of original prevalent cases; no mention was made of screening the exposures to account for this temporal issue.

From the Swedish Cancer Environmental Registry updated to include 1970 census results and cancers diagnosed in 1971-1989, Boffetta et al. (2001) partitioned the cohort of men and women who were actively employed according to both the 1960 and 1970 censuses into sets with and without occupational exposure to diesel exhaust. Individual exposure to diesel emissions was assessed with a matrix of probabilities and intensities expected for each job title. Having found a high concordance between the occupations reported on the two censuses, the researchers opted to encode diesel exposure from the occupation specified on the 1960 census. Melanoma was not among the cancer sites for which there was any suggestion of an increased risk for either men or women who had held a job in 1960 with any likelihood of exposure to diesel emissions. Roughly half the male cases in the sample would intersect with those in the case-control study below, which was based on melanomas diagnosed in Sweden from 1961 to 1979 (Linet et al. 1995).

Case-Control Studies

In a case-control study of patients at Roswell Park Memorial Institute in 1956-1965, the occupational histories of about 14,000 white cancer cases were compared with those of noncancer patients (Decoufle and Stanislawczyk 1977; Viadana et al. 1976). For all the several exhaust-associated occupations of interest, the estimates of association with melanoma were increased, some of them markedly (for example, locomotive engineers and firemen and excavating, grading, and road-machinery operators). Because no more than four men with melanoma had held any of those occupations and only three who had held only clerical positions were available for comparison, all the associated confidence intervals included unity, and no adjustment for possible confounders was attempted.

Siemiatycki et al. (1988) addressed the 121 interviewed melanoma cases in the Montreal multicancer case-control study in seeking associations with various exhaust and combustion-product exposures. They reported that melanoma was associated ($p < 0.05$) with propane exhaust (OR 3.3, 90% CI 1.2-9.0) and there were suggestive increases with jet-fuel exhaust (OR 1.8, 90% CI 0.5-6.4) and liquid-fuel combustion (OR 1.8, 90% CI 0.9-3.4). In a more recent publication on this dataset, Fritschi and Siemiatycki (1996a) found no compelling association between any combustion-products exposure and melanoma. For an exposure to be analyzed (with adjustment for age, education, and ethnicity), there had to be at least four exposed cases. Estimates hovering about unity were reported for gasoline-engine emissions, PAHs from petroleum, and carbon monoxide. An appendix listed several additional combustion-products-related exposures for which the lower 95% confidence limit of the estimate of association with melanoma did not exceed 0.9: the air-transport, motor-transport, and railway-transport industries, with six, eight, and five exposed cases, respectively; the occupations of mechanic or motor-transport worker, with five and 10 exposed cases, respectively; and diesel-engine emissions, liquid-fuel combustion products, PAHs from any source, and pyrolysis fumes not classified elsewhere, with 10, six, 57, and 11 exposed cases, respectively. There was no explanation of why the number of interviewed melanoma cases considered had decreased by 18 (15%); only inconsequential perturbations resulted in the statistics for the exposures common to the two publications (assuming that "petrol engine emissions" equates to "gasoline exhaust").

Nelemans et al. (1993) compared 140 melanoma cases with 181 controls who had other malignancies, all gathered from a cancer registry in the mideastern part of the Netherlands. After adjustment for age, sex, education, pigmentation factors, and exposure to sunlight, those who had ever worked in the "transport and communications" industry had a greater risk of melanoma than those who had not (OR 1.70, 95% CI 0.84-3.46); the difference was intensified by contrasting this group with those who had never worked in any of 10 hypothetically high-risk industries (OR 1.92, 95% CI 0.84-4.35). For the transportation and communications workers, tar products, cutting oils or coolants, and lubricating oils were among the exposures that were self-reported more frequently than by other workers, but no formal analysis was presented, and there was no attempt at a JEM approach to evaluating exposure. This elementary study provides some weak support for the possibility that exposure to combustion products is associated with the occurrence of cutaneous melanoma.

Using the Swedish Cancer Environment Registry database, Linet et al. (1995) identified 3,850 men diagnosed with melanoma in 1961-1979 who had been listed as occupationally active in the 1960 census; this sample would be expected to coincide with the male portion of the set of 5,003 melanoma cases studied in somewhat less detail by Vagero et al. (1990). The global categories for the "transport and communications" industry or occupation showed no indication of a relationship between melanoma and employment that might involve exposure to vehicle exhaust. Occupational subcategories in this sector, however, did show some increases; the risk for "traffic administration" was 1.6 ($p < 0.05$, adjusted for age and region), and the risk for the more specific classification "traffic enforcement or railroad work" even more pronounced (SIR 3.1, $p < 0.01$).

Conclusion

Data from studies of the large Amoco (Nelson et al. 1985, 1987) and Imperial Oil (Hanis et al. 1979) cohorts suggest an increased risk of death from melanoma with exposure to petroleum-derived materials (such as heavy oils and crude oil), and the smaller study (Jarvholm et al. 1997) is not inconsistent with such an association (Lewis et al. 2000b). In all the fuel cohort studies, the peak of melanoma risk occurred with latency (Jarvholm et al. 1997; Nelson et al. 1987) or duration (Lewis et al. 2000b) of around 15 years, rather than showing a dose–response relationship. The studies, however, did not adjust for sun exposure, a major risk factor for melanoma, and the workers—particularly the exploration, drilling, and pipeline workers—may have received considerable sun exposure while performing their jobs. But the one case-control study with fairly reliable exposure analysis (Fritschi and Siemiatycki 1996a) did not support such a conclusion.

The studies addressing exposure to combustion products also failed to adjust for exposure to sunlight. The Montreal case-control study, which had the best exposure assessment, and the record-linkage study of Linet et al. (1995) found isolated effects of specific exposures (propane exhaust and being a traffic administrator, respectively) that were not among the major ones considered by the present committee in evaluating possible effects of combustion products.

> **The committee concludes, from its assessment of the epidemiologic literature, that there is inadequate/insufficient evidence to determine whether an association exists between exposure to fuels or combustion products and cutaneous malignant melanoma.**

NON-MELANOMA SKIN CANCERS

Nonmelanoma skin cancers (basal-cell and squamous-cell carcinomas) (ICD-9 173) are common but rarely fatal. As for cutaneous malignant melanoma, the main risk factor for nonmelanoma skin cancers is exposure to the sun and other sources of UV radiation. Other risk factors for nonmelanoma skin cancer are sex, family history, some specific inherited conditions (for example, basal-cell nevus syndrome and xeroderma pigmentosum), radiation treatment, exposure to some chemicals (such as arsenic, industrial tar, coal, paraffin, and oils), chronic or severe skin problems (such as burns), a weakened immune system, viral infection, and smoking (ACS 2004u).

Fuels

Table 4.23 presents the most relevant findings reviewed by the committee in drawing its conclusion on the possibility of an association between exposure to fuels and nonmelanoma skin cancers.

Cohort Studies

Jarvholm et al. (1997) investigated cancer incidence in a cohort of workers assembled from the personnel records of 26 companies in the Swedish petroleum industry. The study generated a somewhat stronger, yet still weak, estimate of an association of exposure to fuels with nonmelanoma skin cancers (SIR 1.3, 90% CI 0.61-2.4) than it had with melanoma.

Retrieval from the cancer registry generated an identical number (seven) of melanoma and nonmelanoma skin cancers; this suggests that records were incomplete.

Case-Control Studies

Kubasiewicz and Starzynski (1989) described the methods used to identify and interview men who had incident cases of skin cancer from 1982 through 1988 in the registry for Lodz, Poland, and age-matched sets of population and hospital controls. With selection for "all skin lesions suspected to have a neoplastic origin", they reported that the 374 interviewed cases (of the 520 identified cases born after 1900) had 278 basal-cell carcinomas, 70 "carcinomas planoepitheliale", 13 cases of Bowen's disease (carcinoma in situ, precancerous), and 13 cases of Arning's carcinoid (superficial basal-cell carcinoma). In an analysis that focused on occupational exposure to PAHs, Kubasiewicz et al. (1991) reported on a final set of 376 cases and their 752 population and 752 hospital controls. Full work histories were gathered, but the exposures analyzed consisted of self-reports on each of 17 possible agents, three of which would fit in our fuels classification: petroleum, petrol, and gasoline. The distinction between petrol and gasoline was not stated, but the results for gasoline exposure were said to be too sparse to analyze. Minor increases in crude risks of skin cancer were reported for both petroleum and petrol (ORs 1.17 and 1.30, respectively). The definition of skin cancer used in the study clearly excluded melanoma, but it did encompass some skin lesions that do not coincide with the malignant classification the present committee intended to address.

Using the Alberta (Canada) Cancer Registry, Gallagher et al. (1996) identified all men with squamous-cell carcinoma and basal-cell carcinoma who were 20-79 years old when diagnosed in 1983-1984. All 225 subjects with a first primary squamous-cell carcinoma were eligible. For first primary basal-cell carcinoma, only one-fourth of the cases with the lesion on the head or neck were retained, but all subjects with such a tumor elsewhere were kept; the total was 314 eligible cases of basal-cell carcinoma. During home interviews, 180 men with squamous-cell carcinoma and 226 men with basal-cell carcinoma completed a questionnaire that included a complete work history and a list of specific exposures of interest. Of 573 age-matched controls with no history of skin cancer drawn from men in the Alberta Health Care Insurance Plan (which includes everyone resident in the province for more than 3 months), 406 men completed the same questionnaire. The sets of squamous-cell carcinoma and basal-cell carcinoma cases were compared with the controls separately. With adjustment for age, skin pigmentation (for example, fair skin), ethnicity, and exposure to sunlight, but not smoking, the risk of squamous-cell carcinoma after exposure to petroleum products (specified to be gasoline and oil) was increased (OR 1.3, 95% CI 1.0-2.0), but not the risk of basal-cell carcinoma (OR 0.9, 95% CI 0.6-1.3). Although the response rates were low and the exposure data came only from self-reports, the results of the study suggest a potential relationship between exposure to petroleum-derived fuels and squamous-cell carcinoma.

Combustion Products

Table 4.24 presents the most relevant findings reviewed by the committee in drawing its conclusion on the possibility of an association between exposure to combustion products and nonmelanoma skin cancers.

Case-Control Studies

Hannukesela-Svahn et al. (1999) analyzed basal-cell carcinomas and other nonmelanoma skin cancers assembled in the Finnish Cancer Registry over 4 decades by linking to subjects' stated occupations in the 1970 census. For "transportation and communication" (a nonspecific, self-reported occupation code at a single time), the estimated risk of basal-cell carcinoma among men was 1.0 (95% CI 1.0-1.1), which suggests that the risk was not increased. There were only about 15% as many cases of the other types of nonmelanoma skin cancers (predominantly squamous-cell carcinomas) as there were cases of basal-cell carcinoma, so the confidence intervals associated with the estimated risks were wider; the estimated risk in men was slightly below unity, that in women somewhat above.

As discussed above in connection with exposures to fuels, Kubasiewicz et al. (1991) presented an analysis of occupational exposure of 376 skin-cancer subjects (primarily with basal-cell carcinoma) and their 752 population and 752 hospital controls to PAHs. Full work histories had been gathered, but exposure to PAHs was determined on the basis of self-reported exposure to each of 17 possible sources of PAHs. The cases were compared independently (apparently without adjustment beyond matching on age) with both the population and hospital controls, and the results were virtually identical (the statistics related to the population controls are reported here). There was a slight increase in risk in those who had ever been exposed to any of the sources of PAHs (OR 1.15, 95% CI 0.90-1.51; 95% CI calculated with standard methods from the observed and expected numbers presented in the original paper), but there was no indication of a dose–response relationship with duration of exposure.

In the case-control study of squamous-cell carcinoma and basal-cell carcinoma from the Alberta Cancer Registry, Gallagher et al. (1996) presented the results related to several potentially PAH-containing exposures (determined by self-report) in addition to the fuel-related exposure reported above. After adjustment for age, pigmentation, ethnicity, and exposure to sunlight, but not smoking, the risk of squamous-cell carcinoma after exposure to diesel fumes was increased (OR 1.7, 95% CI 1.1-2.5). For basal-cell carcinoma, only a modestly increased PAH-related risk was seen after exposure to diesel fumes (OR 1.1, 95% CI 0.8-1.6).

Conclusion

The committee recognizes that PAHs (present in soot and numerous similar complex mixtures, mostly originating from combustion processes) have long been accepted to be skin carcinogens in animals and humans (ATSDR 1995; IARC 1985). IARC limited the scope of its consideration to chimney soot, so the subjects of the studies on which its conclusions were based were all chimney sweeps. Similarly, the epidemiologic bases of the Agency for Toxic Substances and Disease Registry (ATSDR) conclusions were shale-oil workers and chimney sweeps. As explained in Chapter 2, in planning its approach to its task, the committee considered those types of exposure as too dissimilar to the exposure scenarios in the Persian Gulf to base its conclusions on combustion products and nonmelanoma skin cancers on the conclusions of IARC and ATSDR.

Dermal application of individual PAHs to animals has been shown to lead to skin tumors in a number of studies. Mechanistic studies have demonstrated that some PAHs are genotoxic and can act as initiators, promoters, and complete carcinogens. Despite strong evidence that PAHs are carcinogenic in animal models and that they are genotoxic, the committee used toxicologic information only in a supportive role; that is, it did not base its conclusions solely on toxicologic information.

Of the available epidemiologic studies that met the committee's criteria, the Gallagher et al. (1996) study appears to be the most reliable and well conducted. It reported one borderline association between fuel exposure and squamous-cell carcinoma and several somewhat stronger associations between self-reported exposure to PAH-containing agents and squamous-cell carcinoma. For the more common type of nonmelanoma skin cancer (basal cell carcinoma), however, the findings with both types of exposure were largely negative. The committee concluded that without inclusion of epidemiologic studies regarding occupations that it had determined were dissimilar to exposures experienced during the Gulf War, a consistent and convincing picture of increased risk of nonmelanoma skin cancer did not emerge.

The committee concludes, from its assessment of the epidemiologic literature, that there is inadequate/insufficient evidence to determine whether an association exists between exposure to fuels and non-melanoma skin cancers.

FEMALE BREAST CANCER

Breast cancer (ICD-9 174) is about 100 times more common among women than men (ACS 2003e). There are a number of known or suspected risk factors for breast cancer in women; some major ones are aging, genetics, family history, years of ovulation, parity, and use of hormone-replacement therapy after menopause.

In 2000, there were 135.1 new cases of breast cancer per 100,000 women in the US and 26.7 deaths per 100,000 (Ries et al. 2004).

Fuels

Table 4.25 presents the most relevant findings reviewed by the committee in drawing its conclusion on the possibility of an association between exposure to fuels and breast cancer in women.

Cohort Studies

The risk of breast cancer in women was assessed in two cohorts of workers at petroleum companies (Divine et al. 1999b; Lewis et al. 2000b, 2003). Exposure was assessed in the Texaco cohort by using work histories in company records (Divine et al. 1999b), and no increased risk of breast cancer in women was found (SMR 0.71, 95% CI 0.40-1.18). In the Canadian Imperial Oil cohort, exposure was assessed in the same way (Lewis et al. 2000b, 2003), and neither breast cancer mortality nor incidence was markedly increased (SMR 1.08, 95% CI 0.66-1.67; SIR 1.02, 95% CI 0.80-1.28, respectively).

Lagorio et al. (1994) tracked the mortality experience of 357 women who had been managers of Italian service stations in 1980-1992. The effort complemented a detailed assessment of exposure at service stations by monitoring 111 attendants in 1992 (Lagorio et al. 1993). The OR for female breast-cancer risk was 1.04 (90% CI 0.18-3.28) on the basis of two cases.

Combustion Products

Table 4.26 presents the most relevant findings reviewed by the committee in drawing its conclusion on the possibility of an association between exposure to combustion products and breast cancer in women.

Case-Control Studies

Petralia et al. (1999) conducted a case-control study of 301 women who had premenopausal breast cancer and 316 controls from western New York state. JEMs were used to determine occupational exposure to PAHs and benzene, and the researchers endeavored to separate their individual roles. In comparison with women exposed to neither PAHs nor benene, the adjusted risk of breast cancer among women exposed only to PAHs (six cases) was neutral (RR 1.01, 95% CI 0.55-3.45), whereas the equivalent result for the 24 cases exposed only to benzene was 1.70 (95% CI 1.17-2.92). Smaller numbers of subjects in subcategories made separating the agent-specific contributions to estrogen-receptor-positive or -negative types of breast cancer more ambiguous.

Lewis-Michl et al. (1996) conducted a case-control study of the relationship between breast cancer and residence near industry or traffic on Long Island, New York. Among the women who had premenopausal breast cancer (93 in Nassau County and 70 in Suffolk County), the crude risks gave no indication of a relationship with those factors. In the larger group of 627 postmenopausal cases, crude ORs for high traffic density were not impressively increased among Nassau county subjects and did not exceed unity among women in Suffolk County; these results were essentially unchanged by adjustment for proximity to industry. The relevance to Gulf War exposures of the metric—distance from potential sources of vehicular combustion products—is limited by the ecologic nature of the exposure assessment.

Conclusion

No increased risk of breast cancer was found in a cohort of female petroleum workers (Divine et al. 1999b), and only a modest increase was found in another cohort of female petroleum workers (Lewis et al. 2003) and a cohort of female service-station workers in Italy (Lagorio et al. 1994). The two studies of breast cancer and exposure to combustion products evaluated by the committee (Lewis-Michl et al. 1996, Petralia et al. 1999) had essentially negative results.

The committee concludes, from its assessment of the epidemiologic literature, that there is inadequate/insufficient evidence to determine whether an association exists between exposure to fuels or combustion products and breast cancer in women.

MALE BREAST CANCER

Breast cancer occurs in men (ICD-9 175), although only rarely. Breast cancer accounts for about 0.22% of cancer deaths among men (ACS 2004t). Risk factors include aging, family history, radiation exposure, liver disease, estrogen treatment, physical inactivity, obesity, and the congenital condition Klinefelter syndrome.

In 2000, there were 1.3 new cases of breast cancer per 100,000 men and 0.4 deaths per 100,000 in the United States (Ries et al. 2004).

Fuels

Table 4.27 presents the findings reviewed by the committee in drawing its conclusion on the possibility of an association between exposure to fuels and breast cancer in men.

Case-Control Study

A population-based study of male breast cancer was conducted by using the Danish cancer registry (Hansen 2000). Exposure to gasoline vapors and PAHs (combined) was estimated from trade codes; blue-collar workers who had at least 3 months of employment in service stations, vehicle maintenance, the wholesale gasoline trade, or car-repair shops were classified as exposed. Exposure defined in that way was associated with a greater risk of breast cancer (OR 2.2, 95% CI 1.4-3.6), when birth year and socioeconomic status were controlled for. When a 10-year exposure lag was considered, the risk of breast cancer remained increased (OR 2.5, 95% CI 1.3-4.5). Men younger than 40 years old at the time of first employment had an OR of 3.7, which increased to 5.4 (95% CI 2.4-11.9) for a lag time of 10 years. The study did not control for smoking.

Combustion Products

Table 4.28 presents the most relevant findings reviewed by the committee in drawing its conclusion on the possibility of an association between exposure to combustion products and breast cancer in men.

Case-Control Studies

There are few case-control studies of the relationship between male breast cancer and exposure to combustion products or occupations with combustion-product exposure. As discussed in the previous section on fuel exposure, Hansen (2000) explored the relationship between male breast cancer and occupational exposure to gasoline and vehicle combustion products, including PAHs. Because the exposures were combined in the analysis, it is not possible to determine whether the increased risk of male breast cancer was due to fuel or combustion-product exposure.

Cocco et al. (1998) conducted a case-control study of male breast cancer and occupational exposure. They assessed occupational exposure to PAHs, high temperature, electromagnetic fields, herbicides, pesticides, and organic solvents by applying JEMs based on US census occupation and industry codes. The OR for the association between exposure to PAHs and male breast cancer was not increased. Taxicab drivers and subjects working in the motor-vehicle and equipment industry were at increased risk for male breast cancer.

Conclusion

Hansen (2000) reported positive findings regarding exposure to fuels and combustion products and male breast cancer; but the method used to assess exposure in that study is limited. Cocco et al. (1998) used a JEM and did not find an association between PAH exposure and male breast cancer.

The committee concludes, from its assessment of the epidemiologic literature, that there is inadequate/insufficient evidence to determine whether an association exists between exposure to fuels or combustion products and male breast cancer.

FEMALE GENITAL CANCERS (CERVICAL, ENDOMETRIAL, UTERINE, AND OVARIAN)

Cervical cancer (ICD-9 180) has a number of risk factors, the most important of which is human papillomavirus infection. Other important factors are smoking, immune deficiency, and poor nutrition. Oral contraceptives, multiple pregnancies, maternal diethylstilbestrol use, family history, and socioeconomic status may also contribute to risk (ACS 2004b).

Endometrial cancer (ICD-9 182), which occurs in the inner lining of the uterus, is the most common female reproductive system cancer. A major risk factor in endometrial cancer is exposure to estrogen, which may occur because of early menarche or late menopause (both can lead to longer span of menstruation), infertility, nulliparity, obesity, use of tamoxifen or estrogen-replacement therapy, and some ovarian diseases. Other risk factors are diabetes, diet, age, family history, breast or ovarian cancer, hereditary nonpolyposis colorectal cancer syndrome, and pelvic radiation therapy (ACS 2004c).

Ovarian cancer (ICD-9 183) leads to more deaths than any other cancer of the female reproductive system. Risk factors include age, reproductive history, fertility drugs, estrogen or hormone-replacement therapy, family history, and history of breast cancer. Mutations in the BRCA1 and BRCA2 genes may also increase risk of ovarian cancer (ACS 2004i).

In 2000, there were 32.0 new cases of cervical, uterine, and endometrial cancer per 100,000 women and 6.9 deaths per 100,000 in the US (Ries et al. 2004), and there were 16.3 new cases of ovarian cancer per 100,000 and 8.9 deaths per 100,000 in the US (Ries et al. 2004).

Fuels

Table 4.29 presents the most relevant findings reviewed by the committee in drawing its conclusion on the possibility of an association between exposure to fuels and cervical, endometrial, uterine, and ovarian cancers.

Cohort Studies

Exposure to fuels did not lead to increased risk of cervical cancer or of uterine cancer in either the Texaco or Imperial Oil cohort of petroleum workers (Divine et al. 1999b; Lewis et al. 2003). There was no notable increase in the risk of cancer of the ovary, fallopian tube, or broad ligaments among the women in the Imperial Oil cohort (SMR 1.74, 95% CI 0.70-3.58) (Lewis et al. 2003), but no information on ovarian cancer was available on female workers in the Texaco cohort (Divine et al. 1999b).

A Finnish study used a record-linkage approach to explore the relationship between occupational exposures and ovarian cancer (Vasama-Neuvonen et al. 1999). Gasoline exposure, derived with a JEM based on job titles, was found not to be associated with ovarian cancer.

Combustion Products

Table 4.30 presents the most relevant findings reviewed by the committee in drawing its conclusion on the possibility of an association between exposure to combustion products and cervical, endometrial, uterine, and ovarian cancers.

Case-Control Studies

A study explored the relationship between burning wood in the kitchen and the risk of cervical neoplasia in women in Honduras (Velema et al. 2002). Although the risk of grade III cervical intraepithelial neoplasia (CIN) showed a trend with increasing duration of exposure to wood smoke ($p = 0.022$), women with low or intermediate exposure (up to 25 years) had lower estimated risks than the reference group of women, who said they had never used wood in the kitchen.

Finnish women born in 1906-1945 and active according to the 1970 census were linked to the national cancer registry for 1971-1995. The Finnish JEM applied to the census job titles was used to define exposure to selected occupational agents. Even in the highest exposure categories, Weiderpass et al. (2001) did not find the risk of cervical cancer to be increased by exposure to exhaust from diesel engines (RR 1.7, 95% CI 0.4-6.8) or gasoline engines (RR 1.3, 95% CI 0.7-2.2) or by exposure to PAHs (RR 1.2, 95% CI 0.3-4.8). Weiderpass et al. (2001) found no increase in risk of endometrial cancer associated with any of those three agents. Vasama-Neuvonen et al. (1999) reported on the results of this record-linkage study for ovarian cancer. Risk was not found to be increased by overall exposure to gasoline-engine exhaust, diesel-engine exhaust, or PAHs; there were, however, suggestions of dose–response trends related to exposure to each type of engine exhaust.

Conclusion

Overall, the studies provide inadequate support for an association between exposure to fuels or combustion products and cervical, endometrial, uterine, or ovarian cancer (Divine et al. 1999b; Lewis et al. 2003; Vasama-Neuvonen et al. 1999; Velema et al. 2002; Weiderpass et al. 2001). The association between wood smoke and CIN observed in the study by Velema et al. should be explored further.

The committee concludes, from its assessment of the epidemiologic literature, that there is inadequate/insufficient evidence to determine whether an association exists between exposure to fuels or combustion products and cervical, endometrial, uterine, or ovarian cancer.

MALE GENITAL CANCERS (PROSTATIC OR TESTICULAR)

Factors that increase the risk of developing prostatic cancer (ICD-9 185) include increasing age, race, family history, diet, and physical inactivity (ACS 2004v). Testicular cancer (ICD-9 186) is an uncommon but highly treatable cancer. Known or suspected risk factors include cryptorchidism, family history, some occupational exposures, multiple atypical nevi, HIV infection, race and ethnicity, body size, and maternal hormone use during pregnancy (ACS 2004j).

In 2000, there were 176.9 new cases of prostatic cancer per 100,000 men and 30.6 deaths per 100,000 in the US (Ries et al. 2004), and there were 5.7 new cases of testicular cancer per 100,000 men and 0.2 death per 100,000 (Ries et al. 2004).

Fuels

Table 4.31 presents the most relevant findings reviewed by the committee in drawing its conclusion on the possibility of an association between exposure to fuels and prostatic cancer and the only results on testicular cancer.

Cohort Studies

In a cohort of uranium-processing workers, an industrial-hygiene survey was done to categorize exposure to kerosene (Ritz 1999). At the lowest kerosene exposure, there was no hint of an association with prostatic cancer mortality; while for the six cases with moderate kerosene exposure, the most extreme risk estimate occurred for more than 5 years of exposure and no lag (RR 3.69, 95% CI 0.91-15.0). No workers had the highest exposure to kerosene.

Risk of prostaticcancer was not increased in two cohorts of petroleum-company workers: the Canadian Imperial Oil cohort (Hanis et al. 1979) and the Texaco cohort (Divine et al. 1999b; Lewis et al. 2000b, 2003; Schnatter et al. 1993). Only Lewis et al. (2003) reported on testicular cancer, again with negative findings.

Case-Control Study

In a hospital-based case-control study conducted in Montreal, there was an association between diesel-fuel exposures, as assessed with a JEM based on occupational history, and prostatic cancer (OR 1.7, 90% CI 1.2-2.5) (Siemiatycki et al. 1987a). Modest increases were in association with kerosene, heating oil, and crude oil. No increased risk of prostatic cancer was observed after exposure to automotive gasoline, aviation gasoline, or jet fuel.

Combustion Products

Table 4.32 presents the most relevant findings reviewed by the committee in drawing its conclusion on the possibility of an association between exposure to combustion products and prostatic cancer.

Case-Control Studies

A case-control study in Germany assessed the relationship between occupational factors and prostatic cancer (Seidler et al. 1998). Two JEMs were used to estimate dose-years of exposure, the product of estimates of intensity, duration, and probability of exposure. One of the JEMs yielded estimates of exposure to exhaust fumes that resulted in an increased risk for more than 25 dose-years vs no exposure (OR 2.4, 95% CI 1.2-4.7) but a less pronounced risk for 25 dose-years or fewer (OR 1.2, 95% CI 0.8-1.9). A similar pattern was seen when the other matrix was used to estimate exposure to diesel fumes and fuel; for more than 25 dose-years, the risk was clearly increased (OR 3.7, 95% CI 1.4-9.8), but for 25 dose-years or fewer, the OR was only 1.1 (95% CI 0.7-1.8). For PAH exposure, results contrary to a dose–response relationship were seen: exposure for 25 dose-years or fewer led to an OR of 1.6 (95% CI 1.0-2.4), but for more than 25 dose-years, the OR was 1.4 (95% CI 0.4-4.7).

In another case-control study, the relationship between occupational risk factors and prostatic cancer was examined on the basis of job history obtained by interview (Krstev et al. 1998). An increased risk of prostatic cancer was reported in firefighters (OR 3.34, 95% CI 1.13-9.91) and railroad-transportation workers (OR 1.66, 95% CI 1.13-2.44). A dose–response trend was observed in the railroad-transportation workers; those working in railroad transportation for fewer than 5 years had an OR of 1.47, for 5-19 years an OR of 1.43, and for 20 years or more an OR of 6.47. No increased risk was associated with other transportation or trucking workers.

Aronson et al. (1996) conducted a population-based case-control study of occupational risk factors in a study that included 449 prostatic cancer cases and over 2,000 controls. A JEM was applied to occupational histories to categorize various exposures as “substantial” or “nonsubstantial” for comparison with nonexposed subjects. Nonsubstantial exposure to diesel-engine emissions or to PAHs from coal was associated with increased risks of prostatic cancer; substantial exposure to the agents was associated with less pronounced risks. Substantial exposure to combustion products of liquid fuel or to PAHs from any source was associated with higher estimated risks than nonsubstantial exposure, but still not markedly increased.

A population-based case-control study in Montreal evaluated exposure to combustion products and prostatic cancer. An industrial hygienist reviewed occupational histories to derive the intensity and probability of various exposures (Siemiatycki et al. 1988). The report presented 90% CIs. Increased risks of prostatic cancer were reported for exposure to combustion products of liquid fuel (OR 1.6, 90% CI 1.2-2.1) or of coal (OR 1.6, 90% CI 1.2-2.2) but not of propane, natural gas, or wood or to any of the types of exhaust considered.

Conclusion

There were not enough relevant data to draw any sort of conclusion about exposure to fuels or their combustion products and testicular cancer.

The evidence is inconsistent regarding an association between fuel exposure and prostatic cancer. Only one study (Siemiatycki et al. 1987a) of the several reviewed by the committee reported a positive association between a fuel-related exposure and prostatic cancer.

Although the studies by Siemiatycki et al. (1987a), Aronson et al. (1996), Seidler et al. (1998), and Krstev et al. (1998) reported several positive associations between occupations having potential for exposure to combustion products or PAHs or having more rigorously derived estimates of exposure to such agents and prostatic cancer, the committee noted that the results were not consistently positive.

The committee concludes, from its assessment of the epidemiologic literature, that there is inadequate/insufficient evidence to determine whether an association exists between exposure to fuels or combustion products and prostatic cancer.

NERVOUS SYSTEM CANCERS

This section summarizes what is known about the relationship between exposure to fuels and combustion products and cancers of the nervous system (ICD-9 191-192). Most nervous system tumors are not associated with known risk factors. The few known risk factors associated with those cancers are radiation, immune system disorders, and family history.

In 2000, there were 6.6 new cases of brain and other nervous system cancers per 100,000 people (8.0 among men and 5.4 among women) and 4.5 deaths per 100,000 (5.6 among men and 3.7 among women) in the United States (Ries et al. 2004).

Fuels

Table 4.33 presents the most relevant findings reviewed by the committee in drawing its conclusion on the possibility of an association between exposure to fuels and brain cancer.

Cohort Studies

A series of studies described mortality among refinery, petrochemical, and research workers employed by Texaco (Divine and Barron 1986; Divine et al. 1985, 1999a, 1999b) for at least 5 years, with at least 1 day falling after January 1, 1947. Two of the studies presented the results of followup through 1977 for about 19,077 workers in the three categories, of when only refinery workers were of primary interest to the present committee (Divine and Barron 1986; Divine et al. 1985). With followup through 1993, addition of employees at three refineries acquired after 1977, and the inclusion of workers hired after 1977 (all with at least 5 years of employment), Divine et al. (1999b) considered a total of 28,840 workers, 738,454 person-years, and 9,575 deaths. Mortality from brain tumors (benign or malignant) was somewhat increased among white men who were ever employed in the motor-oil unit (SMR 1.78, 95% CI 0.88-3.19) and more intensely among those who had been employed in that unit for at least 5 years (SMR 3.26, 95% CI 1.40-6.43).

A cohort mortality study of 1,583 workers employed in an oil refinery near Milan, Italy that converted crude oil into a variety of hydrocarbons (solvents, fuel, and lubricants) was conducted to evaluate cancer risk (Bertazzi et al. 1989). Followup on workers was originally from 1949 to 1982; Consonni et al. (1999) extended it to 1991, for a total of 39,857 person-years and 352 deaths. There was an increased mortality from brain cancers, but the number of cases observed was low (five) and the 95% CI included the null value (SMR 2.08, 95% CI 0.67-4.85). Furthermore, the cancer excess was confined to workers employed for less than 15 years and no cases were observed among longer-term workers. Similarly, the largest increase was among workers who died from brain cancer within 9 years of first employment and no cases were observed 20 years after initial employment. No information was provided on brain cancer by type of job. The authors also reported that internal comparisons (using Poisson regression) were noninformative.

A series of cohort studies of petroleum workers at Imperial Oil Limited in Canada was conducted to assess cancer risk (Lewis et al. 2000b, 2003; Schnatter et al. 1993). There wase no notable increase in deaths from nervous system tumors overall (benign or malignant) through 1994 among workers employed in 1964-1983. Minor increases in the estimated risks of malignant brain tumors were found in refinery, upstream (exploration, drilling, production or pipeline), and office workers, whereas the estimate of this risk was less than unity (SMR 0.68, 95% CI 0.31-1.29) among marketing and distribution workers, who would be expected to have greater exposures to petroleum products than workers in other operating segments (Lewis et al. 2000b). In a study of workers hired more recently (1964-1994) by Imperial, the estimated incidence of or mortality from brain malignancies or any other nervoius system tumors were not remarkably increased in either men or women (Lewis et al. 2003).

A nationwide survey of service stations in Italy defined a cohort of 2,665 managers alive at the beginning of 1981. Following their mortality through 1992, the study authors found 250 deaths among the 2,308 men and 20 among the 357 women (Lagorio et al. 1994). The SMR for nervous system cancer was 2.14 (90% CI 0.93-4.21) for all service-station mangers. For small stations, where sales per employee (a surrogate of exposure) were greater, the risk (based on five observed cases, one of them a woman) was more pronounced (SMR 2.66, 90% CI 1.05-5.59); the observation of a single case among men who attended large service stations just exceeded the expectation of 0.9. The authors note that the station employees were exposed to a combination of hydrocarbons from fuels and combustion products.

Case-Control Studies

A case-control study was conducted to evaluation the relationship between glioma and occupational title (De Roos et al. 2003). Four hundred and eighty-nine cases were identified at three US hospitals. Controls were selected from patients admitted to the same hospitals for nonmalignant conditions. Exposure was assessed by questionnaire which was reviewed by an industrial hygienist. No increased risk was observed for gasoline station attendants (ever worked: OR 0.5, 95% CI 0.3-0.9).

A population-based case-control study of glioma, the most common form of primary malignant brain tumor in adults, was conducted in the San Francisco Bay area (Carozza et al. 2000). The estimated risk of glioma in those ever employed as petroleum or gas workers was 4.9 (95% CI 0.6-42.2), but no increase in the risk of glioma was found in service-station workers. For both occupational categories, the estimated ORs and CIs were virtually identical with or without a 10-year latent period.

Combustion Products

Table 4.34 presents the most relevant findings reviewed by the committee in drawing its conclusion on the possibility of an association between exposure to combustion products and brain cancer.

Case-Control Studies

The study by De Roos et al. (2003) that evaluated the relationship between glioma and occupational title did not find increased risk for car and light truck drivers (ever worked: OR 0.9, 95% CI 0.5-1.7) and heavy truck drivers (ever worked: OR 0.7, 95% CI 0.4-1.1). Railroad workers had a slight increase in risk (ever worked: OR 1.1, 95% CI 0.4-3.3), but the CI included the null and there were only 6 cases.

The case-control study of glioma in the San Francisco Bay area discussed above (Carozza et al. 2000) had similar negative findings for mechanics and motor-vehicle operators whether or not provision was made for a 10-year latent period. For occupations that entailed exposure to combustion products that the committee considered relevant to Gulf War veterans, the most increased risk estimate was for motor-vehicle operators exposed for at least 10 years without the requirement of a latent period (OR 2.1, 95% CI 0.7-6.2). Firefighters had an OR of 2.7 (95% CI 0.3-26.1), but they were presumed to be largely urban.

Conclusion

Several studies reported sporadic associations between fuel exposure and brain cancer (Carozza et al. 2000; Consonni et al. 1999; Divine et al. 1999a; Lagorio et al. 1994; Lewis et al. 2003), but none could be considered a high-quality study supported by an adequate exposure assessment. Data on combustion products and brain cancer were too sparse to determine whether an association exists.

The committee concludes, from its assessment of the epidemiologic literature, that there is inadequate/insufficient evidence to determine whether an association exists between exposure to fuels or combustion products and nervous system cancers.

OCULAR MELANOMA

Ocular melanoma (ICD-9 190) is a rare type of eye cancer that usually develops in the choroids, although 10% occur within the iris. Risk factors include coloration (particularly blue eye color), such inherited conditions as dysplastic nevus syndrome and oculodermal melanocytosis (nevus of Ota), and possibly sun exposure (ACS 2004d).

In 2000, there were 0.7 new case of ocular melanoma per 100,000 people (0.9 among men and 0.6 among women) and 0.1 death per 100,000 (0.1 among men and 0.1 among women) in the United States (Ries et al. 2004).

Fuels

The committee did not identify any relevant studies that examined the relationship between exposure to fuels and ocular melanoma.

Combustion Products

Table 4.35 presents the most relevant findings reviewed by the committee in drawing its conclusion on the possibility of an association between exposure to combustion products and ocular melanoma.

Case-Control Studies

Three studies of ocular melanoma were reviewed by the committee (Ajani et al. 1992; Guenel et al. 2001; Monarrez-Espino et al. 2002) all assessed exposure by using self-reported job titles. Each of these modest-size studies reported that occupations or industries involving exposure to combustion products were associated with increased risks of ocular melanoma with imprecise confidence intervals. Ajani et al. (1992) reported an OR of 1.23 (95% CI 0.55-2.74) in transportation, communications, and other public-utilities workers. Guenel et al. (2001) reported an OR of 1.4 (95% CI 0.5-3.8) in male transport equipment operators. Monarrez-Espino et al. (2002) reported an OR of 1.5 (95% CI 0.66-3.23) in male transportation-equipment operators and an OR of 2.5 (95% CI 0.94-6.58) in female station, engine, heavy equipment operators, and freight handlers.

Conclusion

No studies were identified that evaluated exposure to fuels and an association between increased risk of ocular melanoma. Three studies, all lacking adequately specific exposure assessment, reported increased, but imprecise risks of ocular melanoma in occupations related to transportation (Ajani et al. 1992; Guenel et al. 2001; Monarrez-Espino et al. 2002).

The committee concludes, from its assessment of the epidemiologic literature, that there is inadequate/insufficient evidence to determine whether an association exists between exposure to combustion products and ocular melanoma.

BLADDER CANCER

The bladder is lined with transitional and squamous cells. More than 90% of bladder cancers (ICD-9 188) arise in transitional cells, and squamous-cell carcinomas represent only about 8% (NCI, 2002). Because cells that line the renal pelvis and ureter are histologically similar to bladder epithelial cells, tumors of the renal pelvis (ICD-9 189.1), ureters (ICD-9 189.2), and urethra (ICD-9 189.3) are considered urothelial-cell tumors, as are primary tumors of the bladder. Renal-cell carcinomas are histologically distinct from tumors that arise from urothelial tissues, such as those in the renal pelvis. This section, however, addresses only bladder cancer (ICD-9 188) unless it is otherwise stated.

The major risk factor for bladder cancer is smoking. Demographic factors that have some influence on the occurrence of bladder cancer are race (highest in whites, lowest in Asians), increasing age, sex (males at higher risk), and family history. Chronic bladder inflammation due to infections, bladder or kidney stones, or parasites has been associated with bladder cancer. Known occupational risk factors include use of the drug cyclophosphamide, and exposure to aromatic amines, arsenic, and organic chemicals associated with manufacture of rubber, leather, textiles, and paint (ACS 2004o).

In 2000, there were 21.3 new cases of bladder cancer per 100,000 people (37.8 among men and 9.4 among women) and 4.3 deaths per 100,000 (7.6 among men and 2.3 among women) in the United States (Ries et al. 2004).

Fuels

Table 4.36 presents the most relevant findings reviewed by the committee in drawing its conclusion on the possibility of an association between exposure to fuels and bladder cancer. In the text below, the studies are discussed in roughly chronologic order, whereas more recent studies (with publications on a given study population grouped) are generally presented first in the table.

Case-Control Studies

In the earliest case-control study of bladder cancer reviewed by the committee (Cole et al. 1972), an industrial-hygiene-derived group of occupations associated with petroleum products was among 13 occupational classes into which subjects were categorized. When smoking and age were controlled for, no excess risk was observed among men ever or usually working in this petroleum-product group. Some later case-control studies of bladder cancer considered employment in petroleum-related industries or occupations, as abstracted from work histories, among the possible exposures analyzed. Several found associations between petroleum-related entries in work histories and the occurrence of bladder cancer (Howe et al. 1980; Iscovich et al. 1987; Najem et al. 1982), and two found only imprecise indications of increased risks related to such industrial or occupational categories (Risch et al. 1988; Teschke et al. 1997). Using exposures to specific agents as recalled and reported by the subjects themselves, Mommsen and Aagard (1984) reported an increase associated with "work with oil or gasoline" (RR 2.71, 95% CI 1.18-6.17) but a less compelling increase associated with "work with kerosene or asphalt" (RR 3.12, 95% CI 0.88-11.00) (Mommsen et al. 1982). The committee did not regard the exposure assessments conducted in these case-control studies as sufficiently specific or reliable to be indicative themselves of an association between exposure to fuels and bladder cancer. The committee gave more weight to larger studies that included exposure analyses guided by expert understanding of the potential exposures involved in various industrial processes, as described below.

Participants in the National Cancer Institute (NCI) National Bladder Cancer Study (NBCS) were drawn from 10 centers and studied with a common protocol (Hartge et al. 1984). There were several reports from the individual centers—for example, Detroit (Silverman et al. 1983), New Jersey (Schoenberg et al. 1984), and Utah (Schumacher et al. 1989)—or from specific perspectives, such as mechanics (Smith et al. 1985), motor-vehicle exhaust-related occupations (Silverman et al. 1986), the chemical industry (Zahm et al. 1987), and racial differences (Schairer et al. 1988). The summary reports by (Silverman et al. 1989a, 1990, 1989b) on nonwhite men, white women, and white men are focused on analyses by industry and occupational titles with adjustment for smoking.

The analyses of the multicenter dataset with the most power were conducted on the large subsample of 2,100 white males who had bladder cancer and 3,874 white male population controls (Silverman et al. 1989b). For those ever employed in petroleum-processing, the increase in risk was marginally increased (RR 1.3, 95% CI 1.0-1.8); the largest risk was associated with the extraction of crude oil (RR 2.4, 95% CI 1.1-5.5). Three center-specific publications presented reanalyses involving about 62% of the white male subjects; the results were consistent with those above for petroleum-processing and a suggestion of increased risk among service-station workers, a category that had not been reported on in (Silverman et al. 1989b). In the publication on the 332 white men from the Utah study center (Schumacher et al. 1989), a slightly more increased risk of bladder cancer was reported for those who had worked at least 10 years in the "fuel industry", but the estimate for this small subset was imprecise. In the New Jersey subset of 658 white men, Schoenberg et al. (1984) found virtually the same risk as seen in the full NBCS sample for refinery workers (again imprecise in the smaller sample) and a strong association in garage or gas-station workers (OR 2.35, 95% CI 1.47-3.78). In analyzing the Detroit subset of 303 white men, Silverman et al. (1983) found a large refining-related risk based on only six exposed subjects who had bladder cancer (RR 6.0, 95% CI 0.7-49.8) and a more modest increase in those ever employed in gasoline service (RR 1.6, 95% CI 0.8-3.5), which was further reduced when adjusted for smoking (RR 1.3).

In the NBCS subsample of 126 bladder-cancer cases in nonwhite men and their 383 controls, the risk of bladder cancer among petroleum workers (RR 2.1, 95% CI 0.5-9.2) or service-station workers (RR 1.6, 95% CI 0.5-4.9) was somewhat higher (Silverman et al. 1989a). Although the subsample of white women was larger (652 cases and 1,266 controls), there were too few subjects employed in fuel-related jobs for analysis (Silverman et al. 1990). All the results from the NBCS are less compelling because the analyses were based only on industry or job title.

In a study of several types of cancer, Siemiatycki et al. (1987b) investigated the relationship between exposure to various fuels and 486 incident cases of bladder cancer in 29 Montreal hospitals and 2,196 other-cancer controls (excluding lung and kidney cancer). Exposure was categorized on the basis of industrial-hygiene review of occupational history. No increased risk of bladder cancer was attributable to exposure to aviation gasoline, jet fuel, diesel fuel, or heating oil; the risks posed by exposure to automotive gasoline, kerosene, and crude oil were only slightly above unity (Siemiatycki et al. 1987a). In a later analysis of this dataset focused specifically on bladder cancer (Siemiatycki et al. 1994), employment in the petroleum or coal-products industry was the sole exposure pertinent to fuels, and it showed no association with bladder cancer.

Using a record-linkage approach on the Swedish Cancer Environment Registry, Steineck et al. (1989) constructed a case-control study by identifying the 10,123 male bladder-cancer cases diagnosed in 1961-1979 that had also been listed in the 1960 national census. Controls were selected from that census. A JEM was applied to the job reported by each subject in that census with a note on the likelihood that the given job was predictive of exposure to a particular agent. There was no association of exposure with the risk of bladder cancer in men who had reported jobs deemed moderately or highly likely to involve exposure to gasoline.

Steineck et al. (1990a) gathered cases of cancer of the lower urinary tract (bladder, ureter, renal pelvis, and urethra) diagnosed in Stockholm County from 1985 to 1987 and population-based controls. Gasoline and various combustion products were among the occupational exposures assessed by an industrial hygienist on the basis of each participant's work history. The 254 male subjects who had urothelial cancer were compared with 287 age-matched controls (Steineck et al. 1990b). After adjustment for age and smoking, the estimated risk of cancer associated with having worked with gasoline was somewhat increased (RR 1.4, 95% CI 0.7-2.9); the effect on risk apparently was more concentrated in the group considered to have the highest exposure (RR 2.5, 95% CI 0.8-7.5).

Of 1,716 incident bladder-cancer cases in people 40-85 years old identified in the State Health Registry of Iowa in 1986-1989, 1,135 men and 317 women were interviewed (Zheng et al. 2002); next of kin completed the questionnaires for 156 cases. Interviews were completed with 2,434 controls frequency-matched by sex and age group. A detailed occupational history was obtained for each job held for 5 years or more. Analyses were adjusted for smoking status, age, and family history of bladder cancer. On the basis of only seven exposed cases, men who had worked in the petroleum and coal-products industry or the petroleum-refining industry did not have an increased risk of bladder cancer. The estimated risk in garage and service-station workers was a bit high (OR 1.7, 95% CI 0.9-3.1). It was not possible to include the women in the analysis because of a lack of occupational exposure.

The European Merged Bladder Cancer Study (EMBCS) was a large effort that pooled data gathered at 11 European centers according to similar protocols in 1976-1996. There was one center each in Denmark and Greece; two each in France, Italy, and Spain; and three in Germany. Nine centers generated individual publications that considered employment in petroleum-related fields: Denmark (Jensen et al. 1987), France (1) (Clavel et al. 1994; Cordier et al. 1993), France (2) (Hours et al. 1994), Germany (1) (Claude et al. 1988; Kunze et al. 1992), Germany (3) (Pesch et al. 2000b), Greece (Rebelakos et al. 1985), Italy (1) (Vineis and Magnani 1985), Italy (2) (Porru et al. 1996), and Spain (1) (Gonzalez et al. 1989). The overall EMBCS sample was made more uniform by limiting it to people 30-79 years old and to incident cases (only cases in those interviewed within 2 years of their diagnosis); this resulted in the exclusion of 755 male cases and 525 of their controls (Kogevinas et al. 2003) and 253 female cases and 357 of their controls (‘t Mannetje et al. 1999). To take advantage of the greater statistical power provided by the overall large sample, the committee decided to consider the findings in the pooled analyses on the 3,346 male cases and their 6,840 controls (Kogevinas et al. 2003) and on the 700 female cases and their 2,425 controls (‘t Mannetje et al. 1999). Occupations were recoded from the original work histories, and a JEM was applied to assess exposures to specific substances. On the basis of three exposed cases, the risk of bladder cancer was found not to be increased (when adjusted for age, smoking, and study center) in men ever employed as petroleum-refining workers (OR 0.52, 95% CI 0.10-2.69), the only fuel-related exposure presented; for the women, not even this occupational category was reported.

Reporting on fuel-related exposures was also quite sparse in publications concerning the individual study centers. In reporting on 658 male cases at the first French center (of whom 97 were excluded from the pooled study), Cordier et al. (1993) reported a heightened risk estimate (OR 4.04, 95% CI 0.78-21.03, based on seven exposed cases, p = 0.10) in men who had worked in the petroleum-refining industry. In the first German center’s sample of 531 male cases (of whom 168 were excluded from the pooled study), Claude et al. (1988) reported no association between bladder cancer and having ever been employed as a service-station attendant (OR 0.33, 95% CI 0.04-2.87, based on one exposed case) or as an oil refinery worker (OR 1.50, 95% CI 0.25-8.87, based on three exposed cases). In the same German sample, however, Kunze et al. (1992) found that exposure to petroleum in the workplace (self-reported by 26% of the sample) was associated with an increased crude risk (OR 1.4, 95% CI 1.1-1.9); when adjusted for smoking, the risk increased (p for trend = 0.01), although not monotonically, over duration of exposure. Despite its overall size, the pooled EMBCS sample analyzed by (Kogevinas et al. 2003) for men and by ‘t Mannetje et al. (1999) for women actually contains little information on fuel-related occupational exposures and bladder cancer.

Combustion Products

Table 4.37 presents the most relevant findings considered by the committee in drawing its conclusion on the possibility of an association between exposure to combustion products and bladder cancer.

Cohort Studies

Boffetta et al. (2001) used the Swedish Cancer Environment Registry developed by linking the Swedish Cancer Registry of all cancers diagnosed in 1971-1989 with records from the 1960 and 1970 Swedish censuses. According to industrial-hygiene criteria, each occupation and industry listed on the 1960 census was categorized for intensity and likelihood of exposure to diesel emissions. The rates of several cancers (including bladder cancer) in 1971-1989 in the diesel-exhaust cohort thus defined were compared with their incidences in the complementary non-diesel-exposed cohort. In both men and women, there was no indication of an association with bladder cancer.

The Netherlands Cohort Study was established to obtain detailed information on cancer risk factors, including occupational history, in a set of 58,279 men 55-69 years old in 1986 assembled from 204 municipal registries. Zeegers et al. (2001) conducted a nested case-control study of this cohort by linking with cancer registries to identify 532 cohort members diagnosed through 1992 with urothelial cancer (including cancers of the ureter, renal pelvis, and urethra along with bladder cancers). A randomly selected subset of 1,630 men from the cohort (after elimination of those who had cancer other than skin cancer in 1986) served as controls. Industrial hygienists reviewed the occupational histories and derived cumulative estimates of exposure to PAHs and diesel exhaust and exposure to paints and aromatic amines. In the highest tertiles for both PAH and diesel-exhaust exposure, there were small increased risks (RR 1.18, 95% CI 0.62-2.24; RR 1.17, 95% CI 0.74-1.84, respectively). There was no evidence of dose–response relationships for bladder-cancer risk over the tertiles of PAH and diesel-exhaust exposure.

Case-Control Studies

As for fuel-related exposure, a number of case-control studies investigated the possibility of an association between exposure to combustion products and bladder or urothelial-cell cancers. Studies that approached exposure assessment only by addressing industry or occupation reported some suggestive findings, but they are too nonspecific as to exposure agent to be relied on in drawing a conclusion about a possible association with bladder cancer. For the transport occupations and industries related to driving and the railroads, there were reports of increased risk (Hoar and Hoover 1985; Howe et al. 1980; Iscovich et al. 1987) and reports of possibly less stable estimates of increased risk (Brownson et al. 1987; Decoufle and Stanislawczyk 1977; Notani et al. 1993; Risch et al. 1988). This situation was similar for mechanics. Brownson et al. (1987) had a positive finding, and several other researchers reported less certain increased risks of bladder cancer in those working in this field (Decoufle and Stanislawczyk 1977; Teschke et al. 1997). The findings on even these "core" combustion product occupations were not consistent across all studies, and they were found among a clutter of results for diverse types of ill-defined employment that might involve some exposure to combustion products.

NCI's NBCS included 2,100 white men with bladder cancer at 10 US Surveillance, Epidemiology, and End Results centers whose exposure was categorized by industry and occupation (Silverman et al. 1989b). There were modest increases in risk among those who had ever been railroad workers (RR 1.3, 95% CI 0.9-2.0), mechanics (RR 1.2, 95% CI 1.0-1.4), or drivers (RR 1.2, 95% CI 1.1-1.4). In comparing the professional drivers among the white men with those who had never held an exhaust-related job, Silverman et al. (1986) found stronger results when the occupation was the subject's "usual" occupation rather than merely one that he had "ever" held; dose–response relationships by duration of employment were demonstrated in those who had ever worked as truck or taxi drivers. Among nonwhite men (Silverman et al. 1989a), neither mechanics nor drivers had an increased risk, but an increased risk was observed in automobile mechanics (RR 1.4, 95% CI 0.4-4.4) and taxicab drivers or chauffers (RR 1.3, 95% CI 0.5-3.2). For white women (Silverman et al. 1990), the only occupation with exposure to combustion products that had enough subjects for analysis was motor-vehicle driver, for which the estimated risk was not meaningfully increased (RR 1.1, 95% CI 0.4-3.0). The size of this multicenter study compensates in part for its being limited to an analysis of occupations.

In the Iowa case-control study of bladder cancer (Zheng et al. 2002), men who had ever worked in 10 years or more in the railroad-transportation industry showed an increased risk of bladder cancer (OR 1.7, 95% CI 1.0-3.1). The "general automotive repair shops" industry and the occupation of mechanic or repairer also showed associations with bladder cancer in men, especially for those employed for more than 10 years (OR 3.4, 95% CI 1.3-9.0; OR 1.4, 95% CI 1.0-1.8, respectively). The estimated risks observed in men who had worked in the transportation-services industry (OR 2.8, 95% CI 0.7-11.8) or held the job of driver (OR 1.3, 95% CI 0.9-1.8) were less certain. As for fuel exposure, there were no industries or occupations likely to have combustion-product exposure in which enough women had worked to merit analysis.

Considered from the perspective of individual industries or occupations, many classifications could involve exposure to combustion products, so a standard unifying approach for converting an entire work history into exposure (such as a JEM) would be extremely useful. Several studies reported equivocal increases in the risk of bladder cancer posed by exposure to diesel exhaust, either determined by self-reports (Howe et al. 1980; Risch et al. 1988) or derived from self-reports of "usual" occupation (Iyer et al. 1990). More-reliable risk estimates were generated in several studies, described below, that used more-comprehensive exposure-assessment methods informed by industrial hygienists' understanding of the likelihood of exposure to particular substances in various jobs at different times.

Bonassi et al. (1989) contrasted the work histories of 121 men in Italy's Bromida Valley who had been diagnosed with bladder cancer over a 10-year period with those of 342 age-matched community controls. Eleven occupations were categorized as having high risk on the basis of previous studies, and at least a year of work was required to be regarded as exposed. After adjustment for smoking, auto mechanic and truck driver had almost identical increased but imprecise risks. A JEM was used to partition the subjects into "definite", "possible", and unexposed classes for PAHs. After adjustment for smoking, the risk of bladder cancer was increased with possible PAH exposure (OR 1.63, 95% CI 0.95-2.83) and even more certain with definite PAH exposure (OR 2.20, 95% CI 1.12-4.38). Simultaneous adjustment for exposure to aromatic amines, however, slightly reduced the risk estimate for definite PAH exposure and diminished its precision (OR 2.14, 95% CI 0.82-5.60).

Steineck et al. (1990b) compared 254 Swedish men who had urothelial cancer (including an unspecified number of tumors of the renal epithelium) with 287 age-matched controls. An industrial hygienist estimated eight types of combustion product exposures on the basis of the subjects' work histories: diesel or petrol exhaust and soot or combustion gases from coal, oil, or wood. The results (adjusted for age and smoking) were most suggestive for exposure to diesel exhaust (RR 1.7, 95% CI 0.9-3.3). There were patterns of increasing risk with greater exposure to petrol and diesel exhausts individually, and the effect appeared to be concentrated in the seven people who had been exposed moderately or highly to both agents (RR 7.1, 95% CI 0.9-58.8).

In the Montreal multicancer case-control study Siemiatycki et al. (1988) found no association between exposure to products of combustion of gasoline, diesel, jet fuels, coke, or liquid fuel and bladder cancer, but an association was seen between products of combustion of natural gas bladder cancer (OR 1.6, $p < 0.05$). More-detailed analyses (Siemiatycki et al. 1994) yielded similar findings. For natural-gas combustion, all partitions of exposure scales (except duration) suggested a dose–response relationship, and the effect was most specifically associated with higher concentration. For the other industrial-hygiene-coded occupational exposures (to diesel exhaust, benzo[a]pyrene, or coal tar and pitch), no relationships with bladder cancer were found. The strongest association was for the motor-transport industry, but the effect was about the same whether employment had been for less than 10 years (OR 1.9, 95% CI 1.2-2.8) or for more than 10 years (OR 1.7, 95% CI 1.2-2.5).

The Swedish Cancer-Environment Registry (CER), which was used by Boffetta et al. (2001) as described above to define a diesel-exposure cohort, has also been the source for developing case-control studies. People employed in specific occupations as of the 1960 census (and later the 1970 census) have been linked with incident cancers reported in the national cancer registry for 1961-1979 (and later for 1971-1989). Steineck et al. (1989) applied a JEM to 10,000 men whose bladder cancer was newly diagnosed in 1961-1979 and who had been reported as employed in 1960 census. They also reported results of 714 cancers of the renal epithelial tissues (cancers of the renal pelvis) separately, which would be expected to be included in the set of 824 cancers of the renal pelvis that McLaughlin et al. (1987) reported on by occupation in an article on this version of the CER, which also presented separate analyses on a set of renal-cell carcinomas (RCCs).

The original work histories from the 11 studies pooled in the EMBCS were coded according to a Finnish JEM aimed at estimating occupational exposures to PAHs and diesel exhaust. In contrasting the 3,346 male cases with their 6,840 controls, Kogevinas et al. (2003) found that each of the tertiles for PAH exposure had ORs greater than 1, demonstrating a dose–response relationship, culminating in an estimate of 1.23 for the high-exposure category (95% CI 1.07-1.40). Those who had ever worked as motor-vehicle drivers or mechanics showed slightly increased risks (adjusted for age, smoking, and study center); a subgroup of automobile mechanics had a more definitively increased risk (OR 1.38, 95% CI 1.02-1.87). The findings from the considerably smaller set of 700 female bladder-cancer subjects and their 2,425 controls were more limited ('t Mannetje et al. 1999) because occupational exposures were minimal. Kogevinas et al. (2003) noted that higher risks were found in the earlier studies, perhaps implying an improvement in occupational exposure conditions in 1976-1996. The combination of those datasets into a unified analysis supports an association between exposure to the products combustion of petroleum-derived fuels and bladder cancer.

Some of the urothelial cases presented in Pesch et al. (2000b) were incorporated into the EMBCS (Kogevinas et al. 2003; 't Mannetje et al. 1999). However, nearly 30% of the 704 male cases and 50% of the 331 female cases had been excluded from the pooled analyses because they were prevalent cases or fell outside the age range. The publication was of particular interest to the committee because Pesch et al. used British, German, and their own task-defined JEMs to conduct detailed extractions of occupational exposure to combustion products. Again, there were not enough occupationally exposed women for the results to be precise. Only for "tar, pitch, and related products" among the men were all three JEMs applied; the British JEM appeared to be most liberal in attributing exposure (as was also the case for PAHs), and the task-based JEM most conservative. Nonetheless, the resulting risk estimates were similar in the two systems; the highest exposure category in each showed an effect to be likely (British JEM OR 1.6, 95% CI 1.1-2.3; task-based JEM OR 1.8, 95% CI 1.0-3.4). For PAHs, the British JEM, but not the task-based JEM, yielded increased risk estimates with a dose–response relationship, but for exhaust there was no clear indication of increased risk of bladder cancer. Where a contrast could be shown, the JEMs applied to subjects' work histories inferred more exposure than did the self-assessments.

Similarly, with 97 case-control pairs eliminated for not meeting the eligibility criteria for the pooled study, the dataset of Clavel et al. (1994) was one of the two French studies incorporated into the EMBCS (Kogevinas et al. 2003). An extensive analysis of PAH exposure was performed for all 658 pairs of male bladder-cancer cases and hospital controls assembled and interviewed in 1984-1987. With adjustment for age, hospital, residence, ethnicity, smoking, and coffee consumption, exposure to PAHs was associated overall with bladder cancer (OR 1.3, 95% CI 1.0-1.7). Dose–response relationships were evident over most classifications of PAH exposure. For cumulative PAH exposure, however, the lowest category (containing almost 50%

of the exposed cases) had an increased risk (OR 1.7, 95% CI 1.2-2.4), almost as large as that for the much smaller highest exposure group (OR 1.8, 95% CI 0.8-3.9), whereas the intermediate cumulative exposure groups had lower estimated risks.

Additional Studies on Cancers of the Renal Pelvis

Of the analyses discussed above, Steineck et al. (1990b), Pesch et al. (2000b), and Zeegers et al. (2001) merged cancers of the renal epithelium with bladder cancers, and the others addressed only bladder cancers. The two studies discussed below conducted separate analyses of sets of cancers of the renal epithelium.

In conjunction with the bladder-cancer cases in Denmark that were pooled into the EMBCS (Kogevinas et al. 2003; 't Mannetje et al. 1999), Jensen et al. (1988) gathered a set of 96 cancers of the renal pelvis or ureter (none of the urethra) and hospital controls. A broad grouping (chemical, petrochemical, or plastics industry or exposure to gasoline or petroleum), which was related at least in part to fuel exposures, showed a risk for men and women combined. For the 60 male cases, increased smoking-adjusted risks were obtained for occupational exposure to coke or coal (RR 4.0, 95% CI 1.2-13.6) or to asphalt or tar (RR 5.5, 95% CI 1.6-19.6). Similarly, during the process of assembling the set of RCCs in Australia that were incorporated into the International Renal-Cell Cancer Study (IRCCS), McCredie and Stewart (1993) gathered 58 male and 89 female cases of renal pelvic cancer. With the exception of the PAH-related exposure related to having ever been employed in blast-furnace or coke-oven work, the exposures of interest are fuel-related. The age- and sex-adjusted risk associated with having been exposed to gasoline was increased, and the risks in two more categories were also increased: having ever been employed in the petroleum-refining industry (RR 2.97, 95% CI 1.10-8.02) and having ever been occupationally exposed to "other petroleum products", which were said to include jet fuel, heating oil, kerosene, or diesel fuel (RR 2.16, 95% CI 1.44-4.08).

McLaughlin et al. (1987) and Steineck et al. (1989) reported on renal pelvic cancer cases diagnosed in 1961-1979 among men reported as employed in the 1960 census, as culled from the Swedish CER. The analysis of McLaughlin et al. (1987) was limited to industries and occupations listed in 1960 for 821 cases, whereas Steineck et al. (1989) performed a more rigorous exposure analysis by applying a JEM to this information for a set of about 100 fewer cases (probably because of the constraint that they were required to have been 20-64 years old in 1960). Some modest increases in risk were reported by both these record-linkage studies in association with exposures related to combustion products. Compared with the risk estimates associated with the same JEM-derived exposures on the much larger set of only bladder cancers (Steineck et al. 1989), only the estimates of an association with soot from oil, coal, or wood were somewhat higher (but still uncertain) for renal pelvic cancer; the risks of renal pelvic cancers posed by exposure to combustion gases from oil or coal were less than unity, whereas those of bladder cancer had suggested possible increases.

Conclusion

Although there was a suggestion of a relationship between fuel exposure and bladder cancer in some of the case-control studies that categorized exposure on the basis of expert review of job history, the relationship was not consistently increased in any study with detailed and specific exposure assessment. Associations were reported with work in petroleum-related industries and occupations in the NBCS (Silverman et al. 1989b), but these results were based on broad occupational and industrial categories, and the true exposure to fuels is unknown. The large EMBCS, which pooled data from 11 European study centers, overall yielded a negative finding for petroleum refining as an occupation (Kogevinas et al. 2003). The individual northern German center (Kunze et al. 1992) reported an association with petroleum as an occupational exposure, but 32% of the cases in the sample were excluded from the pooled EMBCS because they were prevalent cases or fell outside the permissible age range. The committee concludes that the available epidemiologic data on exposure to fuels, which may be difficult to segregate entirely from exposure to combustion products in some studies, and bladder cancer is insufficient to conclude that there is a relationship between fuels and the occurrence of bladder cancer.

The committee concludes, from its assessment of the epidemiologic literature, that there is inadequate/insufficient evidence to determine whether an association exists between fuels and bladder cancer.

Studies assessing the relationship between exposure to combustion products and bladder cancer have also not been consistently positive, and no studies assessed exposure on the basis of measurements. However, a pooled analysis of occupation and bladder cancer in western Europe (Kogevinas et al. 2003) included 3,346 men who had bladder cancer and 6,840 controls. With adjustment for smoking, questionably increased risks were noted in exhaust-related occupations. A JEM was applied to the occupational histories to derive measures of exposure to PAHs, benzopyrene, and diesel-engine exhaust. Exposure was evaluated as the product of the prevalence of exposure and the average magnitude of exposure in each occupation. The risk increased with higher exposures to PAHs (OR 1.23, 95% CI 1.07-1.4 in the highest tertile and benzopyrene (OR 1.27, 95% CI 1.04-1.54) in the highest tertile. A slightly increased risk was observed for diesel exhaust. In a related study by Pesch et al. (2000b), which included some of the cases pooled in the European study, similar findings were noted with some of the JEM-derived exposures to exhausts and PAHs. Clavel et al. (1994), in cases also included in the pooled European study, carried out a more detailed assessment of PAH exposures based on expert review of work-history information and found apparently stable associations with average and cumulative PAH exposures and total duration of PAH exposures. The results taken together constitute limited or suggestive evidence of an association between combustion products and bladder cancer, but the lack of exposure measurements and the heterogeneity of results precludes classifying this association as sufficient.

The committee concludes, from its assessment of the epidemiologic literature, that there is limited/suggestive evidence to determine whether an association exists between combustion products and bladder cancer.

KIDNEY CANCER

Over 90% of kidney cancers (ICD-9 189) in adults are renal-cell carcinomas (RCCs) or adenocarcinomas (ICD-9 189.0) (ACS 2004r). Most other malignant kidney tumors are transitional-cell carcinomas that arise in the renal pelvis (ICD-9 189.1), ureter (ICD-9 189.2), or urethra (ICD-9 189.3); these are jointly referred to as urothelial carcinomas or cancers of the renal pelvis. Because they resemble bladder tumors in their behavior and microscopically, the studies that assess risk factors for cancers of the renal pelvis separately were considered with bladder cancers in the previous section. In this section, if researchers specifically addressed only

RCCs, that is indicated; otherwise, cancers of the renal pelvis were included in a more global class of kidney cancers that would have been dominated by RCCs.

Smoking and obesity are the major risk factors for kidney cancer. Other risk factors are diet, increasing age, male sex, some hereditary conditions (such as Von Hippel-Lindau disease and hereditary papillary renal-cell carcinoma), and dialysis treatment for kidney disease. Such medications as phenacetin and diuretics (or the high blood pressure that they are used to treat) have also been associated with RCC, as has occupational exposure to asbestos, cadmium, and some organic solvents (ACS 2004r).

In 2000, there were 12.1 new cases of cancer of the renal pelvis and kidney per 100,000 (16.9 among men and 8.3 among women) and 4.2 deaths per 100,000 (6.2 among men and 2.8 among women) in the United States (Ries et al. 2004).

During the 1980s, it was noted that kidney tumors in male rats occurred after chronic gasoline exposure by inhalation. Considerable attention was directed toward monitoring human populations exposed to gasoline for similar tumors. Detailed toxicologic investigations later determined that the carcinogenicity in male rats was attributable to a protein peculiar to them, so gasoline would not be a human renal carcinogen, at least by the same mechanism.

Fuels

Table 4.38 presents the most relevant findings considered by the committee in drawing its conclusion on the possibility of an association between exposure to fuels and kidney cancer. In the text below, the studies are discussed in roughly chronologic order, whereas more recent studies (with publications on a given population grouped) are generally presented first in the table's sections by study design.

Cohort Studies

Wong et al. (1993) conducted a cohort mortality study in 18,135 US petroleum-distribution workers potentially exposed to gasoline. The assessment of exposure to hydrocarbons (HCs), both aromatic and aliphatic, was calibrated in parts per million for each job category in four periods (Smith et al. 1993). Several exposure variables (duration of exposure, time since first employment, job category, cumulative exposure, cumulative frequency of peak exposure, and year of first exposure) were analyzed separately for land-based and marine workers. The risk of kidney cancer was not increased overall (RR 0.73, 95% CI 0.47-1.09) nor did it show any sort of a dose–response relationship. A nested case-control study was conducted to investigate further whether this cancer might be associated with gasoline exposure in the land-based subpopulation of these distribution workers (Wong et al. 1999). The 12 cases of kidney cancer were each matched by age, sex, and company with up to five controls selected from the remainder of the cohort. Again, no relationship was found between kidney cancer and specific jobs ever held, duration of employment, duration of exposure, cumulative exposure, cumulative frequency of peak exposure, or year of first exposure.

A nested case-control study of whether kidney cancer is associated with exposure to HCs was conducted by identifying 100 cases of primary RCC in six petroleum-company cohorts at 36 refinery locations (Poole et al. 1993). The cases were identified by review of all 18,323 death certificates associated with the cohorts. For each case, four refinery-worker controls were selected who were alive and kidney-cancer-free at the time of the case's diagnosis and who matched by employer, refinery location, and decade of birth. A team of industrial hygienists assessed exposure by evaluating every job with respect to five classes of HCs associated with various refinery processes; they used three-point scales for intensity and for frequency (daily, weekly, and monthly) of exposure to each HC class. By apply the scales to the individual work-history records, they derived cumulative exposure scores for each HC class for every subject. RCC was not associated with having ever been exposed to any of the five specific petroleum-refinery HC classes or with cumulative exposure score or exposure duration.

Suggestive findings on kidney cancer in a cohort mortality study of workers at Exxon refineries in Louisiana, New Jersey, and Texas (Shallenberger et al. 1992) motivated conduct of a nested case-control study of kidney cancer diagnosed by 1990 among workers with at least 1 month of service in 1970-1982 (Gamble et al. 1996). A total or 37 confirmed RCCs or renal-cell adenocarcinomas occurred in 1970-1990; 32 of the patients had died by the time the study began. (Nine of the 32 cases, diagnosed at the Louisiana refinery in 1979-1992 and first reported by Hanis et al. (1982), were also included in the analysis of Poole et al. (1993) discussed above. Four controls per case were selected from among cohort members "at risk" (alive and cancer-free) on the date of the case's diagnosis and frequency-matched on sex, race, and dates of birth and hire. A JEM constructed with the assistance of plant industrial hygienists was used to assess the potential intensity and duration of exposure to various classes of petroleum products, defined in terms of chain length, saturation, and whether aromatic. The cases had slightly higher mean cumulative exposure scores for the various HC categories. Workers exposed at the highest level had a 4- to 5-fold increase in risk of developing kidney cancer, but all the 95% CIs included the null value (with the lower limits ranging from 0.65 to 0.88 and the upper limits from 20.8 to 32.9 for various HC groups), and none of the HC categories showed a consistent dose–response relatoinship over quartiles of cumulative exposure. When analyses were adjusted for other risk factors—such as smoking, blood pressure, and body-mass index (BMI)—the risk estimates for each HC class generally increased, but the confidence intervals also widened. The risk associated with long tenure (over 38 years) was substantially increased but imprecise; the authors asserted that the trend over tenure was "close to significance" but gave no statistics.

Lewis et al. (2000b) found that the 41 kidney-cancer deaths observed in 1964-1994 among men who work for Imperial Oil in Canada any time in 1964-1983 were associated overall with a neutral SMR of 0.96 (95% CI 0.69-1.30); a somewhat increased risk was observed among distribution workers (SMR 1.14, 95% CI 0.64-1.88). Similarly, the 15 incident cases of kidney cancer diagnosed in 1969-1994 in the younger cohort of men who were hired in all sectors of the company in 1964-1994 (Lewis et al. 2003) corresponded closely to the incidence expected on the basis of rates in the general Canadian population (SIR 1.00, 95% CI 0.56-1.65).

Case-Control Studies

A population-based case-control study included 495 white residents (313 men and 182 women) of the Minneapolis-St. Paul standard metropolitan statistical area diagnosed with RCC in 1974-1979 and 714 controls selected from the general population matched on age and sex. Only exposures experienced before 1973 were analyzed. For 251 cases, the questionnaire eliciting occupational history and other possible risk characteristics had to be administered to proxies, so the "self-reports" of 25 suspected occupational exposures might be unreliable. McLaughlin et al. (1984) reported that exposure to "petroleum, tar, or pitch products" was the only one of them that showed an apparent association with renal cancer when adjusted only for age and smoking; the association remained high (OR for men 1.6, 95% CI 0.9-2.7; OR for women 4.6, 95% CI 0.4-51) when adjusted for all other risk factors considered (demographic, medical, and dietary). In a later publication, McLaughlin et al. (1985) addressed petroleum-related occupational risks of the male subjects (313 cases and 428 controls) in greater detail. They controlled for potential confounding by age, smoking, BMI, drinking, country of ancestry, and phenacetin use. No trend in RCC was seen by years of employment in the petroleum occupations as a whole. In the subgroup of gasoline-station attendants, however, a modest trend with years of employment was observed.

In the Montreal multicancer case-control study, 181 men who had kidney cancer of any kind (ICD 189) were compared with the other 2,196 cancer cases remaining after the exclusion of lung and bladder cancers (Siemiatycki et al. 1987b). Siemiatycki et al. (1987a) addressed occupational exposures to petroleum-derived fuels, as coded from work histories. Adjusting for age, socioeconomic status, ethnicity, smoking, and blue- or white-collar job history led to imprecise estimates of increased risk posed by automotive gasoline, kerosene, diesel fuel, heating oil, and crude oil. Statistically significant screening results motivated more detailed logistic analysis of aviation gasoline (OR 3.1, 90% CI 1.5-6.5) and of jet fuel (OR 3.1, 90% CI 1.5-6.6); both showed increased risk, concentrated among six persons who had "substantial" exposure. The subset of 142 men who had RCC specifically was analyzed more intensely with respect to those two fuel exposures in comparison with population and cancer controls (Parent et al. 2000a). The adjusted ORs for RCC were 3.5 (95% CI 1.4-8.7) for jet fuel and 3.5 (95% CI 1.4-8.6) for aviation gasoline; and they were slightly higher for RCC than for kidney cancer in general.

Sharpe et al. (1989) conducted a case-control study of 164 male and female RCC cases diagnosed from January 1982 to June 1987 in nine hospitals in Montreal; they probably included many of the 181 male kidney-cancer (142 RCC) cases in the Montreal multicancer case-control study (Parent et al. 2000a, Siemiatycki et al. 1987a, Siemiatycki et al. 1988). In an effort to minimize recall bias, the control subjects were selected from patients who had hematuria but in whom urinary cancer had been ruled out. Having found no association between smoking history and RCC, the authors did not adjust other analyses for this factor. Self-reported occupational exposure to gasoline was associated with a slightly increased estimated risk of RCC (OR 1.09, 95% CI 0.55-2.15), and the risk estimate for kerosene exposure was higher but still imprecise (OR 2.04, 95% CI 0.69-6.28). Both findings are concordant with the results of Siemiatycki et al. (1987a) for those fuels.

Kadamani et al. (1989) gathered 210 RCC cases (142 male and 68 female) from 29 hospitals in Oklahoma City and Tulsa, Oklahoma that were newly diagnosed from July 1981 to August 1983. Controls matched by age and sex were recruited from the general population by random-digit dialing. Work histories were reviewed by two industrial hygienists who scored each job for its likely degree of HC exposure. From the job scores, a lifetime time-weighted average HC exposure index was derived for each subject; those who had any HC exposure were subdivided into low, moderate, and high groups. With adjustment only for weight, the women showed no increase in risk related to HC exposure (OR 0.7, 95% CI 0.3-1.4). An apparent increase in RCC (adjusted for weight and education) was found in the moderately exposed men (OR 2.7, 95% CI 1.2-6.5), but a clear increase was not observed among the highly exposed men (OR 1.6, 95% CI 0.7-3.6). Of the moderately exposed men, those under 60 years old were at the greatest risk for RCC (OR 3.0, $p < 0.05$).

Asal et al. (1988a, 1988b) drew from the same source population with an additional six hospitals and 1 more year of observation to study 315 RCC cases. The cases were matched to both hospital and population controls. An analysis by industry with adjustment for age, smoking, and weight found increases in the risk of RCC in both men (OR 4.3, 95% CI 1.7-10.9) and women (OR 1.6, 95% CI 0.4-6.5) who worked at least a year in petroleum refining and distribution (Asal et al. 1988a). In the full logistic model for RCC in males, the second-most predictive factor (after weight) was "petroleum work" (OR 6.6, 95% CI 2.3-19.2).

Partanen et al. (1991) interviewed 338 ever-employed people who had newly diagnosed RCC (the partition between males and females was not stated) in the Finnish Cancer Registry in 1977 and 1978. Each case had been matched by year of birth, sex, and survival status at the time of data-gathering to one or two responding controls drawn from the Population Register Centre, for a total of 484 controls. Job histories and other risk factors were obtained with mailed questionnaires completed by subjects or next of kin for deceased subjects. For both cases and controls, only about one-fourth of the subjects were alive. Industry and occupation were coded by international and Nordic standards, respectively, for each year from 1920 to 1968 (allowing a 10-year latent period). From that information, an industrial hygienist derived duration, magnitude, and cumulative amount of exposure to gasoline, diesel fuel (and other distilled fuel oils), PAHs, and six other agents. Exposed status was defined as at least 5 years of low-level exposure or at least 1 year of high-level exposure. There was good control for potential confounding by age, sex, obesity, smoking, and caffeine consumption. An increased OR for men and women combined was reported for gasoline (OR 1.72, 95% CI 1.03-2.87), but the increased estimate for "diesel fuels and other distilled fuel oils" was more uncertain (OR 1.20, 95% CI 0.63-2.27). ORs for men alone were slightly lower (1.63 and 1.15 for gasoline and diesel, respectively); 95% confidence limits included the null. The highest OR for men was for those exposed to gasoline without exposure to diesel (OR 2.05, 95% CI 1.05-3.98); the risk in men exposed to both categories of fuel was lower (OR 1.29), and the risk in men exposed only to diesel was not increased (OR 0.68). The authors concluded that they had found evidence of an association between exposure to gasoline and RCC.

Mandel et al. (1995) presented the overall results on occupational exposures and RCC from the IRCCS. This multicenter case-control study involved 1,732 RCC cases in men and women diagnosed in 1989-1991 in five countries. Controls were all population-based, but they were identified in different ways in the separate centers. The questionnaires used by the different study centers to determine exposures also varied somewhat in level of detail. The pooled analysis considered only occupations and exposures that were common to all centers, and it controlled for age, smoking, BMI, study center, and subjects' level of education. Mandel et al. (1995) reported comprehensive adjusted RRs among all the men in the IRCCS (1,050 cases and 1,429 controls) for several types of exposure to petroleum: oil-refinery workers (RR 1.3, 95% CI 0.6-2.4), gas-station attendants (RR 1.3, 95% CI 0.9-1.9), and those who had self-reported exposure to gasoline (RR 1.6, 95% CI 1.2-2.0) or to jet fuel, heating oil, kerosene, or diesel fuel (RR 1.6, 95% CI 1.3-2.1, and a positive dose–response relationship). The risk of RCC was not associated with number of years worked in occupations involving gasoline exposure, and the gasoline-related risks were substantially diminished by adjusting for the other petroleum products noted above, so the authors concluded that the study was negative for an association between gasoline and RCC.

Pesch et al. (2000a) identified RCC cases newly diagnosed in 1991-1995 in five regions of Germany. The sample consisted of 570 male cases and 365 female cases interviewed in the hospital (representing a response rate of 88%) and 2,650 male and 1,648 female controls (71% response rate) matched on sex, age, and region and interviewed at home. In addition to applying both the British and German JEMs, the researchers derived a third matrix for exposure estimation that incorporated information on tasks performed within jobs. For every subject, separate exposure indexes were derived for the exposure agents of interest on the basis of duration, probability, and intensity as characterized with each of the three JEMs. For analysis, the cases' indexes were partitioned into four groups at the 30th, 60th, and 90th percentiles of the exposed controls' distribution. For the occupational category "production and use of petroleum products", which was said to include "transport and use of mineral oils and fuel", the males were found to have slight increases in risk associated with the higher two categories of duration (OR 1.1, 95% CI 0.3-1.1; and OR 1.3, 95% CI 0.6-2.9, respectively).

Combustion Products

Table 4.39 presents the most relevant findings considered by the committee in drawing its conclusion on the possibility of an association between exposure to combustion products and kidney cancer.

Cohort Studies

As described in connection with bladder cancer, Boffetta et al. (2001) used the Swedish CER of all cancers diagnosed in 1971-1989 and records from the 1960 and 1970 Swedish censuses and applied industrial-hygiene criteria to occupations and industries listed on the 1960 census to define a cohort occupationally exposed to diesel emissions. The incidences of several cancers (including kidney cancer) in 1971-1989 in this cohort were compared with incidences in the complementary non-diesel-exposed cohort. In the small set (1,479) of women exposed to diesel exhaust, there was no indication of an association with the occurrence of kidney cancer. In the large sample (54,404) of men exposed to diesel exhaust, however, there was a slight but seemingly real increase in the risk of kidney cancer (SIR 1.06, 95% CI 1.02-1.11, adjusted only for age).

Case-Control Studies

McLaughlin et al. (1987) also used the Swedish CER to define a cohort of men employed in 1960. A search for them in the Swedish tumor registry in 1961-1979 revealed 7,405 RCC cases. There was an increased crude risk of RCC among men employed in the automobile-transportation industry in 1960 (OR 1.33, 95% CI 1.03-1.70, calculated by the committee from numbers in the article), but the overall ORs for industries and occupations with the potential for combustion-product exposure were not consistently increased.

Associations with several occupational exposures involving exhaust and combustion products were also investigated in the Montreal multicancer case-control dataset (Siemiatycki et al. 1988). No definitive associations were found between any of the agents and kidney cancer (in general). The most common exposure (to gasoline exhaust) yielded the strongest indication of increased risks (OR 1.2, 90% CI 0.9-1.4), but the pattern observed in connection with duration and intensity did not suggest a dose–response relationship. Jet-fuel exhaust showed the strongest association (OR 1.4, 90% CI 0.5-3.9). On the basis of the same four cases (which probably also constitute a subset of the people exposed to aviation gasoline and jet fuel), the reanalysis of the dataset for RCC specifically (Parent et al. 2000a) found a somewhat more intense risk for jet-fuel exhaust (OR 2.7, 95% CI 0.9-8.1). Parent et al. (2000a) reported that there was little to suggest an association between motor transport as an industry and RCC (OR 1.0, 95% CI 0.6-1.8) or between motor transport as an occupation and RCC (OR 1.1, 95% CI 0.7-1.8).

The study of 164 RCC cases in Montreal reported by Sharpe et al. (1989) appears to overlap with the Montreal multicancer study discussed above (Parent et al. 2000a; Siemiatycki et al. 1987a, 1988). There was a strong signal for exposure to PAH-laden tar or pitch (OR 9.29, 95% CI 1.16-74.20, $p < 0.02$). The risks posed by occupational exposure to burning coke (OR 2.0, 95% CI 0.49-8.14) or burning coal (OR 2.54, 95% CI 0.96-6.99) were somewhat increased. When integrated with domestic exposure, however, a fairly strong dose–response relationship ($p < 0.025$) was found for exposure to burning coal.

The Finnish population-based case-control study of RCCs of Partanen et al. (1991) reported mildly increased risks among men who worked for more than 5 years in the "transportation and storage" industry (OR 1.13, 95% CI 0.63-2.02) or in transportation occupations (OR 1.09, 95% CI 0.59-2.00) compared with those who never held such jobs in 1920-1968. A small increase in risk was observed among men who had been occupationally exposed to PAHs (OR 1.21, 95% CI 0.43-3.45). Those results provide some slight evidence of a combustion-product effect in association with RCC.

The finding in male gas-station attendants (RR 1.3, 95% CI 0.9-1.9) reported by Mandel et al. (1995) for the entire IRCCS, as discussed above in conjunction with fuels, could also be interpreted as evidence of a relationship between motor-vehicle exhaust and RCC. And the finding in men who had worked in the blast-furnace and coke-oven industry (RR 1.7, 95% CI 1.1-2.7) is evidence of a relationship between PAH exposure and RCC.

Mellemgaard et al. (1994) reported on occupational risk factors in the Danish subpopulation of the IRCCS, which comprised 368 RCC cases (226 men and 142 women) diagnosed in 1989-1992. Controls matched on sex and age in 5-year intervals were drawn from the Central Population Register. Exposures were determined with an interview conducted in a subject's home; occupation was encoded according to the International Standard Classification of Occupation and Industry (ISCOI) by the Standard Industrial Classification. The analysis controlled for age, BMI, and smoking history. In addition to occupational risks similar to those reported on by Mandel et al. (1995) for the entire IRCCS, Danish men who were truck drivers for at least a year (at least 10 years before being interviewed) had an increased risk of RCC (OR 3.1, 95% CI 1.3-7.7).

Schlehofer et al. (1995) reported on the occupational risks observed for the 185 male RCC cases and 192 controls selected from among the residents of Heidelberg, Germany, the site of another participating center in the IRCCS. In addition to the exposure reported on by Mandel et al. (1995), this group reported an apparent increase in the risk of RCC in men who worked in jobs with exposure to exhaust gas for at least 5 years (RR 1.82, 95% CI 1.03-3.22).

The population-based case-control study of RCC in five regions of Germany (Pesch et al. 2000a) used three JEMs (including one that went down to the level of tasks within jobs) to generate estimates of considerably more combustion-related exposures than the single result reported above in the section on exposures to fuels. The grouping "railway brakemen, signalmen, and shunters" was among the seven occupations that had positive results (OR 6.2, 95% CI 1.6-23.4), but, in contrast with the other six positive occupations, too few women had the jobs to permit a comparison that might be informative about the stability of the result. The findings for the occupation of motor-vehicle driver were essentially negative for both men and women. There was a suggestion of a dose–response relationship for exposure of both men and women to "tar, pitch, mineral oil" in the British JEM, but only for women at the highest exposure was the increased risk marginally stable (OR 2.1, 95% CI 1.0-4.5). For PAHs, the British JEM indicated somewhat increased risks of RCC in both men and women but task-JEM-generated risk estimates uniformly less than 1.0 in men (no results were presented for women). In several additional case-control studies, the risk of kidney cancer (or specifically RCC) was examined in relation to various exposures associated with combustion products without addressing in isolation any possible risks posed by fuels.

Several other case-control studies reviewed by the committee contained results of interest but were considered less reliable, largely because of the self-reported or less agent-specific nature of their exposure assessments. Exposures to a mélange of possibly PAH-containing substances were reported by two of these additional case-control studies.

McLaughlin et al. (1984) conducted a traditional case-control study of RCC cases gathered in the Minneapolis-St. Paul area of Minnesota. They reported increased age- and smoking-adjusted risks in both women (OR 4.6, 95% CI 0.4-125.3) and men (OR 1.7, 95% CI 1.0-2.9) who had self-reported exposure to the rather nonspecific agent "petroleum, tar, and pitch products". When adjusted for other potential confounding factors, the estimated risk in men exposed to the PAH-containing products was reduced (OR 1.6, 95% CI 0.9-2.7). The sample of working men was large enough to permit analysis by duration of exposure, which showed the increased risk to be concentrated among those who had 20 years or more of self-reported exposure (OR 2.6, 95% CI 1.2-5.7).

As part of Canada's National Enhanced Cancer Surveillance System (NECSS), Hu et al. (2002) obtained completed questionnaires from 1,279 people (691 men and 588 women) who had newly diagnosed RCC in 1994-1997 in eight provinces (excluding Quebec). A total of 5,380 cancer-free controls (2,704 men and 2,676 women) were assembled from the provinces, frequency matched on age and sex to the overall distribution in the NECSS database of 18 cancer types. The grouping "coal tar, soot, pitch, creosote, asphalt" was one of 17 occupational exposures about which the respondents were asked. Adjusted for age, province, education, BMI, tobacco and alcohol use, and meat consumption, an association between this collection of PAH-bearing agents and RCC was evident in men (OR 1.4, 95% CI 1.1-1.8); in women, an estimated increase of similar magnitude was not nearly as certain (OR 1.3, 95% CI 0.7-2.3).

Four of the additional studies reported risks of renal cancer in association with having worked as a vehicle driver.

The male RCC subjects in the Oklahoma case-control study were also contrasted with their population controls by longest-held occupation with adjustment for age, smoking, and weight. Having a longest-held occupation of "operative", a category noted to have a high prevalence of truck drivers, was found to be associated with the occurrence of RCC (OR 2.0, 95% CI 1.1-3.5) (Asal et al. 1988a).

Hospitals that report newly diagnosed cancers to the Missouri Cancer Registry follow a standardized protocol to gather information on smoking, alcohol use, and occupational history, but the details of the procedure were not reported. Brownson (1988) assembled the 205 white male RCC cases diagnosed from July 1984 to June 1986 and compared them with the 615 white men reported to have cancers not related to smoking (that is, excluding oral, pancreatic, laryngeal, lung, and bladder cancers). Analyses of usual occupation vs all other occupations—adjusted for age, smoking, and alcohol use—found increased risks in automobile mechanics (OR 1.8, 95% CI 0.4-2.0), machinists (OR 2.2, 95% CI 0.5-10.3), and drivers of heavy trucks (OR 3.1, 95% CI 1.1-8.5). The available data apparently were not detailed enough to permit investigation of a full spectrum of demographic and medical factors in conjunction with occupation or to pursue dose–response issues.

Auperin et al. (1994) matched 138 male RCC cases diagnosed in 10 French hospitals in 1987-1991 with 107 cancer controls and 128 noncancer controls, matching by sex, age, hospital, and interviewer. Complete occupational histories were blindly converted into ISCOI codes. After further adjustment for education, smoking, and the Quetelet index of height to weight before diagnosis, no increase in risk (OR 0.5, 95% CI 0.2-1.6) was found in men who had ever been transport-equipment operators, the only combustion-product-related occupation reported on, compared with the pooled cancer and noncancer hospital controls.

Delahunt et al. (1995) compared 710 men who had RCC entered with an active occupation code into the New Zealand Cancer Registry in 1978-1986 with 12,756 employed men who had non-urinary-tract cancers diagnosed during the same period. A crude increase in risk of RCC in firefighters (urban or forest application not specified) was intensified by adjusting for age and smoking status (RR 4.69, 95% CI 2.47-8.93). In transportation-equipment operators, however, there was no observed increase in risk (RR 0.91, 95% CI 0.63-1.32, unadjusted).

Conclusion

No key study that was positive for an association between exposure to fuels and kidney cancer was identified, but the uniformly negative results of the nested case-control study (Poole et al. 1993) of a comprehensive sample of RCC cases in the petroleum industry with excellent exposure assessment were compelling.

Although some studies of exposure to combustion products and kidney cancer suggested a possible association based on job title, the results were not consistently positive.

The committee concludes, from its assessment of the epidemiologic literature, that there is inadequate/insufficient evidence to determine whether an association exists between fuels or combustion products and kidney cancer.

NON-HODGKIN'S LYMPHOMA

Non-Hodgkin's lymphoma (NHL, ICD-9 200, 202) is a cancer originating in the B cells or, less frequently, the T cells of the lymphatic tissue (ACS 2004k). It encompasses the many types of lymphoma that remain after the exclusion of the B-cell lymphoma known as Hodgkin's disease (HD) and is characterized by Reed-Sternberg cells (ICD-9 201). Within the evolving classification systems for lymphohematopoietic cancers overall, there have been a series of systems just for NHL. In ICD-9 coding, those cancers are subdivided within ICD-9 200 and ICD-9 202. The nonconstancy in the terminology and coding for reporting diagnoses of or deaths from this family of diseases complicates epidemiologic research on their etiology. Many risk factors have been identified for NHL: genetic or acquired defects of the immune system; infection by HIV, related T-cell viruses, or Epstein-Barr virus or by some bacteria (such as *Heliobacter pylori*); aging; obesity, the only recognized "lifestyle" factor; radiation; chemotherapy drugs; and possibly some chemicals, with benzene, herbicides, and insecticides most often implicated.

In 2000, there were 19.0 new cases of non-Hodgkin's lymphoma per 100,000 (23.4 among men and 15.4 among women) and 8.2 deaths per 100,000 (10.3 among men and 6.7 among women) in the US (Ries et al., 2004).

Fuels

Table 4.40 presents the most relevant findings considered by the committee in drawing its conclusion on the possibility of an association between exposure to fuels and NHL, presented in reverse chronologic order within type of study design.

Cohort Studies

In conjunction with a detailed exposure assessment of service-station attendants in Italy, Lagorio et al. (1993, 1994) tracked the mortality experience through 1992 of 2,308 men who had been service-station managers in 1980. With only three cases of death due to NHL, the estimated increase in mortality risk was imprecise (SMR 1.73, 90% CI 0.47-4.48).

Jarvholm et al. (1997) investigated cancer morbidity and mortality in a cohort of 4,128 male Swedish petroleum-industry workers by screening the Swedish cancer registry and death certificates. Statistics broken down by site were not presented for cancer mortality, and the incidence information was grouped for all lymphomas (ICD-9 200-202). Exposures were determined from job titles and supported by limited air monitoring of work areas and personal-exposure monitoring, which used benzene concentration as an index rather than a more global measure of HC concentrations. With nine lymphomas observed, the risk was not increased overall (SIR 0.93, 90% CI 0.48-1.6), and there was no suggestion of an increase with duration and latency.

A large cohort of Canadian workers for Imperial Oil did not show an increase in overall mortality from NHL through 1994 among men or women who had worked there any time from 1964 to 1983 (Lewis et al. 2000b). A slight increase among men in the marketing and distribution sector (SMR 1.12, 95% CI 0.65-1.79) showed no relationship to cumulative exposure to total HCs in a nested case-control study (Schnatter et al. 1996). Similarly, among the younger, overlapping cohort of 17,230 men in the entire company who had been first hired in 1964-1994, the incidence of NHL in 1969-1994 was not increased on the basis of 20 incident cases (Lewis et al. 2003).

On the basis of a positive finding for lymphohaematopoietic malignancies in a cohort-mortality study, Lewis et al. (2000a) and Huebner et al. (2000) followed up the incidence of such cancers among 8,942 employees who worked at an Exxon Corporation facility (a combined refinery and chemical plant) in Baton Rouge, Louisiana, in 1970-1992. Work histories from company payroll records were reviewed to assign workers to the occupation and unit where each spent most of his working time. Information on potential confounding factors was not consistently available. Cancers newly diagnosed in 1983-1994 were ascertained from the Louisiana cancer registry. There were 22 cases of NHL in men (SIR 1.06, 95% CI 0.67-1.61) with an indication that any excess occurred among those first employed before 1950 (SIR 1.44, 95% CI 0.85-2.27).

Case-Control Studies

In the Montreal multicancer case-control study of 206 men who had NHL, Siemiatiycki et al. (1987a) found no relationship between exposure to any of seven petroleum-derived fuels and this form of cancer.

Franceschi et al. (1989) interviewed 208 patients who had histologically confirmed NHL and were treated at a hospital in northeast Italy from June 1985 to March 1988. Their self-reported exposures were compared with those of 401 hospital controls who had acute conditions.

Adjusted for age and sex, the estimated risk of NHL in "petrochemical workers" ("chemical workers" were reported on separately) was somewhat increased (RR 1.83, 95% CI 0.87-3.84).

Blair et al. (1993) assembled white, male NHL cases diagnosed in 1980-1983 from the Iowa State Health Registry and from a surveillance network of hospitals in Minnesota. They interviewed 622 of them (or next of kin of 13% who were deceased) and 820 population controls (or next of kin) who were free of lymphohematopoietic cancer and matched by state, age, and year of death. With adjustment for age, state, smoking, family history of lymphoproliferative diseases, exposure to agricultural pesticides, hair-dye use, and response by next of kin, the risk associated with having worked in the petroleum-refining industry for at least 1 year was questionable (SIR 1.6, 95% CI 0.5-5.8).

Combustion Products

Table 4.41 presents the most relevant findings considered by the committee in drawing its conclusion on the possibility of an association between exposure to combustion products and NHL, presented in reverse chronologic order within type of study design.

Cohort Study

Boffetta et al. (1988) tracked the vital status of participants in the ACS II prospective cohort 2 years after enrollment, when detailed information that included a detailed occupational history had been gathered. With adjustment for age, smoking, and other occupational exposure, lymphomas considered together (ICD-9 200-202) showed no increase in risk (RR 0.92) associated with self-reported exposure to diesel-engine exhaust in men 40-79 years old at the time of enrollment.

Case-Control Studies

An early occupational case-control study was constructed by reviewing medical records of patients in 1956-1965 at Roswell Park Memorial Institute (Decoufle and Stanislawczyk 1977; Viadana et al. 1976). When all lymphomas were considered together, locomotive engineer or fireman was the only exhaust-related occupation that showed an intensified (but still imprecise) risk when limited to those with at least 5 years of exposure (RR 2.13).

The Montreal multicancer case-control study's analysis of 206 men who had NHL showed only a modest increased risk posed by exposure to jet-fuel exhaust (OR 1.7, 95% CI 0.5-5.2) on the basis of four exposed cases (Siemiatycki et al. 1988).

The case-control study of NHL in Iowa and Minnesota (Blair et al. 1993) focused on agricultural exposure, but it also reported on some exposures related to combustion products derived by application of a JEM to each subject's work history. The risk estimates for NHL associated with exposure to gasoline or diesel exhaust, to asphalt or creosote, or to oils or greases showed little deviation from unity; for each of these, the risk was slightly greater for high-intensity exposure.

Using the NECSS, Mao et al. (2000) identified histologically confirmed cases of NHL diagnosed in eight Canadian provinces in 1994-1997. Completed mailed questionnaires were received from 764 male cases, 705 female cases, and 5,073 cancer-free population controls that were frequency-matched for age and sex. The analyses of the self-reported exposures were adjusted for age, province, and BMI. Both the men (OR 1.2, 95% CI 0.9-1.5) and the women (OR 1.3, 95% CI 0.7-2.3) had somewhat increased estimated risks of NHL in association with self-reported exposure to coal tar, soot, pitch, creosote, or asphalt. Exposure to mineral, cutting, or lubricating oils (which are often considered vehicles for PAH exposure) posed a marginally increased risk among the men (OR 1.3, 95% CI 1.0-1.5), but not among the women (OR 0.8, 95% CI 0.4-1.4).

In the study of 12 areas of Italy, the only exposure reported by Costantini et al. (2001) of possible relevance to a relationship of exposure to combustion products with NHL was having worked as a transport operator. The occurrence of NHL, also including chronic lymphocytic leukemia (CLL), in men was not related to having worked in this capacity (OR 0.9, 95% CI 0.7-1.3).

Several studies linking national censuses with tumor registries have given some suggestion of a relationship between the transport occupations reported in the census and NHL. In Sweden, the risk in male truck drivers was increased (SIR 1.4, $p < 0.05$) (Linet et al. 1993), but the risk in women employed in the transport industry was not increased (Linet et al. 1994). A similar study in Denmark (Skov and Lynge 1991) found less-certain increases in both men (RR 1.12, 95% CI 0.91-1.38) and women (RR 1.24, 95% CI 0.40-2.90) who were unskilled transport workers.

Conclusion

Although some risk estimates were greater than unity, the reasonably well-conducted studies on NHL had no firmly positive findings. In the petroleum-refining and -distribution cohort with the most thorough quantitative exposure assessment, a nested case-control study found no indication of a dose–response relationship (Schnatter et al. 1996). Similarly, in the case-control study with the most objective exposure assessment, there was no indication of an association with any of the fuels (Siemiatycki et al. 1987a) or their combustion products (Siemiatycki et al. 1988).

> **The committee concludes, from its assessment of the epidemiologic literature, that there is inadequate/insufficient evidence to determine whether an association exists between exposure to fuels or combustion products and NHL.**

HODGKIN'S DISEASE

Hodgkin's disease (HD, also called Hodgkin's lymphoma) (ICD-9 201) is a cancer that originates in the lymphatic tissue (ACS 2004k) . HD is a B-cell lymphoma characterized by microscopically identifiable Reed-Sternberg cells; all other cancers of the lymphatic tissues are called non-Hodgkin's lymphoma. The only known risk factors for HD are infectious mononucleosis (caused by the Epstein-Barr virus) and lowered immunity. HD has not been associated with family history, diet, or environmental exposure.

In 2000, there were 2.7 new cases of Hodgkin's disease per 100,000 people (3.3 among men and 2.3 among women) and 0.5 death per 100,000 (0.6 among men and 0.4 among women) in the United States (Ries et al. 2004).

Fuels

Table 4.42 presents the most relevant findings considered by the committee in drawing its conclusion on the possibility of an association between exposure to fuels and HD, in reverse chronologic order within type of study design.

Cohort Studies

As noted above in the section on NHL, in their investigation of cancer morbidity among Swedish petroleum industry workers, Jarvholm et al. (1997) found no association between exposure to fuels and the incidence of all types of lymphoma combined.

A cohort study of mortality in 1949-1982 was conducted to evaluate cancer risk among 1,583 workers employed in an oil refinery near Milan, Italy, that converted crude oil into a variety of HCs (solvents, fuel, and lubricants) (Bertazzi et al. 1989). A later study extended followup to 1991 (for a total of 39,857 person-years and 352 deaths) (Consonni et al. 1999). The observation of two deaths from HD in 1949-1991 resulted in an increased but imprecise estimate of risk (SMR 1.51, 95% CI 0.17-5.44).

On the basis of a finding of lymphohematopoietic malignancies in a cohort mortality study (Lewis et al. 2000a), Huebner et al. (2000) followed up the incidence of such cancers among 8,942 employees working at an Exxon Corporation facility (a combined refinery and chemical plant) in Baton Rouge, Louisiana, in 1970-1992. Work histories from company payroll records were reviewed to assign each worker to the occupation and unit where he spent most of his working time. Information on potential confounding factors was not consistently available. A search of the Louisiana cancer registry for newly diagnosed cancers in 1983-1994 found four cases of HD among the men in this cohort (SIR 1.54, 95% CI 0.42-3.95), without any clear relationship to job title or year first employed.

Mortality and morbidity associated with HD have been assessed among the petroleum workers of Imperial Oil Limited in Canada (Hanis et al. 1979; Lewis et al. 2000b; Schnatter et al. 1993). In considering mortality from 1964 to 1994, Lewis et al. (2000b) found no increase in the risk of HD for men or women (SMR 0.68, 95% CI 0.28-1.41; SMR 0.79, 95% CI 0.02-4.42; respectively). There was no association between working in any particular division of the industry and HD. Lewis et al. (2003) studied cancer incidence in a younger, overlapping cohort of 17,230 men who had been first hired into any sector of the company in 1964-1994; on the basis of 11 incident cases, the incidence of HD in 1969-1994 was not notably increased (SIR 1.05, 95% CI 0.52-1.88).

Case-Control Study

In the Canadian multicancer case-control study, Fritschi and Siemiatiycki (1996b) reported no fuel-related results related to the small set of 54 HD cases.

Combustion Products

Table 4.43 presents the most relevant findings considered by the committee in drawing its conclusion on the possibility of an association between exposure to combustion products and HD.

Cohort Study

As noted above in the section on NHL, the 2-year followup of the ACS prospective cohort yielded negative findings on an association between self-reported diesel exposure and all lymphomas; a nonspecified number of HD deaths were included in that category (Boffetta et al. 1988).

Case-Control Studies

Similarly, the negative results related to combustion-product-related occupations of the case-control study of patients at the Roswell Park Memorial Institute concerned all lymphomas analyzed together (Decoufle and Stanislawczyk 1977; Viadana et al. 1976).

With only 54 male HD cases, the only finding from the Canadian multicancer case-control study that was at all related to combustion products was an imprecise increased risk posed by exposure to cooking fumes (Fritschi and Siemiatycki 1996b).

In the study of 12 areas of Italy (Costantini et al. 2001), the only reported exposure of possible relevance to the influence of combustion products on HD was the occupation of transport operator. The finding in men was entirely negative (OR 0.8, 95% CI 0.4-1.7).

Conclusion

Overall, the studies described here are limited by their small numbers of cases and the nonspecificity of their exposure assessments. The studies of workers at the Exxon chemical and refinery plant in Baton Rouge (Huebner et al. 2000) and of Italian refinery workers (Consonni et al. 1999) reported similar 50% increases in the estimated risk of HD after exposure to petroleum-related products, but both were imprecise, and neither showed a clear relationship to a specific job or to duration of employment.

In the case of combustion products, there is virtually no information beyond what is shared with NHL in analyses of all lymphomas together.

The committee concludes, from its assessment of the epidemiologic literature, that there is inadequate/insufficient evidence to determine whether an association exists between exposure to fuels or combustion products and Hodgkin's disease.

MULTIPLE MYELOMA

Multiple myeloma (ICD-9 203) is a type of cancer formed by malignant plasma cells (ACS 2004l). The overgrowth of plasma cells can produce tumors in several sites, including the soft interior of the bone marrow. So far, few risk factors for multiple myeloma have been identified. Known risk factors include increased age, race, radiation exposure, family history, some plasma-cell diseases, and some occupational exposures.

In 2000, there were 5.5 new cases of multiple myeloma per 100,000 people (6.8 among men and 4.5 among women) and 3.8 deaths per 100,000 (4.7 among men and 3.3 among women) in the United States (Ries et al. 2004).

Fuels

Table 4.44 presents the most relevant findings considered by the committee in drawing its conclusion on the possibility of an association between exposure to fuels and multiple myeloma (in reverse chronologic order within type of study design).

Cohort Studies

A retrospective cohort study examined mortality through 1989 in 9,026 petroleum-product distribution workers who worked for at least 1 year in land-based terminals for four US companies in 1946-1985 (Wong et al. 1993). Using available industrial-hygiene data, Smith et al. (1993) derived a detailed JEM in terms of total HCs for the tasks performed by distribution workers throughout this period and used it to estimate cumulative lifetime and peak exposures for the people in the cohort. Cases of myeloma were not noted separately, but there was no relationship to total HC exposure for the 18 deaths from cancers of "other lymphatic tissues" (ICD-8 203-203, 208) among land-based distribution workers. The 11 multiple-myeloma deaths in the group were carried into a nested case-control study (Wong et al. 1999), in which they were matched with as many as five controls who were still alive at the time of the cases' deaths and did not die from myeloma, leukemia, or kidney cancer (the subjects of simultaneous nested investigations). The quantitative exposure information was used only to compare the mean values without measures of variance. The authors noted that the cases' averages were "similar or slightly lower" compared with those of the controls; that was the case for duration of employment, duration of exposure, and cumulative exposure, but the cases' mean peak exposure was 28% higher than the controls'. When specific jobs ever held were analyzed, the risk was highest in foremen and supervisors (OR 1.92, 95% CI 0.43-8.59).

On the basis of a positive finding for lymphohematopoietic malignancies in a cohort mortality study (Huebner et al. 2000; Lewis et al. 2000a) followed up the incidence of such cancers among 8,942 employees who worked at an Exxon Corporation facility (a combined refinery and chemical plant) in Baton Rouge in 1970-1992. Work histories from company payroll records were reviewed to assign each worker to the occupation and unit where he spent most of his working time. Information on potential confounding factors was not consistently available. Newly diagnosed cancers in 1983-1994 were ascertained from the Louisiana cancer registry. There were nine cases of multiple myeloma (SIR 1.39, 95% CI 0.64-2.64) without any obvious pattern related to length of work or job title. A formal case-control study was not done.

A series of epidemiologic studies (Hanis et al. 1979; Lewis et al. 2000b, 2003; Schnatter et al. 1992, 1993) have been conducted on workers for Imperial Oil in Canada. Schnatter et al. (1996) conducted a nested case-control study on seven deaths from multiple myeloma among male fuel-distribution workers in the Imperial Oil cohort with followup through 1983 (Schnatter et al. 1993). Four controls from the cohort were selected who were alive after a respective case's death and matched on decade of birth. A panel of industrial hygienists estimated quantitative HC and benzene exposures by considering loading and unloading technology at each location during various periods, types of materials handled, typical tasks performed by workers and job title, typical environmental conditions, and historical industrial-hygiene surveys at some of the sites. There was no association between exposure to HCs or benzene and multiple myeloma.

The most recent update on the Canadian Imperial Oil cohort checked vital status through 1994 (Lewis et al. 2000b). All-causes mortality was lower than that in the general population, and there was no association between working in refineries and multiple myeloma (SMR 0.70,

95% CI 0.30-1.37). In marketing and distribution workers, the SMR was 1.94 (95% CI 1.11-3.15), with a more pronounced risk in workers who had 25-34 years of employment (SMR 3.06, 95% CI 1.47-5.63). In the younger, overlapping cohort of 17,230 men in the entire company who had been first hired in 1964-1994, the incidence of multiple myeloma between 1969 and 1994 was not increased, on the basis of three incident cases (Lewis et al. 2003).

Case-Control Studies

Incident cases of multiple myeloma in 1977-1981were identified in NCI's Surveillance, Epidemiology, and End Results tumor registries in four geographic areas (Washington state, Utah, Atlanta, and Detroit) (Demers et al. 1993; Morris et al. 1986). Controls were selected with random-digit dialing or similar methods. Interviews were conducted to gather information on 698 cases and 1,683 controls; for 221 deceased or severely ill cases the interview was completed with a proxy, whereas proxies were needed for only 1% of the controls. Respondent-selected chemical exposures were grouped into exposure categories by a toxicologist. After adjustment for sex, age, race, and geographic area, the risk of multiple myeloma did not exceed unity in those exposed to aliphatic HCs (including gasoline, diesel, and kerosene exposures), whether or not proxy responses were excluded from the sample. Demers et al. (1993) revisited the dataset's work histories to determine risks associated with various occupations and industries. There was no association with multiple myeloma among those who had worked as gas-station attendants (OR 0.8, 95% CI 0.4-1.5). The only suggestion of a relationship with fuel exposure was seen in those said to have worked in the petroleum-refining and coal-product manufacturing industries (OR 1.2, 95% CI 0.4-3.1), but the increase vanished when the analysis was limited to self-respondents.

Linet et al. (1987) interviewed 100 cases of multiple myeloma diagnosed at seven Baltimore hospitals in 1975-1982. They were individually paired with hospital controls by sex, age, year of diagnosis, and hospital. Inquiries about occupational and environmental exposures were part of the telephone interviews conducted with each subject or next of kin. According to discordant-pair analysis with adjustment for whether the respondent was a subject or a proxy, exposure to petroleum was most strongly related with multiple myeloma (OR 3.7, 95% CI 1.3-10.3) of all the risk factors considered in the study (medical and pharmaceutical, as well as occupational). In a study this small, discordant-pair analysis is unwieldy for adjusting for confounders.

Men diagnosed with multiple myeloma (1,098 cases) in Denmark in 1970-1984 as listed in the Danish Cancer Registry were each matched to four controls (who were alive in the year of diagnosis) on the basis of sex and year of birth (Heineman et al. 1992). Work history since 1964 was obtained by linkage to the Danish Supplemental Pension Fund, and this information was abstracted by industrial hygienists to derive whether (and how long) each subject had been experienced to a variety of workplace exposures. Workers ever employed in the fuel, oil, or gas industry did not have an increased risk of multiple myeloma (OR 0.8, 95% CI 0.4-1.6). Among workers considered exposed to gasoline or oil products, the estimated ORs were consistently slightly increased. The same protocol generated data on 1,010 Danish women who had multiple myeloma and 4,040 population controls, but the analyses of interest were limited to the 363 cases and 1,517 controls who had been in the workforce at any time after 1964. Exposure to coal or oil products was the only exposure pertaining to fuels reported for the women, and there was no suggestion that it was related to multiple myeloma.

Combustion Products

Table 4.45 presents the findings considered most relevant by the committee in drawing its conclusion on the possibility of an association between exposure to combustion products and multiple myeloma, presented in reverse chronologic order within type of study design.

Nested Case-Control Studies

On the basis of self-reported exposure to diesel-engine exhaust, Boffetta et al. (1988) defined a cohort of men who were 40-79 years old at the time of enrollment in the ACS prospective cohort study. Persons who had an extant cancer diagnosis at the time of enrollment were not excluded. After 2 years of followup, comparison of multiple-myeloma mortality in the diesel-exhaust-exposed cohort with that in the complementary nonexposed cohort yielded a mildly increased estimated risk (RR 1.21). After 4 years of followup on the ACS cohort, Boffetta et al. (1989) conducted a more conventionally designed nested case-control study that considered only people who had been cancer-free at the time of enrollment. Exposure to combustion products was addressed in self-reports and the even less specific surrogate of main occupation. The risks posed by the three categories of combustion-product-related agents (coal tar, pitch, or asphalt; diesel exhaust; and gasoline exhaust) showed no consistent pattern. Fully adjusted risks of multiple myeloma were increased but imprecise in truck drivers (OR 2.8, 95% CI 0.5-16.1) but more emphatically increased in railroad workers (OR 7.1, 95% CI 1.2-43.6), although both estimates were based on only three exposed cases.

Wong et al. (1999) matched each of 11 multiple-myeloma deaths observed among 9,026 land-based petroleum-distribution workers with up to five controls on sex, year of birth, and company. None of the occupational groups (mechanics, drivers, and loaders) that might be expected to have job-related exposure to diesel exhaust had an increased rate of multiple myeloma. None of the available surrogates of dose (cumulative and peak HC exposures, duration of employment or of exposure, and year of first exposure) was found to be associated with multiple myeloma in logistic regressions.

Lee et al. (2003) contrasted the occupational exposure of 446 people who had primary incident multiple-myeloma cases in 1971-1999 in a cohort of 365,424 male Swedish construction workers with that of the remainder of the cohort. A JEM was developed on the basis of exposure monitoring conducted from 1971 to 1976 and used to determine each worker's exposure to several substances, including diesel exhaust and asphalt. There was no association between asphalt exposure and multiple myeloma. With adjustment for age, BMI, and the other occupational exposures, the risk associated with diesel exhaust exposure was slightly increased (OR 1.3, 95% CI 1.00-1.77), but a dose–response relationship was not apparent over the three exposure levels used.

Case-Control Studies

In the set of 698 multiple-myeloma cases gathered from the SEER system in 1977-1981, working as a vehicle mechanic, the occupation most closely associated with combustion-product exposure, showed no association with multiple myeloma, with or without the proxy cases included (Demers et al. 1993). Self-reported exposures to diesel, jet-fuel, or automobile exhaust; coal fumes; and smoke were grouped as "carbon monoxide" (Morris et al. 1986). After adjustment for age, sex, race, and study site, the adjusted OR for all cases was 1.8 (95% CI 1.0-3.2); the reliability of this finding was increased by the fact that the result was a bit stronger when proxy respondents were excluded from the analysis (OR 1.9, 95% CI 1.1-3.2). Williams et al. (1989) focused specifically on 69 "light-chain" multiple-myeloma cases in this case group, 46 of whom had completed the interview themselves. Adjusted for age, sex, race, residence, and educational attainment, the RR for all light-chain respondents was 2.9 (95% CI 1.0-8.4); for self-respondents, the relationship was considerably stronger (RR 6.1, 95% CI 2.0-18.2). When the light-chain multiple-myeloma cases were removed, the risk for all other multiple-myeloma cases became uncertain (OR 1.3, 95% CI 0.7-2.7) and led the authors to conclude that diesel exhaust was most strongly associated with the light-chain variety of multiple myeloma. However, there apparently has been no more research into this intriguing possibility.

Flodin et al. (1987) enrolled 131 cases (75 men and 56 women) of multiple myeloma identified at hospitals and clinics in six Swedish cities. They had been diagnosed in 1973-1983, but interviewing did not start until 1981, so short-term survivors were underrepresented; cross-checking with cancer registers suggested that the researchers had enlisted only about one-third of the cases occurring in the nominal study period. The 431 population-based controls, selected with no matching criteria beyond residence in the catchment areas, were the same people used in the authors' case-control study of CLL (Flodin et al. 1988). After adjustment for smoking and other potential confounders in a Mantel-Haenszel analysis, the risk of multiple myeloma in men exposed to engine exhaust remained fairly firmly established (OR 2.1, 95% CI 1.2-3.9) on the basis of 35 exposed cases.

Heineman et al. (1992) identified 1,098 men diagnosed with multiple myeloma in 1970-1984 in the Danish Cancer Registry and drew 4,169 age- and sex-matched population controls from the Danish Central Population Registry. Work histories since 1964 were accessed from the Danish Supplementary Pension Fund, and from them industrial hygienists determined possible or probable exposure to various agents and duration of exposure. Ever having worked in the transportation industry (OR 1.3, 95% CI 1.0-1.6) was associated with an increased risk of multiple myeloma, but there was little evidence of a dose–response relationship (p for trend = 0.24) when those who worked less than 5 years were compared with those who worked 5 years or more. No increased risk was associated with exposure to tar, asphalt, or soot. Exposure to engine exhaust was associated with a modest increase in estimated risk (OR for "possible" exposure 1.3, 95% CI 1.0-1.6; OR for "probable" exposure 1.2, 95% CI 0.9-1.6). Possible exposure to engine exhaust was the one exposure that retained borderline statistical significance when included in a logistic model simultaneously adjusted for exposure to gasoline, phthalates, and vinyl chloride. The exhaust findings are less convincing because "possible" exposure showed a stronger effect than "probable" exposure, and the results for duration also were contrary to dose–response expectations. A companion study of Danish women who had multiple myeloma analyzed 363 cases and 1,517 controls on whom work information was available from the files of the pension fund (Pottern et al. 1992). The increases in the risk of multiple myeloma associated with possible or probable exhaust exposure (OR 1.4, 95% CI 0.6-3.2; OR 1.6, 95% CI 0.4-5.5, respectively) were imprecise in this smaller sample.

In the study of 12 areas of Italy, the only exposure reported by Costantini et al. (2001) of possible relevance with respect to an association between exposure to combustion products and multiple myeloma was the occupation of transport operator. In men, the estimated risk was totally negative (OR 0.5, 95% CI 0.2-1.1).

Conclusion

No consistent relationship between exposure to fuels and multiple myeloma was detected in the studies described above; most studies reported no association. On the basis of small numbers of cases considered to have fuel exposure and the imprecision of the exposure assessments accompanying the case-control and cohort studies considered, there was a limited ability to detect an association between exposure to fuels and multiple myeloma.

Sizable studies of Swedish construction workers (Lee et al. 2003) and of Danish men (Heineman et al. 1992) both used industrial-hygiene methods to derive exposures from work histories, but their estimated risks of multiple myeloma after exposure to exhaust were just barely suggestive. Furthermore, the magnitude of the risks was fairly uniform, showing indications of a dose–response relationship with intensity, duration, or likelihood of exposure. The risk posed by carbon monoxide in the US SEER study (Morris et al. 1986), in which industrial hygienists grouped self-reports, was similarly marginal. Imprecise estimates of increased multiple-myeloma risk in association with exhaust exposure have been reported among Danish working women (Pottern et al. 1992) and in a study in which exposure was declared prospectively (Boffetta et al. 1989), whereas the most stable positive result, reported in a small study of Swedish men (Flodin et al. 1987), was based on self-reported exposure.

> **The committee concludes, from its assessment of the epidemiologic literature, that there is inadequate/insufficient evidence to determine whether an association exists between fuels or their combustion products and multiple myeloma.**

LEUKEMIAS

Leukemias [ICD-9 204-208] are malignant diseases that arise from precursor cells of white blood cells. As for the lymphomas, characterizing cases gathered retrospectively for epidemiologic studies and integrating the results of studies conducted over several decades is particularly challenging because a succession of diagnostic criteria, with corresponding groupings and nomenclature, have been used. Individual leukemias may have unique etiologic factors (for example, T-cell leukemia is caused by the virus HTLV-I), but the recognized risk factors for leukemias in general include exposure to radiation or certain chemicals (for instance, occupational exposure to benzene or chemotherapy with alkylating agents), some genetic conditions (such as some chromosomal abnormalities including, Down syndrome), and particular acquired blood diseases (for example, myelodysplastic syndromes may develop into acute myeloid leukemia) (NCI 2004).

Although all leukemias originate in the bone marrow, there are 4 main types, classified by the type and developmental stage of the cells involved. Leukemias can be either acute — in which the cells grow rapidly and are not able to mature — or chronic — in which the cells grow and accumulate slowly, and look mature. Classification also depends on which cell type is affected. Lymphocytic leukemias affect the lymphocytes, a type of white blood cell that makes up lymphoid tissue; myeloid leukemias affect granulocytes or monocytes, both of which are white blood cells that circulate and protect the body against infection (ACS 2004n). Acute lymphocytic leukemia (ALL) affects children more frequently than adults, while chronic lymphocytic leukemia (CLL) affects only adults, mostly over the age of 40 (ACS 2004e, 2004g). Acute myeloid leukemia (AML), also called acute non-lymphocytic leukemia (ANLL) is the most common leukemia and usually affects adults, particularly men, although it can occur in children (ACS 2004f). Chronic myeloid leukemia (CML) mostly affects adults and is rare in children (ACS 2004h). These 4 types of leukemias can be further divided into sub-types, based on progression of the cancer and cell sub-types.

In 2000, there were 11.9 new cases of leukemia per 100,000 people (15.2 among men and 9.4 among women) and 12.4 deaths per 100,000 (15.9 among men and 9.8 among women) in the US (Ries et al. 2004).

Fuels

The second Gulf War committee found sufficient evidence to conclude that benzene is associated with leukemia, AML in particular. Benzene is a component of all the petroleum-derived fuels under consideration by the current committee and of their exhaust. For example, gasoline contains 0.5-2.5% benzene, and kerosene and the related jet fuels contain 0.1-1% benzene (Ritchie et al. 2003). This committee, therefore, did not revisit the literature related to the possibility of an association between fuels and leukemia.

Combustion Products

Table 4.46 presents the most relevant findings considered by the committee in drawing its conclusion on the possibility of an association between exposure to combustion products and leukemia, in reverse chronologic order within type of study design.

Cohort Study

Boffetta et al. (1988) tracked the vital status of participants in the ACS II prospective cohort 2 years after enrollment, when information that included detailed occupational histories had been gathered. After adjustment for age, smoking, and other occupational exposures, all leukemias considered together (ICD-9 204-208) had an imprecisely estimated risk (RR 1.29) associated with self-reported exposure to diesel-engine exhaust among men who were 40-79 years old at the time of enrollment. The deaths analyzed include those of persons newly diagnosed during the followup period and any occurring among those already diagnosed with leukemia at the time of the cohort's inception; this introduces the possibility of recall bias into the exposure factor defining the cohort in this nominally prospective study.

Nested Case-Control Study

Wong et al. (1999) conducted a nested case-control study of leukemia in a cohort of US land-based petroleum-distribution workers. The entire group of 35 leukemias and the subgroup of 13 AMLs were analyzed for association with several relevant occupational subcategories (mechanics, drivers, and loaders). None of those occupational groups was associated with increased rates of leukemia or AML.

Case-Control Studies

The early case-control study of patients at the Roswell Park Memorial Institute yielded no clearly positive findings on all leukemias in association with occupations that had likely exposure to combustion products (Decoufle and Stanislawczyk 1977). The most increased risk estimates were in small sets of taxi drivers and mine workers (RR 2.08 and 2.16, respectively), but when analysis was limited to those with at least 5 years in these jobs the risks were below unity.

Flodin et al. (1988) conducted a case-control study of CLL (ICD-9 204.15) by identifying cases at hospitals and clinics in five Swedish cities. The resulting 71 male and 40 female cases were compared with 431 population-based controls that were selected on the basis of no matching criteria beyond residence in the catchment areas. Most of the cases were diagnosed in 1975-1984, but some were survivors who had been diagnosed as early as 1964. There was a detailed assessment of radiation exposure, but it and smoking were found to have no influence on the occurrence of CLL. After adjustment for age, sex, farm work, and exposure to horses, DDT, fresh wood, or solvents, the authors found an association between self-reported occupational exposure to engine exhaust and CLL (Mantel-Haenszel incidence rate ratio 2.2, 95% CI 1.2-4.2). The authors noted that benzene is present in exhaust, but they speculated that other leukemogenic agents were involved because the benzene concentratios would be very low. Methodologic weaknesses in sample assembly and in assessment of exposures of interest to this committee reduce the confidence that can be placed in the result.

Lindquist et al. (1991) interviewed 125 patients (76 men and 49 women) who had acute leukemia, classified according to the French-American-British (FAB) system. They were compared with 125 neighborhood controls matched for age and sex. The data were analyzed as exposure-discordant matched pairs, thus forcing accounting for other possible confounders to be indirect. Professional drivers had an increased risk of acute leukemia (OR 3.0, 95% CI 1.1-9.2). The same effect was apparent in a smaller number of recreational drivers and was diminished only modestly when drivers who had also worked as painters were excluded. There was evidence of a dose–response relationship in that the risk was higher in those who had a greater duration of exposure (OR 5.0, $p < 0.05$). The authors suggested that this finding might be attributable to the presence of benzene at about 5% in Swedish fuels.

The case-control study conducted by Costantini et al. (2001) interviewed 383 men and 269 women in 12 areas of Italy who were newly diagnosed with leukemia (ICD-9 204-208) in 1991-1993. The 1,779 controls were randomly selected from each of the regions and frequency-matched for sex and age. Work as a transport operator (as abstracted from the work history) was the only reported exposure possibly related to the influence of the combustion products on the occurrence of leukemia. Among men, the risk of that occupation was only modestly increased (OR 1.1, 95% CI 0.7-1.7). The sample was of substantial size, and the interview's coverage was considerable, but there was no attempt to use the available information to adjust occupational exposures for possible confounders.

Conclusion

The studies address leukemias overall and subtypes (AML and CLL), which represent substantial heterogeneity in health outcome in a fairly limited set of evidence. The apparent associations with exposure are related to separate types of leukemia, and the authors of the studies (Flodin et al. 1988; Lindquist et al. 1991) note that any increase in leukemia risk is difficult to attribute specifically to exhaust because of concurrent exposure to fuels and benzene. The exposure assessments in all the studies are based on information from sources of questionable reliability (personal interviews or medical records) or have a low degree of specificity for combustion products.

The committee concludes, from its assessment of the epidemiologic literature, that there is inadequate/insufficient evidence to determine whether an association exists between exposure to combustion products and leukemia.

MYELODYSPLASTIC SYNDROMES

Myelodysplastic syndromes (MDSs) are hematopoietic disorders of uncertain etiology in which the production of blood cells is compromised (ACS 2004a). Some of the syndromes are marked by high frequency of progression to AML. The FAB system of classification has recently been superseded by one from WHO. MDSs are fairly common sequelae of chemotherapy or radiation therapy, in which case they are regarded as secondary MDSs. Other risk factors thought to be related to the development of MDSs included aging, some genetic conditions, environmental or occupational exposure to radiation or chemicals (particularly benzene), and smoking.

Fuels

Table 4.47 presents the most relevant findings considered by the committee in drawing its conclusion on the possibility of an association between exposure to fuels and MDSs, in reverse chronologic order.

Case-Control Studies

In a pilot study, Farrow et al. (1989) interviewed 39 men and 24 women who had an MDS diagnosed in a hospital in Wales from October 1985 through September 1986. Age- and sex-matched controls were recruited from the outpatient clinics on the same day. The researchers used an approach modeled after that used by Siemiatycki's team in the Montreal multicancer case-control study (Gerin et al. 1985) to derive occupational exposures from the interview data. Preliminary adjusted analyses reported associations ($p < 0.01$) with exposure for at least 6 months to "petrol diesel liquids" or to "petrol diesel fumes" (combustion exhaust may have been intended, rather than volatized fuel).

The same group of researchers (West et al. 1995) used the same recruitment procedures and exposure-assessment technique to gather 400 case-control pairs from three areas of the UK, which probably included the 63 pairs described in Farrow et al. (1989). Of 635 newly diagnosed primary MDS cases identified, only 400 were interviewed and paired with noncancer-patient controls matched for age, sex, residence, hospital, and year of diagnosis. The low ascertainment, primarily due to failure to interview subjects before it was no longer possible, is potentially biasing if an etiologic factor influenced the progression of the disease. Analysis was based on discordant pairs, and this limited adjustment to the matching factors. Two of the five classes of "petroleum products" ("diesels and petrols" and "oils and greases") might be considered to fit within the exposures that the present committee is considering. The risk related to "oils and greases" was modestly increased (OR 1.29, 95% CI 0.88-1.89), and neither exposure showed any suggestion of a dose–response relationship with duration or intensity of exposure.

Another pilot study (Nisse et al. 1995) reported on the first 100 cases of MDS diagnosed at the University Hospital of Lille (from September 1991 through July 1993) and suggested associations both with "oils and greases" and with exhaust gases. Collection continued through

February 1996 for the full set of 204 newly diagnosed cases and 204 sex- and age-matched population controls (Nisse et al. 2001). Cases and controls were questioned by a trained interviewer to gather extensive demographic, medical, and occupational information. The resulting data were reviewed and distilled by a group of experts in occupational exposure to estimate lifetime cumulative exposure to various agents according to the approach of the Montreal multicancer case-control study (Gerin et al. 1985). The exposures were classified as exposed or nonexposed and regarded from the perspective of duration and frequency. The risk factors analyzed included gasoline, "oil", exhaust gases, and PAHs. Cases were more likely to have been occupationally exposed to oil (OR 4.2, 95% CI 2.0-9.9), but the risk posed by petrol exposure was less precise (OR 2.5, 95% CI 0.9-7.7). Beyond control provided by the matching variables in a Mantel-Haenzel test, there was apparently no adjustment for possible confounders despite their availability in the detailed database developed.

Several other case-control studies of MDSs (Goldberg et al. 1990; Ido et al. 1996; Nagata et al. 1999; Rigolin et al. 1998) contained no analyses specifically of fuels (or combustion products) but might be considered indirectly related to fuels by virtue of their focus on solvents, primarily benzene, and were reviewed by the second Gulf War committee (IOM 2003). With the exception of the results of Goldberg et al. (1990), the risks associated with solvent exposures (all based on self-reports) were increased.

Combustion Products

Table 4.48 presents the most relevant findings considered by the committee in drawing its conclusion on the possibility of an association between exposure to combustion products and MDSs, in reverse chronologic order.

Case-Control Studies

For their 400 case-control pairs, West et al. (1995) reported that exposure to coal tar (a PAH-containing substance) showed no association with the occurrence of MDSs. The risks posed by exposure to exhaust gases showed minor increases, and there was not a monotonic increase in risk with increasing duration of exposure. For the only occupational grouping possibly characterized by exposure to combustion products ("transport operating, material moving and storing and related"), there was no association with MDSs.

In their case-control study of French subjects, Nisse et al. (2001) found that MDS cases were as likely as controls to have been exposed to exhaust gases (OR 1.0, 95% CI 0.5-1.9), but their estimated risk related to exposure to PAHs was only modestly increased (OR 1.8, 95% CI 0.7–4.6). Machine operators, an occupational group potentially exposed to combustion products, manifested a risk of MDS (OR 2.8, 95% CI 1.3-6.4). Logistic regressions were said to have been performed on variables that were associated with MDSs in univariate comparisons, but the fully adjusted results were not presented systematically.

Conclusion

Nisse et al. (2001) obtained positive findings for exposure to petroleum-related substances. Given the benzene content of fuels, one might have expected a clear picture to emerge, but it did not in the work of West et al. (1995).

For combustion products, only the increased risk estimate for the not particularly substance-specific occupational category of machine operator appeared stable (Nisse et al. 2001).

Despite the apparent rigor of the data-collection methods used, the researchers' analyses were rudimentary, and failed even to adjust for possible confounders when the information was at hand.

The committee concludes, from its assessment of the epidemiologic literature, that there is inadequate/insufficient evidence to determine whether an association exists between fuels or combustion products and myelodysplastic syndromes.

SUMMARY OF CONCLUSIONS

The committee's conclusions about the strength of the evidence between fuels and combustion products and various types of cancers are summarized in Box 4.1.

BOX 4.1
Summary of Findings Regarding the Association Between Specific Cancers and Exposure to Fuels and Combustion Products

Sufficient Evidence of a Causal Relationship

No conclusions

Sufficient Evidence of an Association

Combustion products and lung cancer

Limited/Suggestive Evidence of an Association

Combustion products and:
- Cancers of the oral cavity and oropharynx
- Cancers of the nasal cavity and nasopharynx
- Laryngeal cancer
- Bladder cancer

Inadequate/Insufficient Evidence of an Association

Fuels and:
- Cancers of the oral cavity and oropharynx
- Cancers of the nasal cavity and nasopharynx
- Esophageal cancer
- Stomach cancer
- Colon cancer
- Rectal cancer
- Hepatic cancer
- Pancreatic cancer
- Laryngeal cancer
- Lung cancer
- Melanoma
- Non-melanoma skin cancer
- Female breast cancer

Male breast cancer
Female genital cancers (cervical, endometrial, uterine, and ovarian cancers)
Prostate cancer
Testicular cancer
Nervous system cancers
Kidney cancer
Bladder cancer
Hodgkin's disease
Non-Hodgkin's lymphoma
Multiple myeloma
Myelodysplastic syndromes

Combustion products and:
Esophageal cancer
Stomach cancer
Colon cancer
Rectal cancer
Hepatic cancer
Pancreatic cancer
Melanoma
Female breast cancer
Male breast cancer
Female genital cancers (cervical, endometrial, uterine, and ovarian cancers)
Prostate cancer
Testicular cancer
Nervous system cancers
Ocular melanoma
Kidney cancer
Non-Hodgkin's lymphoma
Hodgkin's disease
Multiple myeloma
Leukemia
Myelodysplastic syndromes

TABLES

TABLE 4.1 Cancers of the Oral Cavity and Oropharynx and Exposure to Fuels—Selected Epidemiologic Studies

Reference	Study Population	Exposed Cases	Estimated Relative Risk (95% CI)
Cohort Studies—Mortality			
Ritz 1999	Uranium-processing workers in Fernald, Ohio (ICD-8 140-149)	9	1.05 (0.48-1.99)
	Kerosene exposure (industrial-hygiene reconstruction)		
	Low exposure (>2 yr, 15-yr lag)	na	1.85 (0.37-9.36)
	Moderate exposure (>2 yr, 15-yr lag)	na	2.87 (0.43-19.2)
Lagorio et al. 1994	Filling-station attendants in Italy (exposure reconstruction using monitoring)	1	0.38 (0.02-1.79)[a]
Cohort Study—Incidence			
Jarvholm et al. 1997	Petroleum-industry workers in Sweden (ICD-9 140-149) (qualitative industrial-hygiene-interpretation of personnel records)		
	≥1-yr duration; ≥1-yr latency	6	1.2 (0.54-2.5)[a]
	≥1-yr duration; ≥20-yr latency	5	2.0 (0.79-4.2)[a]
	≥10-yr duration; ≥20-yr latency	5	2.2 (0.90-4.8)[a]
	Refinery operators		
	≥1-yr duration; ≥1-yr latency	1	0.58 (0.03-2.8)[a]
	≥1-yr duration; ≥20-yr latency	1	1.1 (0.06-5.3)[a]
	≥10 yr-duration; ≥20-yr latency	1	1.3 (0.06-5.9)[a]
	Distribution workers		
	≥1-yr duration; ≥1-yr latency	3	1.8 (0.48-4.6)[a]
	≥1-yr duration; ≥20-yr latency	2	2.3 (0.40-7.0)[a]
	≥10-yr duration; ≥20-yr latency	2	2.5 (0.44-7.9)[a]
Case-Control Studies			
Zheng et al. 1996	41 salivary gland cancer (ICD-9 142) cases among residents of Shanghai, China; self-reported agents (not smoking adjusted)		
	Occupational exposure to petroleum products	14	1.8 (0.8-3.8)
	Kerosene exposure from cooking	13	3.5 (1.6-7.4)
	With multivariate analysis	13	3.0 (1.4-6.8)
	Gas exposure from cooking	28	1.3 (0.6-2.6)
Huebner et al. 1992	762 cancers of oral cavity and pharynx (ICD-9 141, 143-146, 148, 149) among male residents of California, Georgia, and New Jersey; self-reported occupation (smoking adjusted)		
	Petroleum-industry workers	16	1.79 (0.75-4.25)
	Cancer of tongue	8	3.2 (1.15-8.9)
	Cancer of mouth	1	0.41 (0.05-3.46)
	Cancer of pharynx	7	2.31 (0.75-7.15)
	Service-station workers	48	0.85 (0.53-1.36)

NOTE: na=not available.
[a] 90% CIs reported in this paper.

TABLE 4.2 Cancers of the Oral Cavity and Oropharynx and Exposure to Combustion Products—Selected Epidemiologic Studies

Reference	Study Population	Exposed Cases	Estimated Relative Risk (95% CI)
Case-Control Studies—Adjusted for smoking, unless otherwise noted			
Gustavsson et al. 1998	545 cancer cases among male residents of two regions in Sweden; industrial-hygiene-derived agents		
	Oral cavity		
	PAHs (low)	25	0.99 (0.57-1.73)
	PAHs (high)	41	1.39 (0.86-2.25)
	Pharynx		
	PAHs (low)	28	1.06 (0.61-1.82)
	PAHs (high)	44	1.52 (0.94-2.45)
Pintos et al. 1998	784 pharyngeal-cancer cases among residents of three cities in southern Brazil; self-reports		
	Pharynx—use of wood stove	na	3.82 (1.96-7.42)
	Males		2.82 (1.63-4.86)
	Females		5.78 (0.52-64.3)
	Mouth—use of wood stove	na	2.73 (1.76-4.24)
	Males		2.52 (1.69-3.76)
	Females		2.77 (1.09-7.02)
Zheng et al. 1996	41 salivary gland cancer cases among residents of urban Shanghai, China; self-reported agents (not smoking adjusted)		
	Fuel used for cooking		
	Kerosene	13	3.5 (1.6-7.4)
	Coal	38	1.6 (0.5-5.6)
	Gas	28	1.3 (0.6-2.6)
	Wood or straw	6	1.6 (0.6-4.4)
Dietz et al. 1995	Incident cancer cases among residents of Heidelberg, Germany; self-reported agents		
	105 pharyngeal cancer cases		
	Air pollution on job (>20 yr)	21	0.94 (0.53-1.65)[a]
	Traffic jams on way to work (>20 yr)	20	0.85 (0.48-1.50)[a]
	High traffic emissions, residential (>20 yr)	23	0.74 (0.43-1.27)[a]
	Outdoor air pollution, residential (>20 yr)	8	0.48 (0.20-1.07)[a]
	Heating, fossil-fuel stoves (>40 yr)	33	2.60 (1.54-4.37)[a]
	Cooking, fossil-fuel stoves (>20 yr)	24	1.41 (0.81-2.44)[a]
	100 oral cavity cancer cases		
	Air pollution on the job (>20 yr)	22	1.09 (0.62-1.92)[a]
	Traffic jams on way to work (>20 yr)	21	1.03 (0.58-1.82)[a]
	High traffic emissions, residential (>20 yr)	34	1.41 (0.86-2.31)[a]
	Outdoor air pollution, residential (>20 yr)	14	0.67 (0.35-1.29)[a]
	Heating, fossil-fuel stoves (>40 yr)	33	1.60 (0.97-2.65)[a]
	Cooking, fossil-fuel stoves (>20 yr)	34	2.09 (1.26-3.48)[a]

Reference	Study Population	Exposed Cases	Estimated Relative Risk (95% CI)
Huebner et al. 1992	1,114 oral- and pharyngeal-cancer cases among residents of five US locations; self-reported job titles		
	762 men		
	Boiler or furnace operators	20	1.50 (0.68-3.34)
	Heavy-equipment operators	55	1.25 (0.78-2.01)
	Motor-vehicle operators	157	1.01 (0.75-1.35)
	Railroad-transport workers	8	1.00 (0.30-3.35)
	Cooks or other food service workers	83	1.00 (0.67-1.47)
	Mechanics or repairers	207	0.86 (0.66-1.12)
	Transportation worker (industry)	86	1.07 (0.74-1.56)
	Trucking or warehousing workers (industry)	62	0.86 (0.56-1.31)
	352 women		
	Motor-vehicle workers	7	2.80 (0.61-12.9)
	Cooks or other food service workers	44	1.34 (0.78-2.28)
Zheng et al. 1992	204 oral- and pharyngeal-cancer cases among residents of urban Shanghai, China; self-reports (not smoking adjusted)		
	Men		
	Petroleum products, occupational exposure	53	1.76 (1.10-2.82)[a]
	Use of kerosene stove	31	2.24 (1.27-3.97)[a]
	Women		
	Petroleum products, occupational exposure	15	1.63 (0.72-3.72)[a]
	Use of kerosene stove	13	1.01 (0.45-2.26)[a]
Merletti et al. 1991	86 oropharyngeal-cancer cases among residents of Turin, Italy		
	Transportation and communication (occupation)	8	0.7 (0.9-1.5)
	PAHs (JEM-derived agent)		
	Any exposure	56	1.0
	Probable or definite exposure	20	0.6
Decoufle and Stanislawczyk 1977	Buccal-cavity and pharyngeal cancer cases among male patients at Roswell Park Memorial Institute in Buffalo, New York (job history, including durations, from medical charts)		
	Occupations (ever)		
	Deliverymen and routemen	na	1.16, ns
	Machinists	na	1.36, ns
	Mechanics and repairmen	na	0.98
	Bus, taxicab, and truck drivers	na	1.37, ns
	Locomotive engineers and firemen	na	1.64, ns
Viadana et al. 1976	Bus, taxicab, and truck drivers (not smoking adjusted)	89	1.44 , ns
	Exposed 5+ yr	68	1.33, ns
	Locomotive engineers and firemen	18	1.64, ns
	Exposed 5+ yr	17	1.97, ns

NOTE: na=not available; ns=not statistically significant ($p < 0.5$) for a risk estimate above unity.
[a] Unadjusted ORs and 95% CI calculated with standard methods from observed numbers presented in original paper.

TABLE 4.3 Cancers of the Nasal Cavity and Nasopharynx and Exposure to Fuels—Selected Epidemiologic Studies

Reference	Study Population	Exposed Cases	Estimated Relative Risk (95% CI)
Case-Control Studies			
Armstrong et al. 2000	282 nasopharyngeal-cancer cases among Chinese residents of Selangor and Federal Territory, Malaysia; self-reported exposures (smoking adjusted)		
	Motor fuel and oil	83	1.33 (0.81-2.20)
Teschke et al. 1997	48 sinonasal-cancer cases among residents of British Columbia, Canada; self-reported exposures (smoking adjusted)		
	Service-station attendants and managers	4	0.8 (0.2-2.8)
	20-yr latency	4	1.0 (0.2-3.7)

TABLE 4.4 Cancers of the Nasal Cavity and Nasopharynx and Exposure to Combustion Products—Selected Epidemiologic Studies

Reference	Study Population	Exposed Cases	Estimated Relative Risk
Case-Control Studies			
Leclerc et al. 1997	930 sinonasal-cancer cases pooled from 12 studies in seven countries; job titles (not smoking-adjusted)		
	Motor-vehicle driver, males	41	1.13 (0.78-1.63)
	<10 yr		1.15
	≥10 yr		1.22
Armstrong et al. 2000	282 nasopharyngeal-cancer cases among Chinese residents of Selangor and Federal Territory, Malaysia; self-reported agents (smoking-adjusted)		
	Cooking fumes	19	0.93 (0.38-2.27)
	10-fold exposure increase		0.97 (0.78-1.21)
	Engine exhaust fumes	59	1.05 (0.61-1.79)
	10-fold exposure increase		1.00 (0.88-1.14)
	Wood fumes	27	1.65 (0.69-3.92)
	10fold exposure increase		1.08 (0.84-1.38)
	Other fumes	29	1.46 (0.66-3.23)
	10-fold exposure increase		1.12 (0.91-1.39)
Zheng et al. 1994	88 nasopharyngeal-cancer cases among residents of Zangwu County, China; self-reported agents (not smoking-adjusted)		
	Use of wood fuel (adjusted)	80	5.4 (1.5-19.8)
	Use of wood fuel (crude, matched)	80	3.7 ($p = 0.02$)
	With windows in home	73	3.6 ($p = 0.03$)
	Without windows in home	7	7.8 ($p = 0.009$)
	With good ventilation in home	24	3.1 ($p = 0.07$)
	With poor ventilation in home	56	4.7 ($p = 0.01$)
	With kitchen in home	66	3.4 ($p = 0.04$)
	With kitchen outside in shack	14	5.9 ($p = 0.01$)
	With windows in kitchen	59	3.4 ($p = 0.08$)
	Without windows in home	7	5.4 ($p = 0.06$)

Reference	Study Population	Exposed Cases	Estimated Relative Risk
Yu et al. 1990	306 nasopharyngeal cancer cases among residents of Guangzhou City, China; self-reported agents (not smoking-adjusted)		
	Combustion products (univariate)	63	2.4 (1.4-4.2)
	1-9 yr	32	1.6 (0.9-2.9)
	10+ yr	31	7.1 (2.5-20.6)
	Combustion products (multivariate)		
	1-9 yr	32	1.8 (0.9-3.6)
	10+ yr	31	9.0 (2.8-28.8)

TABLE 4.5 Esophageal Cancer and Exposure to Fuels—Selected Epidemiologic Studies

Reference	Study Population	Exposed Cases	Estimated Relative Risk (95% CI)
Cohort Studies—Mortality			
Lewis et al. 2000b	Refinery workers in Toronto, Canada		
	Males	42	0.96 (0.69-1.29)
	Refinery segment	20	1.10 (0.67-1.70)
	Marketing or distribution segment	14	1.04 (0.57-1.74)
	Females	3	1.54 (0.32-4.50)[a]
Ritz 1999	Uranium-processing workers in Fernald, Ohio—esophageal and stomach cancers (analyzed together)		
	Kerosene, light exposure		
	>2-yr duration, no lag	10	1.98 (0.77-5.09)
	>2-yr duration, 15-yr lag	9	3.46 (1.22-9.80)
	>5-yr duration, no lag	5	0.96 (0.32-2.94)
	>5-yr duration, 15-yr lag	3	1.26 (0.31-5.15)
	Kerosene, moderate exposure		
	>2-yr duration, no lag	5	3.00 (0.81-11.2)
	>2-yr duration, 15-yr lag	5	7.71 (2.04-29.1)
	>5-yr duration, no lag	4	2.86 (0.60-13.6)
	>5-yr duration, 15-yr lag	4	10.7 (2.26-50.7)
Lagorio et al. 1994	Filling-station attendants in Italy (exposure reconstruction using monitoring)	4	2.34 (0.80-5.35)[b]
	Men	4	2.41 (0.82-5.51)[b]
	At smaller stations	4	3.51 (1.20-8.03)[b]
	Women	0	0.0 (0.0-36.9)[a]

[a] Risk estimates and 95% CIs calculated with standard methods from observed and expected numbers presented in original paper.
[b] 90% CIs presented.

TABLE 4.6 Esophageal Cancer and Exposure to Combustion Products—Selected Epidemiologic Studies

Reference	Study Population	Exposed Cases	Estimated Relative Risk (95% CI)
Cohort Study—Mortality			
Gustavsson et al. 1990	Male bus-garage workers in Stockholm, Sweden		
	Stockholm referent	4	1.93 (0.53-4.94)
	Sweden referent	4	3.27 (0.89-8.37)
Cohort Study—Incidence			
Chow et al. 1995	Esophageal-cancer cases among male residents of Sweden		
	Transport Industry	143	1.0 (0.84-1.18)[a]
	Locomotive/traffic workers	118	1.1 (0.91-1.32)[a]
	Machine, engine maintenance	46	1.0 (0.74-1.34)[a]
Case-Control Studies			
Parent et al. 2000b	99 esophageal-cancer cases among male residents of Montreal, Canada; industrial-hygiene-derived agents (smoking-adjusted)		
	Nitrogen oxides (any)	21	0.9 (0.6-1.6)
	Gasoline-engine emissions (any)	41	0.9 (0.6-1.5)
	Carbon monoxide (any)	45	0.7 (0.4-1.1)
	PAHs from any source (any)	64	0.9 (0.5-1.5)
	Benzo[a]pyrene (any)	24	1.1 (0.7-1.9)
	Benzo[a]pyrene (nonsubstantial)	19	1.0 (0.5-1.7)
	Benzo[a]pyrene (substantial)	5	2.3 (0.8-6.5)
	PAHs from coal (any)	10	1.2 (0.6-2.5)
	PAHs from coal (nonsubstantial)	4	0.7 (0.2-2.1)
	PAHs from coal (substantial)	6	2.0 (0.8-5.3)
	PAHs from petroleum (any)	64	1.0 (0.6-1.6)
	PAHs from other sources (any)	16	0.7 (0.4-1.2)
	Mononuclear aromatic hydrocarbons (any)	29	0.8 (0.5-1.3)
Gustavsson et al. 1998	122 esophageal-cancer cases among male residents of two regions in Sweden; industrial-hygiene-derived agents (smoking-adjusted)		
	PAHs (low)	32	2.01 (1.16-3.48)
	PAHs (high)	37	1.87 (1.11-3.16)
Siemiatycki et al. 1988	107 esophageal-cancer cases among residents of Montreal, Canada; industrial-hygiene-derived agents (smoking-adjusted)		
	Gasoline exhaust	47	1.0 (0.8-1.4)[b]
	Diesel exhaust	12	0.6 (0.4-0.9)[b]
	Jet-fuel exhaust	2	2.5 (0.4-14.8)[b]
	Propane exhaust	0	0.0 (0.0-1.7)[b]
	Propane combustion	4	1.2 (0.5-3.0)[b]
	Natural-gas combustion	3	0.8 (0.3-2.0)[b]
	Liquid-fuel combustion	5	0.7 (0.3-1.4)[b]
	Coal combustion	4	0.9 (0.4-1.9)[b]
	Coke combustion	2	2.1 (0.5-9.8)[b]
	Wood combustion	8	2.3 (1.2-4.5)

[a] 95% CIs calculated with standard methods from risks and observed numbers presented in original paper.
[b] 90% CIs reported in this paper.

TABLE 4.7 Stomach Cancer and Exposure to Fuels—Selected Epidemiologic Studies

Reference	Study Population	Exposed Cases	Estimated Relative Risk (95% CI)
Cohort Studies—Mortality			
Lewis et al. 2000b	Refinery workers in Toronto, Canada		
	Males	83	0.70 (0.56-0.87)
	Refinery segment	42	0.80 (0.57-1.08)
	Marketing/distribution segment	31	0.86 (0.58-1.22)
	Females	4	0.54 (0.15-1.38)
Ritz 1999	Uranium-processing workers in Fernald, Ohio—esophageal and stomach cancers (analyzed together)		
	Kerosene, light exposure		
	>2-yr duration, no lag	10	1.98 (0.77-5.09)
	>2-yr duration, 15-yr lag	9	3.46 (1.22-9.80)
	>5-yr duration, no lag	5	0.96 (0.32-2.94)
	>5-yr duration, 15-yr lag	3	1.26 (0.31-5.15)
	Kerosene, moderate exposure		
	>2-yr duration, no lag	5	3.00 (0.81-11.2)
	>2-yr duration, 15-yr lag	5	7.71 (2.04-29.1)
	>5-yr duration, no lag	4	2.86 (0.60-13.6)
	>5-yr duration, 15-yr lag	4	10.7 (2.26-50.7)
Lagorio et al. 1994	Filling-station attendants in Italy (exposure reconstruction using monitoring)	6	0.60 (0.26-1.18)[b]
	Men	6	0.64 (0.28-1.27)[b]
	Women	0	0.0 (0.0-5.27)[a]
Nelson et al. 1987	Amoco Oil refinery cohort		
	Maintenance jobs	4	0.86
	Operations jobs	9	2.06
Case-Control Study			
Siemiatycki et al. 1987a	250 stomach cancer cases among residents of Montreal, Canada; industrial-hygiene-derived agents (smoking-adjusted)		
	Automotive gasoline	44	1.5 (1.2-1.9)[b]
	Aviation gasoline	3	0.8 (0.3-2.7)[b]
	Kerosene	24	1.7 (1.2-2.3)[b]
	Jet fuel	1	0.2 (0.0-1.7)[b]
	Diesel fuel	10	1.0 (0.6-1.6)[b]
	Heating oil	15	1.4 (0.9-2.1)[b]
	Crude oil	3	1.4 (0.4-5.0)[b]

[a] Risk estimates and 95% CIs calculated with standard methods from observed and expected numbers presented in original paper.
[b] 90% CIs presented.

TABLE 4.8 Stomach Cancer and Exposure to Combustion Products—Selected Epidemiologic Studies

Reference	Study Population	Exposed Cases	Estimated Relative Risk (95% CI)
Cohort Studies—Incidence			
Chow et al. 1994	Male residents of Sweden		
	Industries		
	Transportation and communication	1162	1.0
	Occupations		
	Transport and communication	1062	1.0
	Machine and engine maintenance	348	1.0 ($p < 0.05$)
	Crane operators	66	1.5 ($p < 0.01$)
	Forklift operators	102	1.0
	Dock workers	134	1.3 ($p < 0.05$)
	Warehouse workers	443	1.1 ($p < 0.05$)
Kneller et al. 1990	Residents of Shanghai, China		
	Fuel suppliers	23	1.33
	Petroleum-refinery workers	5	4.39 ($p < 0.05$)
	Boiler firemen	118	1.59 ($p < 0.01$)
Case-Control Studies			
Cocco et al. 1994	640 stomach-cancer cases among residents of Italy; occupation (not smoking-adjusted)		
	Mechanics, repairmen and allied		
	Ever worked	36	1.0 (0.6-1.5)
	Worked 21+ yr	19	0.8 (0.5-1.5)
	Railroad workers, drivers, and allied		
	Ever worked	51	1.0 (0.7-1.5)
	Worked 21+ yr	30	1.3 (0.8-2.2)
	Nitrogen oxides		
	Ever exposed	453	1.4 (1.0-2.1)
	Exposed 21+ yr	na	0.7 (0.3-1.5)
Siemiatycki et al. 1988	250 stomach-cancer cases among residents of Montreal, Canada; industrial-hygiene-derived agents (smoking-adjusted)		
	Gasoline exhaust	111	1.1 (0.9-1.3)[a]
	Diesel exhaust	41	0.9 (0.7-1.1)[a]
	Jet-fuel exhaust	2	0.8 (0.2-3.5)[a]
	Propane exhaust	7	1.2 (0.6-2.2)[a]
	Propane combustion	12	1.5 (0.9-2.4)[a]
	Natural-gas combustion	11	1.3 (0.8-2.2)[a]
	Liquid-fuel combustion	16	0.9 (0.6-1.3)[a]
	Coal combustion	14	1.3 (0.8-2.0)[a]
	Coke combustion	3	1.5 (0.4-5.8)[a]
Weinberg et al. 1985	178 stomach-cancer cases among residents of four counties in Pennsylvania; next-of-kin reports (not smoking-adjusted)		
	Coal heating	162	
	Digestive-cancer controls		1.69 (0.85-3.36)
	ASHD controls		1.08 (0.49-2.37)
	Neighborhood controls		1.20 (0.52-2.78)

Reference	Study Population	Exposed Cases	Estimated Relative Risk (95% CI)
	Coal cooking	90	
	Digestive-cancer controls		1.00 (0.63-1.57)
	ASHD controls		0.84 (0.55-1.27)
	Neighborhood controls		0.97 (0.59-1.59)
	Gas heating	125	
	Digestive-cancer controls		0.61 (0.36-1.02, p < 0.08)
	ASHD controls		0.62 (0.36-1.06)
	Neighborhood controls		0.64 (0.33-1.24)
	Gas cooking	129	
	Digestive-cancer controls		0.67 (0.40-1.12)
	ASHD controls		0.49 (0.29-0.83, p < 0.005)
	Neighborhood controls		0.54 (0.28-1.06)
Decoufle and Stanislawczyk 1977	Stomach-cancer cases among patients at Roswell Park Memorial Institute in Buffalo, New York		
	Bus drivers	1	2.06
	Taxicab drivers and chauffeurs	1	2.15
	Truck and tractor drivers	8	1.56
	Bus, taxicab, and truck drivers	5	0.89
	Locomotive engineers and firemen	2	1.14
	Machinists	2	0.92
	Mechanics and repairmen	15	1.60

NOTE: na=not available; ASHD=arteriosclerotic heart disease.
[a] 90% CIs reported in this paper

TABLE 4.9 Colon Cancer and Exposure to Fuels—Selected Epidemiologic Studies

Reference	Study Population	Exposed Cases	Estimated Relative Risk (95% CI)
Cohort Studies—Mortality			
Lewis et al. 2000b	Imperial Oil workers in Canada—cancer of the large intestine except rectum (ICD 153)		
	Males	183	1.06 (0.91-1.22)
	Refinery segment	65	0.88 (0.68-1.12)
	Marketing-distribution segment	63	1.20 (0.92-1.53)
	Females	19	0.88 (0.53-1.37)
Ritz 1999	Uranium-processing workers in Fernald, Ohio—colon and rectal cancers (analyzed together)		
	Kerosene, light exposure		
	>2-yr duration, no lag	10	1.13 (0.49-2.60)
	>2-yr duration, 15-yr lag	9	1.20 (0.50-2.91)
	>5-yr duration, no lag	9	1.26 (0.52-3.01)
	>5-yr duration, 15-yr lag	7	1.40 (0.52-3.74)
	Kerosene, moderate exposure		
	>2-yr duration, no lag	8	1.80 (0.64-5.06)
	>2-yr duration, 15-yr lag	7	2.11 (0.75-5.97)
	>5-yr duration, no lag	5	1.13 (0.31-4.18)
	>5-yr duration, 15-yr lag	4	1.91 (0.50-7.27)
Nelson et al.	Amoco Oil refinery cohort—cancer of the large intestine		

Reference	Study Population	Exposed Cases	Estimated Relative Risk (95% CI)
1987			
	Maintenance jobs	12	1.11
	Operations jobs	12	1.19
Case-Control Studies			
Gerhardsson de Verdier et al. 1992	352 colon-cancer cases among residents of Stockholm, Sweden; self-reported occupations and agents (not smoking-adjusted)		
	Petrol station and automotive repair (occupation)	12	1.8 (0.6-5.2)
	Self-reported agents		
	Combustion gases from coal, coke, and wood	21	1.3 (0.6-2.5)
	Soot	24	1.7 (0.8-3.4)
	Tar and asphalt	8	0.7 (0.2-1.9)
Siemiatycki et al. 1987a	233 cases among residents of Montreal, Canada—industrial-hygiene-derived agents (smoking-adjusted)		
	Colon cancer		
	Automotive gasoline	39	1.0 (0.7-1.2)[a]
	Aviation gasoline	7	1.7 (0.7-3.6)[a]
	Kerosene	14	0.7 (0.5-1.1)[a]
	Jet fuel	7	2.1 (0.9-5.1)[a]
	Diesel fuel	10	0.7 (0.4-1.1)[a]
	Heating oil	13	0.9 (0.6-1.5)[a]
	Crude oil	3	1.5 (0.3-6.8)[a]
	Rectosigmoid cancer		
	Automotive gasoline	25	0.9 (0.7–1.3)[a]
	Aviation gasoline	3	0.8 (0.2–2.7)[a]
	Kerosene	11	0.9 (0.5–1.4)[a]
	Jet fuel	2	0.8 (0.2–3.8)[a]
	Diesel fuel	4	0.4 (0.2–0.9)[a]
	Heating oil	6	0.6 (0.3–1.2)[a]
	Crude oil	0	—
Spiegelman and Wegman 1985	370 colon cancer cases in seven US metropolitan areas; fuel oil; JEM-derived agents (not smoking-adjusted)		
	Males: colorectal cancer	na	1.53 ($p = 0.01$)
	Colon cancer only	na	1.61 ($p = 0.02$)
	Females: colorectal cancer	na	1.24 ($p = 0.21$)
	Colon cancer only	na	1.34 ($p = 0.12$)

NOTE: na=not available.
[a] 90% CIs reported in this paper.

TABLE 4.10 Colon Cancer and Exposure to Combustion Products—Selected Epidemiologic Studies

Reference	Study Population	Exposed Cases	Estimated Relative Risk (95% CI)
Case-Control Studies			
Goldberg et al. 2001	497 colon cancer cases among residents of Montreal, Canada; industrial-hygiene-derived agent (smoking-adjusted)		
	Diesel-engine emissions		
	Nonsubstantial	45	1.2 (0.8-1.8)
	Substantial	35	1.6 (1.0-2.5)

Reference	Study Population	Exposed Cases	Estimated Relative Risk (95% CI)
Gerhardsson de Verdier et al. 1992	352 colon-cancer cases among residents of Stockholm, Sweden; self-reported occupations, agents (not smoking-adjusted)		
	Railway work	5	1.4 (0.3-6.3)
	Combustion gases from coal, coke, and wood	21	1.3 (0.6-2.5)
	Soot	24	1.7 (0.8-3.4)
	Tar and asphalt	8	0.7 (0.2-1.9)
Siemiatycki et al. 1988	364 colon-cancer cases among residents of Montreal, Canada; industrial-hygiene-derived agents (smoking-adjusted)		
	Gasoline exhaust	147	1.0 (0.9-1.2)[a]
	Diesel exhaust	68	1.3 (1.1-1.6)[a]
	Short, low	6	0.7 (0.3-1.4)[a]
	Short, high	5	0.6 (0.3-1.3)[a]
	Long, low	27	1.5 (1.0-2.2)[a]
	Long, high	30	1.7 (1.2-2.5)[a]
	Jet-fuel exhaust	4	1.3 (0.4-4.2)[a]
	Propane exhaust	7	0.9 (0.5-1.8)[a]
	Propane combustion	12	1.0 (0.6-1.6)[a]
	Natural-gas combustion	6	0.5 (0.2-0.9)[a]
	Liquid-fuel combustion	19	0.9 (0.6-1.4)[a]
	Coal combustion	8	0.5 (0.3-0.8)[a]
	Coke combustion	2	0.7 (0.1-3.5)[a]

[a] 90% CIs reported in this paper.

TABLE 4.11 Rectal Cancer and Exposure to Fuels—Selected Epidemiologic Studies

Reference	Study Population	Exposed Cases	Estimated Relative Risk (95% CI)
Cohort Studies—Mortality			
Lewis et al. 2000b	Refinery workers in Toronto, Canada		
	Males	55	0.87 (0.65-1.13)
	Refinery segment	30	1.09 (0.73-1.55)
	Marketing and distribution segment	12	0.62 (0.32-1.08)
	Females	3	0.60 (0.12-1.74)
Ritz 1999	Uranium-processing workers in Fernald, Ohio—colon and rectal cancers (analyzed together)		
	Kerosene, light exposure		
	>2-yr duration, no lag	10	1.13 (0.49-2.60)
	>2-yr duration, 15-yr lag	9	1.20 (0.50-2.91)
	>5-yr duration, no lag	9	1.26 (0.52-3.01)
	>5-yr duration, 15-yr lag	7	1.40 (0.52-3.74)
	Kerosene, moderate exposure		
	>2-yr duration, no lag	8	1.80 (0.64-5.06)
	>2-yr duration, 15-yr lag	7	2.11 (0.75-5.97)
	>5-yr duration, no lag	5	1.13 (0.31-4.18)
	>5-yr duration, 15-yr lag	4	1.91 (0.50-7.27)
Nelson et al.	Amoco Oil refinery cohort		

Reference	Study Population	Exposed Cases	Estimated Relative Risk (95% CI)
1987			
	Maintenance jobs	5	1.67
	Operations jobs	5	1.78
Case-Control Studies			
Gerhardsson de Verdier et al. 1992	217 rectal-cancer cases among residents of Stockholm, Sweden; self-reported agents (not smoking-adjusted)		
	Petrol station/automotive repair	7	1.5 (0.4-5.6)
	Combustion gases from coal, coke, and wood	21	2.1 (1.0-4.6)
	Soot	21	2.7 (1.2-5.7)
	Tar and asphalt	7	1.0 (0.3-2.8)
Siemiatycki et al. 1987a	190 rectal-cancer cases among residents of Montreal, Canada; industrial-hygiene-derived agents (smoking-adjusted)		
	Automotive gasoline	24	1.1 (0.8-1.6)[a]
	Aviation gasoline	4	2.5 (0.6-10.3)[a]
	Kerosene	11	0.9 (0.6-1.6)[a]
	Jet fuel	4	2.1 (0.6-7.4)[a]
	Diesel fuel	11	1.4 (0.8-2.5)[a]
	Heating oil	11	1.5 (0.8-2.6)[a]
Spiegelman and Wegman 1985	Colon and rectal cancer cases in seven US metropolitan areas		
	Fuel oil: males; colorectal cancer	na	1.53 ($p = 0.01$)
	Colon-cancer only	na	1.61 ($p = 0.02$)
	Females: colorectal cancer	na	1.24 ($p = 0.21$)
	Colon-cancer only	na	1.34 ($p = 0.12$)

NOTE: na=not available.
[a] 90% CIs presented.

TABLE 4.12 Rectal Cancer and Exposure to Combustion Products—Selected Epidemiologic Studies

Reference	Study Population	Exposed Cases	Estimated Relative Risk (95% CI)
Case-Control Studies			
Dumas et al. 2000	257 rectal-cancer cases among residents of Montreal, Canada; industrial-hygiene-derived agents (smoking-adjusted)		
	Soot		
	Any	17	0.8 (0.5-1.3)
	Substantial	4	0.8 (0.3-2.4)
	Coal		
	Any	8	0.6 (0.3-1.3)
	Substantial	6	1.3 (0.5-3.3)
	Wood		
	Any	9	0.7 (0.3-1.4)
	Substantial	4	1.0 (0.3-3.2)
Gerhardsson de Verdier et al. 1992	217 rectal-cancer cases among residents of Stockholm, Sweden; self-reported agents (not smoking-adjusted)		

Reference	Study Population	Exposed Cases	Estimated Relative Risk (95% CI)
	Railway work	5	2.3 (0.5-10.4)
	Combustion gases from coal, coke, and wood	21	2.1 (1.0-4.6)
	Soot	21	2.7 (1.2-5.7)
	Tar and asphalt	7	1.0 (0.3-2.8)
Siemiatycki et al. 1988	190 rectal-cancer cases among residents of Montreal, Canada; industrial-hygiene-derived agents (smoking-adjusted)		
	Gasoline exhaust	89	1.2 (1.0-1.7)[a]
	Short, low	17	1.3 (0.8-2.1)[a]
	Short, high	9	1.0 (0.5-1.8)[a]
	Long, low	27	1.1 (0.7-1.6)[a]
	Long, high	36	1.6 (1.1-2.3)[a]
	Diesel exhaust	35	1.1 (0.9-1.5)[a]
	Jet-fuel exhaust	3	1.7 (0.4-7.8)[a]
	Propane exhaust	3	0.7 (0.2-2.4)[a]
	Propane combustion	10	1.1 (0.6-1.9)[a]
	Natural-gas combustion	5	0.8 (0.3-1.8)[a]
	Liquid-fuel combustion	14	1.1 (0.7-1.8)[a]
	Coal combustion	7	0.7 (0.4-1.3)[a]
	Coke combustion	0	0.0 (0.0-1.7)[a]

[a] 90% CIs reported in this paper.

TABLE 4.13 Hepatic Cancer and Exposure to Fuels—Selected Epidemiologic Studies

Reference	Study Population	Exposed Cases	Estimated Relative Risk (95% CI)
Case-Control Study			
Stemhagen et al. 1983	265 hepatic-cancer cases among residents of New Jersey; industries (not smoking-adjusted)		
	Motor vehicles and equipment manufacturing	11	2.20 (0.95-5.07)
	Gasoline service stations	12	2.88 (1.20-6.88)

TABLE 4.14 Hepatic Cancer and Exposure to Combustion Products—Selected Epidemiologic Studies

Reference	Study Population	Exposed Cases	Estimated Relative Risk (95% CI)
Case-Control Study			
Stemhagen et al. 1983	265 hepatic cancer cases among residents of New Jersey; industries (not smoking-adjusted)		
	Bus lines	7	2.80 (0.93-8.40)
	Gasoline service stations	12	2.88 (1.20-6.88)

TABLE 4.15 Pancreatic Cancer and Exposure to Fuels—Selected Epidemiologic Studies

Reference	Study Population	Exposed Cases	Estimated Relative Risk (95% CI)
Cohort Studies			
Lewis et al. 2003	Petroleum workers in Canada		
	Males, mortality	4	0.51 (0.14-1.31)
	Females, mortality	1	0.48 (0.01-2.69)[a]
	Males, incidence	5	0.59 (0.19-1.39)
	Females, incidence	0	0.00 (0.00-1.63)[a]
Ritz et al. 1999	Uranium-processing workers in Fernald, Ohio		
	Kerosene, light exposure		
	> 5-yr duration, 15-yr lag	na	1.33 (0.31-5.66)
	Kerosene, moderate exposure		
	> 5-yr duration, 15-yr lag	na	2.78 (0.51-15.2)

NOTE: na=not available.
[a] Unadjusted risk estimates and 95% CIs calculated with standard methods from observed and expected numbers presented in original paper.

TABLE 4.16 Pancreatic Cancer and Exposure to Combustion Products—Selected Epidemiologic Studies

Reference	Study Population	Exposed Cases	Estimated Relative Risk (95% CI)
Case-Control Studies			
Alguacil et al. 2000	185 pancreatic-cancer cases among residents of eastern Spain (smoking-adjusted)		
	Industrial-hygiene assessment		
	PAHs	13	0.81 (0.37-1.76)
	Low	10	0.74 (0.31-1.77)
	High	3	1.11 (0.24-5.21)
	Exposed ≥ 10-yr, 10 yr before diagnosis		
	Low	8	1.08 (0.39-3.00)
	High	2	1.73 (0.22-13.8)
	Finnish JEM assessment (substantial vs low exposure)		
	Benzo[a]pyrene	6	3.10 (0.73-13.2)
	Diesel-engine exhaust	4	2.39 (0.50-11.4)
	Gasoline-engine exhaust	4	2.42 (0.51-11.6)
	PAHs	2	0.78 (0.12-5.18)
Kauppinen et al. 1995	595 pancreatic-cancer cases among residents of Finland; JEM-derived agents (smoking-adjusted)		
	Engine exhaust	19	0.89 (0.51-1.53)
	PAHs	14	1.33 (0.69-2.57)
Siemiatycki et al. 1988	117 pancreatic-cancer cases among residents of Montreal, Canada; industrial-hygiene-derived agents (smoking-adjusted)		
	Gasoline exhaust	47	0.9 (0.7-1.2)[a]
	Diesel exhaust	15	0.6 (0.4-0.9)[a]
	Jet-fuel exhaust	2	1.6 (0.3-7.7)[a]
	Propane exhaust	2	0.7 (0.2-2.5)[a]
	Propane combustion	3	0.8 (0.3-2.2)[a]

Reference	Study Population	Exposed Cases	Estimated Relative Risk (95% CI)
	Natural-gas combustion	6	1.5 (0.7-3.1)[a]
	Liquid-fuel combustion	10	1.3 (0.8-2.3)[a]
	Coal combustion	10	2.3 (1.4-4.0)[a]
	Nonsubstantial	2	0.7 (0.2-2.4)[a]
	Substantial	8	3.5 (1.7-7.3)[a]
	Coke combustion	2	2.2 (0.4-10.5)[a]

NOTE: na=not available.
[a] 90% CIs reported in this paper.

TABLE 4.17 Laryngeal Cancer and Exposure to Fuels—Selected Epidemiologic Studies

Reference	Study Population	Exposed Cases	Estimated Relative Risk (95% CI)
Cohort Study–Mortality			
Lagorio et al. 1994	Male filling-station attendants in Italy		
	Stations of all sizes	3	1.05 (0.29–2.72)[a]
	Small stations	3	1.53 (0.42–3.96)[a]
Case-Control Studies			
De Stefani et al. 1998	112 laryngeal-cancer cases among residents of Montevideo, Uruguay (smoking-adjusted)		
	Gasoline fillers (job title)	2	1.4 (0.2-7.7)
	Gasoline (self-reported agent)	22	1.4 (0.8-2.6)
	1-20 yr	6	1.1 (0.4-2.8)
	21+ yr	16	1.7 (0.9-3.5)
	Supraglottic	na	1.3 (0.5-3.4)
	Glottic	na	2.5 (0.8-8.2)
Wortley et al. 1992	235 laryngeal-cancer cases among residents of 13 counties in western Washington; occupation (smoking-adjusted)		
	Vehicle mechanics	32	1.2 (0.6-2.1)
	Garage and service-station work	12	0.8 (0.4-1.8)
Ahrens et al. 1991	100 laryngeal-cancer cases among residents of Bremen, Germany; self-reported agents (smoking-adjusted)		
	Diesel oil	na	1.7 (0.8-3.5)
	Gasoline	na	2.8 (1.0-7.7)
Brown et al. 1988	183 laryngeal-cancer cases among residents along Gulf Coast of Texas; industry (smoking-adjusted)		
	Petroleum refining and chemical manufacturing (ever vs never)	47	0.93 (0.59-1.46)

NOTE: na=not available.
[a] 90% CIs reported.

TABLE 4.18 Laryngeal Cancer and Exposure to Combustion Products—Selected Epidemiologic Studies

Reference	Study Population	Exposed Cases	Estimated Relative Risk (95% CI)
Cohort Study—Incidence			
Boffetta et al. 2001	Cohort exposed to diesel exhausted defined on industrial-hygiene coding of occupation on 1960 Swedish census (not smoking-adjusted)		
	Males	730	1.09 (1.01-1.17)
	Probability of exposure		
	Low	272	1.1 (0.99-1.27)
	Medium	218	0.92 (0.80-1.05)
	High	204	1.1 (0.96-1.28)
	Intensity of exposure		
	Low	473	1.1 (0.95-1.17)
	Medium	127	1.1 (0.88-1.26)
	High	94	0.99 (0.81-1.22)
	Females	5	2.39 (0.78-5.57)
Case-Control Studies			
1,010 cases of laryngeal cancer (ICD-9 161) or hypopharyngeal cancer (ICD-9 146.4, 146.5, 148, 149.8) among male residents of France, Italy, Spain, and Switzerland (IARC six-center study) (smoking-adjusted)			
Boffetta et al. 2003	Railway transport (ever vs never) (industry)	44	1.52 (0.97-2.39)
	Duration		p for trend = 0.02
	1-10 yr	11	1.1
	11-20 yr	5	0.3
	21+ yr	28	2.2 ($p < 0.05$)
	Occupations (ever vs never)		
	Motor-vehicle mechanics	17	1.09 (0.55-2.16)
	Other mechanic	42	1.39 (0.87-2.23)
	Railway-vehicle loaders	14	1.39 (0.61-3.15)
	Lorry drivers, local	42	1.14 (0.73-1.79)
	Lorry drivers, long-distance	37	1.28 (0.78-2.10)
	Other motor-vehicle drivers	12	1.32 (0.58-3.03)
Berrino et al. 2003	695 cases ≥55 yr old		
	PAHs (JEM-derived agent)	na	1.0 (0.7-1.3)
	315 cases <55 yr old		
	PAHs (JEM-derived agent)	263	0.7 (0.3-1.4)
	Likelihood of exposure		
	Possible	107	0.5 (0.2-1.1)
	Probable	156	0.8 (0.3-1.8)
	Duration of exposure		
	<10 yr	na	0.6 (0.2-1.8)
	10-19 yr	na	0.9 (0.4-2.1)
	≥20 yr	na	1.1 (0.5-2.4)
Elci et al. 2003	940 laryngeal-cancer cases among male residents of Istanbul, Turkey (smoking-adjusted)		
	Diesel exhaust (JEM-derived agent)	297	1.5 (1.3-1.9)
	Intensity of exposure		
	Low	161	1.5 (1.1-1.8)
	Medium	91	1.7 (1.2-2.3)
	High	45	1.6 (1.0-2.4)

Reference	Study Population	Exposed Cases	Estimated Relative Risk (95% CI)
	Probability of exposure		
	Low	92	1.6 (1.2-2.2)
	Medium	148	1.5 (1.1-1.9)
	High	57	1.6 (1.1-2.4)
	Gasoline exhaust (JEM-derived agent)	220	1.6 (1.3-2.0)
	Intensity of exposure		
	Low	141	1.5 (1.2-2.0)
	Medium	78	1.8 (1.3-2.5)
	Probability of exposure		
	Low	86	1.6 (1.1-2.2)
	Medium	131	1.7 (1.3-2.2)
	High	3	0.7 (0.2-2.9)
	PAHs (JEM-derived agent)	376	1.3 (1.1-1.6)
	Intensity of exposure		
	Low	189	1.4 (1.1-1.7)
	Medium	138	1.3 (1.0-1.6)
	High	49	1.5 (1.0-2.2)
	Probability of exposure		
	Low	106	1.4 (1.0-1.8)
	Medium	176	1.4 (1.1-1.7)
	High	94	1.3 (1.0-1.7)
Elci et al. 2001	Occupations		
	Drivers	75	1.7 (1.1-2.4)
	Glottis	22	2.2 (1.3-3.8)
	Supraglottis	27	1.2 (0.7-1.9)
	Other	26	1.8 (1.1-3.1)
	Mechanics	28	0.8 (0.5-1.3)
De Stefani et al. 1998	112 laryngeal-cancer cases among male residents of Montevideo, Uruguay (smoking-adjusted)		
	Automobile mechanic (job title)	8	1.1 (0.5-2.8)
	Supraglottic	na	1.3 (0.3-5.9)
	Glottic	na	5.5 (1.3-23.5)
	Truck driver (job title)	8	0.8 (0.3-1.8)
	Supraglottic	na	0.6 (0.1-2.9)
	Glottic	na	2.7 (0.7-10.7)
	Tractor driver (job title)	7	0.6 (0.2-1.5)
	Gasoline fillers (job title)	2	1.4 (0.2-7.7)
	Diesel exhausts (self-reported agent)	17	0.8 (0.4-1.4)
	1-20 yr	3	0.3 (0.1-0.9)
	20+ yr	14	1.4 (0.7-2.8)
	Supraglottic	na	0.7 (0.2-1.9)
	Glottic	na	1.9 (0.6-5.8)
	Gasoline exhausts (self-reported agent)	22	0.9 (0.6-1.8)
	1-20 yr	7	0.8 (0.3-1.9)
	20+ yr	15	1.2 (0.6-2.3)
	Supraglottic	na	0.8 (0.3-2.1)
	Glottic	na	1.8 (0.6-5.7)
Gustavsson et al. 1998	Laryngeal-cancer cases among male residents of two regions in Sweden		
	PAHs (low)	26	0.77 (0.46-1.28)
	PAHs (high)	53	1.47 (0.96-2.24)

Reference	Study Population	Exposed Cases	Estimated Relative Risk (95% CI)
Pintos et al. 1998	Laryngeal-cancer cases among residents of three cities in southern Brazil		
	Use of wood stove	na	2.34 (1.17-4.67)
	Males		2.03 (1.12-3.67)
	Females		16.24 (2.66-99.1)
Goldberg et al. 1997	Laryngeal cancer cases among male residents of France		
	Industry		
	Railway transportation	30	1.4 (0.6-3.1)
	Road transportation	31	1.0 (0.4-2.1)
	Other transportation	16	0.8 (0.3-2.2)
	Repair of motor vehicles	21	0.9 (0.4-2.0)
	Occupation		
	Motor-vehicle mechanics	27	1.2 (0.5-2.5)
	Transport-equipment operators	118	1.4 (0.9-2.3)
Maier and Tisch 1997	Laryngeal-cancer cases among residents of Heidelberg, Germany	na	
	PAH		2.7 (1.2-6.1)
	Fossil-fuel single stove		
	0-20 yr		1.0
	20-40 yr		1.2 (0.8-1.9)
	>40 yr		2.5 (1.5-4.1)
Dietz et al. 1995	Laryngeal-cancer cases among residents of Heidelberg, Germany		
	Air pollution on job (>20 yr)	34	1.44 (0.91-2.26)[a]
	Traffic jams on way to work (>20 yr)	23	0.69 (0.41-1.14)[a]
	High traffic emissions, residential (>20 yr)	39	33.8 (13.34-90.85)[a]
	Outdoor air pollution, residential (>20 yr)	21	1.00 (0.58-1.71)[a]
	Heating, fossil-fuel stoves (>40 yr)	57	2.11 (1.43-3.12)[a]
	Cooking, fossil-fuel stoves (>20 yr)	33	1.47 (0.92-2.33)[a]
	Coal, briquette, or coke heating	138	1.52 (0.94-2.47)[a]
	Gas heating	16	0.52 (0.29-0.93)[a]
Muscat and Wynder 1995	Laryngeal cancer cases among residents of New York, Illinois, Michigan, and Pennsylvania		
	Truck driver	30	1.22 (0.65-2.28)[a]
	Diesel-exhaust jobs	36	0.96 (0.5-1.8)
	Automobile mechanics	13	1.30 (0.4-4.1)
	Diesel exhaust	13	1.47 (0.5-4.1)
	Diesel fumes	16	6.4 (1.8-22.6)
Pollan and Lopez-Abente 1995	Laryngeal-cancer cases among male residents of Madrid, Spain		
	Mechanics and assembly workers	8	1.56 (0.49-4.98)
	1-20 yr	4	1.21 (0.25-5.82)
	>20 yr	4	3.04 (0.52-17.71)
	Transport drivers	8	2.71 (0.85-8.64)
	1-20 yr	3	5.76 (0.71-46.48)
	>20 yr	4	1.96 (0.43-8.96)

Reference	Study Population	Exposed Cases	Estimated Relative Risk (95% CI)
Wortley et al. 1992	Laryngeal-cancer cases among residents of western Washington state		
	Vehicle mechanics	32	1.2 (0.6-2.1)
	<10 yr		0.6
	≥10 yr		3.2
	Motor vehicle operators	54	1.3 (0.8-2.1)
	<10 yr		1.6
	≥10 yr		0.8
	Transportation, motor vehicles	19	1.3 (0.6-2.8)
	<10 yr		1.1
	≥10 yr		0.8
	Diesel fumes—peak		
	None	112	1.0
	Low	58	1.2 (0.7-1.9)
	Medium	65	1.1 (0.7-1.8)
	Diesel fumes—duration		
	<1 yr	118	1.0
	1-9 yr	70	1.0 (0.7-1.6)
	≥10 yr	47	1.0 (0.6-1.8)
	Diesel fumes—exposure scores		
	<5	158	1.0
	5-19	39	1.3 (0.7-2.2)
	≥20	38	1.0 (0.6-1.7)
Ahrens et al. 1991	Laryngeal-cancer cases among male residents of Bremen, Germany (smoking-adjusted)		
	Transportation and communication (industry)	24	1.3 (0.64-2.59)
	Fumes or smoke (self-reported agent)	na	0.7 (0.3-1.4)
Brown et al. 1988	183 laryngeal-cancer cases among residents along gulf coast of Texas (smoking-adjusted)		
	Transportation, communication, utilities, and sanitary services (industry)	63	1.62 (1.04-2.51)
	Transportation (occupation)	39	1.42 (0.86-2.36)
	Specific occupations		
	Driver	15	1.69 (0.75-3.83)
	Mechanic	33	1.06 (0.63-1.77)
	Diesel or gasoline fumes (industrial-hygiene-coded agent)	79	1.50 (1.00-2.26)
	<5 yr	32	1.8 (1.0-3.1)
	5-14 yr	16	1.3 (0.6-2.7)
	≥15 yr	26	1.6 (0.8-2.9)
Decoufle and Stanislawczyk 1977	Laryngeal cancer cases among male patients at Roswell Park Memorial Institute in Buffalo, New York (job history, including durations, from medical charts) (smoking-adjusted)		
	Occupations (ever)		
	Bus, taxicab, and truck drivers	na	0.95
	Delivery and routemen	na	0.68
	Locomotive engineers and firemen	na	1.07, ns
	Machinists	na	1.38, ns

Reference	Study Population	Exposed Cases	Estimated Relative Risk (95% CI)
	Mechanics and repairmen	na	0.95

NOTE: na=not available; ns=not statistically significant ($p < 0.5$) for risk estimate above unity; IARC=International Agency for Research on Cancer.
[a] Unadjusted odds ratios and 95% CIs calculated with standard methods from observed numbers presented in original paper.

TABLE 4.19 Lung Cancer and Exposure to Fuels—Selected Epidemiologic Studies

Reference	Study Population	Exposed Cases	Estimated Relative Risk (95% CI)
Cohort Study—Mortality			
Lewis et al. 2000b	Refinery workers in Toronto, Canada		
	Males	478	0.85 (0.77-0.93)
	Refinery segment	221	0.96 (0.83-1.09)
	Marketing and distribution segment	150	0.87 (0.74-1.02)
	Females	34	1.10 (0.76-1.53)
Case-Control Studies			
Rosamilia et al. 1999	Lung-cancer cases nested among refinery workers at Mobil in Beaumont, Texas		
	Process operations, duration of employment		
	0 yr	50	1.0
	<5 yr	12	0.66 (0.31-1.36)
	5-14 yr	9	0.64 (0.28-1.44)
	15+ yr	41	1.34 (0.82-2.19)
	Maintenance and mechanical operations, duration of employment		
	0 yr	18	1.0
	<5 yr	26	1.12 (0.55-2.31)
	5-14 yr	26	0.70 (0.35-1.42)
	15+ yr	42	1.32 (0.68-2.55)
Siemiatycki et al. 1987a	857 lung-cancer cases among residents of Montreal, Canada; industrial-hygiene-derived agents (smoking-adjusted)		
	Automotive gasoline		
	Oat cell	26	1.2 (0.8-1.6)[a]
	Squamous cell	53	1.0 (0.8-1.3)
	Adenocarcinoma	26	1.1 (0.8-1.5)
	Other cell types	19	0.8 (0.6-1.1)
	Aviation gasoline		
	Oat cell	1	0.4 (0.1-3.2)
	Squamous cell	2	0.4 (0.1-1.6)
	Adenocarcinoma	2	0.9 (0.2-3.8)
	Other cell types	1	0.4 (0.1-3.1)
	Kerosene		
	Oat cell	0	0.9 (0.6-1.5)
	Squamous cell	34	1.4 (1.0-1.9)
	Adenocarcinoma	15	1.5 (1.0-2.3)
	Other cell types	13	1.2 (0.8-1.9)
	Jet fuel		
	Oat cell	2	1.3 (0.2-7.0)

Reference	Study Population	Exposed Cases	Estimated Relative Risk (95% CI)
	Squamous cell	1	0.2 (0.0-2.4)
	Adenocarcinoma	2	1.2 (0.2-6.6)
	Other cell types	1	0.6 (0.1-6.0)
	Diesel fuel		
	Oat cell	10	1.7 (0.9-3.0)
	Squamous cell	20	1.5 (1.0-2.2)
	Adenocarcinoma	7	1.0 (0.5-1.9)
	Other cell types	9	1.4 (0.8-2.5)
	Heating oil		
	Oat cell	13	1.7 (1.0-2.7)
	Squamous cell	25	1.3 (0.9-1.8)
	Adenocarcinoma	11	1.3 (0.8-2.1)
	Other cell types	5	0.6 (0.3-1.1)
	Crude oil		
	Oat cell	1	0.7 (0.1-8.0)
	Squamous cell	7	2.8 (1.0-7.6)
	Adenocarcinoma	1	0.8 (0.1-9.7)
	Other cell types	0	—

[a] 90% CIs calculated.

TABLE 4.20 Lung Cancer and Exposure to Combustion Products—Selected Epidemiologic Studies

Reference	Study Population	Exposed Cases	Estimated Relative Risk (95% CI)
Ambient Air Pollution			
Cohort Study—Incidence			
Nafstad et al. 2003	Male residents of Oslo, Norway (smoking-adjusted)		
	NOx		
	0-9.99 $\mu g/m^3$	18	1.00
	10-19.99 $\mu g/m^3$	17	1.02 (0.75-1.39)
	20-20.99 $\mu g/m^3$	22	1.33 (0.87-2.04)
	30+ $\mu g/m^3$	24	2.22 (1.30-3.79)
	Per 10 $\mu g/m^3$		1.10 (1.03-1.17)
	SO_2		
	0-9.99 $\mu g/m^3$	18	1.00
	10-19.99 $\mu g/m^3$	21	0.84 (0.57-1.23)
	20-20.99 $\mu g/m^3$	20	0.78 (0.53-1.16)
	30+ $\mu g/m^3$	18	0.56 (0.33-0.95)
	Per 10 $\mu g/m^3$		0.96 (0.88-1.04)
Cohort Studies—Mortality			
Hoek et al. 2002	Residents of Netherlands—Netherlands Cohort Study on Diet and Cancer (smoking-adjusted)		
	Black smoke	na	1.06 (0.43-2.63)
	NO_2	na	1.25 (0.42-3.72)
Pope et al. 2002	Residents of US—Cancer Prevention Study II (smoking-adjusted)	na	
	$PM_{2.5}$ mean conc.; per 10 $\mu g/m^3$		1.14 (1.04-1.23)
	SO_4 mean conc.; per 6.5 $\mu g/m^3$		1.10 (1.04-1.15)[a]
	SO_2 mean conc.; per 9.7 ppb		1.03 (0.98-1.07)[a]
	NO_2 mean conc.; per 27.9 ppb		0.96 (0.88-1.05)[a]
	CO mean conc.; per 1.7 ppm		0.97 (0.92-1.03)[a]

Reference	Study Population	Exposed Cases	Estimated Relative Risk (95% CI)
	O_3 mean conc.; per 47.9 ppb		0.96 (0.86-1.06)[a]
Krewski et al. 2003	Residents of the US—Harvard Six Cities Study (smoking-adjusted)	na	
	$PM_{2.5}$ mean conc.; per 18.5 μg/m^3		1.17 (0.67-2.04)
	SO_4 mean conc.; per 7.5 μg/m^3		1.14 (0.66-1.96)
	SO_2 mean conc.; per 19.8 ppb		1.13 (0.66-1.95)
	NO_2 mean conc.; per 15.8 ppb		1.15 (0.65-2.04)
Abbey et al. 1999	Seventh-Day Adventist nonsmokers in California (smoking-adjusted)		
	Males	18 total	
	PM_{10} > 100 μg/m^3; per 43 days/yr		2.38 (1.42-3.97)
	PM_{10} mean conc.; per 24.08 μg/m^3		3.36 (1.57-7.19)
	SO_2 mean conc.; per 3.72 ppb		1.99 (1.24-3.20)
	NO_2 mean conc.; per 19.78 ppb		1.82 (0.93-3.57)
	Females	12 total	
	PM_{10} > 100 μg/m^3; per 43 days/yr		1.08 (0.55-2.13)
	PM_{10} mean conc.; per 24.08 μg/m^3		1.33 (0.60-2.96)
	SO_2 mean conc.; per 3.72 ppb		3.01 (1.88-4.84)
	NO_2 mean conc.; per 19.78 ppb		2.81 (1.15-6.89)
Beeson et al. 1998	Seventh-Day Adventist male nonsmokers in California—Incidence (smoking-adjusted)	16 total	
	PM_{10}, hour in excess of μg/m^3		
	40 μg/m^3		4.50 (1.31-15.44)
	50 μg/m^3		4.96 (1.54-16.00)
	60 μg/m^3		4.72 (1.69-13.18)
	80 μg/m^3		3.43 (1.71-6.88)
	100 μg/m^3		2.95 (1.71-5.09)
	PM_{10} mean conc.; per 24 μg/m^3		5.21 (1.94-13.99)
	SO_2 mean conc.; per 3.7 ppb		2.66 (1.62-4.39)
	NO_2 mean conc.; per 1.98 ppb		1.45 (0.67-3.14)
Case-Control Studies			
Nyberg et al. 2000	1,042 lung-cancer cases among residents of Stockholm, Sweden; residence linked to detailed emission database (smoking-adjusted)		
	Traffic-related air pollution—NO_2; 30-yr averages		
	Per 10 μg/m^3		1.05 (0.93-1.18)
	<15.20 μg/m^3	242	1.0
	15.20-19.84 μg/m^3	276	1.18 (0.93-1.49)
	19.85-25.05 μg/m^3	252	0.90 (0.71-1.14)
	25.06-30.54 μg/m^3	160	1.05 (0.79-1.40)
	≥30.55 μg/m^3	112	1.17 (0.84-1.62)
	Traffic-related air pollution—NO_2; 10-yr averages, 20-yr lag		
	Per 10 μg/m^3		1.10 (0.97-1.23)
	<12.78 μg/m^3	243	1.0
	12.78-17.34 μg/m^3	264	1.15 (0.91-1.46)
	17.35-23.16 μg/m^3	250	1.01 (0.79-1.29)
	23.17-29.25 μg/m^3	165	1.07 (0.81-1.42)
	≥29.26 μg/m^3	120	1.44 (1.05-1.99)
	Air pollution from heating—SO_2; 30-yr averages		
	Per 10 μg/m^3		1.00 (0.96-1.05)

Reference	Study Population	Exposed Cases	Estimated Relative Risk (95% CI)
	<41.30 μg/m^3	245	1.0
	41.30-52.74 μg/m^3	254	1.06 (0.83-1.35)
	52.75-67.13 μg/m^3	272	0.98 (0.77-1.24)
	67.14-78.20 μg/m^3	152	0.90 (0.68-1.19)
	≥78.20 μg/m^3	119	1.00 (0.73-1.37)
	Air pollution from heating—SO_2; 10-yr averages, 20-yr lag		
	Per 10 μg/m^3		1.01 (0.98-1.03)
	<66.20 μg/m^3	239	1.0
	66.20-87.59 μg/m^3	270	1.16 (0.91-1.47)
	87.60-110.29 μg/m^3	259	1.00 (0.79-1.27)
	110.30-129.09 μg/m^3	151	0.92 (0.70-1.21)
	≥129.10 μg/m^3	123	1.21 (0.89-1.66)
Marsh et al. 1998	142 lung-cancer cases among residents of four smelter towns in Arizona; atmospheric-diffusion modeling (smoking-adjusted)		
	Highest exposure level		
	None and background	na	1.00
	Low	na	0.93 (0.51-1.70)
	Medium, high, and very high	na	1.00 (0.53-1.89)
	Duration above background		
	0	na	1.00
	0-13 yr	na	1.31 (0.63-2.74)
	13-26 yr	na	1.20 (0.65-2.20)
	>26 yr	na	0.71 (0.34-1.48)
	Cumulative exposure		
	0	na	1.00
	0-13	na	1.22 (0.56-2.65)
	13-35	na	1.19 (0.62-2.27)
	>35	na	0.90 (0.48-1.71)
	Occupational exposure		
	Definite smelter	na	1.73 (0.99-3.01)
	Potential smelter	na	2.24 (1.27-3.98)
Barbone et al. 1995	755 lung-cancer cases among residents of Trieste, Italy (smoking-adjusted)		
	Level of particulate deposition from fixed-site monitoring stations		
	<0.175 g/m^2-day	188	1.0
	0.176-0.298 g/m^2-day	256	1.1 (0.8-1.5)
	>0.298 g/m^2-day	311	1.4 (1.1-1.8)
			p for trend = 0.022
Jockel et al. 1992	194 lung-cancer cases among residents of five cities in Germany (smoking-adjusted)		
	Emission index of SO_2 from energy-consumption statistics		
	Low air-pollution level	41	1.0
	High air-pollution level	39	1.01 (0.53-1.91)
	Semiquantitative index of B[a]P, TSP, and SO_2 from variety of sources		
	Low air-pollution level	36	1.0
	High air-pollution level	44	1.16 (0.64-2.13)
Katsouyanni et al. 1991	101 lung-cancer cases among female residents of Athens, Greece—Cumulative air-pollution exposure from fixed-site		

Reference	Study Population	Exposed Cases	Estimated Relative Risk (95% CI)
	monitoring stations according to borough (smoking-adjusted)		
	Nonsmokers		
	1st quartile (low)	16	1.0
	2nd quartile	16	1.20
	3rd quartile	8	0.43
	4th quartile (high)	8	0.69
			p for trend = 0.20
	Current and past smokers		
	1st quartile (low)	6	1.0
	2nd quartile	11	2.14
	3rd quartile	14	2.72
	4th quartile (high)	22	8.56
			p for trend = 0.007
Jedrychowski et al. 1990	Lung-cancer cases among residents of Cracow, Poland—air pollution index from fixed-site monitoring stations for TSP and SO_2 and geographically interpolated (smoking-adjusted)		
	Males		
	Low air pollution	650	1.0
	Medium air pollution	129	1.00 (0.75-1.33)
	High air pollution	122	1.46 (1.06-1.99)
	Females		
	Low air pollution	124	1.0
	Medium or high air pollution	74	1.17 (0.70-1.96)
	Nonsmoking males		
	Low air pollution	32	1.0
	High air pollution	17	1.45 (0.74-2.87)
	Nonsmoking females		
	Low air pollution	56	1.0
	High air pollution	23	1.16 (0.48-2.80)
Vena 1982	417 lung-cancer cases among white male residents of Erie County, New York (smoking-adjusted)		
	Years in high or medium air pollution, from 21 fixed-site monitoring stations of TSP, interpolated to town level		
	0-29 yr	54	1.00
	30-49 yr	114	1.03
	>50 yr	249	1.26
Indoor Air Pollution			
Cohort Study—Incidence			
Lan et al. 2002	Farmers in Xuanwei County, China (smoking-adjusted)		
	Males	na	
	No stove improvement		1.0
	Changed to stove with chimney		0.59 (0.49-0.71)
	0-9 yr after improvement		1.79 (1.48-2.18)
	10-19 yr after		0.25 (0.19-0.31)
	≥20 yr		0.07 (0.03-0.17)
	Cooked food <20 yr		1.0
	Cooked ≥ 20 yr		1.42 (1.05-1.93)
	Females	na	
	No stove improvement		1.0
	Changed to stove with chimney		0.54 (0.44-0.65)
	0-9 yr after improvement		1.41 (1.15-1.73)

Reference	Study Population	Exposed Cases	Estimated Relative Risk (95% CI)
	10-19 yr after		0.24 (0.19-0.31)
	≥20 yr		0.17 (0.10-0.31)
Case-Control Studies			
Kleinermann et al. 2002	846 lung-cancer cases among residents of Pingliang and Qingyang, China; self-reported agents (smoking-adjusted)		
	Type of fuel		
	Biomass	554	1.00
	Coal	278	1.29 (1.03-1.61)
	Amount of coal (tertiles)		
	0	325	1.00
	I	146	1.18 (0.92-1.51)
	II	207	1.06 (0.83-1.34)
	III	134	1.29 (0.96-1.73)
			p for trend = 0.173
	% of time coal used		
	No coal use	478	1.00
	0.7-56%	102	1.99 (1.46-2.71)
	57-100%	262	1.51 (1.20-1.91)
			p for trend = 0.024
Lan et al. 2001	97 lung-cancer cases among residents of Xuanwei County, China; self-reported agents (smoking-adjusted)		
	Smoky coal (tons)		
	Total		
	<130	na	1.0
	130-240	na	1.48 (0.73-3.20)
	>240	na	3.21 (1.23-9.03)
			p for trend = 0.01
	Males		
	<130	na	1.0
	130-240	na	1.30 (0.50-3.15)
	>240	na	1.88 (0.54-7.09)
			P for trend = 0.32
	Females		
	<130	na	1.0
	130-240	na	2.21 (0.64-8.14)
	>240	na	7.94 (1.46-60.44)
			p for trend = 0.008
Lan et al. 1993	139 lung-cancer cases among female farmers in Xuanwei County, China; self-reported agents (all subjects smoked) (smoking-adjusted)		
	Use of smoky coal	74	7.53 (3.31-17.17)
	<3 tons/yr	23	8.24 (2.33-29.17)
	≥3 tons/yr	51	7.53 (3.03-18.72)
	Use of smoky coal from Laibin mine		
	Used after 20 yr old	12	1.84 (0.56-6.05)
	Used before 20 yr old	10	5.10 (0.97-26.81)
	Lifetime use	57	9.89 (3.95-24.75)
Simonato et al. 2000	305 lung-cancer cases among residents of Venice, Italy; self-reported agents (smoking-adjusted)		
	Venice islands		

Reference	Study Population	Exposed Cases	Estimated Relative Risk (95% CI)
	Indoor heating	30	1.0
	No heating	39	13.7 (4.2-45.3)
	No coal	19	1.0
	Ever coal	49	1.3 (0.5-3.3)
	Venice inland		
	Indoor heating	67	1.0
	No heating	74	1.4 (0.8-2.2)
	No coal	24	1.0
	Ever coal	119	0.4 (0.2-0.9)
Zhong et al. 1999	504 lung-cancer cases among nonsmoking female residents of Shanghai, China; self-reported agents (smoking-adjusted)		
	Fuel used for cooking		
	Coal	166	1.00
	Coal and gas	123	0.92 (0.63-1.35)
	Gas	312	0.90 (0.66-1.23)
Shen et al. 1998	70 lung-cancer cases among nonsmoking female residents of Nanjing, China; self-reported agents (smoking-adjusted)		
	Single-factor analysis		
	Gaseous fuel in home	na	1.51 (0.47-4.78)
	Coal stove for heating	na	1.78 (0.79-4.02)
Ko et al. 1997	117 lung-cancer cases among nonsmoking female residents of Kaohsiung, Taiwan; self-reported agents (smoking-adjusted)		
	No cooking or gas	172	1.0
	Coal or anthracite	25	1.3 (0.3-5.8)
	Wood or charcoal	113	2.7 (0.9-8.9)
	Presence of fume extractor	108	1.0
	No fume extractor	160	8.3 (3.1-22.7)
Dai et al. 1996	120 lung-cancer cases among nonsmoking female residents of Harbin, China; self-reported agents (smoking-adjusted)		
	Period of coal-stove use in bedroom		
	1-19 yr	na	4.46 (1.61-12.33)
	≥30 yr	na	18.75 (3.94-29.32)
	Period of heating with coal		
	01-24 yr	na	5.81 (1.67-20.22)
	25-34 yr	na	4.70 (1.28-17.18)
Du et al. 1996	849 lung-cancer cases among residents of Guangzhou, China; next-of-kin report (smoking-adjusted)		
	Males—coal-fumes exposure	na	0.89
	Nonsmokers		1.50 (0.69-3.27)
	Smokers		4.29 (2.33-7.88)
	Females—coal-fumes exposure	na	2.21 (1.16-4.21)
	Nonsmokers		1.56 (0.57-4.25)
	Smokers		2.89 (1.09-8.65)
Lei et al. 1996	792 lung-cancer cases among residents of Guangzhou, China; next-of-kin report (smoking-adjusted)		
	Exposure to coal smoke		
	Males		
	Infrequent	350	1.0

Reference	Study Population	Exposed Cases	Estimated Relative Risk (95% CI)
	Regular	196	1.08 (0.84-1.40)[b]
	Females		
	Infrequent	48	1.0
	Regular	177	0.90 (0.55-1.45)[b]
Luo et al. 1996	102 lung-cancer cases among residents of Fuzhou, China; self-reported agents		
	Air pollution due to indoor burning of coal	na	7.6 (3.7-15.7)
	Squamous-cell carcinoma (smoking-adjusted)	na	14.1 (1.37-145.8)[c]
	Adenocarcinoma	na	6.0 (1.96-18.31)[c]
Shen et al. 1996	263 lung-cancer cases among residents of Nanjing, China; self-reported agents		
	Squamous-cell carcinoma—coal stove for heating	na	3.72 (0.88-15.71)
Xu et al. 1996a	1,249 lung-cancer cases among residents of Liaoning Province, China; self-reported agents (smoking-adjusted)		
	Cooking characteristics—males		
	Burning kang (coal)		
	1-19 yr	na	1.7 ($p < 0.05$)
	≥20 yr	na	2.1 ($p < 0.05$)
	Gas fuel for cooking		
	1-9 yr	na	0.9
	≥10 yr	na	0.8
	Cooking characteristics—females		
	Burning kang (coal)		
	1-19 yr	na	1.3
	≥20 yr	na	2.3 ($p < 0.05$)
	Cooking in bedroom (using coal)		
	1-19 yr	na	1.5
	≥20 yr	na	1.8 ($p < 0.05$)
	Gas fuel for cooking		
	1-9 yr	na	0.9
	≥10 yr	na	0.8
	Indoor air-pollution index (based on cooking fuel, place of cooking, and weighted by duration)—males		
	I (low)	na	1.0
	II	na	1.1 (0.8-1.4)
	III	na	1.2 (0.9-1.6)
	IV (high)	na	1.6 (1.2-2.3)
	Indoor air pollution index—females		
	I (low)	na	1.0
	II	na	1.2 (0.9-7.8)
	III	na	1.3 (0.9-1.9)
	IV (high)	na	1.5 (1.0-2.4)
Liu et al. 1993	316 lung-cancer cases among residents of Guangzhou, China; self-reported agents, interviewer measurements (smoking-adjusted)		
	Cooking fuel—males		
	Coal	200	1.0
	Gas	14	0.48 (0.15-1.6)
	Wood	8	0.57 (0.11-3.0)
	Other	2	0

Reference	Study Population	Exposed Cases	Estimated Relative Risk (95% CI)
	Cooking fuel—females		
	Coal	81	1.0
	Gas	8	0.90 (0.24-3.3)
	Wood	3	0.67 (0.04-11.7)
	Other	0	0
	Size of kitchen ventilation opening—males		
	0.0-0.4 m^2	79	1.0
	0.5-0.9 m^2	58	0.77 (0.36-1.7)
	1.0-1.4 m^2	48	0.23 (0.10-0.56)
	1.5-1.9 m^2	19	0.49 (0.16-1.5)
	$\geq$ 2.0 m^2	20	0.15 (0.05-0.44)
			p for trend <0.001
	Size of kitchen ventilation opening—females		
	0.0-0.4 m^2	22	1.0
	0.5-0.9 m^2	27	0.11 (0.02-0.60)
	1.0-1.4 m^2	24	0.13 (0.02-0.74)
	1.5-1.9 m^2	7	0.09 (0.01-0.63)
	$\geq$2.0 m^2	12	0.06 (0.01-0.32)
			p for trend <0.001
Huang et al. 1992	Lung-cancer cases among residents of Sichuan, China		
	Coal-burning indoors	na	1.59 (1.01-2.07)
Chen et al. 1990	135 lung-cancer cases among residents of Taiwan; self-reported agents		
	Cooking fuels: wood and coal		
	Epidermoid carcinoma	na	0.85 (ns)
	Small-cell carcinoma	na	1.08 (ns)
	Adenocarcinoma	na	1.02 (ns)
	Cooking fuels: charcoal, gas, and electricity		
	Epidermoid carcinoma	na	1.00 (ns)
	Small-cell carcinoma	na	1.00 (ns)
	Adenocarcinoma	na	1.00 (ns)
Koo et al. 1983	200 lung-cancer cases among female residents of Hong Kong, China; self-reported agents	na	
	Type of cooking fuel		
	Kerosene		0.75 (0.35-1.58)[d]
	Wood or grass		0.74 (0.37-1.47)[d]
	Liquid-petroleum gas		0.44 (0.29-0.68)[d]
	Gas		1.31 (0.79-2.18)[d]
	Charcoal		0.96 (0.55-1.69)[d]
	Coal		0.32 (0.07-1.32)[d]
	Electricity		3.03 (0.28-76.24)[d]
Occupational Studies of Engine Exhausts			
Cohort Studies—Incidence			
Jarvholm and Silverman 2003	Diesel-exposed construction workers in Sweden (smoking-adjusted)		
	Truck drivers	61	
	SIR reference group: carpenters and electricians		1.29 (0.99-1.65)
	SIR reference group: population		1.14 (0.87-1.46)
	Heavy-construction equipment operators	61	
	SIR reference group: carpenters and electricians		0.87 (0.66-1.11)

Reference	Study Population	Exposed Cases	Estimated Relative Risk (95% CI)
	SIR reference group: population		0.76 (0.58-0.97)
Soll-Johanning et al. 2003	Bus drivers or tramway employees in Copenhagen, Denmark—nested case-control study (smoking-adjusted)		
	No lag time		
	Cumulated employment		
	<3 months	5	0.74 (0.23-2.39)
	3 months-2 yr	29	1.00
	2-<10 yr	54	1.26 (0.69-2.28)
	10-<20 yr	22	1.39 (0.69-2.81)
	20+ yr	43	0.63 (0.32-1.14)
	Diesel-exposed in another job		
	No	80	1.00
	Yes	57	0.85 (0.53-1.36)
	Air-pollution index (ordinal scale—0-10—reflecting level of pollution from bus routes used)		
	Low	14	1.00
	High	41	1.12 (0.40-3.12)
	>10-yr lag time		
	Cumulated employment		
	<3 months	4	0.50 (0.14-1.81)
	3 months - 2 yr	27	1.00
	2 - <10 yr	45	1.03 (0.54-1.95)
	10 - <20 yr	22	1.34 (0.65-2.77)
	20+ yr	43	0.54 (0.28-1.03)
	Diesel-exposed in another job		
	No	74	1.00
	Yes	49	0.80 (0.48-1.32)
	Air-pollution index		
	Low	14	1.00
	High	39	0.99 (0.36-2.75)
Soll-Johanning et al. 1998	Bus drivers or tramway employees in Copenhagen, Denmark		
	Males		
	Denmark reference	473	1.6 (1.5-1.8)
	Copenhagen reference	473	1.2 (1.1-1.3)
	Time since first employment		
	0-14 yr	35	1.2
	15-29 yr	77	1.55 ($p < 0.001$)
	≥30 yr	361	1.7 ($p < 0.001$)
	Females		
	Denmark reference	15	2.6 (1.5-4.3)
	Copenhagen reference	15	2.2 (1.2-3.6)
	Time since first employment		
	0-14 yr	3	1.3
	15-29 yr	10	3.5 ($p < 0.001$)
	≥30 yr	2	3.8
Guberan et al. 1992	Male commercial drivers in Geneva, Switzerland	64	1.61 (1.29-1.98)
Netterstrom 1988	Male bus drivers in Denmark	15	0.55 (0.33-0.99)

Reference	Study Population	Exposed Cases	Estimated Relative Risk (95% CI)
Cohort Studies—Mortality			
Jarvholm and Silverman 2003	Diesel-exposed construction workers in Sweden (smoking-adjusted)		
	Truck drivers	57	
	SMR reference group: carpenters and electricians		1.37 (1.04-1.78)
	SMR reference group: population		1.18 (0.89-1.53)
	Heavy-construction equipment operators	49	
	SMR reference group: carpenters and electricians		0.83 (0.61-1.09)
	SMR reference group: population		0.70 (0.51-0.92)
Borgia et al. 1994	Male taxi drivers in Rome, Italy	76	1.23 (0.97-1.55)[e]
	Age at first enrollment		
	18-44 yr	24	1.30 (0.83-1.93)[e]
	45-54 yr	22	1.16 (0.76-1.83)[e]
	55+ yr	30	1.23 (0.83-1.76)[e]
	Duration of membership		
	0-9 yr	35	1.18 (0.83-1.66)[e]
	10-19 yr	35	1.50 (1.06-2.10)[e]
	20+ yr	6	0.68 (0.25-1.48)[e]
	Time since first enrollment		
	0-9 yr	25	1.37 (0.88-2.02)[e]
	10-19 yr	40	1.44 (1.04-1.98)[e]
	20+ yr	11	0.70 (0.35-1.25)[e]
Alfredsson et al. 1993	Male bus drivers in five counties in Sweden	64	1.0 (0.8-1.3)
Hansen 1993	Male truck drivers in Denmark (compared with other employed men; SES adjusted)		
	All respiratory cancers	84	1.60 (1.28-1.98)
	Lung cancer	76	1.60 (1.26-2.00)
Guberan et al. 1992	Commercial drivers in Geneva, Switzerland (compared with active unskilled workers)	77	1.50 (1.23-1.81)
	Time from first exposure		
	0-14 yr	2	0.67 (0.08-2.41)[e]
	15-24 yr	11	1.18 (0.59-2.12)[e]
	25-34 yr	24	1.30 (0.83-1.93)[e]
	35-44 yr	21	1.35 (0.84-2.07)[e]
	45+ yr	21	2.59 (1.60-3.96)[e]
			p for trend <0.02
Rafnsson and Gunnarsdottir 1991	Taxi and truck drivers in Reykjavik, Iceland		
	Truck drivers only (no other occupation)	24	2.14 (1.37-3.18)
	Duration of employment (ever worked)		
	<2 yr	na	2.70 (0.74-6.92)
	2-10 yr	na	2.46 (0.99-5.08)
	11-30 yr	na	0.68 (0.01-3.76)
	>30 yr	na	2.32 (0.85-5.04)
	Any	na	2.09 (1.32-3.13)
	Taxi drivers only (no other occupation)	12	1.39 (0.72-2.43)
	Duration of employment (ever worked)		

Reference	Study Population	Exposed Cases	Estimated Relative Risk (95% CI)
	<2 yr	na	0
	2-10 yr	na	0.59 (0.02-3.30)
	11-30 yr	na	0
	>30 yr	na	1.60 (0.33-4.66)
	Any	na	0.84 (0.23-2.16)
Paradis et al. 1989	Male bus drivers in Montreal, Canada	78	0.92 (0.73-1.14)
	<30 yr duration	34	1.01 (0.70-1.38)
	≥30 yr duration	44	0.85 (0.62-1.13)
Stern et al. 1981	Motor vehicle examiners in New Jersey—respiratory-system cancer	16	1.02 (0.58-1.65)[e]
Kaplan 1959	Baltimore and Ohio Railroad workers		
	Directly exposed occupations	49	0.88 (0.65-1.16)[f]
	Less-exposed occupations	67	0.72 (0.56-0.91)[f]
	Rarely exposed occupations	38	0.89 (0.64-1.24)[f]
Case-Control Studies			
Menvielle et al. 2003	228 lung-cancer cases among residents of New Caledonia; self-reported job titles and industrial-hygienist-assigned exposure to specific agents (smoking-adjusted)		
	Dockers	22	1.1 (0.5-2.3)
	<5 yr	10	0.5 (0.2-1.4)
	5+ yr	12	3.3 (1.0-10.7)
	Transportation-equipment managers	23	1.0 (0.5-2.0)
	<5 yr	18	0.8 (0.4-1.6)
	5+ yr	5	5.8 (1.1-30.7)
	Motor-bus, lorry, and van drivers	13	2.7 (1.1-7.0)
	<15 yr	8	2.1 (0.7-22.1)
	15+ yr	5	4.7 (1.0-22.1)
	Diesel-engine emissions	88	0.8 (0.5-1.2)
	PAHs from any source	124	0.8 (0.5-1.4)
Bruske-Hohlfeld et al. 2000	3,498 pooled lung-cancer cases among residents of East and West Germany; self-reported agents and job titles (smoking-adjusted)		
	Transport worker and freight handler	1,203	1.28 (1.13-1.45)
	Diesel-engine exhaust, ever exposed	716	1.43 (1.23-1.67)
	>0-3 yr	132	1.28 (0.95-1.73)
	>3-10 yr	155	1.21 (0.91-1.61)
	>10-20 yr	165	1.84 (1.34-2.52)
	>20-30 yr	148	1.62 (1.16-2.24)
	>30 yr	116	1.35 (0.95-1.93)
	PAHs, ever exposed	181	1.53 (1.14-2.04)
	>0-3 yr	40	1.16 (0.68-1.98)
	>3-10 yr	58	2.02 (1.17-3.48)
	>10-20 yr	36	2.03 (0.96-4.31)
	>20-30 yr	23	1.40 (0.65-3.01)
	>30 yr	24	1.16 (0.54-2.52)
	Cumulative PAH exposure		
	>0-20 benzo[a]pyrene-yr	80	1.15 (0.77-1.71)
	>20 benzo[a]pyrene-yr	101	2.09 (1.36-3.22)

Reference	Study Population	Exposed Cases	Estimated Relative Risk (95% CI)
Bruske-Hohlfeld et al. 1999	3,498 pooled lung-cancer cases among residents of East and West Germany; professional drivers, self-reported job titles (smoking-adjusted)		
	West Germany, ever exposed	412	1.44 (1.18-1.76)
	>0-3 yr	89	1.69 (1.13-2.53)
	>3-10 yr	94	1.09 (0.76-1.58)
	>10-20 yr	102	2.02 (1.32-3.08)
	>20-30 yr	68	1.15 (0.74-1.80)
	>30 yr	59	1.51 (0.90-2.52)
	East Germany, ever exposed	122	0.83 (0.60-1.14)
	>0-3 yr	17	0.60 (0.30-1.20)
	>3-10 yr	24	1.02 (0.51-2.04)
	>10-20 yr	28	1.02 (0.52-2.00)
	>20-30 yr	28	0.95 (0.48-1.86)
	>30 yr	25	0.67 (0.34-1.30)
Jockel et al. 1998	1,004 lung-cancer cases among residents of Bremen and Frankfurt, West Germany; self-reported job titles (smoking-adjusted)		
	Docker and freight handler	53	1.95 (1.11-3.42)
Matos et al. 2000	199 lung-cancer cases among male residents of Buenos Aires, Argentina (adjusted for other occupations); self-reported job titles (smoking-adjusted)		
	Motor-vehicle drivers	28	0.7 (0.4-1.2)
	Truck drivers	13	1.5 (0.6-3.4)
	Railway transport	8	0.9 (0.4-2.3)
	PAH exposure		
	Ever		
	Any duration of exposure	70	0.9 (0.6-1.4)
	10+ yr of exposure	49	1.2 (0.7-2.1)
	Probable		
	Any duration of exposure	26	0.6 (0.3-1.2)
	10+ yr of exposure	19	1.2 (0.6-2.6)
	Definite		
	Any duration of exposure	50	1.0 (0.6-1.6)
	10+ yr of exposure	34	1.2 (0.7-2.2)
Hansen et al. 1998	28,744 lung-cancer cases among male residents of Denmark (adjusted for SES, not smoking); job titles		
	Lorry and bus drivers		
	Duration of employment, no lag		
	<0.5 yr	na	1.0 (0.8-1.3)
	0.5-1 yr	na	1.3 (0.9-1.7)
	1-5 yr	na	1.4 (1.1-1.6)
	>5 yr	na	1.4 (1.1-1.7)
	Duration of employment, 10-yr lag		
	<0.5 yr	na	1.1 (0.9-1.4)
	0.5-1 yr	na	1.2 (0.8-1.6)
	1-5 yr	na	1.4 (1.1-1.7)
	>5 yr	na	1.4 (1.1-1.8)
	Taxi drivers		
	Duration of employment, no lag		
	<0.5 yr	na	0.7 (0.4-1.2)

Reference	Study Population	Exposed Cases	Estimated Relative Risk (95% CI)
	0.5-1 yr	na	1.6 (0.8-3.2)
	1-5 yr	na	1.7 (1.0-2.9)
	>5 yr	na	2.2 (1.1-4.7)
	Duration of employment, 10-yr lag		
	<0.5 yr	na	1.0 (0.5-1.7)
	0.5-1 yr	na	1.6 (0.8-3.4)
	1-5 yr	na	1.8 (1.0-3.2)
	>5 yr	na	3.0 (1.2-6.8)
Steenland et al. 1998	996 lung-cancer cases among male truck drivers in US Teamsters Union (smoking-adjusted)		
	Assumed emissions in 1970; 5-yr lag		
	0-169 μg/m^3-yr	na	1.08 (0.72-1.63)
	169-257 μg/m^3-yr	na	1.10 (0.74-1.65)
	257-331 μg/m^3-yr	na	1.36 (0.90-2.04)
	331+ μg/m^3-yr	na	1.64 (1.09-2.49)
	Increase across interquartile range (169-331 μg/m^3-yr)	na	1.71 (1.08-2.34)[f]
	Occupation category (geometric mean exposure to elemental carbon, μg/m^3), next-of-kin report		
	Dockworkers (1.3)	na	0.93 (0.55-1.55)
	Long-haul drivers (3.8)	na	1.27 (0.83-1.93)
	Short-haul drivers (4.0)	na	1.31 (0.81-2.11)
	Mechanics (12.1)	na	1.69 (0.92-3.09)
Steenland et al. 1990	996 lung-cancer cases among male truck drivers in the US Teamsters Union (smoking-adjusted)		
	Diesel-truck driver		
	1-24 yr employment	48	1.27 (0.70-2.27)
	25-34 yr employment	72	1.26 (0.74-2.16)
	35+ yr employment	56	1.89 (1.04-3.42)
	Gasoline-truck driver		
	1-24 yr employment	72	1.24 (0.74-2.16)
	25-34 yr employment	87	1.10 (0.67-1.80)
	35+ yr employment	86	1.34 (0.81-2.22)
	Drove both truck types		
	1-24 yr employment	50	1.27 (0.71-2.26)
	25-34 yr employment	95	1.15 (0.70-1.90)
	35+ yr employment	102	1.34 (0.81-2.20)
	Diesel-exposed, non-truck drivers		
	Teamster data	na	1.44 (0.88-2.39)
	Next-of-kin data	na	1.54 (0.93-2.15)
Bovenzi et al. 1993	756 lung-cancer cases among male residents of northeastern Italy; next-of-kin reports (smoking-adjusted)		
	Shipyard workers	74	2.40 (1.54-3.74)
	Dockworkers	32	2.13 (1.13-4.04)
Swanson et al. 1993	3,792 lung-cancer cases among male residents of Detroit, Michigan; self-reported job titles (smoking-adjusted)		
	White males		
	Drivers of heavy trucks		
	0 yr employed	88	1.0
	1-9 yr	78	1.4 (0.8-2.4)
	10-19 yr	38	1.6 (0.8-3.5)

Reference	Study Population	Exposed Cases	Estimated Relative Risk (95% CI)
	20+ yr	121	2.5 (1.4-4.4) p for trend <0.05
	Drivers of light trucks		
	0 yr employed	88	1.0
	1-9 yr	46	1.7 (0.9-3.3)
	10+ yr	36	2.1 (0.9-4.6) p for trend <0.05
	Garage and service-station workers		
	0 yr employed	88	1.0
	1-9 yr	47	2.2 (1.1-4.4)
	10+ yr	7	2.3 (0.5-10.8)
	Black males		
	Drivers of heavy trucks		
	0 yr employed	12	1.0
	1-9 yr	27	2.7 (0.8-9.2)
	10-19 yr	16	1.9 (0.5-7.2)
	20+ yr	16	2.1 (0.5-9.2)
	Drivers of light trucks		
	0 yr employed	12	1.0
	1-9 yr	11	1.7 (0.4-7.7)
	10+ yr	8	1.4 (0.3-7.7)
	Garage and service-station workers		
	0 yr employed	12	1.0
	1-9 yr	8	1.7 (0.3-8.7)
	10+ yr	9	6.8 (0.7-70.8)
Hayes et al. 1989	1,444 lung-cancer cases among residents pooled from case-control studies in Florida, New Jersey, and Louisiana; job titles (smoking-adjusted)		
	Driver or operator: truck		
	No employment	1,099	1.0
	<10 yr employment	196	0.9 (0.8-1.2)
	10+ yr employment	147	1.5 (1.1-1.9)
	Driver or operator: heavy equipment		
	No employment	1,413	1.0
	<10 yr employment	17	1.0 (0.5-2.1)
	10+ yr employment	14	1.3 (0.6-3.1)
	Driver or operator: bus		
	No employment	1,368	1.0
	<10 yr employment	38	1.1 (0.6-1.7)
	10+ yr employment	38	1.6 (0.9-2.8)
	Driver or operator: taxi and chauffeur		
	No employment	1,386	1.0
	<10 yr employment	40	2.5 (1.4-4.8)
	10+ yr employment	16	1.2 (0.5-2.6)
	Driver or operator: other		
	No employment	1,429	1.0
	<10 yr employment	13	1.0 (0.4-2.3)
	10+ yr employment	2	0.2 (0.0-1.6)
Vineis et al. 1988	2,973 lung-cancer cases among residents pooled from case-control studies in Louisiana, Florida, Pennsylvania, Virginia, and New Jersey; job titles (smoking-adjusted)		
	Truck drivers	433	1.1 (0.9-1.3)

Reference	Study Population	Exposed Cases	Estimated Relative Risk (95% CI)
Zahm et al. 1989	4,431 lung-cancer cases among white male residents of Missouri; job titles (smoking-adjusted)		
	Motor-vehicle drivers	186	1.5 (1.2-1.8)
	Railroad and sea occupations	30	1.4 (0.8-2.3)
	Freight, stock, and garbage handlers	19	1.9 (0.9-4.0)
Benhamou et al. 1988	1,625 lung-cancer cases among residents of France; self-reported job titles (smoking-adjusted)		
	Transport-equipment operators	157	1.35 (1.05-1.75)
	Motor-vehicle drivers	128	1.42 (1.07-1.89)
Damber and Larsson 1987	456 lung-cancer cases among male residents of northern Sweden; self-reported job titles (smoking-adjusted)		
	Professional drivers		
	≥1 yr	63	1.0 (0.7-1.6)
	≥20 yr	33	1.1 (0.6-2.2)
Lerchen et al. 1987	506 lung-cancer cases among residents of New Mexico; self-reported job titles or exposures (smoking-adjusted)		
	Diesel-engine mechanics, ever worked	5	0.6 (0.2-2.0)
	Engineers and firemen, ever worked	2	0.6 (0.1-3.3)
	Diesel-exhaust fumes	7	0.6 (0.2-1.6)
Buiatti et al. 1985	376 lung cancer cases among residents of Florence, Italy; self-reported job titles (smoking-adjusted)		
	Transportation, ever worked	45	1.1 (0.7-1.6)
	Taxi driving, ever worked	20	1.8 (1.0-3.4)
	Train conductor, ever worked	7	1.4 (0.5-3.9)
Diesel Exhaust and PAHs			
Cohort Studies—Incidence			
Boffetta et al. 2001	Residents of Sweden—diesel-engine emissions		
	Males	6,266	1.09 (1.06-1.12)
	Probability of exposure		
	Low	2,222	1.1 (1.04-1.13)
	Medium	1,881	0.90 (0.86-0.94)
	High	1,841	1.2 (1.10-1.21)
	Intensity of exposure		
	Low	3,705	0.95 (0.92-0.98)
	Medium	1,181	1.1 (1.08-1.21)
	High	1,058	1.3 (1.26-1.42)
	Females	57	1.09 (0.83-1.42)
	Probability of exposure		
	Low	32	0.85 (0.60-1.20)
	Medium	6	0.62 (0.28-1.39)
	High	13	1.1 (0.61-1.82)
	Intensity of exposure		
	Low	38	0.80 (0.58-1.10)
	Medium-high	13	1.1 (0.62-1.84)
Van Loon et al. 1997	Residents of Netherlands—Netherlands Cohort Study on Diet and Cancer		

Reference	Study Population	Exposed Cases	Estimated Relative Risk (95% CI)
	Occupational exposure to PAHs—adjusted for age only		
	No exposure	487	1.0
	1 tertile (low)	10	1.44 (0.67-3.09)
	2 tertile	12	1.61 (0.78-3.34)
	3 tertile (high)	12	1.35 (0.66-2.76)
			p for trend = 0.07
	Occupational exposure to PAHs—adjusted for age and other occupational exposures		
	No exposure	487	1.0
	1 tertile (low)	10	1.32 (0.60-2.89)
	2 tertile	12	1.09 (0.49-2.40)
	3 tertile (high)	12	0.63 (0.25-1.58)
			p for trend = 0.45
	Occupational exposure to PAHs—adjusted for age, other occupational exposures, smoking, and vitamin intake (smoking-adjusted)		
	No exposure	487	1.0
	1 tertile (low)	10	0.53 (0.13-2.14)
	2 tertile	12	0.83 (0.32-2.20)
	3 tertile (high)	12	0.28 (0.09-0.89)
			p for trend <0.01
Van Den Eeden and Friedman 1993	Residents of northern California—engine-exhaust fumes (smoking-adjusted)		
	Past year	na	1.13 (0.93-1.36)
	Past year and before	na	1.02 (0.81-1.29)
Cohort Studies—Mortality			
Baris et al. 2001	Male firefighters in Philadelphia, Pennsylvania	162	1.13 (0.97-1.32)
	Cumulative runs (emergency response to a fire or false-alarm) with diesel exposure		
	Low (1-259 runs)	12	0.97 (0.53-1.79)
	Medium (260-1,422 runs)	17	1.17 (0.68-2.02)
	High (≥ 1,423 runs)	12	1.01 (0.51-2.01)
Larkin et al. 2000	Railroad workers in US—diesel exhaust-exposed (vs unexposed workers with indirect adjustment for smoking) (smoking-adjusted)	na	
	40-44 yr old at time of entry into cohort		1.44 (1.01-2.05)
	45-49 yr old at time of entry into cohort		1.12 (0.81-1.54)
	50-54 yr old at time of entry into cohort		1.04 (0.77-1.41)
	55-59 yr old at time of entry into cohort		1.18 (0.92-1.51)
Garshick et al. 1988	Railroad workers in the US—Diesel exhaust exposed (vs. unexposed workers)	na	
	40-44 yr old at time of entry into cohort		1.45 (1.11-1.89)
	45-49 yr old		1.33 (1.03-1.73)
	50-54 yr old		1.12 (0.88-1.42)
	55-59 yr old		1.18 (0.94-1.50)
	60-64 yr old		0.99 (0.74-1.33)
Saverin et al. 1999	Potash miners in South Harz Mountains of Germany—Exposure to diesel exhaust (smoking distributed evenly across		

Reference	Study Population	Exposed Cases	Estimated Relative Risk (95% CI)
	exposure groups)		
	East Germany reference	38	0.78 (0.55-1.07)
	Internal workshop reference	38	2.17 (0.79-5.99)
	Rate ratio for exposure increase of 4.9 mg-yr/m^3 of elemental carbon: Cohort	38	1.68 (0.49-5.8)
	Rate ratio for exposure increase of 4.9 mg-yr/m^3 of elemental carbon: Subcohort of underground workers with stable jobs and >10 yr employment	21	2.70 (0.52-14.1)
Gustavsson et al. 1990	Bus-garage workers in Stockholm, Sweden		
	General-population reference, Stockholm	17	1.15 (0.67-1.84)
	Occupationally active reference, Stockholm	17	1.22 (0.71-1.96)
	Cumulative exposure index to diesel exhaust		
	0-10	5	0.97 (0.31-2.27)[e]
	10-30	5	1.52 (0.49-3.54)[e]
	> 30	7	1.27 (0.51-2.62)[e]
	Cumulative exposure index to diesel exhaust; nested case-control analysis		
	0-10	5	1.0
	10-20	2	1.34 (1.09-1.64)
	20-30	3	1.81 (1.20-2.71)
	> 30	10	2.43 (1.32-4.47)
Boffetta et al. 1988	Male enrollees in American Cancer Society's Cancer Prevention II Study (smoking-adjusted)	174	1.18 (0.97-1.44)
	Duration of diesel-exhaust exposure		
	1-15 yr	na	1.05 (0.80-1.39)
	16+ yr	na	1.21 (0.94-1.56)
	Ever exposed to diesel exhausts		
	Nonsmokers	7	1.73 (0.60-4.95)
	Ex-smokers	85	11.06 (6.27-19.53)
	Current smokers	78	19.82 (11.20-35.07)
	Occupations with presumptive diesel-exhaust exposure		
	Railroad workers	14	1.59 (0.94-2.69)
	Truck drivers	48	1.24 (0.93-1.66)
	Heavy-equipment operators	5	2.60 (1.12-6.06)
Magnani et al. 1988	Residents of England and Wales (adjusted for social class)		
	Diesel fumes, greater than background	na	0.97 (0.94-0.99)
	PAHs, greater than background	na	0.99 (0.97-1.01)
Wong et al. 1985	Members of International Union of Operating Engineers		
	Lung cancer	309	0.99 (0.88-1.10)
	Duration of union membership		
	<5 yr	10	0.45 (0.22-0.83)[e]
	5-9 yr	25	0.75 (0.48-1.11)[e]
	10-14 yr	53	1.08 (0.81-1.42)[e]
	15-19 yr	58	1.02 (0.78-1.33)[e]
	≥20 yr	163	1.07 (0.91-1.25)[e]
	Time since first employment		
	<10 yr	28	0.66 (0.44-0.95)[e]
	10-19 yr	90	0.90 (0.73-1.11)[e]

Reference	Study Population	Exposed Cases	Estimated Relative Risk (95% CI)
	≥20 yr	191	1.12 (0.97-1.29)[e]
Howe et al. 1983	Male pensioners of Canadian National Railway Company—cancers of trachea, bronchus, and lung	933	1.06 (0.99-1.13)[e]
	Diesel fumes		
	Nonexposed	239	1.00
	Possibly exposed	407	1.20 ($p = 0.013$)
	Probably exposed	279	1.35 ($p < 0.001$)
	Conductor	50	1.52 (1.14-2.02)[e]
	Porter	11	2.13 (1.06-3.81)[e]
	Yard helper	14	1.93 (1.05-3.24)[e]
	Unspecified foreman	31	1.62 (1.11-2.32)[e]
	Cook	15	2.09 (1.17-3.45)[e]
Case-Control Studies			
Gustavsson et al. 2000	1,042 lung-cancer cases among residents of Stockholm County, Sweden; industrial-hygienist assigned occupational exposures from self-reported job titles (smoking-adjusted)		
	Diesel exhaust—exposure intensity (μg NO_2/m^3)		
	None	842	1.00
	40-119	134	1.16 (0.90-1.49)
	120-399	43	1.40 (0.90-2.19)
	≥400	3	0.61 (0.16-2.28)
	Motor exhaust (mixed gasoline/diesel)—exposure intensity (mg CO/m^3)		
	None	833	1.00
	1.1-3.3	101	1.22 (0.91-1.63)
	3.4-11.3	60	1.03 (0.72-1.47)
	≥11.4	33	1.31 (0.78-2.19)
	Combustion products—exposure intensity (μg benzo[a]pyrene/m^3)		
	None	824	1.00
	0.05-0.4	46	1.07 (0.72-1.60)
	0.5-4.9	48	1.33 (0.89-2.00)
	≥5	35	2.10 (1.25-3.53)
	Diesel exhaust—cumulative exposure (mg-yr/m^3 of NO_2)		
	None	842	1.00
	>0-0.53	29	0.65 (0.40-1.04)
	0.54-1.41	54	1.13 (0.77-1.66)
	1.42-2.37	45	1.05 (0.70-1.60)
	≥2.38	72	1.63 (1.14-2.33)
	Motor exhaust (mixed gasoline and diesel)—cumulative exposure (mg-yr/m^3 of CO)		
	None	833	1.00
	>0-13.5	19	0.43 (0.25-0.74)
	13.6-38.8	47	1.10 (0.74-1.65)
	38.9-113.6	78	1.32 (0.92-1.90)
	≥113.7	65	1.09 (0.74-1.61)
	Combustion products—cumulative exposure (μg-yr/m^3 of benzo[a]pyrene)		
	None	824	1.00
	>0-2.9	47	1.20 (0.80-1.80)
	3.0-6.6	51	1.05 (0.71-1.57)
	6.7-23.8	47	1.05 (0.69-1.59)

Reference	Study Population	Exposed Cases	Estimated Relative Risk (95% CI)
	≥23.9	73	1.60 (1.09-2.34)
	Diesel exhaust—duration of exposure	na	
	None		1.00
	>0-9 yr		0.76 (0.51-1.13)
	10-29 yr		1.21 (0.88-1.65)
	≥30		1.38 (0.97-1.97)
	Motor exhaust, mixed—duration of exposure	na	
	None		1.00
	> 0-9 yr		0.69 (0.48-0.99)
	10-29 yr		1.15 (0.85-1.57)
	≥30		1.64 (1.14-2.36)
	Combustion products—duration of exposure	na	
	None		1.00
	>0-9 yr		1.42 (0.96-2.10)
	10-29 yr		1.37 (1.01-1.85)
	≥30		1.37 (0.98-1.91)
Muscat et al. 1998	550 lung-cancer cases among black residents of New York, Illinois, Michigan, Pennsylvania, and District of Columbia; self-reported agents and occupations		
	Males		
	Gas fumes	32	0.7 (0.4-1.2)
	Diesel exhaust	11	0.9 (0.3-2.6)
	Coal dust	28	2.8 (1.1-7.0)
	Drivers	59	1.5 (0.9-2.5)
	Highway	39	0.9 (0.4-1.2)
	Mechanics	7	0.6 (0.2-2.1)
	Railroad workers	3	0.7 (0.1-4.1)
	Females		
	Gas fumes	6	7.1 (1.2-41.8)
	Diesel exhaust	0	0
	Coal dust	2	0.5 (0.1-4.8)
	Drivers	2	0
	Highway	1	0.9 (0.0-32.9)
Xu et al. 1996b	610 lung-cancer cases among active or retired employees of Anshan Iron-Steel Complex in Liaoning province, China (smoking-adjusted)		
	Cumulative total B[a]P (mg/m^3-yr)		
	<0.85	72	1.1 (0.8-1.7)
	0.85-1.96	117	1.6 (1.2-2.3)
	1.97-3.2	96	1.6 (1.1-2.3)
	>3.2	105	1.8 (1.2-2.5)
			p for trend = 0.004
Boffetta et al. 1990	2,584 lung-cancer cases among residents of six US cities		
	Self-reported diesel-exhaust exposure		
	None	442	1.00
	Ever	35	1.21 (0.73-2.02)
	1-15 yr	11	0.90 (0.40-1.99)
	16-30 yr	12	1.04 (0.44-2.48)
	31+ yr	12	2.39 (0.87-6.57)
			p for trend = 0.12

Reference	Study Population	Exposed Cases	Estimated Relative Risk (95% CI)
Nadon et al. 1995	857 lung cancer cases among residents of Montreal, Canada—PAH exposures from occupational sources (smoking-adjusted)		
	Benzo[a]pyrene		
	Nonexposed	622	1.0
	Low	160	0.9 (0.7-1.2)
	High	75	1.0 (0.7-1.4)
	Coal		
	Nonexposed	766	1.0
	Low	63	1.1 (0.8-1.6)
	High	28	1.0 (0.6-1.8)
	Petroleum		
	Nonexposed	269	1.0
	Low	395	1.0 (0.8-1.2)
	High	193	1.0 (0.8-1.3)
	Wood		
	Nonexposed	814	1.0
	Low	32	1.3 (0.8-2.0)
	High	11	0.9 (0.4-1.9)
	Other		
	Nonexposed	662	1.0
	Low	141	1.1 (0.8-1.4)
	High	54	0.8 (0.6-1.2)
	Total		
	Nonexposed	230	1.0
	Low	418	1.0 (0.8-1.3)
	High	209	1.0 (0.8-1.3)
Emmelin et al. 1993	50 lung-cancer cases among dock workers in Sweden, surrogate exposures to diesel exhaust (smoking-adjusted)		
	Machine time		
	Low	9	1.0
	Medium	27	1.2 (0.4-4.2)
	High	14	1.3 (0.3-5.6)
	Fuel		
	Low	10	1.0
	Medium	25	1.1 (0.4-3.2)
	High	15	1.7 (0.5-5.9)
	Exposed time		
	Low	12	1.0
	Medium	19	1.6 (0.5-5.1)
	High	19	2.9 (0.8-10.7)
Garshick et al. 1987	1,256 lung-cancer cases among US railroad workers; industrial-hygiene-derived agents (smoking-adjusted)		
	Diesel-yr (continuous variable)		
	Age ≤ 64	215	1.41 (1.06-1.88)
	Age ≥ 65	441	0.91 (0.71-1.17)
Gulf War Veterans			
Smith et al. 2002	US Gulf War veterans—oil-well fire smoke (exposed vs nonexposed)	49	1.10 (0.56-2.17)

NOTE: na=not available.
All SMRs and SIRs adjusted for age and calendar year unless otherwise noted.
[a] Data provided by Pope from Figure 5.

[b] Unadjusted ORs and 95% CIs calculated with standard methods from observed numbers presented in original paper.
[c] 95% CIs calculated with standard methods from regression-model parameters presented in original paper.
[d] 95% CIs calculated with standard methods from observed numbers presented in the original paper.
[e] 95% CIs calculated with standard methods from observed and expected numbers presented in the original paper.
[f] Unadjusted risk estimates and 95% CI were calculated with standard methods from observed and expected numbers presented in original paper.

TABLE 4.21 Melanoma Skin Cancer and Exposure to Fuels—Selected Epidemiologic Studies

Reference	Study Population	Exposed Cases	Estimated Relative Risk (95% CI)
Cohort Studies			
Workers for Imperial Oil, Canada; total HCs from solvents or fuels industrial-hygiene-derived from job histories (ppm-yr)			
Lewis et al. 2000b	Melanoma deaths in 1964-1994 among 34,560 workers employed any time during 1964-1983		
	Females	1	0.39 (0.01-2.16)[a]
	Males	22	1.32 (0.83-2.00)
	Refinery	4	0.65 (0.18-1.66)
	Marketing or distribution	8	1.59 (0.69-3.14)
	5-14 yr, ≥20-yr latency	1	2.70 (0.07-15.05)[a]
	15-24 yr, ≥20-yr latency	3	3.45 (0.71-10.08)[a]
	25-34 yr, ≥20-yr latency	2	1.27 (0.15-4.60)[a]
	>34 yr, ≥20-yr latency	0	0.00 (0.0-4.19)[a]
	Upstream (exploration, drilling, production, or pipeline)		
		7	2.82 (1.13-5.81)
Schnatter et al. 1992	Melanoma deaths in 1964-1983	16	1.87 (1.07-3.04)
	Females	1	0.91
	Males	15	
	Refinery	3	1.00 (0.21-2.92)[a]
	Marketing/distribution	6	2.56 (0.94-5.57)
	Upstream	6	6.00 (2.19-13.06)
	Unexposed	2	6.62 (0.80-23.92)
	Exposed to HCs	3	5.48 (1.13-16.03)
	Unknown exposure status	1	6.64 (0.17-36.90)
Lewis et al. 2003	Incident melanoma cases in 1969-1994 among 25,292 workers hired in 1964-1983		
	Females	16	1.46 (0.83-2.37)
	Males	26	1.25 (0.82-1.83)
	Unexposed to HCs	10	1.0
	>0->2.5 ppm-yr	6	1.1 (0.4-3.0)
	≥2.5->30.0 ppm-yr	6	1.2 (0.4-3.4)
	≥30.0 ppm-yr	4	0.6 (0.2-2.1)
Jarvholm et al. 1997	4,128 male workers in Swedish petroleum industry for at least 1 yr (qualitative industrial-hygiene-interpretation of personnel records)		
	Incident cases of melanoma (1958-1991) (all <20 yr latency)	7	1.1 (0.49-2.0)[b]
Nelson et al. 1987	Skin-cancer deaths through 1982 among 9,187 white male workers employed at 10 Amoco refineries in	11	2.01 (1.00-3.60)

Reference	Study Population	Exposed Cases	Estimated Relative Risk (95% CI)
	1970-1980; exposures by industrial-hygiene review of personnel records described in Nelson et al. (1985)		
	By job type		
	Administrative	1	0.89
	Maintenance	8	3.78, $p < 0.05$
	Operations	2	0.95
	Exposure to refinery processes		
	Occasional	1	1.59, ns
	Routine	10	2.68, $p < 0.05$
	By latenct period		
	<15 yr	na	5.24, $p < 0.05$
	≥15 yr	na	1.53, ns

NOTE: HC=hydrocarbon; na=not available; ns=estimated risk greater than unity not significant at 0.05 level.
[a] Risk estimates and 95% CIs calculated with standard methods from observed and expected numbers presented in original paper.
[b] This article reported 90% CIs.

TABLE 4.22 Melanoma Skin Cancer and Exposure to Combustion Products—Selected Epidemiologic Studies

Reference	Study Population	Exposed Cases	Estimated Relative Risk (95% CI)
Cohort Studies			
Boffetta et al. 2001	Cohort defined as those exposed to diesel emissions within Swedish Cancer Environment Registry of occupationally active residents of Sweden, 1960 and 1970—record-linkage approach (agent coded by JEM from 1960 occupation)		
	Melanoma cases (1971-1989)		
	Men	1,272	0.88 (0.83-0.93)
	Women	37	0.87 (0.61-1.19)
Cohort of ACS Cancer Prevention II Study			
Boffetta et al. 1988	Melanoma deaths among 369,943 male enrollees 40-79 yr old at 2-yr followup— Diesel engine exhaust (self-reported agent)	11	1.67, ns
Pion et al. 1995	2,780 melanoma cases among male and female enrollees at 6-yr followup		
	Self-reported agents		
	Coal tar, pitch, asphalt	na	0.90 (0.64-1.25)
	Diesel-engine exhaust	na	0.97 (0.82-1.15)
	Gasoline exhaust	na	0.99 (0.87-1.13)
	Occupation, males only		
	Truck driver	14	0.72 (0.40-1.30)
	Fireman	7	2.29 (0.85-6.16)
Case-Control Studies			
Multicancer case-control study in Montreal, Canada (industrial-hygiene-coded agents from interview)			
Siemiatycki et al. 1988	121 male melanoma cases vs 2,737 cancer controls		
	Gasoline exhaust	43	0.9 (0.7-1.2) [a]
	Diesel exhaust	17	1.1 (0.7-1.7) [a]

Reference	Study Population	Exposed Cases	Estimated Relative Risk (95% CI)
	Jet-fuel exhaust	3	1.8 (0.5-6.4)[a]
	Liquid-fuel combustion	8	1.8 (0.9-3.4)[a]
	Coke combustion	0	0.0 (0.0-1.9)[a]
	Propane exhaust	5	3.3 (1.2-9.0)[a]
Fritschi and Siemiatycki 1996a	103 male melanoma cases vs 533 cancer and 533 population controls pooled		
	Gasoline engine emissions	37	1.1 (0.7–1.8)
	Carbon monoxide	42	1.0 (0.6–1.5)
	PAHs from petroleum	54	0.9 (0.6–1.4)
Linet et al. 1995	3,850 male melanoma cases (1961-1979) from Swedish Cancer Environment Registry of occupationally active residents of Sweden in 1960—record-linkage approach (occupation and industry from 1960 census)		
	Transportation (industry)	327	1.0
	Transport	251	1.0
	Transport-associated	31	0.9
	Post office and telecommunications	45	0.9
	Transport and communications (occupation)	281	0.9
	Ship's officers	17	1.0
	Deck and machine-crew work	13	1.0
	Aeronautics	4	2.7, ns
	Locomotive engineers and other railroad or highway	168	0.8
	Traffic administration	23	1.6, $p < 0.05$
	Traffic enforcement and railroad work	18	3.1, $p < 0.01$
	Post office and telecommunications	14	1.6, ns
	Postal and other messenger work	34	1.9, ns
	Other transport and communications	7	1.0
Nelemans et al. 1993	140 melanoma cases among residents of mideastern part of Netherlands (industry from interview work history)		
	Petrochemical	1	–
	Transportation or communication		
	Ever vs never this industry	44	1.70 (0.84-3.46)
	Ever vs never any high-risk industry	44	1.92 (0.84-4.35)
Decoufle and Stanislawczyk 1977	Male melanoma cases among patients at Roswell Park Memorial Institute in Buffalo, New York		
	Bus drivers	0	–
	Taxicab drivers and chauffeurs	1	3.51
	Truck and tractor drivers	2	1.24
	Bus, taxicab, or truck drivers, exposed 5+ yr	2	1.68
	Delivery and routemen	1	1.92
	Locomotive engineers and firemen	3	9.70
	Exposed 5+ yr	2	9.07
	Mechanics and repairmen	4	1.81
	Exposed 5+ yr	4	2.33
	Mine operatives and laborers	3	6.78

Reference	Study Population	Exposed Cases	Estimated Relative Risk (95% CI)
	Exposed 5+ yr	2	5.10
	Excavating, grading, and road machinery operators	2	9.92

NOTE: na=not available; ns=risk estimate greater than unity not significant at 0.05 level.
[a] This article reported 90% CIs.

TABLE 4.23 Non-Melanoma Skin Cancer and Exposure to Fuels—Selected Epidemiologic Studies

Reference	Study Population	Exposed Cases	Estimated Relative Risk (95% CI)
Cohort Study—Incidence (not smoking-adjusted)			
Jarvholm et al. 1997	Male workers in the Swedish petroleum industry ≥1 yr (qualitative industrial-hygiene-interpretation of personnel records)		
	Cases of nonmelanoma skin cancer	7	1.3 (0.61-2.4)[a]
	With ≥20-yr latency	6	1.8 (0.77-3.5)[a]
	With ≥10-yr duration	3	0.97 (0.26-2.5)[a]
Case-Control Studies-Incidence (none smoking-adjusted)			
Gallagher et al. 1996	Nonmelanoma skin cancers among male residents of Alberta, Canada; self-reported agents		
	226 BCCs-ever exposed to petroleum products (gasoline and oil)	88	0.9 (0.6-1.3)
	180 SCCs-ever exposed to petroleum products (gasoline and oil)	91	1.3 (1.0-2.0)
Kubasiewicz et al. 1991	376 skin cancer cases among male residents of Lodz, Poland; self-reported agents		
	Petrol ever exposed	71	1.30, ns
	Petroleum ever exposed	57	1.17, ns
	Gasoline ever exposed	Too sparse to report	–

NOTE: ns=estimated risk greater than unity not significant at 0.05 level.
[a] This article reported 90% CIs.

TABLE 4.24 Non-Melanoma Skin Cancer and Exposure to Combustion Products—Selected Epidemiologic Studies

Reference	Study Population	Exposed Cases	Estimated Relative Risk (95% CI)
Case-Control Studies (none smoking-adjusted)			
Hannuksela-Svahn et al. 1999	Nonmelanoma skin cancers diagnosed in 1971-1995 among residents of Finland born in 1906-1945—record linkage approach (main occupation from 1970 census)		
	Basal-cell carcinoma		
	49,910 male		
	Transportation and communication	1,910	1.0 (1.0-1.1)
	Engine drivers	na	1.6
	70,320 female		
	Transportation and communication	542	1.0 (0.9-1.1)
	Other non-melanoma skin cancer cases (predominantly squamous cell carcinomas)		
	8,380 male		

Reference	Study Population	Exposed Cases	Estimated Relative Risk (95% CI)
	Transportation and communication	232	0.9 (0.8-1.0)
	9,395 female		
	Transportation and communication	61	1.1 (0.9-1.4)
Gallagher et al. 1996	Nonmelanoma skin cancers among male residents of Alberta, Canada (self-reported agents)		
	226 basal-cell carcinomas—ever exposed to:		
	Diesel fumes	85	1.1 (0.8-1.6)
	Pitch tar and tar products	32	1.2 (0.7-2.1)
	Grease	84	0.9 (0.6-1.3)
	Coal dust	67	1.4 (0.9-2.1)
	180 squamous-cell carcinomas—ever exposed to:		
	Diesel fumes	83	1.7 (1.1-2.5)
	Pitch tar and tar products	27	0.9 (0.5-1.7)
	Grease	94	1.4 (0.9-2.1)
	Coal dust	69	1.6 (1.0-2.4)
Kubasiewicz et al. 1991	376 skin-cancer cases among male residents of Lodz, Poland		
	PAHs (composite of self-reports on 17 agents)		
	None	160	1.0
	Any (vs population controls)	216	1.15 (0.90-1.51)[a]
	>0-9 yr	49	1.43, ns
	10-19 yr	42	1.20, ns
	20-29 yr	36	0.78
	30+ yr	89	1.29, ns
	Ever exposed to source of PAHs (self-reported agents)		
	Grease	172	1.15, ns
	Tar	28	1.09, ns
	Pitch	15	0.93
	Soot	29	1.22, ns
	Mineral oils	99	1.46 (1.06-2.05)
	Coke	32	1.29, ns
	Paraffin	24	1.81, ns
	Paraffin oils	8	1.45, ns
	Bituminous mass	13	2.03, ns

NOTE: na=not available; ns=estimated risk greater than unity not statistically significant at 0.05%.
[a] 95% CIs calculated with standard methods from observed and expected numbers presented in original paper.

TABLE 4.25 Female Breast Cancer and Exposure to Fuels—Selected Epidemiologic Studies

Reference	Study Population	Exposed Cases	Estimated Relative Risk (95% CI)
Cohort Studies			
Lewis et al. 2003	Imperial Oil workers in Canada		
	Mortality	20	1.08 (0.66-1.67)
	Incidence	76	1.02 (0.80-1.28)
Divine et al. 1999b	Texaco mortality study	15	0.71 (0.40-1.18)
Lagorio et al.	Filling-station attendants in Italy (exposure	2	1.04 (0.18-3.28)

Reference	Study Population	Exposed Cases	Estimated Relative Risk (95% CI)
1994	reconstruction using monitoring)		

TABLE 4.26 Female Breast Cancer and Exposure to Combustion Products—Selected Epidemiologic Studies

Reference	Study Population	Exposed Cases	Estimated Relative Risk (95% CI)
Case-Control Studies (not adjusted for smoking)			
Petralia et al. 1999	301 cases among premenopausal female residents of western New York state; JEM-derived agents		
	PAHs (with or without benzene exposure)	38	1.82 (1.02-3.16)
	PAHs (without benzene exposure)	6	1.01 (0.55-3.45)
	PAHs (with benzene exposure)	32	2.01 (1.08-3.75)
	Duration		
	< 4 yr	19	2.25 (0.99-5.09)
	≥ 4 yr	18	1.49 (0.70-3.18)
	Average probability		
	Low	23	1.56 (0.78-3.12)
	Medium to high	14	2.40 (0.96-6.01)
	Intensity		
	Low	26	1.65 (0.85-3.21)
	Medium to high	11	2.25 (0.82-6.13)
	Cumulative exposure		
	Low	26	2.10 (1.07-4.53)
	Medium to high	11	1.30 (0.54-3.17)
	Latency		
	10-19 yr	12	1.48 (0.59-3.71)
	≥ 20 yr	13	1.78 (0.70-4.52)
Lewis-Michl et al. 1996	627 cases among postmenopausal female residents of Nassau and Suffolk counties, New York; geographic-information-system-derived exposures (fully adjusted)		
	Nassau—401 cases		
	Chemical or other facilities in residence grid	127	1.11 (0.83-1.48)
	Chemical facilities in residence grid	58	1.61 (1.06-2.43)
	Only other facilities in residence grid	69	1.08 (0.80-1.46)
	High-density traffic	33	1.29 (0.77-2.15)
	Suffolk—226 cases		
	Chemical or other facilities in residence grid	44	1.12 (0.72-1.74)
	Chemical facilities in residence grid	14	1.58 (0.71-3.51)
	Only other facilities in residence grid	30	0.99 (0.62-1.56)
	High-density traffic	11	0.89 (0.40-1.99)

TABLE 4.27 Male Breast Cancer and Exposure to Fuels—Selected Epidemiologic Studies

Reference	Study Population	Exposed Cases	Estimated Relative Risk (95% CI)
Case-Control Study (not adjusted for smoking)			
Hansen 2000	230 cases among male residents of Denmark; exposure derived from job title and white- or blue-collar worker status		
	Gasoline and combustion products		
	No lag	19	2.2 (1.4-3.6)
	Period of first exposure		
	<1965	10	2.6 (1.3-4.9)
	1965-1974	8	2.0 (1.0-4.2)
	1975-1989	1	1.5 (0.2-10.1)
	Age at first exposure		
	<40 yr	9	3.7 (1.7-7.9)
	40-66 yr	10	1.7 (0.9-3.4)
	10 yr lag	12	2.5 (1.3-4.5)
	Period of first exposure		
	<1965	8	2.8 (1.4-5.5)
	1965-1974	4	2.0 (1.0-4.0)
	1975-1989	0	—
	Age at first exposure		
	<40 yr	8	5.4 (2.4-11.9)
	40-66 yr	4	1.2 (0.4-3.3)

TABLE 4.28 Male Breast Cancer and Exposure to Combustion Products—Selected Epidemiologic Studies

Reference	Study Population	Exposed Cases	Estimated Relative Risk (95% CI)
Case-Control Studies			
Hansen 2000	230 cases among male residents of Denmark; exposure derived from job title and white- or blue-collar worker status (not smoking-adjusted)		
	Gasoline and combustion products		
	No lag time	19	2.2 (1.4-3.6)
	Period of first exposure		
	<1965	10	2.6 (1.3-4.9)
	1965-1974	8	2.0 (1.0-4.2)
	1975-1989	1	1.5 (0.2-10.1)
	Age at first exposure		
	<40 yr	9	3.7 (1.7-7.9)
	40-66 yr	10	1.7 (0.9-3.4)
	10-yr lag time	12	2.5 (1.3-4.5)
	Period of first exposure		
	<1965	8	2.8 (1.4-5.5)
	1965-1974	4	2.0 (1.0-4.0)
	Age at first exposure		
	<40 yr	8	5.4 (2.4-11.9)
	40-66 yr	4	1.2 (0.4-3.3)
Cocco et al. 1998	178 cases among male residents of US; job titles, JEM-derived agents (smoking-adjusted)		
	PAHs		
	Nonexposed	135	1.0

Reference	Study Population	Exposed Cases	Estimated Relative Risk (95% CI)
	Probability of exposure		
	Low	13	1.3 (0.7-2.6)
	Medium	7	0.6 (0.3-1.5)
	High	23	0.7 (0.4-1.2)
	Intensity of exposure		
	Low	25	0.7 (0.5-1.2)
	Medium	12	1.0 (0.5-2.1)
	High	6	1.0 (0.4-2.5)
	Taxicab drivers	3	4.8 (1.1-20.1)
	Motor vehicles and equipment (industry)	7	3.1 (1.2-8.2)
	Railways (industry)	3	1.0 (0.3-3.7)

TABLE 4.29 Female Genital Cancers and Exposure to Fuels—Selected Epidemiologic Studies

Reference	Study Population	Exposed Cases	Estimated Relative Risk (95% CI)
Cohort Studies (not adjusted for smoking)			
Lewis et al. 2003	Cancers 1969-1994 among female Canadian Imperial Oil workers hired in 1964-1994		
	Cervical cancer		
	Incidence	7	0.42 (0.17-0.86)
	Mortality	3	1.01 (0.21-2.95)[a]
	Uterine cancer		
	Incidence	3	0.31 (0.06-0.89)
	Mortality	0	0.00 (0.00-7.24)[a]
	Cancers of the ovary, fallopian tubes, and broad ligaments		
	Incidence	15	1.40 (0.78-2.30)
	Mortality	7	1.74 (0.70-3.58)
Divine et al. 1999b	Texaco mortality study		
	Cervical cancer	1	0.30 (0.00-1.67)
	Uterine cancer	4	1.43 (0.39-3.67)
Nested Case-Control Study (not adjusted for smoking)			
Vasama-Neuvonen et al. 1999	5,072 ovarian-cancer cases nested among occupationally active female residents of Finland; JEM-derived agents		
	Gasoline	na	0.8 (0.2-3.4)
	Low		0.8 (0.4-1.8)
	Medium and high		0.8 (0.2-3.4)

NOTE: na=not available.

[a] Unadjusted risk estimates and 95% CIs calculated with standard methods from observed and expected numbers presented in original paper.

TABLE 4.30 Female Genital Cancers and Exposure to Combustion Products—Selected Epidemiologic Studies

Reference	Study Population	Exposed Cases	Estimated Relative Risk (95% CI)
Case-Control Studies (not adjusted for smoking)			
Velema et al. 2002	366 cervical-cancer cases among female residents of Honduras		
	Exposure to wood smoke (self-reported agent)		
	Grade I neoplasia		
	0 yr	9	1.00
	1-14 yr	20	0.61 (0.20-1.90)
	15-24 yr	10	0.45 (0.13-1.55)
	25+ yr	5	0.32 (0.06-1.58)
			p for trend = 0.105
	Grade II neoplasia		
	0 yr	9	1.00
	1-14 yr	11	0.28 (0.07-1.15)
	15-24 yr	10	0.90 (0.19-4.25)
	25+ yr	6	0.66 (0.08-5.63)
			p for trend = 0.152
	Grade III neoplasia		
	0 yr	9	1.00
	1-14 yr	11	0.36 (0.11-1.18)
	15-24 yr	8	0.35 (0.09-1.39)
	25-34 yr	8	1.34 (0.20-91.8)
	35+ yr	9	4.89 (0.51-47.1)
			p for trend = 0.022
Weiderpass et al. 2001	Finnish women born in 1906-1945 employed according to 1970 census (excluding managerial, clerical, and agricultural); agent exposure determined with Finnish JEM		
	1,101 cervical cancers		
	Diesel-engine exhaust		
	Low	15	1.0 (0.6-1.7)
	High	2	1.7 (0.4-6.8)
	Gasoline-engine exhaust		
	Low	15	1.4 (0.8-2.3)
	High	13	1.3 (0.7-2.2)
	PAHs		
	Low	20	1.3 (0.8-2.1)
	High	2	1.2 (0.3-4.8)
	2,833 endometrial cancers		
	Diesel-engine exhaust		
	Low	20	0.8 (0.5-1.2)
	High	2	0.8 (0.2-3.0)
	Gasoline-engine exhaust		
	Low	22	0.9 (0.6-1.4)
	High	17	0.9 (0.6-1.5)
	PAHs		
	Low	35	1.0 (0.7-1.5)
	High	2	0.6 (0.1-2.2)
Vasama-Neuvonen et al. 1999	5,072 ovarian cancers		
	Diesel-engine exhaust	na	1.3 (0.8-2.2)
	Low		1.3 (0.9-1.8)

Reference	Study Population	Exposed Cases	Estimated Relative Risk (95% CI)
	Medium and high		1.7 (0.7-4.1)
	Gasoline-engine exhaust	na	1.2 (0.8-1.6)
	Low		0.7 (0.4-1.1)
	Medium and high		1.5 (1.0-2.0)
	PAHs	na	0.7 (0.4-1.5)
	Low		0.9 (0.6-1.3)
	Medium and high		0.3 (0.0-2.1)
	Maintenance crew and supervisor	18	1.9 (1.1-3.0)
	Motor vehicle and streetcar driver	6	0.9 (0.3-2.0)

NOTE: na=not available.

TABLE 4.31 Prostatic Cancer and Exposure to Fuels—Selected Epidemiologic Studies

Reference	Study Population	Exposed Cases	Estimated Relative Risk (95% CI)
Cohort Studies (not adjusted for smoking)			
Lewis et al. 2003	Cancers 1969-1994 among male Canadian Imperial Oil workers hired in 1964-1994		
	Prostate cancer		
	Incidence	20	0.67 (0.41-1.03)
	Mortality	1	0.22 (0.01-1.21)[a]
	Testicular cancer		
	Incidence	14	0.82 (0.45-1.37)
	Mortality	3	1.86 (0.38-5.45)[a]
Ritz et al. 1999	Prostatic-cancer cases among white male uranium-processing workers in Fernald, Ohio	24	1.40 (0.90-2.08)
	Kerosene (exposure reconstruction by industrial-hygienists)		
	Light exposure		
	>2 yr duration, no lag	7	0.76 (0.29-2.02)
	>2 yr duration, 15 yr lag	7	0.88 (0.33-2.36)
	>5 yr duration, no lag	6	0.92 (0.32-2.63)
	>5 yr duration, 15 yr lag	6	1.10 (0.37-3.23)
	Moderate exposure		
	>2 yr duration, no lag	6	2.00 (0.54-7.34)
	>2 yr duration, 15 yr lag	6	2.44 (0.69-2.36)
	>5 yr duration, no lag	6	3.69 (0.91-15.0)
	>5 yr duration, 15 yr lag	5	3.40 (0.78-14.8)
Case-Control Study (adjusted for smoking)			
Siemiatycki et al. 1987a	452 prostatic cancer cases among residents of Montreal, Canada; industrial-hygiene-derived agents		
	Automotive gasoline	56	1.0 (0.8-1.2)[b]
	Aviation gasoline	6	0.9 (0.4-2.0)[b]
	Kerosene	34	1.1 (0.8-1.5)[b]
	Jet fuel	4	0.7 (0.2-2.1)[b]
	Diesel fuel	25	1.7 (1.2-2.5)[b]
	Heating oil	26	1.4 (1.0-1.9)[b]
	Crude oil	6	2.3 (0.7-7.1)[b]

[a] Risk estimates and 95% CIs calculated with standard methods from observed and expected numbers presented in original paper.
[b] 90% CIs presented.

TABLE 4.32 Prostatic Cancer and Exposure to Combustion Products—Selected Epidemiologic Studies

Reference	Study Population	Exposed Cases	Estimated Relative Risk (95% CI)
Case-Control Studies (adjusted for smoking, unless noted otherwise)			
Krstev et al. 1998	Prostate cancer cases among residents of Atlanta, GA; Detroit, MI; and 10 counties in NJ; job titles, occupation (not adjusted for smoking)		
	Firefighting (occupation)	10	3.34 (1.13-9.91)
	Railroad transportation (industry)	65	1.66 (1.13-2.44)
	<5 yr	41	1.47 (0.92-2.34)
	5-19 yr	14	1.43 (0.66-3.09)
	≥20 yr	10	6.47 (1.40-29.9)
Aronson et al. 1996	449 prostatic-cancer cases among residents of Montreal, Canada; job titles, industrial-hygiene-derived agents (not adjusted for smoking)		
	Railway transport (industry)		
	<10 yr	19	1.51 (0.88-2.61)
	≥10 yr	32	1.27 (0.83-1.94)
	Mechanics		
	<10 yr	16	1.02 (0.57-1.80)
	≥10 yr	32	1.29 (0.84-1.97)
	Railway-transport workers		
	<10 yr	5	4.47 (1.26-15.83)
	≥10 yr	7	1.81 (0.71-4.58)
	Diesel-engine emissions		
	Nonsubstantial	44	1.54 (1.04-2.27)
	Substantial	32	1.05 (0.68-1.64)
	Propane-engine emissions		
	Nonsubstantial	5	1.88 (0.61-5.75)
	Substantial	8	1.83 (0.77-4.38)
	Liquid-fuel combustion products		
	Nonsubstantial	19	1.51 (0.85-2.70)
	Substantial	20	1.77 (0.98-3.19)
	Soot		
	Nonsubstantial	40	1.25 (0.78-2.01)
	Substantial	10	1.20 (0.52-2.81)
	PAHs from any source		
	Nonsubstantial	238	0.84 (0.63-1.12)
	From coal	40	1.99 (1.24-3.20)
	Substantial	62	1.21 (0.68-2.17)
	From coal	20	1.08 (0.40-2.95)
	Benzo[a]pyrene, substantial	22	0.63 (0.28-1.39)
Siemiatycki et al. 1988	452 prostate cancer cases among residents of Montreal, Canada; industrial-hygiene-derived agents		
	Exhausts		
	Gasoline	197	1.1 (0.9-1.2)[a]
	Diesel	86	1.2 (1.0-1.5)
	Jet fuel	2	0.7 (0.1-5.1)
	Propane	13	1.5 (0.9-2.7)
	Combustion products		
	Propane	17	1.3 (0.8-2.0)
	Natural gas	9	0.8 (0.4-1.4)
	Liquid fuel	39	1.6 (1.2-2.1)

Reference	Study Population	Exposed Cases	Estimated Relative Risk (95% CI)
	Coal	35	1.6 (1.2-2.2)
	Coke	5	1.0 (0.3-2.6)
Seidler et al. 1998	192 prostatic-cancer cases among residents of Hamburg and Frankfurt, Germany		
	Diesel fuel (self-reports)		
	Never	142	1.0
	Occasionally	26	1.0 (0.6-1.9)
	Frequently	24	0.9 (0.5-1.6)
	Diesel fuel and fumes (JEM-derived)		
	0 dose-yr	118	1.0
	>0-25 dose-yr	53	1.1 (0.7-1.8)
	>25 dose-yr	17	3.7 (1.4-9.8)
	PAHs (JEM-derived)		
	0 dose-yr	118	1.0
	>0-25 dose-yr	64	1.6 (1.0-2.4)
	>25 dose-yr	6	1.4 (0.4-4.7)
	Exhaust fumes (JEM-derived)		
	0 dose-yr	48	1.0
	>0-25 dose-yr	102	1.2 (0.8-1.9)
	>25 dose-yr	38	2.4 (1.2-4.7)

NOTE: na=not available; dose-yr = product of intensity, probability, and duration.
[a] 90% CIs reported in this paper.

TABLE 4.33 Brain/CNS Cancers and Exposure to Fuels—Selected Epidemiologic Studies

Reference	Study Population	Exposed Cases	Estimated Relative Risk (95% CI)
Cohort Studies—Mortality (not adjusted for smoking)			
Divine et al. 1999a	Deaths through 1993 among Texaco refinery, petrochemical, or research workers employed for at least 5 yr (with at least 1 day after 1976)		
	Tumors (benign or malignant) of brain and CNS		
	White men	85	1.13 (0.90-1.40)
	Date of hire		
	Before 1950	62	1.13 (0.86-1.45)
	1950 or after	23	1.13 (0.72-1.70)
	Motor-oil unit		
	Ever	11	1.78 (0.88-3.19)
	>5 yr	8	3.26 (1.40-6.43)
Divine et al. 1999b	Cancers of brain and CNS (ICD-8 191-192)		
	White men	64	1.08 (0.83-1.37)
	Duration of employment		
	5-10 yr	8	1.25 (0.54-2.46)
	10-19 yr	14	1.25 (0.68-2.10)
	20-29 yr	16	1.00 (0.57-1.62)
	>30 yr	26	1.00 (0.66-1.47)
	Date of hire		
	Before 1950	48	1.13 (0.83-1.50)
	1950 or after	16	0.95 (0.54-1.54)

Reference	Study Population	Exposed Cases	Estimated Relative Risk (95% CI)
	Motor oil units, >5 yr	6	3.14 (1.15-6.84)
	Nonwhite men	4	2.87 (0.77-7.35)
	Women	1	0.40 (0.01-2.21)
Consonni et al. 1999	Oil-refinery workers in Milan vicinity, Italy	5	2.08 (0.67-4.85)
	Duration of employment		
	0-4 yr	3	3.97 (0.80-11.61)
	5-14 yr	2	2.26 (0.25-8.17)
	15+ yr	0	0.00 (0.00-4.77)
	Time since first hire		
	0-9 yr	3	9.60 (1.93-28.04)
	10-19 yr	2	3.41 (0.38-12.31)
	20-29 yr	0	0.00 (0.00-4.01)
	30+ yr	0	0.00 (0.00-6.18)
Lagorio et al. 1994	Filling-station attendants in Italy—xervous system cancer (exposure reconstruction using monitoring)	6	2.14 (0.93-4.21)
	Subset of smaller stations	5	2.66 (1.05-5.59)
	Men	5	1.95 (0.77-4.11)
	Employed at small stations	4	2.33 (0.79-5.32)
	Women	1	4.00 (0.20-18.98)
	Employed at small stations	1	6.25 (0.32-29.65)
Case-Control Studies (not adjusted for smoking)			
De Roos et al. 2003	479 glioma cases from three US hospitals		
	Gas station attendants	14	0.5 (0.3-0.9)
	> 5 years total	3	0.8 (0.2-3.6)
Carozza et al. 2000	476 glioma cases among residents of six San Francisco Bay counties in California; occupation		
	No latency		
	Petroleum and gas workers		
	Ever	5	4.9 (0.6-42.2)
	< 10 yr		3.8 (0.4-34.4)
	Service station attendants		
	Ever	17	0.5 (0.3-1.0)
	< 10 yr		0.4 (0.2-0.9)
	10-yr latency		
	Petroleum and gas workers		
	Ever		4.9 (0.6-42.2)
	< 10 yr		3.8 (0.4-34.4)
	Service station attendants		
	Ever		0.5 (0.3-1.1)
	< 10 yr		0.4 (0.2-0.9)

TABLE 4.34 Brain/CNS Cancers and Exposure to Combustion Products—Selected Epidemiologic Studies

Reference	Study Population	Exposed Cases	Estimated Relative Risk (95% CI)
Case-Control Studies (not adjusted for smoking)			
De Roos et al. 2003	479 glioma cases from three US hospitals		
	Drivers (car and light trucks)	20	0.9 (0.5-1.7)
	> 5 years total	3	0.6 (0.2-2.3)
	Truck drivers (heavy)	31	0.7 (0.4-1.1)
	> 5 years total	13	0.7 (0.3-1.3)
	Railroad occupations	6	1.1 (0.4-3.3)
	> 5 years total	0	0.0 (0.0-∞)
Carozza et al. 2000	476 glioma cases among residents of six San Francisco Bay counties in California; occupation		
	No latency		
	Motor-vehicle operators, ever employed	42	1.0 (0.6-1.6)
	<10 yr		0.8 (0.5-1.4)
	≥10 yr		2.1 (0.7-6.2)
	Vehicle mechanics, ever employed	24	0.4 (0.2-0.7)
	< 10 yr		0.5 (0.2-0.9)
	≥10 yr		0.4 (0.2-1.0)
	Mechanics, not elsewhere classified, ever employed	18	0.7 (0.4-1.4)
	<10 yr		0.9 (0.4-1.8)
	≥10 yr		0.4 (0.1-1.7)
	10-yr latency		
	Motor-vehicle operators, ever employed		1.0 (0.6-1.8)
	<10 yr		0.8 (0.4-1.6)
	≥10 yr		1.8 (0.6-5.3)
	Vehicle mechanics, ever employed		0.5 (0.3-0.8)
	<10 yr		0.6 (0.3-1.1)
	≥10 yr		0.4 (0.2-1.0)
	Mechanics, not elsewhere classified, ever employed		0.7 (0.3-1.4)
	<10 yr		0.8 (0.4-1.7)
	≥10 yr		0.3 (0.0-2.5)

TABLE 4.35 Ocular Melanoma and Exposure to Combustion Products—Selected Epidemiologic Studies

Reference	Study Population	Exposed Cases	Estimated Relative Risk (95% CI)
Case-Control Studies (not adjusted for smoking)			
Monarrez-Espino et al. 2002	118 pooled uveal melanoma cases from two studies among residents of Germany; self-reported job titles		
	Men		
	Transport equipment operators	11	1.5 (0.66-3.23)
	Women		
	Station, engine, heavy-equipment operators, freight handlers	9	2.5 (0.94-6.58)
Guenel et al. 2001	50 ocular melanoma cases among residents of 10 administrative areas in France; self-reported job titles		

Reference	Study Population	Exposed Cases	Estimated Relative Risk (95% CI)
	Transport-equipment operators		
	Males	5	1.4 (0.5-3.8)
	Females	0	—
Ajani et al. 1992	197 uveal melanoma cases among white residents of six New England states; self-reported job titles		
	Transportation, communications, and other public utilities	13	1.23 (0.55-2.74)

TABLE 4.36 Bladder Cancer and Exposure to Fuels—Selected Epidemiologic Studies

Reference	Study Population	Exposed Cases	Estimated Relative Risk (95% CI)
Case-Control Studies (adjusted for smoking, unless noted otherwise)			
Kogevinas et al. 2003	3,346 incident bladder cancer cases in men 30-79 yr old in six countries pooled in EMBCS		
	Petroleum-refining occupation (ISCO code 745) (ever)	3	0.52 (0.10-2.69)
Cordier et al. 1993	658 male bladder-cancer cases in France (561 included in EMBCS sample + 97 men excluded from pooled study)		
	Petroleum-refining industry (ever)	7	4.04 (0.78-21.03)
Claude et al. 1988	531 male bladder cancer cases in Germany (363 included in EMBCS sample + 168 men excluded from pooled study)		
	Occupation (ever) (not adjusted for smoking)		
	Gas station attendant and garage	1	0.33 (0.04-2.87)
	Oil refinery worker	3	1.50 (0.25-8.87)
Kunze et al. 1992	Petroleum (self-reported agent) (not adjusted for smoking)	156	1.4 (1.1-1.9)
	Duration		
	1-9 yr	20	1.2
	10-19 yr	26	1.0
	20-29 yr	30	1.3
	≥30 yr	80	1.8 ($p < 0.05$)
Zheng et al. 2002	1,135 male bladder-cancer cases among residents of Iowa		
	Industries		
	Petroleum and coal products	7	1.0 (0.4-2.9)
	<10 yr	2	3.2 (0.3-40.9)
	≥10 yr	5	0.8 (0.2-2.6)
	Petroleum refining	7	1.1 (0.4-3.2)
	<10 yr	2	3.2 (0.3-40.9)
	≥10 yr	5	0.8 (0.3-2.8)
	Occupation		
	Garage and service station	27	1.7 (0.9-3.1)
	<10 yr	10	1.8 (0.7-4.8)
	≥10 yr	17	1.6 (0.8-3.5)

Reference	Study Population	Exposed Cases	Estimated Relative Risk (95% CI)
Steineck et al. 1990b	254 male urothelial-cancer cases among residents of Stockholm, Sweden		
	Petrol (industrial-hygiene integration of self-reports of occupation, industry, and specific exposures)	18	1.4 (0.7-2.9)
	Low annual dose	na	0.7 (0.2-2.7)
	Medium annual dose	na	0.9 (0.2-4.3)
	High annual dose	na	2.5 (0.8-7.5)
Steineck et al. 1989	10,123 bladder-cancer cases (1961-1979) among men employed in 1960 Swedish census (record-linkage approach, not adjusted for smoking) (JEM used to derive exposure from census occupation)		
	Gasoline—moderate-high likelihood	245	0.87 (0.76-1.00)
	Gasoline—high likelihood	70	1.00 (0.79-1.27)
Multicancer case-control study in Montreal, Canada			
Siemiatycki et al. 1987a	486 male bladder cancer cases vs cancer controls,		
	Agents—ever exposed (industrial-hygienist-derived)		
	Automotive gasoline	64	1.2 (0.9-1.4)[a]
	Aviation gasoline	6	1.0 (0.5-2.2)[a]
	Kerosene	31	1.1 (0.8-1.5)[a]
	Jet fuel	4	0.7 (0.3-1.8)[a]
	Diesel fuel	13	0.7 (0.5-1.1)[a]
	Heating oil	18	0.9 (0.6-1.3)[a]
	Crude oil	1	0.2 (0.1-2.0)[a]
Siemiatycki et al. 1994	484 male bladder-cancer cases vs pooled cancer and population controls		
	Petroleum and coal products (industry)		
	<10 yr	4	0.9 (0.3-2.7)
	≥10 yr	2	0.4 (0.1-1.6)
	NCI NBCS, exposure classification by industry and occupation		
Silverman et al. 1989a	126 nonwhite male bladder-cancer cases in 10 US SEER centers		
	Petroleum worker (ever)	4	2.1 (0.5-9.2)
	Garage and/or gas-station worker (ever)	6	1.6 (0.5-4.9)
Silverman et al. 1989b	2,100 white male bladder cancer cases in 10 US SEER centers		
	Petroleum-processing occupation (ever)	71	1.3 (1.0-1.8)
	Crude extraction	16	2.4 (1.1-5.5)
	Refining	39	1.3 (0.8-2.0)
	Products	22	1.2 (0.7-2.1)
Silverman et al. 1983	303 white male bladder-cancer cases in Detroit subset of NBCS		
	Industry (ever)	6	6.0 (0.7-49.8)
	Petroleum extracting and refining (not adjusted for smoking)		
	Gasoline service (adjusted for smoking and age)	18	1.3 (0.8-3.5)
	Garage and/or gas-station occupation (ever) (not	18	1.2 (0.6-2.4)

Reference	Study Population	Exposed Cases	Estimated Relative Risk (95% CI)
	adjusted for smoking)		
Schoenberg et al. 1984	658 white male bladder-cancer cases in New Jersey-subset of NBCS		
	Petroleum-refinery worker (ever)	13	1.34 (0.64-2.82)
	Garage and/or gas-station worker (ever)	43	2.35 (1.47-3.78)
Schumacher et al. 1989	332 white male bladder cancer cases in Utah subset of NBCS		
	Fuel industry (>10 yr)	15	1.54 (0.77-3.11)

NOTE: EMBCS=European Merged Bladder Cancer Study; na=not available; NBCS=National Bladder Cancer Study.
[a] 90% CIs reported in this paper.

TABLE 4.37 Bladder Cancer and Exposure to Combustion Products—Selected Epidemiologic Studies

Reference	Study Population	Exposed Cases	Estimated Relative Risk (95% CI)
Cohort Studies (adjusted for smoking, unless noted otherwise)			
Zeegers et al. 2001	Nested case-control study of 532 male urothelial-cancer cases from Netherlands Cohort Study		
	PAHs (industrial-hygiene integration of probability and duration of exposure)		
	Low exposure tertile	7	0.51 (0.22-1.19)
	Medium exposure tertile	13	0.97 (0.49-1.90)
	High exposure tertile	19	1.18 (0.62-2.24)
			p for trend = 0.85
	Diesel exhaust (industrial-hygiene integration of probability and duration of exposure)		
	Low exposure tertile	35	1.00 (0.65-1.54)
	Medium exposure tertile	31	0.96 (0.60-1.53)
	High exposure tertile	32	1.17 (0.74-1.84)
			p for trend = 0.76
Boffetta et al. 2001	Cohort exposed to diesel emissions (industrial-hygiene-derived agent from job on 1960 Swedish census) defined among occupationally active residents of Sweden, 1960 and 1970—record-linkage approach, not adjusted for smoking		
	Bladder-cancer (ICD-7 181) cases (1971-1989)		
	Men	4,018	1.00 (0.97-1.03)
	Women	38	1.02 (0.72-1.41)
Case-Control Studies (adjusted for smoking, unless noted otherwise)			
European Merged Bladder Cancer Study (EMBCS) pooling results from 11 studies in six countries			
Kogevinas et al. 2003	3,346 incident bladder-cancer cases in men 30-79 yr old		
	Occupations (ever)		
	Firefighters, urban not distinguished from forest	7	0.66 (0.27-1.62)
	Motor-vehicle mechanic	108	1.16 (0.90-1.50)
	Automobile mechanic	78	1.38 (1.02-1.87)
	Selected transport occupations		
	Railway-engine drivers and firemen	34	1.41 (0.87-2.28)

Reference	Study Population	Exposed Cases	Estimated Relative Risk (95% CI)
	Railway brakemen, signalmen, and shunters	18	1.43 (0.77-2.63)
	Motor-vehicle drivers	302	1.14 (0.97-1.33)
	Agents (Finnish JEM)—highest tertile vs unexposed		
	PAHs	na	1.23 (1.07-1.40)
	Benzo[a]pyrene	na	1.27 (1.04-1.54)
't Mannetje et al. 1999	700 incident bladder-cancer cases in women 30-79 yr old		
	Motor-vehicle drivers (occupation ever)	2	1.15 (unadjusted)
	PAHs (Finnish JEM)		
	Low	17	1.5 (0.8-2.9)
	Medium	4	1.1 (0.4-3.5)
	High	7	1.0 (0.4-2.5)
	PAHs (British JEM)		
	Low	42	0.9 (0.6-1.4)
	Medium	5	1.1 (0.4-3.4)
	High	5	1.2 (0.4-3.3)
Pesch et al. 2000b	Urothelial-carcinoma cases among residents of five regions in Germany (508 men and 176 women in EMBCS sample, plus 196 male and 155 female cases excluded from pooled study)		
	704 male cases		
	Motor-vehicle driver (occupation)		
	Medium duration	43	1.0 (0.7-1.4)
	Long duration	54	1.7 (1.2-2.4)
	Very long duration	21	1.5 (0.9-2.6)
	Production of tar, pitch, or bitumen (occupation)		
	Medium duration	1	0.8 (0.1-8.2)
	Long duration	1	0.6 (0.1-5.0)
	Very long duration	3	4.8 (0.9-26.0)
	Tar, pitch, and related products (agent)		
	Self-report		
	Medium duration	14	0.6 (0.4-1.2)
	Long duration	27	1.1 (0.7-1.7)
	Very long duration	8	1.0 (0.4-2.2)
	British JEM		
	Medium	111	1.1 (0.9-1.4)
	High	112	1.2 (0.9-1.5)
	Substantial	50	1.6 (1.1-2.3)
	German JEM		
	Medium	71	0.7 (0.5-0.9)
	High	87	0.8 (0.6-1.1)
	Substantial	27	1.0 (0.7-1.7)
	Task-based JEM		
	Medium	18	0.6 (0.4-1.0)
	High	36	1.2 (0.8-1.8)
	Substantial	18	1.8 (1.0-3.4)
	PAHs (agent)		
	British JEM		
	Medium	97	1.0 (0.8-1.3)
	High	123	1.3 (1.0-1.7)
	Substantial	47	1.6 (1.1-2.3)

Reference	Study Population	Exposed Cases	Estimated Relative Risk (95% CI)
	Task-based JEM		
	Medium	70	0.7 (0.5-1.0)
	High	92	0.8 (0.6-1.1)
	Substantial	47	1.2 (0.9-1.8)
	Exhaust (agent)		
	Self-assessed		
	Medium	38	0.6 (0.4-0.9)
	High	74	1.0 (0.8-1.3)
	Substantial	19	0.8 (0.5-1.4)
	German JEM		
	Medium	157	1.0 (0.8-1.3)
	High	173	1.3 (1.0-1.6)
	Substantial	57	1.2 (0.9-1.7)
	331 female cases		
	Tar, pitch, and related products—British JEM (agent)		
	Medium	14	1.1 (0.6-2.0)
	High	16	1.3 (0.7-2.3)
	Substantial	7	1.6 (0.6-4.3)
	PAHs—British JEM (agent)		
	Medium	17	1.0 (0.6-1.8)
	High	17	1.3 (0.7-2.3)
	Substantial	4	1.3 (0.4-4.2)
	Exhaust (agent)		
	Self-assessed		
	Medium	2	0.6 (0.1-2.9)
	High	1	0.3 (0.04-2.2)
	Substantial	2	1.2 (0.2-6.0)
	German JEM		
	Medium	21	1.3 (0.7-2.2)
	High	18	1.0 (0.6-1.8)
	Substantial	2	0.7 (0.2-3.2)
Clavel et al. 1994	658 male bladder-cancer cases among male residents of France (561 in EMBCS sample, plus 97 cases excluded from pooled study)		
	Motor-vehicle mechanics (occupation)	26	1.1 (0.6-2.1)
	Motor-vehicle driver (occupation)	52	0.8 (0.6-1.2)
	PAHs (from expert review of job history)		
	Exposed	231	1.3 (1.0-1.7)
	Maximal exposure		p for trend <0.05
	Low	129	1.2 (0.9-1.7)
	Medium	64	1.3 (0.9-2.1)
	High	29	1.8 (0.9-3.6)
	Average exposure to PAHs		p for trend <0.05
	Low	127	1.2 (0.9-1.7)
	Medium	64	1.4 (0.9-2.2)
	High	26	1.8 (0.8-3.9)
	Cumulative exposure to PAHs (ng/m^3 x yr)		p for trend, ns
	<100	108	1.7 (1.2-2.4)
	100-499	37	0.8 (0.5-1.3)
	500-14,999	48	1.3 (0.8-2.0)
	≥15,000	24	1.8 (0.8-3.9)
	Total duration (yr)		p for trend, ns

Reference	Study Population	Exposed Cases	Estimated Relative Risk (95% CI)
	≤5	46	1.3 (0.9-2.1)
	5-15	50	1.5 (0.9-2.4)
	16-30	74	2.3 (1.3-4.2)
	>30	47	0.8 (0.5-1.3)
	Time since starting exposure (yr)		p for trend = 0.09
	≤20	18	1.4 (0.7-2.8)
	20-29	26	1.8 (0.9-3.5)
	30-39	74	1.3 (0.8-1.9)
	40-49	56	1.2 (0.8-1.9)
	>50	43	1.3 (0.7-2.2)
	Age at beginning of exposure		p for trend <0.05
	≤25	157	1.2 (0.9-1.6)
	>25	60	1.7 (1.1-2.7)
	Time since cessation of exposure		
	≤15 yr	101	1.1 (0.8-1.6)
	16-25	76	1.9 (1.2-2.8)
	>35	40	1.3 (0.8-2.2)
Jensen et al. 1987	281 male and 91 female bladder-cancer cases among residents of Copenhagen, Denmark (subset with complete information of 288 men and 96 women contributed to EMBCS sample)		
	Land transport (industry) ever	51	1.55 (1.06-2.28)
	Land transport (occupation) for 10 yr	na	1.28 (1.04-1.45)
	Bus, taxi, or truck driver (occupation)-for 10 yr	na	1.29 (1.05-1.59)
Zheng et al. 2002	1,135 male bladder-cancer cases among residents of Iowa		
	Industries (≥5 yr)		
	Railroad transportation (40)	33	1.4 (0.8-2.3)
	<10 yr	4	0.6 (0.2-2.0)
	≥10 yr	29	1.7 (1.0-3.1)
	Railroads (401)	11	1.5 (0.6-3.9)
	<10 yr	3	2.1 (0.3-13.3)
	≥10 yr	8	1.4 (0.5-4.0)
	Transportation services (47)	6	2.8 (0.7-11.8)
	<10 yr	2	2.9 (0.2-35.4)
	≥10 yr	4	2.7 (0.5-15.8)
	General automotive repair shops	20	3.0 (1.3-6.7)
	<10 yr	4	2.0 (0.4-9.3)
	≥10 yr	16	3.4 (1.3-9.0)
	Occupations (≥5 yr)		
	Mechanics and repairers (61)	118	1.3 (1.0-1.8)
	<10 yr	21	1.2 (0.6-2.1)
	≥10 yr	97	1.4 (1.0-1.9)
	Automobile mechanics (6111)	44	1.6 (1.0-2.6)
	<10 yr	8	1.4 (0.5-3.7)
	≥10 yr	36	1.7 (1.0-2.8)
	Miscellaneous mechanics and repairers (617)	32	1.8 (1.0-3.1)
	<10 yr	8	1.0 (0.4-2.7)
	≥10 yr	24	2.4 (1.2-4.7)
	Drivers	78	1.3 (0.9-1.8)
	<10 yr	21	1.3 (0.7-2.4)
	≥10 yr	57	1.3 (0.9-2.0)

Reference	Study Population	Exposed Cases	Estimated Relative Risk (95% CI)
Steineck et al. 1990b	254 male urothelial-cancer cases among residents of Stockholm, Sweden		
	Occupation		
	Railway	8	0.4 (0.2-1.0)
	Petrol station and automobile repair	17	1.3 (0.6-2.8)
	Agents (self-reported)		
	Combustion gases from coal, coke, or wood	53	1.0 (0.7-1.6)
	Tar or asphalt	19	0.9 (0.5-1.7)
	Agents (industrial-hygiene integration of self-reports of occupation, industry, and specific exposures)		
	Combustion gases from coal	27	0.8 (0.5-1.4)
	Low annual dose	na	0.9 (0.3-2.2)
	Medium annual dose	na	0.8 (0.3-2.2)
	High annual dose	na	0.9 (0.4-1.9)
	Combustion gases from oil	10	0.9 (0.4-2.3)
	Combustion gases from wood	23	1.2 (0.6-2.3)
	Diesel exhausts	25	1.7 (0.9-3.3)
	Low annual dose	na	1.3 (0.6-3.1)
	Medium annual dose	na	2.2 (0.7-6.6)
	High annual dose	na	2.9 (0.3-30.0)
	Petrol exhausts	24	1.0 (0.5-1.9)
	Low annual dose	na	0.6 (0.3-1.3)
	Medium annual dose	na	1.4 (0.5-3.7)
	High annual dose	na	3.9 (0.4-35.5)
	Both diesel and petrol exhausts (moderate/high)	7	7.1 (0.9-58.8)
Steineck et al. 1989	10,123 male bladder-cancer cases (1961-1979) among men employed in 1960 Swedish census—record-linkage approach, not adjusted for smoking (JEM used to derive exposure from census job, linked to Swedish Cancer Registry)		
	Diesel exhausts	332	0.98 (0.87-1.10)
	Gasoline exhausts	567	0.95 (0.87-1.03)
	Combustion gases from oil	88	1.17 (0.95-1.44)
	Combustion gases from coal	112	1.19 (0.99-1.43)
	Soot from oil or coal	19	1.28 (0.82-2.01)
	Combustion gases from wood	72	1.16 (0.92-1.46)
	Soot from wood	56	1.19 (0.91-1.54)
	Coal tar	2	1.60 (0.40 -6.29)
NCI National Bladder Cancer Study (NBCS); occupational history from interview			
Silverman et al. 1986, 1989b	2,100 bladder-cancer cases among white male residents of 10 US SEER locations		
	Railroad workers (ever)	57	1.3 (0.9-2.0)
	Mechanics (ever)	353	1.2 (1.0-1.4)
	Motor-vehicle drivers (ever)	556	1.2 (1.1-1.4)
	Motor-vehicle drivers vs those never holding exhaust-related occupation		
	Truck driver or deliveryman (usual)	99	1.5 (1.1-2.0)
	Truck driver or deliveryman (ever)	488	1.3 (1.1-1.4)
	Duration (yr)		p for trend <0.001
	<5	208	1.1

Reference	Study Population	Exposed Cases	Estimated Relative Risk (95% CI)
	5-9	102	1.3
	10-14	58	1.7
	15-24	59	2.2
	25+	54	1.1
	Taxicab driver or chauffeur (usual)	10	6.3 (1.6-29.3)
	Taxicab driver or chauffeur (ever)	77	1.6 (1.2-2.2)
	Duration (yr)		p for trend = 0.014
	<5	44	1.9
	5-9	14	1.0
	10+	16	2.0
	Bus driver (usual)	9	1.5 (0.6-3.9)
	Bus driver (ever)	49	1.3 (0.9-1.9)
	Duration (yr)		p for trend, ns
	<5	21	1.3
	5-9	11	1.2
	10+	16	1.3
Silverman et al. 1989a	126 bladder-cancer cases among nonwhite male residents of 10 US SEER locations		
	Mechanics (ever)	13	1.1 (0.5-2.5)
	Auto mechanic (ever)	6	1.4 (0.4-4.4)
	Motor vehicle drivers (ever)	40	1.0 (0.6-1.5)
	Taxicab driver or chauffer (ever)	10	1.3 (0.5-3.2)
Silverman et al. 1990	652 bladder-cancer cases among white female residents of 10 US SEER locations		
	Motor vehicle drivers (ever)	9	1.1 (0.4-3.0)
Bonassi et al. 1989	121 male bladder-cancer cases among residents of Bormida Valley, Italy		
	Auto mechanics	3	1.84 (0.43-7.84)
	Truck drivers	3	1.88 (0.44-8.00)
	PAHs (JEM-derived agent)		
	Possible	74	1.63 (0.95-2.83)
	Also adjusted for aromatic amine exposure		1.05 (0.45-2.44)
	Definite	25	2.20 (1.12-4.38)
	Also adjusted for aromatic amine exposure		2.14 (0.82-5.60)
Multicancer case-control study in Montreal, Canada			
Siemiatycki et al. 1988	486 male bladder-cancer cases vs cancer controls		
	Agents—ever exposed (industrial-hygiene-derived)		
	Gasoline exhaust	208	1.0 (0.9-1.1)[a]
	Diesel exhaust	82	1.0 (0.8-1.2)[a]
	Jet-fuel exhaust	1	0.2 (0.0-1.2)[a]
	Liquid-fuel combustion	28	0.9 (0.7-1.2)[a]
	Coke combustion	3	0.7 (0.2-2.5)[a]
	Natural-gas combustion	22	1.6 (1.1-2.3)[a], $p < 0.05$
Siemiatycki et al. 1994	484 male bladder-cancer cases vs pooled cancer and population controls		
	Industries		
	Motor transport		
	<10 yr	34	1.9 (1.2-2.8)
	≥10 yr	40	1.7 (1.2-2.5)

Reference	Study Population	Exposed Cases	Estimated Relative Risk (95% CI)
	Motor-vehicle sales and service		
	<10 yr	25	1.8 (1.1-3.0)
	≥10 yr	13	0.9 (0.5-1.6)
	Occupations		
	Motor-transport workers		
	<10 yr	40	1.4 (0.9-2.0)
	Truck drivers	25	1.1 (0.7-1.8)
	≥10 yr	46	1.3 (0.9-1.9)
	Truck drivers	26	1.2 (0.8-1.9)
	Air-transport workers (all <10 yr)	6	3.3 (1.2-9.1)
	Industrial-hygiene-derived agents		
	Benzo[a]pyrene	106	
	Nonsubstantial	91	1.0 (0.8-1.3)
	Substantial	15	0.6 (0.3-1.1)
	Coal tar and pitch	13	
	Nonsubstantial	7	0.7 (0.3-1.7)
	Substantial	6	1.3 (0.5-3.3)
	Diesel-engine emissions	78	
	Nonsubstantial	46	1.3 (0.9-1.9)
	Substantial	32	1.0 (0.6-1.4)
	Probable	28	1.0 (0.7-1.6)
	Definite	50	1.2 (0.9-1.7)
	Low concentration	27	1.2 (0.8-1.9)
	High concentration	51	1.1 (0.8-1.5)
	Low frequency	48	1.1 (0.8-1.5)
	High frequency	30	1.3 (0.8-1.9)
	1-10-yr duration	22	1.2 (0.7-1.9)
	≥11-yr duration	56	1.3 (0.8-1.5)
	Natural gas combustion products	22	
	Nonsubstantial	14	1.2 (0.6-2.2)
	Substantial	8	3.0 (1.2-7.5)
	Probable	5	1.3 (0.5-3.6)
	Definite	17	1.5 (0.8-2.6)
	Low concentration	11	0.9 (0.5-1.8)
	High concentration	11	2.9 (1.4-6.2)
	Low frequency	7	1.0 (0.4-2.2)
	High frequency	15	1.9 (1.0-3.5)
	1-10 yr duration	9	1.9 (0.9-4.3)
	≥11 yr duration	13	1.2 (0.6-2.3)

NOTES: na=not available; ns=not statistically significant ($p < 0.5$) for risk estimate above unity.
[a] 90% CIs reported in this paper.
[b] Number of exposed cases and controls.
[c] Risk estimates and 95% CIs calculated with standard methods from observed and expected numbers in original paper.

TABLE 4.38 Kidney Cancer and Exposure to Fuels—Selected Epidemiologic Studies

Reference	Study Population	Exposed Cases	Estimated Relative Risk (95% CI)
Cohort Studies (not adjusted for smoking, unless otherwise noted)			
Imperial Oil, Canada			
Lewis et al. 2000b	Kidney-cancer (ICD-9 189.0-189.2) deaths in 1964-1994 among petroleum workers employed any time during 1964-1983		
	Males	41	0.96 (0.69-1.30)
	Refinery segment	16	0.91 (0.52-1.48)
	Marketing and distribution segment	15	1.14 (0.64-1.88)
	Females	3	0.91 (0.19-2.67)[a]
Lewis et al. 2003	Incident cases of kidney cancer in 1969-1994 among male petroleum workers hired in 1964-1994	15	1.00 (0.56-1.65)
Exxon refineries in Louisiana, New Jersey, and Texas			
Shallenberger et al. 1992	Kidney-cancer (ICD-8 189) deaths in LA (1970-1982)	18	1.92 ($p < 0.05$)
Hanis et al. 1982	Kidney-cancer (ICD-8 189) deaths in LA (1970-1977)	9	1.55 (0.71- 2.94)
Gamble et al. 1996	Nested case-control study of 37 incident kidney cancer (ICD-8 189) cases (1970-1990)	(32 dead and 5 alive)	
	By duration of employment (adjusted for smoking)		
	<25 yr	10	1.0
	25-32 yr	9	1.34 (0.23-7.77)
	32-38 yr	9	3.26 (0.27-39.72)
	≥38 yr	9	4.08 (0.24-68.72)
Poole et al. 1993	Nested case-control study of 100 RCC deaths among petroleum industry workers from 36 US locations		
	Ever (vs never) exposed above background:		
	Nonaromatic, liquid gasoline distillates	87	1.00 (0.51-1.94)
	Aromatic hydrocarbons	80	0.95 (0.50-1.80)
	Volatile hydrocarbons	85	1.31 (0.72-2.39)
	Higher boiling hydrocarbons	86	0.95 (0.49-1.84)
	PAHs	76	0.69 (0.40-1.21)
Wong et al. 1993	Kidney-cancer (ICD-8 189) deaths among US petroleum-distribution workers	24	0.73 (0.47-1.09)
	Marine distribution workers	12	0.84 (0.46-1.41)
	Land-based distribution workers	12	0.65 (0.34-1.14)
	Total hydrocarbons (JEM-derived)—cumulative exposure		
	<500 ppm-yr	4	1.19
	500-1,000 ppm-yr	1	0.40
	1,000-2,000 ppm-yr	4	0.95
	>2,000 ppm-yr	3	0.37

Reference	Study Population	Exposed Cases	Estimated Relative Risk (95% CI)
Case-Control Studies (adjusted for smoking, unless otherwise noted)			
Pesch et al. 2000a	570 male RCC cases among residents of five regions in Germany		
	Production and use of petroleum products (grouped over job tasks)—duration		
	Medium	9	0.5 (0.3-1.0)
	Long	10	1.1 (0.3-1.1)[b]
	Very long	8	1.3 (0.6-2.9)
Mandel et al. 1995	1,050 male RCC cases in five countries pooled in International Renal Cell Cancer Study		
	Oil refinery (industry)	21	1.3 (0.6-2.4)
	Gas-station attendants (occupation)	56	1.3 (0.9-1.9)
	Gasoline (self-reported agent)	164	1.6 (1.2-2.0)
	1-5 yr	56	1.6 (1.1-2.4)
	6-27 yr	56	1.4 (0.9-2.1)
	28-62 yr	52	1.6 (1.1-2.5)
	Jet fuel, heating oil, kerosene, or diesel fuel (self-reported agent)	195	1.6 (1.3-2.1)
	1-9 yr	49	1.5 (1.0-2.2)
	10-24 yr	75	1.6 (1.1-2.3)
	25-60 yr	71	1.9 (1.8-2.7)
Partanen et al. 1991	338 RCC cases among residents of Finland (industrial-hygiene-coded agents)		
	Diesel or fuel oils (not adjusted for smoking)	21	1.20 (0.63-2.27)
	Gasoline (≥1 yr high or ≥5 yr low) (not adjusted for smoking, but all of following estimates are)	39	1.72 (1.03-2.87)
	Level (ppm equivalent of benzene)		
	0.1-0.19	4	0.63 (0.19-2.12)
	0.2-0.9	25	1.55 (0.83-2.91)
	1.0-2.0	10	7.39 (1.58-34.6)
	Duration (yr)		
	5-11	13	1.39 (0.61-3.13)
	12-20	13	2.02 (0.83-4.90)
	21-51	13	1.58 (0.69-3.63)
	Cumulative exposure (ppm-yr)		
	0.5-1.9	7	1.28 (0.45-3.65)
	2.0-13	23	1.39 (0.75-2.58)
	14-102	9	4.34 (1.15-16.4)
	Latency (yr)		
	17-26	10	1.23 (0.51-2.96)
	27-33	17	2.82 (1.17-6.80)
	34-58	12	1.28 (0.56-2.98)
	Men only (<278, exact number not given)		
	Either gasoline or diesel	42	
	Diesel	19[c]	1.15 (0.60-2.20)
	Gasoline	36[c]	1.63 (0.97-2.75)
	Only gasoline	23	2.05 (1.05-3.98)

Reference	Study Population	Exposed Cases	Estimated Relative Risk (95% CI)
	Only diesel	6	0.68 (0.23-2.01)
	Both	13	1.29 (0.55-3.02)
Kadamani et al. 1989	210 RCC cases among patients at 23 hospitals in Oklahoma City and Tulsa, Oklahoma (not adjusted for smoking)		
	68 women		
	Any hydrocarbon exposure (industrial-hygiene-coded agent)	28	0.7 (0.3-1.4)
	142 men		
	Any hydrocarbon exposure (industrial-hygiene-coded agent)	121	1.6 (0.8-3.2)
	Low	29	1.3 (0.5-3.0)
	Moderate	53	2.7 (1.2-6.5)
	High	39	1.6 (0.7-3.6)
	Duration of hydrocarbon exposure (yr)		
	1-15	35	1.2 (0.6-2.4)
	16-30	31	2.4 (1.0-6.2)
	>30	55	2.3 (1.0-5.2)
Siemiatycki et al. 1987a	181 kidney-cancer (ICD 189) cases in multi-cancer study among male residents of Montreal, Canada (1979-1985)—industrial-hygiene-coded agents		
	Adjusted for age, socioeconomic status, ethnicity, and blue- vs white-collar jobs, in addition to smoking		
	Crude oil	2	1.2 (0.2-6.3)[d]
	Automotive gasoline	24	1.2 (0.8-1.6)[d]
	Kerosene	12	1.3 (0.8-2.1)[d]
	Diesel fuel	10	1.4 (0.8-2.3)[d]
	Heating oil	8	1.1 (0.6-2.1)[d]
	Logistic model with adjustment for all identified potential confounders		
	Aviation gasoline	7	3.1 (1.5-6.5)[d]
	Nonsubstantial	1	1.5 (0.3-8.6)[d]
	Substantial	6	3.9 (1.7-8.8)[d]
	Jet fuel	7	3.1 (1.5-6.6)[d]
	Nonsubstantial	1	2.1 (0.3-12.7)[d]
	Substantial	6	3.4 (1.5-7.6)[d]
McLaughlin et al. 1985	313 RCC cases among male residents of Minneapolis-St. Paul, Minnesota		
	Petroleum-related (occupation—ever)	116	1.0 (0.7-1.4)
	1-2 yr	32	0.9 (0.5-1.6)
	3-10 yr	39	1.0 (0.6-1.6)
	>10 yr	45	1.1 (0.7-1.7)
	Gasoline station attendants (occupation)	20	1.2 (0.6-2.3)
	1-2 yr	8	0.9 (0.3-2.4)
	3-5 yr	6	1.3 (0.3-4.5)
	>5 yr	6	1.7 (0.4-6.5)

NOTE: na=not available; RCC=renal-cell cancer.

[a] Risk estimate and 95% CI calculated with standard methods from observed and expected numbers presented in

original paper.
[b] Error evident in original publication (Pesch et al., 2000) which gave identical value for both odds ratio and upper confidence limit.
[c] Error evident in exposed cases listed for men in Table 6 from comparison with Tables 5 and 7 (Partanen et al., 1991).
[d] 90% CIs reported in this paper.

TABLE 4.39 Kidney Cancer and Exposure to Combustion Products—Selected Epidemiologic Studies

Reference	Study Population	Exposed Cases	Estimated Relative Risk (95% CI)
Cohort Study (not adjusted for smoking)			
Boffetta et al. 2001	Kidney cancer [ICD-7 180] cases (1971-1989) among occupationally active residents of Sweden, 1960 and 1970 from data in Swedish Cancer-Environment Registry established by record linkage		
	Diesel emissions (industrial-hygiene-coded agent from 1960 occupation and industry)		
	Men	2,243	1.06 (1.02-1.11)
	Women	33	0.82 (0.57-1.16)
Case-Control Studies (adjusted for smoking, unless otherwise noted)			
Pesch et al. 2000a	RCC cases among residents of five regions in Germany		
	570 male RCC cases		
	Railway brakemen, signalmen, and shunters (longest-held job, 3-digit occupation)	5	6.2 (1.6-23.4)
	Motor-vehicle driver (occupation)—duration		
	Medium	27	0.9 (0.6-1.4)
	Long	28	0.9 (0.6-1.4)
	Very long	7	0.6 (0.3-1.4)
	Tar, pitch, and mineral oil—British JEM		
	Medium	86	1.1 (0.9-1.5)
	High	96	1.2 (0.9-1.6)
	Substantial	34	1.4 (0.9-2.1)
	PAHs		
	British JEM		
	Medium	71	0.9 (0.7-1.2)
	High	96	1.3 (1.0-1.6)
	Substantial	32	1.2 (0.8-1.9)
	Task approach—JEM		
	Medium	80	0.9 (0.7-1.2)
	High	67	0.8 (0.6-1.0)
	Substantial	26	0.9 (0.6-1.4)
	365 female RCC cases		
	Motor vehicle drivers (occupation)—duration		
	Medium	0	—
	Long	1	0.9 (0.1-7.7)
	Very long	1	1.9 (0.2-21.3)
	Tar, pitch, mineral oil - British JEM		
	Medium	15	1.0 (0.6-1.7)
	High	16	1.2 (0.7-2.0)
	Substantial	10	2.1 (1.0-4.5)
	PAHs—British JEM		
	Medium	17	1.1 (0.6-1.8)

Reference	Study Population	Exposed Cases	Estimated Relative Risk (95% CI)
	High	21	1.5 (0.9-2.4)
	Substantial	6	1.3 (0.5-3.3)
Mandel et al. 1995	1,050 male RCC cases in five countries pooled in International Renal Cell Cancer Study		
	Blast furnace and coke ovens (occupation)	57	1.7 (1.1-2.7)
Partanen et al. 1991	338 RCC cases (including at least 60 women) among residents of Finland; results from analyses on men only		
	Transport and storage (industry)	23	1.13 (0.63-2.02)
	Transportation (occupation)	21	1.09 (0.59-2.00)
	PAHs (industrial-hygienist-coded agent)	7	1.21 (0.43-3.45)
Multicancer study among male residents of Montreal, Canada (1979-1985)			
Siemiatycki et al. 1988	181 kidney cancer (ICD 189) cases vs cancer controls		
	Gasoline exhaust (industrial-hygienist-coded agent)	80	1.2 (0.9-1.4)[a]
	Short, low	15	1.5 (0.9-2.3)[a]
	Short, high	7	0.7 (0.4-1.4)[a]
	Long, low	24	1.1 (0.8-1.7)[a]
	Long, high	34	1.4 (1.0-2.0)[a]
	Diesel exhaust (industrial-hygienist-coded agent)	29	0.9 (0.7-1.3)[a]
	Jet-fuel exhaust (industrial-hygienist-coded agent)	4	1.4 (0.5-3.9)[a]
	Liquid-fuel combustion (industrial-hygienist-coded agent)	10	0.8 (0.5-1.4)[a]
	Coke combustion (industrial-hygienist-coded agent)	1	0.6 (0.0-7.4)[a]
Parent et al. 2000a	142 RCC (ICD 189.0) cases (subset of cases in Siemiatycki et al. 1988) vs. pooled cancer and population controls		
	Jet-fuel engine emissions (industrial-hygiene-coded agent)	4	2.7 (0.9-8.1)
	Motor transport		
	Industry	14	1.0 (0.6-1.8)
	Occupation	21	1.1 (0.7-1.8)
Sharpe et al. 1989	164 RCC cases among residents of Montreal, Canada (men and women, but partition not given; about 65% of men were probably in Siemiatycki dataset) (not adjusted for smoking after smoking history found to be unrelated to cancer status)—self-reported agents		
	Occupational exposures		
	Tar or pitch	9	9.29 (1.16-74.2)
	Burning coke	6	2.00 (0.49-8.14)
	Burning coal	17	2.54 (0.96-6.99)
	Any exposure to burning coal (in order of assumed increasing exposure)		
	House with coal fuel but no handling	53	1.07 (0.58-1.96)
	Domestic handling only	56	1.41 (0.76-2.62)

Reference	Study Population	Exposed Cases	Estimated Relative Risk (95% CI)
	Occupational handling	14	2.42 (0.81-7.46)
	Occupational and domestic handling	3	8.45 (0.42-168.7)
McLaughlin et al. 1987	7,405 male RCCs (1961-1979) employed in Sweden in 1960 from data in Swedish Cancer-Environment Registry established by record linkage (not adjusted for smoking)		
	Transport and communication (industry)	606	1.04 (0.96-1.13)[b]
	Automobile transportation	65	1.33 (1.03-1.70)[b]
	Transport and communication (occupation)	532	1.00 (0.92-1.09)[b]
	Craftsmen, production workers, and laborers (occupation)—code 8	965	0.94 (0.88-1.00)[b]
	Stationary engine and equipment operators—code 87	170	1.15 (0.99-1.34)[b]
	Stationary engine and equipment operators—code 88	233	0.93 (0.82-1.06)[b]

NOTE: RCC=renal-cell cancer.
[a] 90% CIs reported in this paper.
[b] 95% CIs calculated with standard methods from risks and observed numbers presented in original paper.

TABLE 4.40 Non-Hodgkin's Lymphoma and Exposure to Fuels—Selected Epidemiologic Studies

Reference	Study Population	Exposed Cases	Estimated Relative Risk (95% CI)
Cohort Studies			
Imperial Oil, Canada			
Lewis et al. 2000b	NHL (ICD-9 200, 202.0, 202.2) deaths (1964-1994) among petroleum workers employed anytime in 1964-1983		
	Females	5	0.82 (0.27-1.91)
	Males	49	0.98 (0.72-1.29)
	Refinery segment	22	1.09 (0.68-1.65)
	Marketing and distribution segment	17	1.12 (0.65-1.79)
Schnatter et al. 1996	Nested case-control study of 8 NHL deaths occurring before 1984 (with 5-yr lag); total hydrocarbons (ppm-yr)		
	0.0-11.6	3	1.0
	11.7-29.9	2	1.73 (0.02-137)
	30.0-549	2	0.52 (0.01-12.1)
	550-6,721	1	1.22 (0.01-137)
Lewis et al. 2003	Incident NHL (ICD-9 200.0-200.2, 202.0, 202.2) cases (1969-1994) among male petroleum workers hired 1964-1994		
	Females	7	1.19 (0.48-2.46)
	Males	20	0.97 (0.59-1.50)
Huebner et al. 2000	Incident NHL (ICD-9 200.0-200.2, 200.8, 202.0-202.2, 202.8-202.9) cases (1983-1994) among men working in 1970-1992 at Exxon facility in Baton Rouge, Louisiana	22	1.06 (0.67-1.61)
	First employed		

Reference	Study Population	Exposed Cases	Estimated Relative Risk (95% CI)
	≥1950	4	0.49 (0.13-1.26)
	<1950	18	1.44 (0.85-2.27)
	Latency ≥40 yr	17	1.40 (0.82-2.24)
	Duration of employment		
	20-39 yr	13	1.27 (0.68-2.18)
	≥40 yr	4	2.07 (0.56-5.31)[a]
Jarvholm et al. 1997	Male workers in the Swedish petroleum industry ≥1 yr (qualitative industrial-hygienist-interpretation of personnel records)		
	Incident cases of all types of lymphoma (ICD-9 200-202)	9	0.93 (0.48-1.6)[b]
	With ≥20-yr latency	3	0.65 (0.18-1.7)[b]
	With ≥10-yr duration	2	0.48 (0.08-1.5)[b]
Lagorio et al. 1994	NHL (ICD-9 200, 202) deaths among male filling-station attendants in Italy (exposure reconstruction using monitoring)		
	At stations of all sizes	3	1.73 (0.47-4.48)[b]
	At small stations	2	1.71 (0.30-5.38)[b]
Case-Control Studies			
Blair et al. 1993	622 NHL cases among white male residents of Iowa and Minnesota; self-reported industry		
	Petroleum refining	5	1.6 (0.5-5.8)
Franceschi et al. 1989	208 NHL cases among residents of northeast Italy; self-reported occupation		
	Petrochemical worker	15	1.83 (0.87-3.84)
Siemiatycki et al. 1987a	206 NHL cases vs cancer controls among male residents of Montreal, Canada; industrial-hygiene-derived agents		
	Automotive gasoline	20	0.8 (0.5-1.1)[b]
	Aviation gasoline	1	0.4 (0.1-2.5)[b]
	Kerosene	5	0.4 (0.2-0.7)[b]
	Jet fuel	2	0.7 (0.2-3.2)[b]
	Diesel fuel	10	1.1 (0.7-1.8)[b]
	Heating oil	6	0.7 (0.4-1.3)[b]
	Crude oil	1	0.5 (0.1-3.8)[b]

NOTE: NHL=non-Hodgkin's lymphoma.
[a] Risk estimate and 95% CI calculated with standard methods from observed and expected numbers presented in original paper.
[b] 90% CIs reported in this paper.

TABLE 4.41 Non-Hodgkin's Lymphoma and Exposure to Combustion Products—Selected Epidemiologic Studies

Reference	Study Population	Exposed Cases	Estimated Relative Risk (95% CI)
Cohort Study—Mortality			
Boffetta et al. 1988	All lymphoma deaths (ICD-9 200-202) among male 40- to 79-yr-old enrollees of ACS Cancer Prevention Study at 2-yr followup		
	Diesel-engine exhaust (self-reported agent)	20	0.92
Case-Control Studies			
Costantini et al. 2001	811 NHL (ICD-9 200, 202) and CLL (ICD-9 204.1) cases among men in 12 areas of Italy; occupation (not smoking-adjusted)		
	Transport operators (occupation)	74	0.9 (0.7-1.3)
Mao et al. 2000	764 male and 705 female incident NHL cases from Canada's National Enhanced Cancer Surveillance System in eight provinces (self-reported exposures on mailed questionnaire)		
	Coal tar, soot, pitch, creosote, or asphalt		
	Men	122	1.2 (0.9-1.5)
	Women	19	1.3 (0.7-2.3)
	Mineral, cutting, or lubricating oil		
	Men	177	1.3 (1.0-1.5)
	Women	14	0.8 (0.4-1.4)
Blair et al. 1993	622 NHL cases among white male residents of Iowa and Minnesota		
	Transportation by air (industry)	7	1.8 (0.6-5.5)
	Air transport on certified carriers	4	3.1 (0.6-16.9)
	Oils and greases (JEM-derived agent)	280	1.1 (0.9-1.4)
	Lower intensity	168	1.1 (0.8-1.4)
	Higher intensity	112	1.2 (0.9-1.7)
	Gasoline and diesel exhausts (JEM-derived agent)	265	1.0 (0.8-1.3)
	Lower intensity	230	1.0 (0.8-1.2)
	Higher intensity	35	1.1 (0.7-1.7)
	Asphalt and creosote (JEM-derived agent)	53	1.0 (0.7-1.5)
	Lower intensity	49	1.0 (0.7-1.5)
	Higher intensity	4	1.1 (0.3-4.0)
Siemiatycki et al. 1988	206 NHL cases vs cancer controls among male residents of Montreal, Canada		
	Gasoline exhaust (industrial-hygienist-coded agent)	83	0.9 (0.8-1.1)[a]
	Diesel exhaust (industrial-hygienist-coded agent)	29	0.7 (0.5-1.0)[a]
	Jet-fuel exhaust (industrial-hygienist-coded agent)	4	1.7 (0.5-5.2)[a]
	Liquid-fuel combustion (industrial-hygienist-coded agent)	11	0.8 (0.5-1.3)[a]
	Coke combustion (industrial-hygienist-coded agent)	2	1.4 (0.3-7.3)[a]
Decoufle and	Male lymphoma cases of all types among patients at		

Reference	Study Population	Exposed Cases	Estimated Relative Risk (95% CI)
Stanislawczyk 1977	Roswell Park Memorial Institute in Buffalo, New York (smoking-adjusted)		
	Bus drivers	2	0.71
	Taxicab drivers and chauffeurs	3	0.44
	Truck and tractor drivers	23	0.63
	Bus, taxicab, or truck drivers (combined)—exposed 5+ yr	17	0.72
	Delivery and routemen	13	1.20, ns
	Exposed 5+ yr	4	0.86
	Locomotive engineers and firemen	8	1.23, ns
	Exposed 5+ yr	8	2.13, ns
	Mechanics and repairmen	37	0.83
	Exposed 5+ yr	18	0.77
	Mine operatives and laborers	4	0.45, ns
	Exposed 5+ yr	3	0.54

NOTE: na=not available; ns=risk estimate greater than unity not statistically significant at 0.05 level.
[a] 90% CIs reported in this paper.

TABLE 4.42 Hodgkin's Disease and Exposure to Fuels—Selected Epidemiologic Studies

Reference	Study Population	Exposed Cases	Estimated Relative Risk (95% CI)
Cohort Studies			
Imperial Oil, Canada			
Lewis et al. 2000b	HD (ICD-9 201) deaths (1964-1994) among petroleum workers employed any time during 1964-1983		
	Females	1	0.79 (0.02-4.42)[a]
	Males	7	0.68 (0.28-1.41)
	Refinery segment	1	0.25 (0.01-1.41)[a]
	Marketing and distribution segment	3	0.97 (0.20-2.83)[a]
Lewis et al. 2003	Incident HD (ICD-9 201) cases (1969-1994) among male petroleum workers hired in 1964-1994		
	Females	3	0.90 (0.19-2.63)[a]
	Males	11	1.05 (0.52-1.88)
Huebner et al. 2000	Incident HD (ICD-9 201) cases (1983-1994) among men working in 1970-1992 at Exxon facility in Baton Rouge, Louisiana	4	1.54 (0.42-3.95)[a]
Consonni et al. 1999	Oil-refinery workers in Milan vicinity, Italy	2	1.51 (0.17-5.44)
Jarvholm et al. 1997	Male workers in the Swedish petroleum industry ≥1 yr (qualitative industrial-hygienist-interpretation of personnel records)		
	Incident cases of all types of lymphoma (ICD 200-202)	9	0.93 (0.48-1.6)[b]
	With ≥20-yr latency	3	0.65 (0.18-1.7)[b]
	With ≥10-yr duration	2	0.48 (0.08-1.5)[b]

[a] Risk estimates and 95% CI were calculated with standard methods from observed and expected numbers presented in original paper.
[b] 90% CIs reported in this paper.

TABLE 4.43 Hodgkin's Disease and Exposure to Combustion Products—Selected Epidemiologic Studies

Reference	Study Population	Exposed Cases	Estimated Relative Risk (95% CI)
Cohort Study			
Boffetta et al. 1988	All lymphoma deaths (ICD-9 200-202) among male 40- to 79-yr-old enrollees of ACS Cancer Prevention Study at 2-yr followup		
	Diesel-engine exhaust (self-reported agent)	20	0.92
Case-Control Studies			
Costantini et al. 2001	193 HD (ICD-9 201) cases among men in 12 areas of Italy		
	Transport operators (occupation)	10	0.8 (0.4-1.7)
Decoufle and Stanislawczyk 1977	Male lymphoma cases of all types among patients at Roswell Park Memorial Institute in Buffalo, New York		
	Bus drivers	2	0.71
	Taxicab drivers and chauffeurs	3	0.44
	Truck and tractor drivers	23	0.63
	Bus, taxicab, or truck drivers (combined)—exposed 5+ yr	17	0.72
	Delivery and routemen	13	1.20, ns
	Exposed 5+ yr	4	0.86
	Locomotive engineers and firemen	8	1.23, ns
	Exposed 5+ yr	8	2.13, ns
	Mechanics and repairmen	37	0.83
	Exposed 5+ yr	18	0.77
	Mine operatives and laborers	4	0.45, ns
	Exposed 5+ yr	3	0.54

NOTE: ns=risk estimate greater than unity not statistically significant at 0.05 level.

TABLE 4.44 Multiple Myeloma and Exposure to Fuels—Selected Epidemiologic Studies

Reference	Study Population	Exposed Cases	Estimated Relative Risk (95% CI)
Cohort Studies			
Imperial Oil, Canada			
Lewis et al. 2000b	Multiple myeloma (ICD-9 203) deaths (1964-1994) among petroleum workers employed any time in 1964-1983		
	Females	2	0.71 (0.09-2.58)[a]
	Males	30	1.10 (0.75-1.58)
	Refinery segment	8	0.70 (0.30-1.37)
	Marketing and distribution segment	16	1.94 (1.11-3.15)
	Duration		

Reference	Study Population	Exposed Cases	Estimated Relative Risk (95% CI)
	<25 yr	4	1.88 (0.51-4.81)[a]
	25-34 yr	10	3.06 (1.47-5.63)
	≥35 yr	2	0.82 (0.10-2.96)[a]
Schnatter et al. 1996	Nested case-control study of seven multiple myeloma deaths occurring before 1984 (with 5-yr lag)		
	Total hydrocarbons (ppm-yr)		
	0.0-29.9	3	1.0
	30.0-549	1	1.41 (0.02-118)
	550-6,721	3	0.86 (0.10-7.48)
Lewis et al. 2003	Incident multiple myeloma (ICD-9 203.0) cases (1969-1994) among male petroleum workers hired in 1964-1994	3	0.89 (0.17-2.40)[a]
Huebner et al. 2000	Incident multiple myeloma (ICD-9 203.0) cases (1983-1994) among men working in 1970-1992 at Exxon facility in Baton Rouge, Louisiana	9	1.39 (0.64-2.64)
US land-based oil-distribution workers			
Wong et al. 1993	Deaths (1946-1989) from cancers of "other lymphatic tissue" (ICD-8 202-203, 208)	18	0.92 (0.54-1.45)
	Total hydrocarbon exposure (ppm-yr) (JEM-derived)		
	<500	4	1.12, ns
	500-1,000	2	0.76
	1,000-2,000	4	0.90
	≥2,000	8	0.90
Wong et al. 1999	Nested case-control study of 11 multiple myeloma (ICD-8 203) deaths		
	Job (company records, ever vs never)		
	Plantmen	na	0.55 (0.15-2.10)
	Warehousemen	na	1.82 (0.32-10.4)
	Clerks and office workers	na	0.29 (0.04-2.28)
	Foremen and supervisors	na	1.92 (0.43-8.59)
Case-Control Studies			
Multiple myeloma cases from Danish Cancer Registry (1970-1984)			
Heineman et al. 1992	1,098 male multiple myeloma cases		
	Industry, ever (from Danish Pension Fund)		
	Wholesale trade in fuel, oil, or gas	12	0.8 (0.4-1.6)
	Industrial-hygiene-derived exposures		
	Gasoline		
	Possible exposure	146	1.2 (1.0-1.5)
	1 months-5 yr	48	1.3 (0.9-1.9)
	≥5 yr	85	1.2 (0.9-1.5)
	Probable exposure	41	1.4 (0.9-2.1)
	1 months-5 yr	14	1.5 (0.8-2.9)
	≥5 yr	24	1.4 (0.9-2.4)
	Oil products		

Reference	Study Population	Exposed Cases	Estimated Relative Risk (95% CI)
	Possible exposure	200	1.1 (0.9-1.3)
	1 months-5 yr	57	1.1 (0.8-1.6)
	≥5 yr	131	1.1 (0.9-1.4)
	Probable exposure	57	1.4 (1.0-1.9)
	1 months-5 yr	19	1.5 (0.8-2.6)
	≥5 yr	32	1.4 (0.9-2.1)
Pottern et al. 1992	363 female multiple myeloma cases employed after 1964		
	Coal and oil products (industrial-hygiene-derived agent)		
	Possible exposure	39	1.0 (0.7-1.5)
	Probable exposure	2	0.8 (0.1-3.9)
Linet et al. 1987	100 multiple myeloma cases among residents of Baltimore		
	Petroleum (self-reported agent)	na	3.7 (1.3-10.3)
698 multiple myeloma cases (477 cases responded for self; next of kin responded for 221 cases) from four US SEER registries (1977-1981)			
Morris et al. 1986	Exposures grouped from interview lists of exposure agents		
	Aliphatic hydrocarbons	109	0.9 (0.7-1.2)
	Self-respondents only	85	1.1 (0.8-1.5)
Demers et al. 1993	Occupations and industries from work history in interview		
	Garage and service station	13	0.8 (0.4-1.5)
	Self-respondents only	9	0.8 (0.3-1.7)
	Petroleum and coal refining and manufacturing industries	8	1.2 (0.4-3.1)
	Self-respondents only	2	0.4 (0.1-1.9)

NOTE: na=not available

[a] Risk estimates and 95% CIs calculated with standard methods from observed and expected numbers presented in original paper.

TABLE 4.45 Multiple Myeloma and Exposure to Combustion Products—Selected Epidemiologic Studies

Reference	Study Population	Exposed Cases	Estimated Relative Risk (95% CI)
Nested Case-Control Studies			
Lee et al. 2003	466 male multiple myeloma cases diagnosed 1971-1999 among Swedish construction workers		
	JEM-derived agents		
	Diesel exhaust (ever)	79	1.3 (1.00-1.77)
	Low	52	1.4 (0.99-1.92)
	Medium	10	1.1 (0.56-2.04)
	High	17	1.4 (0.77-2.59)
	Asphalt (ever)	6	0.8 (0.35-1.85)
Wong et al. 1999	11 multiple myeloma deaths in nested case-control study of cohort of land-based US distribution workers		

Reference	Study Population	Exposed Cases	Estimated Relative Risk (95% CI)
	(Wong et al. 1993, which presented no separate results for multiple myeloma)		
	Job (company records–ever vs never)		
	Mechanic	na	0.45 (0.05-3.81)
	Loader	na	1.00 (0.11-9.51)
	Driver	na	0.91 (0.21-3.96)
Boffetta et al. 1989	128 multiple myeloma deaths among cancer-free enrollees in ACS Cancer Prevention Study II cohort during 4-yr followup		
	Agents (self-report)		
	Diesel exhaust	14	1.4 (0.7-2.7)
	Gasoline exhaust	14	0.9 (0.5-1.6)
	Coal tar, pitch, or asphalt	4	1.7 (0.5-5.6)
	Main occupation (self-report)		
	Truck driver	3	2.8 (0.5-16.1)
	Railroad worker	3	7.1 (1.2-43.6)
Case-Control Studies			
Costantini et al. 2001	133 multiple myeloma cases among men in 12 areas of Italy		
	Transport operators (self-reported occupation)	7	0.5 (0.2-1.1)
Multiple myeloma cases from Danish Cancer Registry (1970-1984)			
Heineman et al. 1992	1,098 male multiple myeloma cases		
	Industry, ever (from Danish Pension Fund)		
	Transportation	100	1.3 (1.0-1.6)
	1 month-5 yr	41	1.1 (0.8-1.6)
	≥5 yr	59	1.2 (0.9-1.6)
	Industrial-hygiene-derived exposures		
	Tar, asphalt, or soot		
	Possible exposure	49	1.1 (0.8-1.6)
	Probable exposure	17	0.6 (0.3-1.0)
	Engine exhaust		
	Possible exposure		
	1 month-5 yr	52	1.5 (1.0-2.1)
	≥5 yr	76	1.3 (1.0-1.7)
	Probable exposure		
	1 month-5 yr	25	1.4 (0.9-2.4)
	≥5 yr	52	1.3 (0.9-1.8)
Pottern et al. 1992	363 female multiple cases employed after 1964		
	Industry, ever (from Danish Pension Fund)		
	Transportation	13	1.0 (0.5-1.9)
	Industrial-hygiene-derived exposures		
	Exhaust gases		

Reference	Study Population	Exposed Cases	Estimated Relative Risk (95% CI)
	Possible exposure	8	1.4 (0.6-3.2)
	Probable exposure	4	1.6 (0.4-5.5)
Flodin et al. 1987	75 prevalent multiple myeloma cases among male residents of Sweden		
	Exposure to engine exhaust >1 yr (self-report)	35	2.1 (1.2-3.9)
698 multiple myeloma cases from four US SEER registries (1977-1981) (477 cases responded for themselves; next of kin responded for 221 cases)			
Morris et al. 1986	Exposures grouped from interview lists of exposure agents		
	Carbon monoxide (surrogate for exhausts and smokes)	27	1.8 (1.0-3.2)
	Self-respondents only	24	1.9 (1.1–3.2)
Williams et al. 1989	69 cases with light-chain myeloma	5	2.9 (1.0-8.4)
	Self-respondents only	5	6.1 (2.0-18.2)
	629 cases with non-light-chain myeloma	19	1.3 (0.7-2.7)
Demers et al. 1993	Occupations and industries from work history in interview		
	Vehicle mechanics	24	0.8 (0.5–1.4)
	Self-respondents only	16	0.9 (0.5–1.6)

NOTE: na=not available; ns=risk estimate greater than unity not statistically significant at 0.05 level.

TABLE 4.46 Leukemias and Exposure to Combustion Products—Selected Epidemiologic Studies

Reference	Study Population	Exposed Cases	Estimated Relative Risk (95% CI)
Cohort Study			
Boffetta et al. 1988	All leukemia deaths (ICD-9 204-208) occurring during 2-yr followup in cohort of 62,800 men 40-79 yr old at enrollment in ACS Cancer Prevention Study with self-reported exposure to diesel engine exhaust; expectations based on experience of 307,143 nonexposed counterparts	17	1.29, ns
Nested Case-Control Study			
Wong et al. 1999	Nested case-control study on cohort of land-based US distribution workers (Wong et al. 1993) Jobs from company records (ever vs never)		
	Total leukemia (ICD-8 204-207) deaths	35	
	Mechanic	na	0.83 (0.30-2.34)
	Loader	na	0.79 (0.09-6.82)
	Drivers	na	0.77 (0.35-1.71)
	AML (ICD-8 205.0)	13	
	Mechanic	na	0.91 (0.17-4.80)
	Loader	0	–
	Drivers	na	0.42 (0.13-1.44)

Reference	Study Population	Exposed Cases	Estimated Relative Risk (95% CI)
Case-Control Studies			
Costantini et al. 2001	383 leukemias (ICD-9 204-208) cases among men in 12 areas of Italy		
	Transport operators (occupation)	34	1.1 (0.7-1.7)
Lindquist et al. 1991	125 acute leukemia cases among residents of Sweden		
	Professional drivers (>1 month)	18	3.0 (1.1-9.2)
	Exposed >5 yr during lifetime or >1 yr during period 5-20 yr before diagnosis	10	5.0 ($p < 0.05$)
	Less exposure	8	0.75
Flodin et al. 1988	111 chronic lymphocytic leukemia cases (ICD-9 204.15) among residents of Sweden		
	Engine exhaust (self-reported agent)	31	2.2 (1.2-4.2)
Decoufle and Stanislawczyk 1977	Male leukemia cases among patients at Roswell Park Memorial Institute in Buffalo, New York (job history, including durations, from medical charts)		
	Bus drivers	0	–
	Taxicab drivers and chauffeurs	4	2.08, ns
	Truck and tractor drivers	6	0.51
	Bus, taxicab, or truck drivers (combined), duration 5+ yr	7	0.71
	Delivery and routemen	2	0.60
	Duration 5+ yr	1	0.51
	Locomotive engineers and firemen	2	0.99
	Duration 5+ yr	2	1.35, ns
	Mechanics and repairmen	10	0.75
	Duration 5+ yr	6	0.64
	Mine operatives and laborers	6	2.16, ns
	Duration 5+ yr	2	0.87

NOTE: na=not available; ns=risk estimate greater than unity not statistically significant at 0.05 level.

TABLE 4.47 Myelodysplastic Syndromes and Exposure to Fuels—Selected Epidemiologic Studies

Reference	Study Population	Exposed Cases	Estimated Relative Risk (95% CI)
Case-Control Studies (none adjusted for smoking)			
Nisse et al. 2001	204 MDS cases among residents of northern France; industrial-hygiene-derived agents		
	Petrol	15	2.5 (0.9–7.7)
	Oil	44	4.2 (2.0–9.9)
West et al. 1995	400 MDS cases among residents of three regions in UK; industrial-hygiene-derived agents		
	Petroleum products (≥low intensity)	203	1.09 (0.79-1.50)[a]
	Diesels and petrols (≥low intensity)	123	1.01 (0.72-1.44)[a]
	>50 hr (≥medium intensity)	na	1.02 (0.67-1.56)[a]
	>2,500 hr (≥medium intensity)	na	1.09 (0.66-1.81)[a]

Reference	Study Population	Exposed Cases	Estimated Relative Risk (95% CI)
	Oils and greases (≥low intensity)	123	1.29 (0.88–1.89)
	>50 hr (≥medium intensity)	na	0.92 (0.60-1.40)[a]
	>2,500 hr (≥medium intensity)	na	1.22 (0.77-1.95)[a]
Farrow et al. 1989	63 MDS cases among residents of Wales; industrial-hygiene-derived agents; pilot for and likely subset of sample in West et al. 1995		
	Petrol-diesel liquids	29	2.99 (1.29-6.98)[a]
	Petrol-diesel fumes	35	2.17 (1.00-4.74)[a]

NOTE: na=not available; ns=risk estimate greater than unity not statistically significant at 0.05 level.
[a] Unadjusted ORs and 95% CIs calculated with standard methods from observed numbers presented in original paper.

TABLE 4.48 Myelodysplastic Syndromes and Exposure to Combustion Products—Selected Epidemiologic Studies

Reference	Study Population	Exposed Cases	Estimated Relative Risk (95% CI)
Case-Control Studies (none adjusted for smoking)			
Nisse et al. 2001	204 MDS cases among residents of northern France		
	Industrial-hygiene-derived agents		
	Exhaust gases	33	1.0 (0.5–1.9)
	PAHs	17	1.8 (0.7–4.6)
	Machine operator (occupation, ≥6 mo)	na	2.8 (1.3-6.4)
West et al. 1995	400 MDS cases among residents of three regions in UK		
	Industrial-hygiene-derived agents		
	Exhaust gases (≥low intensity)	79	1.26 (0.86–1.86)
	>50 hr (≥medium intensity)	na	1.72 (0.93-3.20)
	>2,500 hr (≥medium intensity)	na	1.57 (0.77-3.23)
	Coal tar (≥low intensity)	35	1.07 (0.62-1.84)[a]
	>50 hr (≥medium intensity)	na	1.00 (0.47-2.14)[a]
	>2,500 hr (≥medium intensity)	na	0.88 (0.27-2.76)[a]
	Transport operating, material moving and storing, and so on (occupation, ≥6 mo)	32	0.78 (0.46-1.31)[a]

NOTE: na=not available; ns=risk estimate greater than unity not statistically significant at 0.05 level.
[a] Unadjusted ORs and 95% CIs calculated with standard methods from observed numbers presented in original paper.

REFERENCES

Abbey DE, Nishino N, McDonnell WF, Burchette RJ, Knutsen SF, Beeson WL, Yang JX. 1999. Long-term inhalable particles and other air pollutants related to mortality in nonsmokers. *American Journal of Respiratory and Critical Care Medicine* 159(2):373-382.

ACS (American Cancer Society). 2003a. *ACS: Laryngeal and Hypopharyngeal Cancer Detailed Guide*. [Online]. Available: http://www.cancer.org/docroot/CRI/content/CRI_2_4_7x_CRC_Laryngeal_and_Hypopharyngeal_Cancer_PDF.asp [accessed January 28, 2004].

ACS. 2003b. *ACS: Nasal Cavity and Paranasal Cancer*. [Online]. Available: http://www.cancer.org/docroot/CRI/CRI_2_3x.asp?dt=75 [accessed January 28, 2004].

ACS. 2003c. *ACS: Nasospharyngeal Cancer*. [Online]. Available: http://www.cancer.org/docroot/CRI/CRI_2_3x.asp?dt=17 [accessed January 28, 2004].

ACS. 2003d. *ACS: Oral Cavity and Oropharyngeal Cancer Detailed Guide*. [Online]. Available: http://www.cancer.org/docroot/CRI/content/CRI_2_4_7x_CRC_Oral_Cavity_and_Oropharyngeal_Cancer_PDF.asp [accessed January 28, 2004].

ACS. 2003e. *ACS: What Are the Risk Factors for Breast Cancer?* [Online]. Available: http://www.cancer.org/docroot/CRI/content/CRI_2_4_2X_What_are_the_risk_factors_for_breast_cancer_5.asp?sitearea= [accessed June 9, 2004].

ACS. 2003f. *ACS: What Are the Risk Factors for Liver Cancer?* [Online]. Available: http://www.cancer.org/docroot/CRI/content/CRI_2_4_2X_What_are_the_risk_factors_for_liver_cancer_25.asp?sitearea= [accessed June 4, 2004].

ACS. 2003g. *Cancer Facts and Figures 2003*. [Online]. Available: http://www.cancer.org/docroot/STT/content/STT_1x_Cancer_Facts__Figures_2003.asp [accessed January 14, 2003].

ACS. 2004a. *ACS: All About Myelodysplastic Syndrome*. [Online]. Available: http://www.cancer.org/docroot/cri/cri_2x.asp [accessed September 7, 2004].

ACS. 2004b. *ACS: Detailed Guide: Cervical Cancer*. [Online]. Available: http://www.cancer.org/docroot/CRI/CRI_2_3x.asp?rnav=cridg&dt=8 [accessed June 10, 2004].

ACS. 2004c. *ACS: Detailed Guide: Endometrial Cancer*. [Online]. Available: http://www.cancer.org/docroot/CRI/CRI_2_3x.asp?dt=11 [accessed June 10, 2004].

ACS. 2004d. *ACS: Detailed Guide: Eye Cancer*. [Online]. Available: http://www.cancer.org/docroot/CRI/content/CRI_2_4_1x_What_is_eye_cancer_74.asp?rnav=cri [accessed April 22, 2004].

ACS. 2004e. *ACS: Detailed Guide: Leukemia - Acute Lymphocytic (ALL)*. [Online]. Available: http://www.cancer.org/docroot/CRI/CRI_2_3x.asp?dt=57 [accessed November 5, 2004].

ACS. 2004f. *ACS: Detailed Guide: Leukemia - Acute Myeloid (AML)*. [Online]. Available: http://www.cancer.org/docroot/CRI/CRI_2_3x.asp?dt=82 [accessed November 5, 2004].

ACS. 2004g. *ACS: Detailed Guide: Leukemia - Chronic Lymphocytic (CLL)*. [Online]. Available: http://www.cancer.org/docroot/CRI/CRI_2_3x.asp?dt=62 [accessed November 5, 2004].

ACS. 2004h. *ACS: Detailed Guide: Leukemia - Chronic Myeloid (CML)*. [Online]. Available: http://www.cancer.org/docroot/CRI/CRI_2_3x.asp?dt=83 [accessed November 5, 2004].

ACS. 2004i. *ACS: Detailed Guide: Ovarian Cancer*. [Online]. Available: http://www.cancer.org/docroot/CRI/CRI_2_3x.asp?dt=33 [accessed June 10, 2004].

ACS. 2004j. *ACS: Detailed Guide: Testicular Cancer*. [Online]. Available: http://www.cancer.org/docroot/CRI/CRI_2_3x.asp?dt=41 [accessed June 10, 2004].

ACS. 2004k. *ACS: Hodgkin's Disease Detailed Guide*. [Online]. Available at: http://www.cancer.org/docroot/CRI/content/CRI_2_4_7x_CRC_Hodgkin_Disease_PDF.asp [accessed February 10, 2004].

ACS. 2004l. *ACS: Multiple Myeloma Detailed Guide*. [Online]. Available: http://www.cancer.org/docroot/CRI/content/CRI_2_4_7x_CRC_Multiple_Myeloma_PDF.asp [accessed February 10, 2004].

ACS. 2004m. *ACS: Overview: Pancreatic Cancer*. [Online]. Available: http://www.cancer.org/docroot/CRI/CRI_2_1x.asp?dt=34 [accessed January 30, 2004].

ACS. 2004n. *ACS: The Different Types of Leukemia*. [Online]. Available: http://www.cancer.org/docroot/CRI/content/CRI_2_2_1X_The_different_types_of_leukemia_57.asp?sitearea= [accessed November 5, 2004].

ACS. 2004o. *ACS: What Is Bladder Cancer?* [Online]. Available: http://www.cancer.org/docroot/CRI/content/CRI_2_4_1X_What_is_bladder_cancer_44.asp?sitearea= [accessed February 4, 2004].

ACS. 2004p. *ACS: What Is Colorectal Cancer?* [Online]. Available: http://www.cancer.org/docroot/CRI/content/CRI_2_2_1X_What_is_colon_and_rectum_cancer_10.asp?sitearea= [accessed January 30, 2004].

ACS. 2004q. *ACS: What Is Esophagus Cancer?* [Online]. Available: http://www.cancer.org/docroot/CRI/content/CRI_2_2_1X_What_is_esophagus_cancer_12.asp?sitearea= [accessed January 30, 2004].

ACS. 2004r. *ACS: What Is Kidney Cancer (Renal Cell Carcinoma)?* [Online]. Available: http://www.cancer.org/docroot/CRI/content/CRI_2_4_1X_What_is_kidney_cancer_22.asp?sitearea= [accessed February 4, 2004].

ACS. 2004s. *ACS: What Is Lung Cancer?* [Online]. Available: http://www.cancer.org/docroot/CRI/content/CRI_2_2_1X_What_is_lung_cancer_26.asp?sitearea= [accessed February 4, 2004].

ACS. 2004t. *ACS: What Is Male Breast Cancer?* [Online]. Available: http://www.cancer.org/docroot/CRI/content/CRI_2_4_1X_What_is_male_breast_cancer_28.asp?sitearea= [accessed February 4, 2004].

ACS. 2004u. *ACS: What Is Melanoma Skin Cancer?* [Online]. Available: http://www.cancer.org/docroot/CRI/content/CRI_2_2_1X_What_is_melanoma_skin_cancer_50.asp?sitearea= [accessed February 4, 2004].

ACS. 2004v. *ACS: What Is Prostate Cancer?* [Online]. Available: http://www.cancer.org/docroot/CRI/content/CRI_2_4_1X_What_is_prostate_cancer_36.asp?sitearea = [accessed February 4, 2004].

ACS. 2004w. *ACS: What Is Stomach Cancer?* [Online]. Available: http://www.cancer.org/docroot/CRI/content/CRI_2_2_1X_What_is_stomach_cancer_40.asp?sitearea = [accessed January 30, 2004].

Ahrens W, Jockel KH, Patzak W, Elsner G. 1991. Alcohol, smoking, and occupational factors in cancer of the larynx: A case-control study. *American Journal of Industrial Medicine* 20(4):477-493.

Ajani UA, Seddon JM, Hsieh CC, Egan KM, Albert DM, Gragoudas ES. 1992. Occupation and risk of uveal melanoma. An exploratory study. *Cancer* 70(12):2891-2900.

Alarie Y, Ulrich CE, Busey WM, Krumm AA, MacFarland HN. 1972. Long-term continuous exposure to sulfur dioxide in cynomolgus monkeys. *Archives of Environmental Health* 24(2):115-128.

Alfredsson L, Hammar N, Hogstedt C. 1993. Incidence of myocardial infarction and mortality from specific causes among bus drivers in Sweden. *International Journal of Epidemiology* 22(1):57-61.

Alguacil J, Kauppinen T, Porta M, Partanen T, Malats N, Kogevinas M, Benavides FG, Obiols J, Bernal F, Rifa J, Carrato A. 2000. Risk of pancreatic cancer and occupational exposures in Spain. *Annals of Occupational Hygiene* 44(5):391-403.

Armstrong RW, Armstrong MJ. 1983. Environmental risk factors and nasopharyngeal carcinoma in Selangor, Malaysia: A cross-ethnic perspective. *Ecology of Disease* 2(3):185-198.

Armstrong RW, Imrey PB, Lye MS, Armstrong MJ, Yu MC, Sani S. 2000. Nasopharyngeal carcinoma in Malaysian Chinese: Occupational exposures to particles, formaldehyde and heat. *International Journal of Epidemiology* 29(6):991-998.

Aronson KJ, Siemiatycki J, Dewar R, Gerin M. 1996. Occupational risk factors for prostate cancer: Results from a case-control study in Montreal, Quebec, Canada. *American Journal of Epidemiology* 143(4):363-373.

Asal NR, Geyer JR, Risser DR, Lee ET, Kadamani S, Cherng N. 1988a. Risk factors in renal cell carcinoma. II. Medical history, occupation, multivariate analysis, and conclusions. *Cancer Detection and Prevention* 13(3-4):263-279.

Asal NR, Risser DR, Kadamani S, Geyer JR, Lee ET, Cherng N. 1988b. Risk factors in renal cell carcinoma: I. Methodology, demographics, tobacco, beverage use, and obesity. *Cancer Detection and Prevention* 11(3-6):359-377.

ATSDR (Agency for Toxic Substances and Disease Registry). 1995. *Toxicological Profile for Polycyclic Aromatic Hydrocarbons (PAHs) (Update)*. Atlanta, GA: US Department of Health and Human Services, Public Health Service, ATSDR

Auperin A, Benhamou S, Ory-Paoletti C, Flamant R. 1994. Occupational risk factors for renal cell carcinoma: A case-control study. *Occupational and Environmental Medicine* 51(6):426-428.

Barbone F, Bovenzi M, Cavallieri F, Stanta G. 1995. Air pollution and lung cancer in Trieste, Italy. *American Journal of Epidemiology* 141(12):1161-1169.

Baris D, Garrity TJ, Telles JL, Heineman EF, Olshan A, Zahm SH. 2001. Cohort mortality study of Philadelphia firefighters. *American Journal of Industrial Medicine* 39(5):463-476.

Beeson WL, Abbey DE, Knutsen SF. 1998. Long-term concentrations of ambient air pollutants and incident lung cancer in California adults: Results from the AHSMOG study. *Environmental Health Perspectives* 106(12):813-823.

Benhamou S, Benhamou E, Flamant R. 1988. Occupational risk factors of lung cancer in a French case-control study. *British Journal of Industrial Medicine* 45(4):231-233.

Berrino F, Richiardi L, Boffetta P, Esteve J, Belletti I, Raymond L, Troschel L, Pisani P, Zubiri L, Ascunce N, Guberan E, Tuyns A, Terracini B, Merletti F, Arduini L, Baldasseroni A, Continenza D, Crosignani P, Ferrario F, Macaluso M, Magnani C, Merler E. 2003. Occupation and larynx and hypopharynx cancer: A job-exposure matrix approach in an international case-control study in France, Italy, Spain and Switzerland. *Cancer Causes and Control* 14(3):213-223.

Bertazzi PA, Pesatori AC, Zocchetti C, Latocca R. 1989. Mortality study of cancer risk among oil refinery workers. *International Archives of Occupational and Environmental Health* 61(4):261-270.

Biggeri A, Barbone F, Lagazio C, Bovenzi M, Stanta G. 1996. Air pollution and lung cancer in Trieste, Italy: Spatial analysis of risk as a function of distance from sources. *Environmental Health Perspectives* 104(7):750-754.

Blair A, Linos A, Stewart PA, Burmeister LF, Gibson R, Everett G, Schuman L, Cantor KP. 1993. Evaluation of risks for non-Hodgkin's lymphoma by occupation and industry exposures from a case-control study. *American Journal of Industrial Medicine* 23(2):301-312.

Boffetta P, Dosemeci M, Gridley G, Bath H, Moradi T, Silverman D. 2001. Occupational exposure to diesel engine emissions and risk of cancer in Swedish men and women. *Cancer Causes & Control* 12(4):365-374.

Boffetta P, Harris RE, Wynder EL. 1990. Case-control study on occupational exposure to diesel exhaust and lung cancer risk. *American Journal of Industrial Medicine* 17(5):577-591.

Boffetta P, Richiardi L, Berino F, Esteve J, Pisani P, Crosignani P, Raymond L, Zubire L, Del Moral A, Lehmann W, Donato F, Terracini B, Tuyns A, Merletti F. 2003. Occupation and larynx and hypopharynx cancer: An international case-control study in France, Italy, Spain, and Switzerland. *Cancer Causes & Control* 14(3):203-212.

Boffetta P, Stellman SD, Garfinkel L. 1988. Diesel exhaust exposure and mortality among males in the American Cancer Society prospective study. *American Journal of Industrial Medicine* 14(4):403-415.

Boffetta P, Stellman SD, Garfinkel L. 1989. A case-control study of multiple myeloma nested in the American Cancer Society prospective study. *International Journal of Cancer* 43(4):554-559.

Bonassi S, Merlo F, Pearce N, Puntoni R. 1989. Bladder cancer and occupational exposure to polycyclic aromatic hydrocarbons. *International Journal of Cancer* 44(4):648-651.

Borgia P, Forastiere F, Rapiti E, Rizzelli R, Magliola ME, Perucci CA, Axelson O. 1994 . Mortality among taxi drivers in Rome: A cohort study. *American Journal of Industrial Medicine* 25(4):507-517.

Bovenzi M, Stanta G, Antiga G, Peruzzo P, Cavallieri F. 1993. Occupational exposure and lung cancer risk in a coastal area of northeastern Italy. *International Archives of Occupational and Environmental Health* 65(1):35-41.

Brown LM, Mason TJ, Williams Pickle L, Stewart PA, Buffler PA, Burau K, Ziegler RG, Fraumeni Jr JF. 1988. Occupational risk factors for laryngeal cancer on the Texas Gulf Coast. *Cancer Research* 48(7):1960-1964.

Brownson RC. 1988. A case-control study of renal cell carcinoma in relation to occupation, smoking, and alcohol consumption. *Archives of Environmental Health* 43(3):238-241.

Brownson RC, Chang JC, Davis JR. 1987. Occupation, smoking, and alcohol in the epidemiology of bladder cancer. *American Journal of Public Health* 77(10):1298-1300.

Bruske-Hohlfeld I, Mohner M, Ahrens W, Pohlabeln H, Heinrich J, Kreuzer M, Jockel KH, Wichmann HE. 1999. Lung cancer risk in male workers occupationally exposed to diesel motor emissions in Germany. *American Journal of Industrial Medicine* 36(4):405-414.

Bruske-Hohlfeld I, Mohner M, Pohlabeln H, Ahrens W, Bolm-Audorff U, Kreienbrock L, Kreuzer M, Jahn I, Wichmann HE, Jockel KH. 2000. Occupational lung cancer risk for men in Germany: Results from a pooled case-control study. *American Journal of Epidemiology* 151(4):384-395.

Buiatti E, Kriebel D, Geddes M, Santucci M, Pucci N. 1985. A case control study of lung cancer in Florence, Italy. I. Occupational risk factors. *Journal of Epidemiology and Community Health* 39(3):244-250.

Carozza SE, Wrensch M, Miike R, Newman B, Olshan AF , Savitz DA, Yost M, Lee M. 2000. Occupation and adult gliomas. *American Journal of Epidemiology* 152(9):838-846.

Chen CJ, Wu HY, Chuang YC, Chang AS, Luh KT, Chao HH, Chen KY, Chen SG, Lai GM, Huang HH. 1990. Epidemiologic characteristics and multiple risk factors of lung cancer in Taiwan. *Anticancer Research* 10(4):971-976.

Chow WH, McLaughlin JK, Malker HS, Linet MS, Weiner JA, Stone BJ. 1995. Esophageal cancer and occupation in a cohort of Swedish men. *American Journal of Industrial Medicine* 27(5):749-757.

Chow WH, McLaughlin JK, Malker HS, Weiner JA, Ericsson JL, Stone BJ, Blot WJ. 1994. Occupation and stomach cancer in a cohort of Swedish men. *American Journal of Industrial Medicine* 26(4):511-520.

Claude JC, Frentzel-Beyme RR, Kunze E. 1988. Occupation and risk of cancer of the lower urinary tract among men. A case-control study. *International Journal of Cancer* 41(3):371-379.

Clavel J, Mandereau L, Limasset JC, Hemon D, Cordier S. 1994. Occupational exposure to polycyclic aromatic hydrocarbons and the risk of bladder cancer: A French case-control study. *International Journal of Epidemiology* 23(6):1145-1153.

Cocco P, Figgs L, Dosemeci M, Hayes R, Linet MS, Hsing AW. 1998. Case-control study of occupational exposures and male breast cancer. *Occupational and Environmental Medicine* 55(9):599-604.

Cocco P, Palli D, Buiatti E, Cipriani F, DeCarli A, Manca P, Ward MH, Blot WJ, Fraumeni Jr JF. 1994. Occupational exposures as risk factors for gastric cancer in Italy. *Cancer Causes & Control* 5(3):241-248.

Cole P, Hoover R, Friedell GH. 1972. Occupation and cancer of the lower urinary tract. *Cancer* 29(5):1250-1260.

Consonni D, Pesatori AC, Tironi A, Bernucci I, Zocchetti C, Bertazzi PA. 1999. Mortality study in an Italian oil refinery: Extension of the follow-up. *American Journal of Industrial Medicine* 35(3):287-294.

Cordier S, Clavel J, Limasset JC, Boccon-Gibod L, Le Moual N, Mandereau L, Hemon D. 1993. Occupational risks of bladder cancer in France: A multicentre case-control study. *International Journal of Epidemiology* 22(3):403-411.

Costantini AS, Miligi L, Kriebel D, Ramazzotti V, Rodella S, Scarpi E, Stagnaro E, Tumino R, Fontana A, Masala G, Vigano C, Vindigni C, Crosignani P, Benvenuti A, Vineis P. 2001. A multicenter case-control study in Italy on hematolymphopoietic neoplasms and occupation. *Epidemiology* 12(1):78-87.

Dai XD, Lin CY, Sun XW, Shi YB, Lin YJ. 1996. The etiology of lung cancer in nonsmoking females in Harbin, China. *Lung Cancer* 14(Suppl 1):S85-S91.

Damber L, Larsson LG. 1985. Professional driving, smoking, and lung cancer: A case referent study. *British Journal of Industrial Medicine* 42(4):246-252.

Damber LA, Larsson LG. 1987. Occupation and male lung cancer: A case-control study in northern Sweden. *British Journal of Industrial Medicine* 44(7):446-453.

De Roos AJ, Stewart PA, Linet MS, Heineman EF, Dosemeci M, Wilcosky T, Shapiro WR, Selker RG, Fine HA, Black PM, Inskip PD. 2003. Occupation and the risk of adult glioma in the United States. *Cancer Causes and Control* 14(2):139-50.

De Stefani E, Boffetta P, Oreggia F, Ronco A, Kogevinas M, Mendilaharsu M. 1998. Occupation and the risk of laryngeal cancer in Uruguay. *American Journal of Industrial Medicine* 33(6):537-542.

Decoufle P, Stanislawczyk K. 1977. *A Retrospective Survey of Cancer in Relation to Occupation*. Cincinnati, OH: Center for Disease Control, National Institute for Occupational Safety and Health.

Delahunt B, Bethwaite PB, Nacey JN. 1995. Occupational risk for renal cell carcinoma. A case-control study based on the New Zealand Cancer Registry. *British Journal of Urology* 75(5):578-582.

Demers PA, Kogevinas M, Boffetta P, Leclerc A, Luce D, Gerin M, Battista G, Belli S, Bolm-Audorf U, Brinton LA, Colin D, Comba P, Hardell L, Hayes RB, Magnani C, Merler E, Morcet JF, Preston-Martin S, Matos E, Rodella S, Vaughan TL, Zheng W, Vainio H. 1995. Wood dust and sino-nasal cancer: Pooled reanalysis of twelve case-control studies. *American Journal of Industrial Medicine* 28(2):151-166.

Demers PA, Vaughan TL, Koepsell TD, Lyon JL, Swanson GM, Greenberg RS, Weiss NS. 1993. A case-control study of multiple myeloma and occupation. *American Journal of Industrial Medicine* 23(4):629-639.

Dietz A, Senneweld E, Maier H. 1995. Indoor air pollution by emissions of fossil fuel single stoves: Possibly a hitherto underrated risk factor in the development of carcinomas in the head and neck. *Otolaryngology - Head & Neck Surgery* 112(2):308-315.

Divine BJ, Barron V. 1986. Texaco Mortality Study: II. Patterns of mortality among white males by specific job groups. *American Journal of Industrial Medicine* 10(4):371-381.

Divine BJ, Barron V, Kaplan SD. 1985. Texaco mortality study. I. Mortality among refinery, petrochemical, and research workers. *Journal of Occupational Medicine* 27(6):445-447.

Divine BJ, Hartman CM, Wendt JK. 1999a. Update of the Texaco mortality study 1947-93: Part II. Analyses of specific causes of death for white men employed in refining, research, and petrochemicals. *Occupational & Environmental Medicine* 56(3):174-180.

Divine BJ, Hartman CM, Wendt JK. 1999b. Update of the Texaco mortality study 1947-93: Part I. Analysis of overall patterns of mortality among refining, research, and petrochemical workers. *Occupational and Environmental Medicine* 56(3):167-173.

Du YX, Cha Q, Chen XW, Chen YZ, Huang LF, Feng ZZ, Wu XF, Wu JM. 1996. An epidemiological study of risk factors for lung cancer in Guangzhou, China. *Lung Cancer* 14(Suppl 1):S9-S37.

Dumas S, Parent ME, Siemiatycki J, Brisson J. 2000. Rectal cancer and occupational risk factors: A hypothesis-generating, exposure-based case-control study. *International Journal of Cancer* 87(6):874-879.

Elci OC, Akpinar-Elci M, Blair A, Dosemeci M. 2003. Risk of laryngeal cancer by occupational chemical exposure in Turkey. *Journal of Occupational and Environmental Medicine* 45(10):1100-1106.

Elci OC, Dosemeci M, Blair A. 2001. Occupation and the risk of laryngeal cancer in Turkey. *Scandinavian Journal of Work, Environment & Health* 27(4):233-239.

Emmelin A, Nystrom L, Wall S. 1993. Diesel exhaust exposure and smoking: A case-referent study of lung cancer among Swedish dock workers. *Epidemiology* 4(3):237-244.

Farrow A, Jacobs A, West RR. 1989. Myelodysplasia, chemical exposure, and other environmental factors. *Leukemia* 3(1):33-35.
Flodin U, Fredriksson M, Persson B. 1987. Multiple myeloma and engine exhausts, fresh wood, and creosote: A case-referent study. *American Journal of Industrial Medicine* 12(5):519-529.
Flodin U, Fredriksson M, Persson B, Axelson O. 1988. Chronic lymphatic leukaemia and engine exhausts, fresh wood, and DDT: A case-referent study. *British Journal of Industrial Medicine* 45(1):33-38.
Franceschi S, Serraino D, Bidoli E, Talamini R, Tirelli U, Carbone A, La Vecchia C. 1989. The epidemiology of non-Hodgkin's lymphoma in the north-east of Italy: A hospital-based case-control study. *Leukemia Research* 13(6):465-472.
Fritschi L, Siemiatycki J. 1996a. Melanoma and occupation: Results of a case-control study. *Occupational and Environmental Medicine* 53(3):168-173.
Fritschi L, Siemiatycki J. 1996b. Lymphoma, myeloma and occupation: Results of a case-control study. *International Journal of Cancer* 67(4):498-503.
Gallagher RP, Bajdik CD, Fincham S, Hill GB, Keefe AR, Coldman A, McLean DI. 1996. Chemical exposures, medical history, and risk of squamous and basal cell carcinoma of the skin. *Cancer Epidemiology, Biomarkers and Prevention* 5(6):419-424.
Gamble JF, Pearlman ED, Nicolich MJ. 1996. A nested case-control study of kidney cancer among refinery/petrochemical workers. *Environmental Health Perspectives* 104(6):642-650.
Garshick E, Schenker MB, Munoz A, Segal M, Smith TJ, Woskie SR, Hammond SK, Speizer FE. 1987. A case-control study of lung cancer and diesel exhaust exposure in railroad workers. *American Review of Respiratory Disease* 135(6):1242-1248.
Garshick E, Schenker MB, Munoz A, Segal M, Smith TJ, Woskie SR, Hammond SK, Speizer FE. 1988. A retrospective cohort study of lung cancer and diesel exhaust exposure in railroad workers. *American Review of Respiratory Disease* 137(4):820-825.
Gerhardsson de Verdier MG, Plato N, Steineck G, Peters JM. 1992. Occupational exposures and cancer of the colon and rectum. *American Journal of Industrial Medicine* 22(3):291-303.
Gerin M, Siemiatycki J, Kemper H, Begin D. 1985. Obtaining occupational exposure histories in epidemiologic case-control studies. *Journal of Occupational Medicine* 27(6):420-426.
Goldberg H, Lusk E, Moore J, Nowell PC, Besa EC. 1990. Survey of exposure to genotoxic agents in primary myelodysplastic syndrome: Correlation with chromosome patterns and data on patients without hematological disease. *Cancer Research* 50(21):6876-6881.
Goldberg MS, Parent ME, Siemiatycki J, Desy M, Nadon L, Richardson L, Lakhani R, Latreille B, Valois MF. 2001. A case-control study of the relationship between the risk of colon cancer in men and exposures to occupational agents. *American Journal of Industrial Medicine* 39(6):531-546.
Goldberg P, Leclerc A, Luce D, Morcet JF, Brugere J. 1997. Laryngeal and hypopharyngeal cancer and occupation: Results of a case control-study. *Occupational and Environmental Medicine* 54(7):477-482.
Gonzalez CA, Lopez-Abente G, Errezola M, Escolar A, Riboli E, Izarzugaza I, Nebot M. 1989. Occupation and bladder cancer in Spain: A multi-centre case-control study. *International Journal of Epidemiology* 18(3):569-577.
Guberan E, Usel M, Raymond L, Bolay J, Fioretta G, Puissant J. 1992. Increased risk for lung cancer and for cancer of the gastrointestinal tract among Geneva professional drivers. *British Journal of Industrial Medicine* 49(5):337-344.
Guenel P, Laforest L, Cyr D, Fevotte J, Sabroe S , Dufour C, Lutz JM, Lynge E. 2001. Occupational risk factors, ultraviolet radiation, and ocular melanoma: A case-control study in France. *Cancer Causes & Control* 12(5):451-459.
Gustavsson P, Jakobsson R, Johansson H, Lewin F, Norell S, Rutkvist LE. 1998. Occupational exposures and squamous cell carcinoma of the oral cavity, pharynx, larynx, and oesophagus: A case-control study in Sweden. *Occupational and Environmental Medicine* 55(6):393-400.

Gustavsson P, Jakobsson R, Nyberg F, Pershagen G, Jarup L, Scheele P. 2000. Occupational exposure and lung cancer risk: A population-based case-referent study in Sweden. *American Journal of Epidemiology* 152(1):32-40.

Gustavsson P, Plato N, Lidstrom EB, Hogstedt C. 1990. Lung cancer and exposure to diesel exhaust among bus garage workers. *Scandinavian Journal of Work, Environment & Health* 16(5):348-354.

Hanis NM, Stavraky KM, Fowler JL. 1979. Cancer mortality in oil refinery workers. *Journal of Occupational Medicine* 21(3):167-174.

Hanis NM, Holmes TM, Shallenberger G, Jones KE. 1982. Epidemiologic study of refinery and chemical plant workers. *Journal of Occupational Medicine* 24(3):203-212.

Hannuksela-Svahn A, Pukkala E, Karvonen J. 1999. Basal cell skin carcinoma and other nonmelanoma skin cancers in Finland from 1956 through 1995. *Archives of Dermatology* 135(7):781-786.

Hansen ES. 1993. A follow-up study on the mortality of truck drivers. *American Journal of Industrial Medicine* 23(5):811-821.

Hansen J. 2000. Elevated risk for male breast cancer after occupational exposure to gasoline and vehicular combustion products. *American Journal of Industrial Medicine* 37(4):349-352.

Hansen J, Raaschou-Nielsen O, Olsen JH. 1998. Increased risk of lung cancer among different types of professional drivers in Denmark. *Occupational and Environmental Medicine* 55(2):115-118.

Hartge P, Cahill JI, West D, Hauck M, Austin D, Silverman D, Hoover R. 1984. Design and methods in a multi-center case-control interview study. *American Journal of Public Health* 74(1):52-56.

Hayes RB, Thomas T, Silverman DT, Vineis P, Blot WJ, Mason TJ, Pickle LW, Correa P, Fontham ETH, Schoenberg JB. 1989. Lung cancer in motor exhaust-related occupations. *American Journal of Industrial Medicine* 16(6):685-695.

He XZ, Chen W, Liu ZY, Chapman RS. 1991. An epidemiological study of lung cancer in Xuan Wei County, China: Current progress. Case-control study on lung cancer and cooking fuel. *Environmental Health Perspectives* 94:9-13.

Heineman EF, Olsen JH, Pottern LM, Gomez M, Raffn E, Blair A. 1992. Occupational risk factors for multiple myeloma among Danish men. *Cancer Causes & Control* 3(6):555-568.

Hoar SK, Hoover R. 1985. Truck driving and bladder cancer mortality in rural New England. *Journal of the National Cancer Institute* 74(4):771-774.

Hoek G, Brunekreef B, Goldbohm S, Fischer P, Van den Brandt PA. 2002. Association between mortality and indicators of traffic-related air pollution in the Netherlands: A cohort study. *Lancet* 360(9341):1203-1209.

Hours M, Dananche B, Fevotte J, Bergeret A, Ayzac L, Cardis E, Etard JF, Pallen C, Roy P, Fabry J. 1994. Bladder cancer and occupational exposures. *Scandinavian Journal of Work, Environment & Health* 20(5):322-330.

Howe GR, Burch JD, Miller AB, Cook GM, Esteve J, Morrison B, Gordon P, Chambers LW, Fodor G, Winsor GM. 1980. Tobacco use, occupation, coffee, various nutrients, and bladder cancer. *Journal of the National Cancer Institute* 64(4):701-713.

Howe GR, Fraser D, Lindsay J, Presnal B, Yu SZ. 1983. Cancer mortality (1965-77) in relation to diesel fume and coal exposure in a cohort of retired railway workers. *Journal of the National Cancer Institute* 70(6):1015-1019.

Hu J, Mao Y, White K. 2002. Renal cell carcinoma and occupational exposure to chemicals in Canada. *Occupational Medicine* 52(3):157-164.

Huang C, Zhang X, Qiao Z, Guan L, Peng S, Liu J, Xie R, Zheng L. 1992. A case-control study of dietary factors in patients with lung cancer. *Biomedical & Environmental Sciences* 5(3):257-265.

Huebner WW, Chen VW, Friedlander BR, Wu XC, Jorgensen G, Bhojani FA, Friedmann CH, Schmidt BA, Sales EA, Joy JA, Correa CN. 2000. Incidence of lymphohaematopoietic malignancies in a petrochemical industry cohort: 1983-94 follow up. *Occupational & Environmental Medicine* 57(9):605-614.

Huebner WW, Schoenberg JB, Kelsey JL, Wilcox HB, McLaughlin JK, Greenberg RS, Preston-Martin S, Austin DF, Stemhagen A, Blot WJ, Winn DM, Fraumeni J, Jr. 1992. Oral and pharyngeal cancer and occupation: A case-control study. *Epidemiology* 3(4):300-309.

IARC (International Agency for Research on Cancer). 1984a. *Polynuclear Aromatic Compounds, Part 2, Carbon Blacks, Mineral Oils and some Nitroarenes.* 33. Lyon, France: IARC.

IARC. 1984b. *Polynuclear Aromatic Compounds, Part 3, Industrial Exposures in Aluminum Production, Coal Gasification, Coke Production, and Iron and Steel Founding.* 34. Lyon, France: IARC.

IARC. 1985. *Polynuclear aromatic Compounds, Part 4, Bitumens, Coal-Tars and Derived Products, Shale-oils and Soots.* 35. Lyon, France: IARC.

Ido M, Nagata C, Kawakami N, Shimizu H, Yoshida Y, Nomura T, Mizoguchi H. 1996. A case-control study of myelodysplastic syndromes among Japanese men and women. *Leukemia Research* 20(9):727-731.

IOM (Institute of Medicine). 2003. *Gulf War and Health, Volume 2: Insecticides and Solvents.* Washington, DC: The National Academies Press.

Iscovich J, Castelletto R, Esteve J, Munoz N, Colanzi R, Coronel A, Deamezola I, Tassi V, Arslan A. 1987. Tobacco smoking, occupational exposure and bladder cancer in Argentina. *International Journal of Cancer* 40(6):734-740.

Iyer V, Harris RE, Wynder EL. 1990. Diesel exhaust exposure and bladder cancer risk. *European Journal of Epidemiology* 6(1):49-54.

Jarvholm B, Silverman D. 2003. Lung cancer in heavy equipment operators and truck drivers with diesel exhaust exposure in the construction industry. *Occupational and Environmental Medicine* 60(7):516-520.

Jarvholm B, Mellblom B, Norrman R, Nilsson R, Nordlinder R. 1997. Cancer incidence of workers in the Swedish petroleum industry. *Occupational and Environmental Medicine* 54(9):686-691.

Jedrychowski W, Becher H, Wahrendorf J, Basa-Cierpialek Z. 1990. A case-control study of lung cancer with special reference to the effect of air pollution in Poland. *Journal of Epidemiology and Community Health* 44(2):114-120.

Jemal A, Murray T, Samuels A, Ghafoor A, Ward E, Thun MJ. 2003. Cancer statistics, 2003. *CA: A Cancer Journal for Clinicians* 53(1):5-26.

Jensen OM, Knudsen JB, McLaughlin JK, Sorensen BL. 1988. The Copenhagen case-control study of renal pelvis and ureter cancer: Role of smoking and occupational exposures. *International Journal of Cancer* 41(4):557-561.

Jensen OM, Wahrendorf J, Knudsen JB, Sorensen BL. 1987. The Copenhagen case-referent study on bladder cancer. Risks among drivers, painters and certain other occupations. *Scandinavian Journal of Work, Environment & Health* 13(2):129-134.

Jockel KH, Ahrens W, Jahn I, Pohlabeln H, Bolm-Audorff U. 1998. Occupational risk factors for lung cancer: A case-control study in West Germany. *International Journal of Epidemiology* 27(4):549-560.

Jockel KH, Ahrens W, Wichmann HE, Becher H, Bolm-Audorff U, Jahn I, Molik B, Greiser E, Timm J. 1992. Occupational and environmental hazards associated with lung cancer. *International Journal of Epidemiology* 21(2):202-213.

Kadamani S, Asal NR, Nelson RY. 1989. Occupational hydrocarbon exposure and risk of renal cell carcinoma. *American Journal of Industrial Medicine* 15(2):131-141.

Kaplan I. 1959. Relationship of noxious gases to carcinoma of the lung in railroad workers. *JAMA* 171:2039-2043.

Katsouyanni K, Trichopoulos D, Kalandidi A, Tomos P, Riboli E. 1991. A case-control study of air pollution and tobacco smoking in lung cancer among women in Athens. *Preventive Medicine* 20(2):271-278.

Kauppinen T, Partanen T, Degerth R, Ojajarvi A. 1995. Pancreatic cancer and occupational exposures. *Epidemiology* 6(5):498-502.

Kleinerman RA, Wang Z, Wang L, Metayer C, Zhang S, Brenner AV, Zhang S, Xia Y, Shang B, Lubin JH. 2002. Lung cancer and indoor exposure to coal and biomass in rural China. *Journal of Occupational and Environmental Medicine* 44(4):338-344.

Kneller RW, Gao YT, McLaughlin JK, Gao RN, Blot WJ, Liu MH, Sheng JP, Fraumeni JF Jr. 1990. Occupational risk factors for gastric cancer in Shanghai, China. *American Journal of Industrial Medicine* 18(1):69-78.

Ko YC, Lee CH, Chen MJ, Huang CC, Chang WY, Lin HJ, Wang HZ, Chang PY. 1997. Risk factors for primary lung cancer among non-smoking women in Taiwan. *International Journal of Epidemiology* 26(1):24-31.

Kogevinas M, 't Mannetje A, Cordier S, Ranft U, Gonzalez C, Vineis P, Chang-Claude J, Lynge E, Wahrendorf J, Tzonou A, Jockel K, Serra C, Porru S, Hours M, Greiser E, Boffetta P. 2003. Occupation and bladder cancer among men in Western Europe. *Cancer Causes & Control* 14(10):907-914.

Koo LC, Lee N, Ho JH. 1983. Do cooking fuels pose a risk for lung cancer? A case-control study of women in Hong Kong. *Ecology of Disease* 2(4):255-265.

Krewski D, Burnett RT, Goldberg MS, Hoover BK, Siemiatycki J, Jerrett M, Abrahamowicz M, White WH. 2003. Overview of the reanalysis of the Harvard Six Cities Study and American Cancer Society Study of Particulate Air Pollution and Mortality. *Journal of Toxicology and Environmental Health - Part A* 66(16-19):1507-1551.

Krewski D, Snyder R, Beatty P, Granville G, Meek B, Sonawane B. 2000. Assessing the health risks of benzene: A report on the Benzene State-of-the-Science Workshop. *Journal of Toxicology and Environmental Health - Part A* 61(5-6):307-338.

Krstev S, Baris D, Stewart P, Dosemeci M, Swanson G, Greenberg R, Schoenberg J, Schwartz A, Liff J, Hayes RB. 1998. Occupational risk factors and prostate cancer in U.S. blacks and whites. *American Journal of Industrial Medicine* 34(5):421-430.

Kubasiewicz M, Starzynski Z. 1989. Case-referent study on skin cancer and its relation to occupational exposure to polycyclic aromatic hydrocarbons: I. Study design. *Polish Journal of Occupational Medicine* 2(3):221-228.

Kubasiewicz M, Starzynski Z, Szymczak W. 1991. Case-referent study on skin cancer and its relation to occupational exposure to polycyclic aromatic hydrocarbons. II. Study results. *Polish Journal of Occupational Medicine and Environmental Health* 4(2):141-147.

Kunze E, Chang-Claude J, Frentzel-Beyme R. 1992. Life style and occupational risk factors for bladder cancer in Germany: A case-control study. *Cancer* 69(7):1776-1790.

Lagorio S, Forastiere F, Iavarone I, Rapiti E, Vanacore N, Perucci CA, Carere A. 1994. Mortality of filling station attendants. *Scandinavian Journal of Work, Environment & Health* 20(5):331-338.

Lagorio S, Forastiere F, Iavarone I, Vanacore N, Fuselli S, Carere A. 1993. Exposure assessment in a historical cohort of filling station attendants. *International Journal of Epidemiology* 22(Suppl 2):S51-S56.

Lan Q, Chapman RS, Schreinemachers DM, Tian L, He X. 2002. Household stove improvement and risk of lung cancer in Xuanwei, China. *Journal of the National Cancer Institute* 94(11):826-835.

Lan Q, Chen W, Chen H, He XZ. 1993. Risk factors for lung cancer in non-smokers in Xuanwei County of China. *Biomedical and Environmental Sciences* 6(2):112-118.

Lan Q, Feng Z, Tian D, He X, Rothman N, Tian L, Lu X, Terry MB, Mumford JL. 2001. p53 gene expression in relation to indoor exposure to unvented coal smoke in Xuan Wei, China. *Journal of Occupational and Environmental Medicine* 43(3):226-30.

Larkin EK, Smith TJ, Stayner L, Rosner B, Speizer FE, Garshick E. 2000. Diesel exhaust exposure and lung cancer: Adjustment for the effect of smoking in a retrospective cohort study. *American Journal of Industrial Medicine* 38(4):399-409.

Leclerc A, Luce D, Demers PA, Boffetta P, Kogevinas M, Belli S, Bolm-Audorff U, Brinton LA, Colin D, Comba P, Gerin M, Hardell L, Hayes RB, Magnani C, Merler E, Morcet JF, Preston-Martin S, Vaughan TL, Zheng W. 1997. Sinonasal cancer and occupation. Results from the reanalysis of twelve case-control studies. *American Journal of Industrial Medicine* 31(2):153-165.

Lee WJ, Baris D, Jarvholm B, Silverman DT, Bergdahl IA, Blair A. 2003. Multiple myeloma and diesel and other occupational exposures in Swedish construction workers. *International Journal of Cancer* 107(1):134-138.

Lei YX, Cai WC, Chen YZ, Du YX. 1996. Some lifestyle factors in human lung cancer: A case-control study of 792 lung cancer cases. *Lung Cancer* 14(Suppl 1):S121-S136.

Lerchen ML, Wiggins CL, Samet JM. 1987. Lung cancer and occupation in New Mexico. *Journal of the National Cancer Institute* 79(4):639-45.

Lewis RJ, Gamble JF, Jorgensen G. 2000a. Mortality among three refinery/petrochemical plant cohorts. I. 1970 to 1982 active/terminated workers. *Journal of Occupational and Environmental Medicine* 42(7):721-729.

Lewis RJ, Schnatter AR, Drummond I, Murray N, Thompson FS, Katz AM, Jorgensen G, Nicolich MJ , Dahlman D, Theriault G. 2003. Mortality and cancer morbidity in a cohort of Canadian petroleum workers. *Occupational and Environmental Medicine* 60(12):918-928.

Lewis RJ, Schnatter AR, Katz AM, Thompson FS, Murray N, Jorgensen G, Theriault G. 2000b. Updated mortality among diverse operating segments of a petroleum company. *Occupational and Environmental Medicine* 57(9):595-604.

Lewis-Michl EL, Melius JM, Kallenbach LR, Ju CL, Talbot TO, Orr MF, Lauridsen PE. 1996 . Breast cancer risk and residence near industry or traffic in Nassau and Suffolk Counties, Long Island, New York. *Archives of Environmental Health* 51(4):255-265.

Lindquist R, Nilsson B, Eklund G, Gahrton G. 1991. Acute leukemia in professional drivers exposed to gasoline and diesel. *European Journal of Haematology* 47(2):98-103.

Linet MS, Harlow SD, McLaughlin JK. 1987. A case-control study of multiple myeloma in whites: Chronic antigenic stimulation, occupation, and drug use. *Cancer Research* 47(11):2978-2981.

Linet MS, Malker HS, Chow WH, McLaughlin JK, Weiner JA, Stone BJ, Ericsson JL, Fraumeni JF Jr. 1995. Occupational risks for cutaneous melanoma among men in Sweden. *Journal of Occupational and Environmental Medicine* 37(9):1127-1135.

Linet MS, Malker HS, McLaughlin JK, Weiner JA, Blot WJ, Ericsson JL, Fraumeni JF Jr. 1993. Non-Hodgkin's lymphoma and occupation in Sweden: A registry based analysis. *British Journal of Industrial Medicine* 50(1):79-84.

Linet MS, McLaughlin JK, Malker HS, Chow WH, Weiner JA, Stone BJ, Ericsson JL, Fraumeni JF Jr. 1994. Occupation and hematopoietic and lymphoproliferative malignancies among women: A linked registry study. *Journal of Occupational Medicine* 36(11):1187-1198.

Liu Q, Sasco AJ, Riboli E, Hu MX. 1993. Indoor air pollution and lung cancer in Guangzhou, People's Republic of China. *American Journal of Epidemiology* 137(2):145-154.

Luce D, Leclerc A, Begin D, Demers PA, Gerin M, Orlowski E, Kogevinas M, Belli S, Bugel I, Bolm-Audorff U, Brinton LA, Comba P, Hardell L, Hayes RB, Magnani C, Merler E, Preston-Martin S, Vaughan TL, Zheng W, Boffetta P. 2002. Sinonasal cancer and occupational exposures: A pooled analysis of 12 case-control studies. *Cancer Causes & Control* 13(2):147-157.

Luo RX, Wu B, Yi YN, Huang ZW, Lin RT. 1996. Indoor burning coal air pollution and lung cancer-a case-control study in Fuzhou, China. *Lung Cancer* 14(Suppl 1):S113-S119.

Magnani C, Pannett B, Winter PD, Coggon D. 1988. Application of a job-exposure matrix to national mortality statistics for lung cancer. *British Journal of Industrial Medicine* 45(1):70-72.

Maier H, Tisch M. 1997. Epidemiology of laryngeal cancer: Results of the Heidelberg case-control study. *Acta Oto-laryngologica. Supplementum* 527:160-164.

Mandel JS, McLaughlin JK, Schlehofer B, Mellemgaard A, Helmert U, Lindblad P, McCredie M, Adami HO. 1995. International renal-cell cancer study. IV. Occupation. *International Journal of Cancer* 61(5):601-605.

Mao Y, Hu J, Ugnat AM, White K. 2000. Non-Hodgkin's lymphoma and occupational exposure to chemicals in Canada. Canadian Cancer Registries Epidemiology Research Group. *Annals of Oncology* 11(Suppl 1):69-73.

Marsh GM, Stone RA, Esmen NA, Gula MJ, Gause CK, Petersen NJ, Meaney FJ, Rodney S, Prybylski D. 1998. A case-control study of lung cancer mortality in four rural Arizona smelter towns. *Archives of Environmental Health* 53(1):15-28.

Matos EL, Vilensky M, Mirabelli D, Boffetta P. 2000. Occupational exposures and lung cancer in Buenos Aires, Argentina. *Journal of Occupational and Environmental Medicine* 42(6):653-659.

McCredie M, Stewart JH. 1993. Risk factors for kidney cancer in New South Wales. IV. Occupation. *British Journal of Industrial Medicine* 50(4):349-354.

McLaughlin JK, Blot WJ, Mehl ES, Stewart PA, Venable FS, Fraumeni JF Jr. 1985. Petroleum-related employment and renal cell cancer. *Journal of Occupational Medicine* 27(9):672-674.

McLaughlin JK, Malker HS, Stone BJ, Weiner JA, Malker BK, Ericsson JL, Blot WJ, Fraumeni JF Jr. 1987. Occupational risks for renal cancer in Sweden. *British Journal of Industrial Medicine* 44(2):119-123.

McLaughlin JK, Mandel JS, Blot WJ, Schuman LM, Mehl ES, Fraumeni JF Jr. 1984. A population-based case-control study of renal cell carcinoma. *Journal of the National Cancer Institute* 72(2):275-284.

Mellemgaard A, Engholm G, McLaughlin JK, Olsen JH. 1994. Occupational risk factors for renal-cell carcinoma in Denmark. *Scandinavian Journal of Work, Environment & Health* 20(3):160-165.

Menvielle G, Luce D, Fevotte J, Bugel I, Salomon C, Goldberg P, Billon-Galland MA, Goldberg M. 2003. Occupational exposures and lung cancer in New Caledonia. *Occupational and Environmental Medicine* 60(8):584-589.

Merletti F, Boffetta P, Ferro G, Pisani P, Terracini B. 1991. Occupation and cancer of the oral cavity or oropharynx in Turin, Italy. *Scandinavian Journal of Work, Environment and Health* 17(4):248-254.

Metayer C, Wang Z, Kleinerman RA, Wang L, Brenner AV, Cui H, Cao J, Lubin JH. 2002. Cooking oil fumes and risk of lung cancer in women in rural Gansu, China. *Lung Cancer* 35(2):111-117.

Michelozzi P, Fusco D, Forastiere F, Ancona C, Dell'Orco V, Perucci CA. 1998. Small area study of mortality among people living near multiple sources of air pollution. *Occupational and Environmental Medicine* 55(9):611-615.

Mommsen S, Aagard J. 1984. Occupational exposures as risk indicator of male bladder carcinoma in a predominantly rural area. *Acta Radiologica - Oncology* 23(2-3):147-152.

Mommsen S, Aagaard J, Sell A. 1982. An epidemiological case-control study of bladder cancer in males from a predominantly rural district. *European Journal of Cancer and Clinical Oncology* 18(11):1205-1210.

Mommsen S, Aagaard J, Sell A. 1983. An epidemiological study of bladder cancer in a predominantly rural district. *Scandinavian Journal of Urology and Nephrology* 17(3):307-312.

Monarrez-Espino J, Stang A, Bromen K, Merzenich H, Anastassiou G, Jockel KH. 2002. Occupation as a risk factor for uveal melanoma in Germany. *Scandinavian Journal of Work, Environment & Health* 28(4):270-277.

Morris PD, Koepsell TD, Daling JR, Taylor JW, Lyon JL, Swanson GM, Child M, Weiss NS. 1986. Toxic substance exposure and multiple myeloma: A case control-study. *Journal of the National Cancer Institute* 76(6):987-994.

Muir C, Waterhouse J, Mack T, Powell J, Whelan S. 1987. *Cancer Incidence in Five Continents, Vol. 5. IARC Scientific Publication.* 88. Lyon, France: IARC; as cited in Yu et al. 1990.

Muscat JE, Wynder EL. 1995. Diesel exhaust, diesel fumes, and laryngeal cancer. *Otolaryngology - Head and Neck Surgery* 112(3):437-440.

Muscat JE, Stellman SD, Richie JP Jr, Wynder EL. 1998. Lung cancer risk and workplace exposures in black men and women. *Environmental Research* 76(2):78-84.

Nadon L, Siemiatycki J, Dewar R, Krewski D, Gerin M. 1995. Cancer risk due to occupational exposure to polycyclic aromatic hydrocarbons. *American Journal of Industrial Medicine* 28(3):303-324.

Nafstad P, Haheim LL, Oftedal B, Gram F, Holme I, Hjermann I, Leren P. 2003. Lung cancer and air pollution: A 27 year follow up of 16,209 Norwegian men. *Thorax* 58(12):1071-1076.

Nagata C, Shimizu H, Hirashima K, Kakishita E, Fujimura K, Niho Y, Karasawa M, Oguma S, Yoshida Y, Mizoguchi H. 1999. Hair dye use and occupational exposure to organic solvents as risk factors for myelodysplastic syndrome. *Leukemia Research* 23(1):57-62.

Najem GR, Louria DB, Seebode JJ, Thind IS, Prusakowski JM, Ambrose RB, Fernicola AR. 1982. Life time occupation, smoking, caffeine, saccharine, hair dyes and bladder carcinogenesis. *International Journal of Epidemiology* 11(3):212-217.

NCI (National Cancer Institute). 2002. *What You Need to Know About Bladder Cancer; Information About Detection, Symptoms, Diagnosis, and Trctment of Bladder Cancer.* [Online]. Available: http://www.lnci.nih.gov/cancerinfo/wyntk/bladder [accessed May 18, 2004].

NCI. 2004. *What You Need to Know About Leukemia.* [Online]. Available: http://www.nci.nih.gov/cancertopics/wyntk/leukemia [accessed August, 2004].

Nelemans PJ, Scholte R, Groenendal H, Kiemeney LA, Rampen FH, Ruiter DJ, Verbeek AL. 1993. Melanoma and occupation: Results of a case-control study in The Netherlands. *British Journal of Industrial Medicine* 50(7):642-646.

Nelson NA, Barker DM, Van Peenen PF, Blanchard AG. 1985. Determining exposure categories for a refinery retrospective cohort mortality study. *American Industrial Hygiene Association Journal* 46(11):653-657.

Nelson NA, Van Peenen PF, Blanchard AG. 1987. Mortality in a recent oil refinery cohort. *Journal of Occupational Medicine* 29(7):610-612.

Netterstrom B. 1988. Cancer incidence among urban bus drivers in Denmark. *International Archives of Occupational and Environmental Health* 61(3):217-221.

Nisse C, Haguenoer JM, Grandbastien B, Preudhomme C, Fontaine B, Brillet JM, Lejeune R, Fenaux P. 2001. Occupational and environmental risk factors of the myelodysplastic syndromes in the North of France. *British Journal of Haematology* 112(4):927-935.

Nisse C, Lorthois C, Dorp V, Eloy E, Haguenoer JM, Fenaux P. 1995. Exposure to occupational and environmental factors in myelodysplastic syndromes. Preliminary results of a case-control study. *Leukemia* 9(4):693-699.

Notani PN, Shah P, Jayant K, Balakrishnan V. 1993. Occupation and cancers of the lung and bladder: A case-control study in Bombay. *International Journal of Epidemiology* 22(2):185-191.

Nyberg F, Gustavsson P, Jarup L, Bellander T, Berglind N, Jakobsson R, Pershagen G. 2000. Urban air pollution and lung cancer in Stockholm. *Epidemiology* 11(5):487-495.

Paradis G, Theriault G, Tremblay C. 1989. Mortality in a historical cohort of bus drivers. *International Journal of Epidemiology* 18(2):397-402.

Parent ME, Hua Y, Siemiatycki J. 2000a. Occupational risk factors for renal cell carcinoma in Montreal. *American Journal of Industrial Medicine* 38(6):609-618.

Parent ME, Siemiatycki J, Fritschi L. 2000b. Workplace exposures and oesophageal cancer. *Occupational & Environmental Medicine* 57(5):325-334.

Partanen T, Heikkila P, Hernberg S, Kauppinen T, Moneta G, Ojajarvi A. 1991. Renal cell cancer and occupational exposure to chemical agents. *Scandinavian Journal of Work, Environment & Health* 17(4):231-239.

Pesch B, Haerting J, Ranft U, Klimpel A, Oeschlagel B, Schill W. 2000a . Occupational risk factors for renal cell carcinoma: Agent-specific results from a case-control study in Germany. *International Journal of Epidemiology* 29(6):1014-1024.

Pesch B, Haerting J, Ranft U, Klimpel A, Oelschlagel B, Schill W. 2000b . Occupational risk factors for urothelial carcinoma: Agent-specific results from a case-control study in Germany. *International Journal of Epidemiology* 29(2):238-247.

Petralia SA, Vena JE, Freudenheim JL, Dosemeci M, Michalek A, Goldberg MS, Brasure J, Graham S. 1999. Risk of premenopausal breast cancer in association with occupational exposure to polycyclic aromatic hydrocarbons and benzene. *Scandinavian Journal of Work, Environment & Health* 25(3):215-221.

Pietri F, Clavel F, Auquier A, Flamant R. 1990. Occupational risk factors for cancer of the pancreas: A case-control study. *British Journal of Industrial Medicine* 47(6):425-428.

Pintos J, Franco EL, Kowalski LP, Oliveira BV, Curado MP. 1998. Use of wood stoves and risk of cancers of the upper aero-digestive tract: A case-control study. *International Journal of Epidemiology* 27(6):936-940.

Pion IA, Rigel DS, Garfinkel L, Silverman MK, Kopf AW. 1995. Occupation and the risk of malignant melanoma. *Cancer* 75(2 Suppl):637-644.

Pollan M, Lopez-Abente G. 1995. Wood-related occupations and laryngeal cancer. *Cancer Detection & Prevention* 19(3):250-257.

Poole C, Dreyer NA, Satterfield MH, Levin L, Rothman KJ. 1993. Kidney cancer and hydrocarbon exposures among petroleum refinery workers. *Environmental Health Perspectives* 101(Suppl 6):53-62.

Pope CA 3rd, Burnett RT, Thun MJ, Calle EE, Krewski D, Ito K, Thurston GD. 2002. Lung cancer, cardiopulmonary mortality, and long-term exposure to fine particulate air pollution. *Journal of the American Medical Association* 287(9):1132-1141.

Pope CA 3rd, Thun MJ, Namboodiri MM, Dockery DW, Evans JS, Speizer FE, Heath CW Jr. 1995. Particulate air pollution as a predictor of mortality in a prospective study of U.S. adults. *American Journal of Respiratory and Critical Care Medicine* 151(3 Pt 1):669-674.

Porru S, Aulenti V, Donato F, Boffetta P, Fazioli R, Cosciani Cunico S, Alessio L. 1996. Bladder cancer and occupation: A case-control study in northern Italy. *Occupational and Environmental Medicine* 53(1):6-10.

Pottern LM, Heineman EF, Olsen JH, Raffn E, Blair A. 1992. Multiple myeloma among Danish women: Employment history and workplace exposures. *Cancer Causes & Control* 3(5):427-432.

Pukkala E, Soderholm AL, Lindqvist C. 1994. Cancers of the lip and oropharynx in different social and occupational groups in Finland. *European Journal of Cancer. Part B, Oral Oncology* 30B(3):209-215.

Raabe GK, Collingwood KW, Wong O. 1998. An updated mortality study of workers at a petroleum refinery in Beaumont, Texas. *American Journal of Industrial Medicine* 33(1):61-81.

Rafnsson V, Gunaarsdottir H. 1991. Mortality among professional drivers. *Scandinavian Journal of Work, Environment & Health* 17(5):312-317.

Rebelakos A, Trichopoulos D, Tzonou A, Zavitsanos X, Velonakis E, Trichopoulos A. 1985. Tobacco smoking, coffee drinking, and occupation as risk factors for bladder cancer in Greece. *Journal of the National Cancer Institute* 75(3):455-461.

Ries, LAG, Eisner, MP, Kosary, CL Hankey BF, Miller, BA, Clegg, L, Mariotto, A, Fay, MP, Feuer, EJ, Edwards, BK, eds. 2003. *SEER Cancer Statistics Review, 1975-2000.* [Online]. Available: http://seer.cancer.gov/csr/1975_2000/ [accessed February 2, 2004].

Ries, LAG, Eisner, MP, Kosary, CL, Hankey BF, Miller, BA, Clegg, L, Mariotto, A, Feuer, EJ, Edwards, BK, eds. 2004. *SEER Cancer Statistics Review, 1975-2001*. [Online]. Available: http://seer.cancer.gov/csr/1975_2001/ [accessed July 15, 2004].

Rigolin GM, Cuneo A, Roberti MG, Bardi A, Bigoni R, Piva N, Minotto C, Agostini P, De Angeli C, Del Senno L, Spanedda R, Castoldi G. 1998. Exposure to myelotoxic agents and myelodysplasia: Case-control study and correlation with clinicobiological findings. *British Journal of Haematology* 103(1):189-197.

Risch HA, Burch JD, Miller AB, Hill GB, Steele R, Howe GR. 1988. Occupational factors and the incidence of cancer of the bladder in Canada. *British Journal of Industrial Medicine* 45(6):361-367.

Ritchie G, Still K, Rossi J3rd, Bekkedal M, Bobb A, Arfsten D. 2003. Biological and health effects of exposure to kerosene-based jet fuels and performance additives. *Journal of Toxicology and Environmental Health B Critical Review* 6(4):357-451.

Ritz B. 1999. Cancer mortality among workers exposed to chemicals during uranium processing. *Journal of Occupational and Environmental Medicine.* 41(7):556-566.

Rosamilia K, Wong O, Raabe GK. 1999. A case-control study of lung cancer among refinery workers. *Journal of Occupational and Environmental Medicine* 41(12):1091-1103.

Saverin R, Braunlich A, Dahmann D, Enderlein G, Heuchert G. 1999. Diesel exhaust and lung cancer mortality in potash mining. *American Journal of Industrial Medicine* 36(4):415-422.

Schairer C, Hartge P, Hoover RN, Silverman DT. 1988. *American Journal of Epidemiology* 128(5):1027-1037.

Schlehofer B, Heuer C, Blettner M, Niehoff D, Wahrendorf J. 1995. Occupation, smoking and demographic factors, and renal cell carcinoma in Germany. *International Journal of Epidemiology* 24(1):51-57.

Schnatter AR, Armstrong TW, Nicolich MJ, Thompson FS, Katz AM, Huebner WW, Pearlman ED. 1996. Lymphohaematopoietic malignancies and quantitative estimates of exposure to benzene in Canadian petroleum distribution workers. *Occupational and Environmental Medicine* 53(11):773-781.

Schnatter AR, Katz AM, Nicolich MJ, Theriault G. 1993. A retrospective mortality study among Canadian petroleum marketing and distribution workers. *Environmental Health Perspectives* 101(Suppl 6):85-99.

Schnatter AR, Theriault G, Katz AM, Thompson FS, Donaleski D, Murray N. 1992. A retrospective mortality study within operating segments of a petroleum company. *American Journal of Industrial Medicine* 22(2):209-229.

Schoenberg JB, Stemhagen A, Mogielnicki AP, Altman R, Abe T, Mason TJ. 1984. Case-control study of bladder cancer in New Jersey. I. Occupational exposures in white males. *Journal of the National Cancer Institute* 72(5):973-981.

Schumacher MC, Slattery ML, West DW. 1989. Occupation and bladder cancer in Utah. *American Journal of Industrial Medicine* 16(1):89-102.

Seidler A, Heiskel H, Bickeboller R, Elsner G. 1998. Association between diesel exposure at work and prostate cancer. *Scandinavian Journal of Work, Environment & Health* 24(6):486-494.

Shallenberger LG, Acquavella JF, Donaleski D. 1992. An updated mortality study of workers in three major United States refineries and chemical plants. *British Journal of Industrial Medicine* 49(5):345-354.

Sharpe CR, Rochon JE, Adam JM, Suissa S. 1989. Case-control study of hydrocarbon exposures in patients with renal cell carcinoma. *Canadian Medical Association Journal* 140(11):1309-1318.

Shen XB, Wang GX, Huang YZ, Xiang LS, Wang XH. 1996. Analysis and estimates of attributable risk factors for lung cancer in Nanjing, China. *Lung Cancer* 14(Suppl 1):S107-S112.

Shen XB, Wang GX, Zhou BS. 1998. Relation of exposure to environmental tobacco smoke and pulmonary adenocarcinoma in non-smoking women: A case control study in Nanjing. *Oncology Reports.* 5(5):1221-1223.

Siemiatycki J, Dewar R, Nadon L, Gerin M. 1994. Occupational risk factors for bladder cancer: Results from a case-control study in Montreal, Quebec, Canada. *American Journal of Epidemiology* 140(12):1061-1080.

Siemiatycki J, Dewar R, Nadon L, Gerin M, Richardson L, Wacholder S. 1987a. Associations between several sites of cancer and twelve petroleum-derived liquids. Results from a case-referent study in Montreal. *Scandinavian Journal of Work, Environment & Health* 13(6):493-504.

Siemiatycki J, Gerin M, Stewart P, Nadon L, Dewar R, Richardson L. 1988. Associations between several sites of cancer and ten types of exhaust and combustion products. Results from a case-referent study in Montreal. *Scandinavian Journal of Work, Environment & Health* 14(2):79-90.

Siemiatycki J, Wacholder S, Richardson L, Dewar R, Gerin M. 1987b. Discovering carcinogens in the occupational environment. Methods of data collection and analysis of a large case-referent monitoring system. *Scandinavian Journal of Work, Environment & Health* 13(6):486-492.
Silverman DT, Hoover RN, Albert S, Graff KM. 1983. Occupation and cancer of the lower urinary tract in Detroit. *Journal of the National Cancer Institute* 70(2):237-245.
Silverman DT, Hoover RN, Mason TJ, Swanson MG. 1986. Motor exhaust-related occupations and bladder cancer. *Cancer Research* 46(4 II):2113-2116.
Silverman DT, Levin LI, Hoover RN. 1989a. Occupational risks of bladder cancer in the United States: II. Nonwhite men. *Journal of the National Cancer Institute* 81(19):1480-1483.
Silverman DT, Levin LI, Hoover RN. 1990. Occupational risks of bladder cancer among white women in the United States. *American Journal of Epidemiology* 132(3):453-461.
Silverman DT, Levin LI, Hoover RN, Hartge P. 1989b. Occupational risks of bladder cancer in the United States: I. White men. *Journal of the National Cancer Institute* 81(19):1472-1480.
Simonato L, Zambon P, Ardit S, Della Sala S, Fila G, Gaborieau V, Gallo G, Magarotto G, Mazzini R, Pasini L, Stracca Pansa V, Sella Della S. 2000. Lung cancer risk in Venice: a population-based case-control study. [Erratum appears in *Eur J Cancer Prev* 2000 9(2):135. Note: Sella Della S corrected to Della Sala S]. *European Journal of Cancer Prevention* 9(1):35-39.
Skov T, Lynge E. 1991. Non-Hodgkin's lymphoma and occupation in Denmark. *Scandinavian Journal of Social Medicine* 19(3):162-169.
Smith EM, Miller ER, Woolson RF, Brown CK. 1985. Bladder cancer risk among auto and truck mechanics and chemically related occupations. *American Journal of Public Health* 75(8):881-883.
Smith TC, Heller JM, Hooper TI, Gackstetter GD, Gray GC. 2002. Are Gulf War veterans experiencing illness due to exposure to smoke from Kuwaiti oil well fires? Examination of Department of Defense hospitalization data. *American Journal of Epidemiology* 155(10):908-917.
Smith TJ, Hammond SK, Wong O. 1993. Health effects of gasoline exposure. I. Exposure assessment for U.S. distribution workers. *Environmental Health Perspectives* 101(Suppl 6):13-21.
Soll-Johanning H, Bach E, Jensen SS. 2003. Lung and bladder cancer among Danish urban bus drivers and tramway employees: A nested case-control study. *Occupational Medicine* 53(1):25-33.
Soll-Johanning H, Bach E, Olsen JH, Tuchsen F. 1998. Cancer incidence in urban bus drivers and tramway employees: a retrospective cohort study. *Occupational & Environmental Medicine* 55(9):594-598.
Spiegelman D, Wegman DH. 1985. Occupation-related risks for colorectal cancer. *Journal of the National Cancer Institute* 75(5):813-821.
Steenland K, Deddens J, Stayner L. 1998. Diesel exhaust and lung cancer in the trucking industry: exposure-response analyses and risk assessment. *American Journal of Industrial Medicine* 34(3):220-228.
Steenland NK, Silverman DT, Hornung RW. 1990. Case-control study of lung cancer and truck driving in the Teamsters Union. *American Journal of Public Health* 80(6):670-674.
Steineck G, Hagman U, Gerhardsson M, Norell SE. 1990a. Vitamin A supplements, fried foods, fat and urothelial cancer. A case-referent study in Stockholm in 1985-87. *International Journal of Cancer* 45(6):1006-1011.
Steineck G, Plato N, Alfredsson L, Norell SE. 1989. Industry-related urothelial carcinogens: Application of a job-exposure matrix to Census data. *American Journal of Industrial Medicine* 16(2):209-224.
Steineck G, Plato N, Gerhardsson M, Norell SE, Hogstedt C. 1990b. Increased risk of urothelial cancer in Stockholm during 1985-87 after exposure to benzene and exhausts. *International Journal of Cancer* 45(6):1012-1017.
Stemhagen A, Slade J, Altman R, Bill J. 1983. Occupational risk factors and liver cancer. A retrospective case-control study of primary liver cancer in New Jersey. *American Journal of Epidemiology* 117(4):443-454.
Swanson GM, Lin CS, Burns PB. 1993. Diversity in the association between occupation and lung cancer among black and white men. *Cancer Epidemiology, Biomarkers and Prevention* 2(4):313-320.

Stern FB, Lemen RA, Curtis RA. 1981. Exposure of motor vehicle examiners to carbon monoxide: A historical prospective mortality study. *Archives of Environmental Health* 36(2):59-65.

't Mannetje A, Kogevinas M, Chang-Claude J, Cordier S, Gonzalez CA, Hours M, Jockel KH, Bolm-Audorff U, Lynge E, Porru S, Donato F, Ranft U, Serra C, Tzonou A, Vineis P, Wahrendorf J, Boffetta P. 1999. Occupation and bladder cancer in European women. *Cancer Causes and Control* 10(3):209-217.

Teschke K, Morgan MS, Checkoway H, Franklin G, Spinelli JJ, van Belle G, Weiss NS. 1997. Surveillance of nasal and bladder cancer to locate sources of exposure to occupational carcinogens. *Occupational and Environmental Medicine* 54(6):443-451.

Vagero D, Swerdlow AJ, Beral V. 1990. Occupation and malignant melanoma: A study based on cancer registration data in England and Wales and in Sweden. *British Journal of Industrial Medicine* 47(5):317-324.

Van Den Eeden SK, Friedman GD. 1993. Exposure to engine exhaust and risk of subsequent cancer. *Journal of Occupational Medicine* 35(3):307-311.

van Loon AJ, Kant IJ, Swaen GM, Goldbohm RA, Kremer AM, van den Brandt PA. 1997. Occupational exposure to carcinogens and risk of lung cancer: Results from The Netherlands cohort study. *Occupational and Environmental Medicine* 54(11):817-824.

Vasama-Neuvonen K, Pukkala E, Paakkulainen H, Mutanen P, Weiderpass E, Boffetta P, Shen N, Kauppinen T, Vainio H, Partanen T. 1999. Ovarian cancer and occupational exposures in Finland. *American Journal of Industrial Medicine* 36(1):83-89.

Vaughan TL. 1989. Occupation and squamous cell cancers of the pharynx and sinonasal cavity. *American Journal of Industrial Medicine* 16(5):493-510.

Velema JP, Ferrera A, Figueroa M, Bulnes R, Toro LA, de Barahona O, Claros JM, Melchers WJ. 2002. Burning wood in the kitchen increases the risk of cervical neoplasia in HPV-infected women in Honduras. *International Journal of Cancer* 97(4):536-541.

Vena JE. 1982. Air pollution as a risk factor in lung cancer. *American Journal of Epidemiology* 116(1):42-56.

Viadana E, Bross ID, Houten L. 1976. Cancer experience of men exposed to inhalation of chemicals or to combustion products. *Journal of Occupational Medicine* 18(12):787-792.

Vineis P, Magnani C. 1985. Occupation and bladder cancer in males: a case-control study. *International Journal of Cancer* 35(5):599-606.

Vineis P, Thomas T, Hayes RB, Blot WJ, Mason TJ, Pickle LW, Correa P, Fontham ET, Schoenberg J. 1988. Proportion of lung cancers in males, due to occupation, in different areas of the USA. *International Journal of Cancer* 42(6):851-856.

Weiderpass E, Pukkala E, Vasama-Neuvonen K, Kauppinen T, Vainio H, Paakkulainen H, Boffetta P, Partanen T. 2001. Occupational exposures and cancers of the endometrium and cervix uteri in Finland. *American Journal of Industrial Medicine* 39(6):572-580.

Weinberg GB, Kuller LH, Stehr PA. 1985. A case-control study of stomach cancer in a coal mining region of Pennsylvania. *Cancer* 56(3):703-713.

West RR, Stafford DA, Farrow A, Jacobs A. 1995. Occupational and environmental exposures and myelodysplasia: A case-control study. *Leukemia Research* 19(2):127-139.

WHO (World Health Organization). 2003. *World Health Report 2003 - Shaping the Future*. [Online]. Available: http://www.who.int/whr/2003/en/Annex2-en.pdf [accessed January 14, 2004].

Williams AR, Weiss NS, Koepsell TD, Lyon JL, Swanson GM. 1989. Infectious and noninfectious exposures in the etiology of light chain myeloma: A case-control study. *Cancer Research* 49(14):4038-4041.

Wong O, Harris F, Rosamilia K, Raabe GK. 2001. An updated mortality study of workers at a petroleum refinery in Beaumont, Texas, 1945 to 1996. *Journal of Occupational and Environmental Medicine* 43(4):384-401.

Wong O, Harris F, Smith TJ. 1993. Health effects of gasoline exposure. II. Mortality patterns of distribution workers in the United States. *Environmental Health Perspectives* 101(Suppl 6):63-76.

Wong O, Morgan RW, Kheifets L, Larson SR, Whorton MD. 1985. Mortality among members of a heavy construction equipment operators union with potential exposure to diesel exhaust emissions. *British Journal of Industrial Medicine* 42(7):435-48.

Wong O, Trent L, Harris F. 1999. Nested case-control study of leukaemia, multiple myeloma, and kidney cancer in a cohort of petroleum workers exposed to gasoline. *Occupational and Environmental Medicine* 56(4):217-221.

Wortley P, Vaughan TL, Davis S, Morgan MS, Thomas DB. 1992. A case-control study of occupational risk factors for laryngeal cancer. *British Journal of Industrial Medicine* 49(12):837-844.

Wu-Williams AH, Dai XD, Blot W, Xu ZY, Sun XW, Xiao HP, Stone BJ, Yu SF, Feng YP, Ershow AG. 1990a. Lung cancer among women in north-east China. *British Journal of Cancer* 62(6):982-987.

Wu-Williams AH, Yu MC, Mack TM. 1990b. Life-style, workplace, and stomach cancer by subsite in young men of Los Angeles County. *Cancer Research* 50(9):2569-2576.

Wu-Williams AH, Xu ZY, Blot WJ, Dai XD, Louie R, Xiao HP, Stone BJ, Sun XW, Yu SF, Feng YP, Fraumeni Jr JF, Henderson BE. 1993. Occupation and lung cancer risk among women in Northern China. *American Journal of Industrial Medicine* 24(1):67-79.

Xu Z, Brown LM, Pan GW, Liu TF, Gao GS, Stone BJ, Cao R-M, Guan DX, Sheng JH, Yan ZS, Dosemeci M, Fraumeni JF Jr, Blot WJ. 1996b. Cancer risks among iron and steel workers in Anshan, China, part II: Case-control studies of lung and stomach cancer. *American Journal of Industrial Medicine* 30(1):7-15.

Xu ZY, Blot WJ, Xiao HP, Wu A, Feng YP, Stone BJ, Sun J, Ershow AG, Henderson BE, Fraumeni JF Jr. 1989. Smoking, air pollution, and the high rates of lung cancer in Shenyang, China. *Journal of the National Cancer Institute* 81(23):1800-1806.

Xu ZY, Brown L, Pan GW, Li G, Feng YP, Guan DX, Liu TF, Liu LM, Chao RM, Sheng JH, Gao GC. 1996a. Lifestyle, environmental pollution and lung cancer in cities of Liaoning in northeastern China. *Lung Cancer* 14(Suppl 1):S149-S160.

Yang CY, Cheng MF, Chiu JF, Tsai SS. 1999. Female lung cancer and petrochemical air pollution in Taiwan. *Archives of Environmental Health* 54(3):180-185.

Yu MC, Garabrant DH, Huang TB, Henderson BE. 1990. Occupational and other non-dietary risk factors for nasopharyngeal carcinoma in Guangzhou, China. *International Journal of Cancer* 45(6):1033-1039.

Zahm SH, Brownson RC, Chang JC, Davis JR. 1989. Study of lung cancer histologic types, occupation, and smoking in Missouri. *American Journal of Industrial Medicine* 15(5):565-578.

Zahm SH, Hartge P, Hoover R. 1987. The National Bladder Cancer Study: Employment in the chemical industry. *Journal of the National Cancer Institute* 79(2):217-222.

Zeegers MP, Swaen GM, Kant I, Goldbohm RA, van den Brandt PA. 2001. Occupational risk factors for male bladder cancer: Results from a population based case cohort study in the Netherlands. *Occupational and Environmental Medicine* 58(9):590-596.

Zheng T, Cantor KP, Zhang Y, Lynch CF. 2002. Occupation and bladder cancer: A population-based, case-control study in Iowa. *Journal of Occupational and Environmental Medicine* 44(7):685-691.

Zheng W, Blot WJ, Shu XO, Diamond EL, Gao YT, Ji BT, Fraumeni JF Jr. 1992. Risk factors for oral and pharyngeal cancer in Shanghai, with emphasis on diet. *Cancer Epidemiology, Biomarkers and Prevention* 1(6):441-448.

Zheng W, Shu XO, Ji BT, Gao YT. 1996. Diet and other risk factors for cancer of the salivary glands: A population-based case-control study. *International Journal of Cancer* 67(2):194-198.

Zheng YM, Tuppin P, Hubert A, Jeannel D, Pan YJ, Zeng Y, De The G. 1994. Environmental and dietary risk factors for nasopharyngeal carcinoma: A case-control study in Zangwu County, Guangxi, China. *British Journal of Cancer* 69(3):508-514.

Zhong L, Goldberg MS, Gao YT, Jin F. 1999. Lung cancer and indoor air pollution arising from Chinese-style cooking among nonsmoking women living in Shanghai, China. *Epidemiology* 10(5):488-494.

5

RESPIRATORY OUTCOMES

This chapter focuses on several long-term respiratory conditions: asthma, chronic bronchitis, emphysema, and chronic obstructive pulmonary disease (COPD). The nature of respiratory symptoms and the reversibility of airway obstruction distinguish asthma from the other respiratory conditions listed above.

Asthma is marked by reversible airway obstruction and airway inflammation. People with asthma manifest symptoms—such as wheezing, coughing, and exertional dyspnea—that are accompanied by increased airflow obstruction. Chronic bronchitis is characterized by chronic cough and sputum production. Pulmonary emphysema (commonly referred to as emphysema) is a pathologic process involving air-space enlargement distal to the terminal bronchioles, accompanied by destruction of the bronchiolar walls. COPD includes chronic bronchitis and emphysema. The diagnosis of COPD requires objective evidence of airflow obstruction with spirometry according to GOLD[1] criteria (Pauwels et al. 2001).

The epidemiologic literature covering environmental agents and respiratory conditions has used varying definitions as knowledge has evolved. Summaries of key studies used by the committee in drawing its conclusions include details of how respiratory conditions were defined. Because of the impracticality of spirometry for large-scale epidemiologic studies, researchers often asked respondents about "physician-diagnosed" respiratory conditions or about respiratory symptoms. The hallmark symptom of asthma is wheezing, and that of chronic bronchitis is persistent cough and phlegm production (usually lasting 3 months/year for more than 2 years). For the last half-century, epidemiologic studies have used standard questions about cough and phlegm or sputum to define chronic bronchitis. Definitive diagnosis of emphysema requires pathologic examination of lung tissue or high-resolution thoracic computed tomography, although it can be inferred from characteristic physiologic changes, such as reduction in diffusion capacity.

The present report focuses on induction rather than exacerbation of disease, so this chapter emphasizes incident cases rather than exacerbation of pre-existing disease (for example, Eisner et al. 2002; Hong et al. 1994). Studies of prevalent disease are also included because they cover both new cases and exacerbation of preexisting conditions. The committee excluded the numerous time-series studies as they examine episodes of daily morbidity or mortality. Time-

[1]World Health Organization Global Initiative for Chronic Obstructive Lung Disease (GOLD).

series studies do not consider pre-existing conditions and report on acute outcomes rather than long-term health effects. For relevance to Gulf War veterans, the committee focused on long-term respiratory effects that persist after exposure ceases (see Chapter 2).

The first section of this chapter will discuss respiratory outcomes related to exposure to fuels, and the next section will discuss outcomes related to exposure to combustion products. The section on combustion products has the benefit of several large epidemiologic studies of Gulf War veterans who had objectively confirmed exposure to smoke from oil-well fires.

FUELS AND RESPIRATORY OUTCOMES

Most studies of fuel exposure reviewed by the committee were cohort-mortality studies. They included Australian petroleum-industry workers (Christie et al. 1987), Chevron petroleum-refinery workers (Dagg et al. 1992), Exxon refinery and chemical-plant workers (Hanis et al. 1985), US petroleum-refinery workers (Kaplan 1986), UK oil-refinery workers (Rushton and Alderson 1981), and petroleum-refinery workers in Beaumont, Texas (Wong et al. 2001a) and Torrance, California (Wong et al. 2001b). The occupational-cohort studies, which had multiple outcomes apart from respiratory disease, are described briefly in Appendix D.

All the occupational studies examined mortality due to noncancer respiratory outcomes among petroleum workers. Generally, the studies failed to indicate specific respiratory outcomes, although some do examine asthma, bronchitis, emphysema, and pneumonia or influenza separately. Most studies group all respiratory outcomes under the broad heading of "diseases of the respiratory system or tract" or "non-malignant respiratory disease".

Nonmalignant Respiratory Disease

The studies that examined nonmalignant respiratory disease (Christie et al. 1987; Dagg et al. 1992; Hanis et al. 1985; Kaplan 1986; Wong et al. 2001a, 2001b) included all respiratory disorders, such as acute infections, diseases of the upper respiratory tract, pneumonia and influenza, asthma, bronchitis, emphysema, COPD, pneumoconiosis and other diseases due to external agents (such as asbestos), and other respiratory diseases. In all of those studies, the standardized mortality ratios (SMRs) were below 1.0 when compared with the general population or those not employed in the petroleum industry; this indicates that persons involved in the petroleum industry are not at greater risk for dying from respiratory diseases than the general population. However, selection bias is a limitation of the studies cited above because of the "healthy-worker" effect.

In addition to the retrospective mortality studies identified above, the committee reviewed a cross-sectional study of Norwegian cable-plant workers exposed to oil mist or kerosene vapors (Skyberg et al. 1986). Seven cases of pulmonary fibrosis were found in 25 workers compared with one case in the control group. In a followup study of those workers (Skyberg et al. 1992), the authors examined whether the progression of pulmonary fibrosis continued after exposure to oil mist and vapors ceased and found that 10 of the 25 workers had pulmonary fibrosis compared with one in the control group. Smoking and exposure to asbestos were possible confounders in both studies.

Asthma

Occupational factors are estimated to account for about 15% of the total burden of adult asthma (Balmes et al. 2003). Asthma is the most commonly reported occupational lung disease in most industrialized countries, and trends from long-standing surveillance in Finland and the UK show little change in incidence of occupational asthma over the last 10 years (Meyer et al. 2001; Reijula et al. 1996).

Four cohort studies of refinery workers (Kaplan 1986); Rushton and Alderson 1981; Wong et al. 2001a, 2001b) did not find an increased risk of asthma compared with that in the general population, however, that may be due to the "healthy worker" effect which might involve self-selection against having asthma specifically. All the SMRs were below 1.0.

The committee reviewed two case reports of asthma due to prolonged exposure to kerosene vapor from accidental domestic oil storage-tank spills (Todd and Buick 2000) and exposure to aviation fuel in an aircraft-engine mechanic (Makker and Ayres 1999). Six adults and three children were exposed to kerosene vapor, and one adult and the three children developed asthma that persisted for 3 years after the incident.

A 42-year-old aircraft-engine mechanic reported being exposed to both high concentrations of aviation-fuel vapors and jet-stream emissions from aircraft engines. He developed symptoms almost immediately on beginning his job and was diagnosed with asthma within 4 years. The man reported that his symptoms improved when he was away from work for periods of at least 2 or 3 days.

A review article by Rodriguez de la Vega et al. (1990) cites a study (Rodriguez de la Vega et al. 1981) in which 286 asthmatic patients who used kerosene for cooking were followed for 5 years. The authors found that 43.9% of those whose asthma did not improve continued to use kerosene as fuel for cooking; this suggests a relationship between exposure to kerosene and asthma.

Chronic Bronchitis and Emphysema

Rushton and Alderson (1981) and Wong et al. (2001a, 2001b) examined rates of bronchitis among refinery workers. Two of the three studies found no increased risk, however, one study found an SMR of 1.32, with a 95% confidence interval (CI) of 0.27-3.84 (Wong et al. 2001b).

Three studies (Kaplan 1986; Wong et al. 2001a, 2001b) examined at emphysema and found SMRs of 1.0 or less, indicating no increased risk among refinery workers compared with the general population. The healthy-worker effect probably contributed to the results.

Summary and Conclusion

A fairly extensive literature describes results of cohort studies designed to examine mortality in workers in the petroleum industry (Table 5.1). Generally, those studies did not provide information about specific respiratory disease outcomes but rather provided SMRs for broad categories of diseases that are designated as "diseases of the respiratory system or tract" or "non-malignant respiratory disease." The studies generally did not report exposure assessment, so it is difficult to reach a conclusion as to a relationship between respiratory disease outcomes and exposure to fuels. Most of the studies indicate a healthy-worker effect, which complicates interpretation of their results.

The committee concludes, from its assessment of the epidemiologic literature, that there is inadequate/insufficient evidence to determine whether an association exists between exposure to fuels and any specific, nonmalignant respiratory outcomes including asthma, bronchitis, and emphysema.

COMBUSTION PRODUCTS AND RESPIRATORY OUTCOMES

The committee divided the epidemiologic literature of respiratory effects and exposure to combustion products into four general types: studies of Gulf War veterans exposed to oil-well fires, community air pollution studies, occupational studies, and studies of biomass fuel, which is burned for heating or cooking primarily in developing countries. Each part of this section begins with the most robust primary studies (that is, studies with strong methods and exposure information), and continues with mortality studies and support studies that add weight to the primary evidence but are not as methodologically robust. Key primary studies used to draw conclusions are also depicted in tables (Tables 5.1 to 5.5). Most studies reported on more than one respiratory condition.

TABLE 5.1 Selected Epidemiologic Studies—Fuel Exposure and Respiratory Outcomes

Reference	Population	Exposed Cases	Estimated Relative Risk (95% CI)
Nonmalignant Respiratory Disease			
Cohort Studies—Mortality			
Christie et al. 1987	Australian petroleum workers (range of ICD-9 codes used)	0	0.00 (0.00-0.44)
Dagg et al. 1992	Chevron petroleum-refinery workers (range of ICD-8 codes used)		
	Richmond Plant	118	0.69 (0.57-0.82)
	El Segundo Plant	59	0.59 (0.45-0.76)
	Total	177	0.65 (0.56-0.75)
Hanis et al. 1985	Exxon refinery and chemical-plant workers (range of ICD-8 codes used)		
	Total	164	0.64 (0.55-0.75)
	Active employees	16	0.27 (0.15-0.44)[a]
	Employees hired before 1956	162	0.65 (0.55-0.75)[a]
	White men	150	0.64 (0.54-0.75)[a]
	Black men	14	0.82 (0.45-1.37)[a]
	Baton Rouge plant	66	0.71 (0.55-0.91)
	Baytown plant	48	0.70 (0.52-0.93)
	Bayway/Bayonne plant	50	0.54 (0.40-0.71)
Kaplan 1986	US petroleum-refinery workers (range of ICD-8 codes used)	167	0.64 (0.54-0.74)

Reference	Population	Exposed Cases	Estimated Relative Risk (95% CI)
Wong et al. 2001a	Beaumont, Texas, refinery workers (range of ICD-8 codes used)		
	Entire cohort	155	0.62 (0.52-0.72) (p<0.01)
	Female employees	1	0.16 (0.004-0.86)
	Male employees	154	0.63 (0.53-0.73) (p<0.01)
	Length of employment, <10 years	14	0.56 (p<0.05)
	Length of employment, 10-29 years	51	0.74 (p<0.05)
	Length of employment, 30+ years	89	0.59 (p<0.01)
	Time since employment, <20 years	4	0.33 (p<0.05)
	Time since employment, 20-39 years	51	0.74 (p<0.05)
	Time since employment, 40+ years	99	0.60 (p<0.01)
Wong et al. 2001b	Torrance, California, refinery workers (range of ICD-8 codes used)		
	Entire cohort	55	0.79 (0.60-1.03)
	Length of employment, <10 years	8	0.77
	Length of employment, 10-29 years	34	0.79
	Length of employment, 30+ years	13	0.86
	Time since employment, <20 years	2	0.35
	Time since employment, 20-39 years	21	0.77
	Time since employment, 40+ years	32	0.90
Cohort Study—Incidence			
Tsai et al. 1992	Shell Deer Park refinery and petroleum workers (range of ICD-9 codes used)	725	1.05 (0.98-1.13)
	Production employees, 1981-1988	646	1.08 (1.00-1.17)
	Staff employees, 1981-1988	79	0.88 (0.69-1.09)
Asthma			
Cohort Studies—Mortality			
Kaplan 1986	US petroleum-refinery workers (range of ICD-8 codes used)	5	0.79 (0.26-1.85)
Rushton and Alderson 1981	UK oil-refinery workers (range of ICD-8 codes used)	15	0.80 (0.45-1.32)[a]
Wong et al. 2001a	Beaumont, Texas, refinery workers (range of ICD-8 codes used)		
	Entire cohort	3	0.78 (0.16-2.28)

Reference	Population	Exposed Cases	Estimated Relative Risk (95% CI)
Bronchitis			
Cohort Studies—Mortality			
Rushton and Alderson 1981	UK oil refinery-workers (range of ICD-8 codes used)	253	0.64 (0.57-0.73)[a]
Wong et al. 2001a	Beaumont, Texas, refinery workers (range of ICD-8 codes used)		
	Entire cohort	3	0.34 (0.07-0.99)
Wong et al. 2001b	Torrance, California, refinery workers (range of ICD-8 codes used)		
	Entire cohort	3	1.32 (0.27-3.84)
Emphysema			
Cohort Studies—Mortality			
Kaplan 1986	US petroleum-refinery workers (range of ICD-8 codes used)	46	0.63 (0.46-0.84)
Wong et al. 2001a	Beaumont, Texas, refinery workers (range of ICD-8 codes used)		
	Entire cohort	42	1.03 (0.74-1.40)
Wong et al. 2001b	Torrance, California, refinery workers (range of ICD-8 codes used)		
	Entire cohort	9	0.82 (0.38-1.56)
Pneumonia and Influenza			
Cohort Studies—Mortality			
Kaplan 1986	US petroleum-refinery workers—pneumonia (range of ICD-8 codes used)	45	0.51 (0.37-0.68)
Rushton and Alderson 1981	UK oil-refinery workers (range of ICD-8 codes used)		
	Pneumonia	157	0.86 (0.73-1.00)[a]
	Influenza	11	0.40 (0.20-0.72)[a]
Wong et al. 2001a	Beaumont, Texas, refinery workers (range of ICD-8 codes used)		
	Entire cohort	60	0.58 (0.44-0.75)
	Female employees	1	0.39 (0.01-2.18)
	Male employees	59	0.59 (0.45-0.76)
	Length of employment, <10 years	4	0.44
	Length of employment, 10-29 years	16	0.54
	Length of employment, 30+ years	39	0.63
	Time since employment, <20 years	2	0.36

Reference	Population	Exposed Cases	Estimated Relative Risk (95% CI)
	Time since employment, 20-39 years	10	0.40
	Time since employment, 40+ years	47	0.68
Wong et al. 2001b	Torrance, California, refinery workers (range of ICD-8 codes used)		
	Entire cohort	15	0.59 (0.33-0.98)
	Length of employment, <10 years	0	0.00 (p<0.05)
	Length of employment, 10-29 years	12	0.75
	Length of employment, 30+ years	3	0.59
	Time since employment, <20 years	0	0.00
	Time since employment, 20-39 years	5	0.59
	Time since employment, 40 + years	10	0.71
Cohort Study—Incidence			
Tsai et al. 1992	Shell Deer Park refinery and petroleum workers (range of ICD-9 codes used)		
	Production employees	168	0.97 (0.83-1.13)
	Staff employees	28	0.74 (0.49-1.08)

NOTE: ICD, International Classification of Diseases.
[a]95% CI calculated by committee with standard methods from observed and expected numbers presented in original study.

Gulf War Studies

In February 1991, retreating Iraqi forces set fire to more than 600 oil wells. Fires burned over a 10-month period, until November 1991, exposing thousands of US troops to combustion products. Several studies of US Gulf War veterans exposed to oil-well fires stand out from most other Gulf War studies by virtue of their focus on a narrow set of respiratory health outcomes and on a single type of exposure (smoke from oil-well fires) and their exposure validation on the basis of models of troop unit movements in relation to air-monitoring data. The vast majority of Gulf War health studies focused on multiple health outcomes, multiple exposures, and self-reporting of exposures without validation. The studies summarized below examined long-term respiratory effects as veterans were surveyed after their deployment to the Persian Gulf. The first indication of possible long-term effects was from an uncontrolled study conducted in Germany, four weeks after deployment, which found that Army veterans that had been stationed near the fires reported coughing more frequently than before the war (Petruccelli et al. 1999). All studies discussed below are summarized in Table 5.2.

Cowan et al. (2002) conducted a case-control study to identify prevalent cases of physician-diagnosed asthma in the Department of Defense (DOD) registry (n = 873) and controls without asthma (n = 2,464). The DOD registry was established for active-duty Gulf War military who wished to receive a comprehensive physical examination. Cases of asthma were defined by physical examination conducted by military physicians (ICD-9-CM [Clinical Modification] codes 493 and 493.91). Exposure to smoke from oil-well fires was estimated by linking troop locations with modeled oil-fire smoke exposure. National Oceanic and Atmospheric Administration (NOAA) researchers modeled exposure on the basis of meteorologic and ground-station air-monitoring data (Draxler et al. 1994; McQueen and Draxler 1994). DOD personnel records were used to ascertain each study subject's unit and dates of service. Only Army personnel were included in the study because their location data were more precise. Two exposure measures were used: cumulative smoke exposure (the sum of the estimated concentration on all days when each subject was in the Gulf War theater) in milligrams per cubic meter per day (mg/m^3 per day), with referent exposure less than 1.0 mg/m^3 per day; and number of days when the subject was exposed at $\mu g/m^3$ or higher.

TABLE 5.2 Gulf War Veteran Health Studies of Oil-Well Fire Smoke

Reference	Type of Study and Population	Exposure Determination	Health Outcome and How Measured	Results	Adjusted OR (95% CI or p)	Limitations
Lange et al. 2002	Population-based cohort study of 1,560 Iowa veterans	Self-reported exposure to "smoke from oil well fires" (5 years after war), duration 1-5, 6-30, or >30 days; exposure modeling via troop positions and air-monitoring data	Self-reported symptoms of bronchitis and asthma (wheezing and coughing) vs control symptoms of major depression and injury	Small correlation between self-reported and modeled exposures ($r = 0.40$-0.48, $p<0.05$); no association between modeled exposure and symptoms of any type (ORs near 1.0, range 0.77-1.26); association found between self-reported exposure and asthma or bronchitis	For modeled exposure, adjusted ORs for symptom groups, including control symptoms, near 1.0, range 0.77-1.26; for self-reported exposure, asthma, OR 1.77-2.83, bronchitis OR 2.14-4.78	Symptom-based case definitions of asthma and bronchitis
Cowan et al. 2002	Case-control study of 873 cases of asthma vs 2,464 controls; DOD registry Army personnel only	Exposure modeling via troop positions and air monitoring data: Cumulative exposure and number of days at high concentration ($\geq 65\ \mu g/m^3$)	Physician-diagnosed asthma 3-6 years after war	Asthma associated with both estimates of exposure, dose-response	Cumulative exposure: OR 1.24 (95% CI 1.00-1.55) for intermediate exposure; 1.40 (95% CI 1.11-1.75) for high exposure; number of days at high levels: OR 1.22 (95% CI 0.99-1.51) for 1-5 days; 1.41 (95% CI 1.12-1.77) for 6-30 days	Self-selected population, pre-exposure asthma status unknown, active-duty military (Army only)
Smith et al. 2002	405,142 active-duty US military deployed to Gulf War	Exposure modeling via troop positions and air-monitoring data used to create seven exposure levels based on average. daily exposure and length of exposure: no exposure; 1-260 $\mu g/m^3$ for: 1-25 days, 26-50 days, >50 days; >260 $\mu g/m^3$ for 1-25 days, 26-50 days, >50 days	Hospitalizations (1991-1999) for any cause, major ICD-9-CM diagnoses and specific diagnoses related to oil-well fires (such as asthma, ischemic heart disease, and emphysema)	With Cox modeling, three of 25 models showed increase in adjusted risk of hospitalization, but no dose-response relationship; when nonexposed and exposed, were compared, none of the adjusted risk ratio for postwar hospitalization		Limited to DOD hospitals, exposures unknown except for oil-well smoke, outpatient data not available

Reference	Type of Study and Population	Exposure Determination	Health Outcome and How Measured	Results	Adjusted OR (95% CI or p)	Limitations
				due to diagnosis related to respiratory system was significant. The seven categories were collapsed into two (exposed and nonexposed) because of relatively small numbers		

NOTE: CI=confidence interval; DOD=Department of Defense; ICD-9-CM=International Classification of Diseases, 9th Edition, Clinical Modification; OR=odds ratio.

Self-reported oil-well fire smoke exposure was associated with a higher risk of asthma (OR [odds ratio] 1.56, 95% CI 1.23-1.97). In addition, modeled cumulative smoke exposure was related to a greater risk of asthma (OR 1.21, 95% CI 0.97-1.51 for the intermediate-exposure group; OR 1.40, 95% CI 1.12-1.76 for the high-exposure group) after controlling for sex, age, race or ethnicity, rank, smoking history, and self-reported exposure. When exposure was classified as number of days with exposure over 65 μg/m3, the risk of asthma also increased. For both exposure metrics, there was evidence of a linear exposure-response trend. Smoking appeared to modify the effect—the effect of oil-well fire smoke exposure was observed among never and former smokers but not among current smokers. Study strengths include the objective exposure assessment and use of physician-diagnosed asthma on the basis of clinical evaluations. Limitations include the self-selection into the DOD registry, which could have introduced selection bias; for example, if the cohort was enriched in persons who both experienced exposure and have respiratory conditions, the risk estimate could be biased upward. Moreover, the study examined prevalent-asthma cases, so a higher incidence of asthma cannot be distinguished from exacerbation or recrudescence of pre-existing disease. The study did not ask about chronic bronchitis or other respiratory effects.

In contrast, the population-based Iowa cohort of 1,560 Gulf War veterans found no association between oil-well fire exposure and the risk of asthma (Lange et al. 2002). Five years after the war, veterans were asked about their exposures and current symptoms. Exposure was modeled with an approach similar to that of Cowan et al. Each veteran's exposure was modeled the basis of the identified unit and its location during the period of oil-well fires (February-October 1991). Cases of asthma were defined by questions assessing wheezing and chest tightness. Cases of bronchitis were assessed by self-reported cough and phlegm production. Both questions pertained to symptoms in the preceding month, so it is not possible to determine whether symptoms were chronic. Self-reported exposure to oil-well fires was associated with a greater risk of asthma and bronchitis. There was no statistical association, however, between modeled exposure and the risk of asthma or bronchitis, when sex, age, race, military rank, smoking history, military service, and level of preparedness for war were controlled for. The three higher exposure quartiles were associated with a similar risk of asthma and bronchitis compared with the lowest-exposure quartile (all ORs near 1.0 with a range of 0.77-1.26). The correlation between self-reported exposure and modeled exposure was moderate (range of 0.40-0.48, $p < 0.05$). The authors ascribed the different results for self-reported vs objective exposure measurement to recall bias. Study strengths include the population-based sampling: findings probably can be generalized to all military personnel in the Persian Gulf; however, the study speaks to the outcome of asthma symptoms rather than an asthma diagnosis. Chronic bronchitis also was not defined with the standard epidemiologic definition, so it was impossible to distinguish between acute and chronic symptoms.

Gray et al. (2000) conducted a study of hospitalizations (1991-1994) at DOD, Department of Veterans Affairs (VA), and used data from the California Office of Statewide Health Planning and Development. Because of the absence of denominator data, the authors compared proportional morbidity ratios (PMRs) of hospitalization discharge diagnoses (14 diagnostic categories from ICD-9) in Gulf War vs nondeployed veterans. PMRs of most disease categories were not increased; however, those of respiratory diseases were increased in veterans (PMR 1.19, 95% CI 1.10-1.29) but not in active-duty military or California residents. Among respiratory diseases, the authors reported increases in asthma, but no data were shown. The study was of hospitalizations, so no data were collected on individual self-reported exposures. The study is reported here because it was antecedent to a more detailed study of respiratory hospitalizations by Smith et al. (2002).

In a historical cohort study of 405,142 active-duty Gulf War veterans, Smith et al. (2002) examined the effect of oil-well fire exposure on the risk of postwar hospitalization. Exposure was estimated by using troop location data and estimated smoke (that is, PM) concentrations based on NOAA modeling (Draxler et al. 1994; McQueen and Draxler 1994). Six exposure categories were created by using average daily exposure and length-of-exposure data (Table 5.3). Hospitalizations were examined for the period 1991-1999, including admissions for any cause, major ICD-9-CM diagnoses, and nine specific diagnoses presumed to be related to oil-well fires. If a subject was hospitalized before the war with one of the specific diagnoses, the subject was excluded from further analysis. The study examined hospitalizations only in DOD hospitals because of the availability of data. Active-duty personnel are rarely hospitalized outside the DOD medical system whereas veterans and National Guard and reserve personnel often use other hospitals. There was no association between exposure to oil-well fires and the risk of hospitalization for asthma (RR [relative risk] 0.90, 95% CI 0.74-1.10), acute bronchitis (RR 1.09, 95% CI 0.62-1.90), or chronic bronchitis (RR 0.78, 95% CI 0.38-1.57). Because most adults who have asthma or chronic bronchitis are never hospitalized for the condition, the study would not be expected to have captured most cases. No information was available on smoking or other exposures that may be related to respiratory symptoms, and although there was an increase in the RR between smoke from oil-well fires and emphysema, the CI included the null value (RR 1.36, 95% CI 0.62-2.98).

TABLE 5.3 Exposure in Smith et al. 2002

Exposure to Smoke from Oil-Well Fires	% of Subjects (n = 405,142) Active-Duty Military During Gulf War	% Hospitalized After War (Feb-Jan 1999) in DOD Hospitals
Not exposed	16.8	19.1
1-260 μg/m^3 for 1-25 days	33.7	20.0
1-260 μg/m^3 for 26-50 days	5.73	19.2
1-260 μg/m^3 for >50 days	0.9	19.3
>260 μg/m^3 for 1-25 days	16.8	20.2
>260 μg/m^3 for 26-50 days	17.0	17.9
>260 μg/m^3 for >50 days	9.0	19.4

NOTE: DOD=Department of Defense.

Several other studies of smoke from oil-well fires in the Persian Gulf were less methodologically robust. A cohort study of Gulf War veterans evaluated self-reported combustion exposure but examined pulmonary symptoms only as a broad class; asthma and bronchitis were not specifically evaluated (Proctor et al. 1998). A prospective study of 125 British Royal Engineer bomb-disposal unit members stationed in Kuwait City found no change in pulmonary function after the oil-well fires were set—forced expiratory flow 25-75% (FEF_{25-75}), the average forced expiratory flow rate over the middle 50% of the forced vital capacity (FVC)—but asthma and bronchitis were not specifically evaluated (Coombe and Drysdale 1993). Finally, an ecologic study of Kuwaiti residents found no increase in the rate of asthma hospitalization after the Gulf War (Al-Khalaf 1998).

Outdoor Air Pollution

Community air-pollution studies typically evaluate the health effects of routinely measured air pollutants, such as nitrogen oxides (NO_x), sulfur dioxides, particles of various sizes (for example, PM_{10}, $PM_{2.5}$)[2] or concentrations (TSP), and in some cases atmospheric transformation products, such as ozone. Some of the studies used single-location measures (or community averages) of air pollutants to characterize exposures of residents of each study community, and a few estimated exposure of individual residents on the basis of interpolation of ambient monitoring data.

Prospective Studies

The Adventist Health Smog study, a prospective cohort study, began in 1976 by following a cohort of 6,000 Seventh-Day Adventists (SDAs) in areas of California with varied air-pollution magnitudes. SDAs are a unique cohort because they are non-smokers (35% of men and 14% of women were smokers before joining the church). The church's prohibition of smoking reduced the confounding effect of current smoking for studying health effects of air pollution.

The following studies of incidence of respiratory outcomes were based on the SDA cohort. Each study used similar methods and confounding and bias controls. Study subjects were over 25 years old, baptized members of the SDA church, non-Hispanic and white, had lived within 5 miles of their permanent residence for more than 10 years, and resided in San Francisco, the Los Angeles Basin, or San Diego. Participants were studied for respiratory and other health outcomes. Respiratory outcomes were studied in a subcohort of nearly 4,000 people. Three respiratory outcomes were analyzed according to responses to a 21-item symptom questionnaire: asthma, chronic bronchitis, and overall airway obstructive disease (AOD). AOD included asthma, chronic bronchitis, and emphysema (there were so few cases of emphysema that it was not analyzed separately). Each subject's symptoms were classified as none, possible, and definite[3] for each respiratory outcome. Exposure to air pollutants was determined for each participant on the basis of ambient monitoring sites in 1977-1987 by interpolating residential ZIP codes and work-location history. The precision of interpolating concentrations was verified. In 1976, each study participant completed a detailed demographic and lifestyle questionnaire about smoking, occupation, hours spent in driving on highways, and other topics. In 1977 and 1987, each participant completed standardized respiratory-symptoms questionnaires (American Thoracic Society, ATS) to ascertain self-reported symptoms of chronic respiratory disease. Most analyses controlled for age, sex, previous smoking, occupational exposure to tobacco smoke, AOD before the age of 16 years, and education. Overall, study findings are informative, particularly because they focus on incident, rather than prevalent, respiratory disease. Study limitations include self-reporting of respiratory symptoms, varying specificity in measures of exposure, and coexposures to ozone and photochemical oxidants. The following paragraphs summarize a series of four reports about the incidence of respiratory outcomes covering various

---

[2]PM_{10} and $PM_{2.5}$ are notations for particulate matter of less than 10 microns in diameter and less than 2.5 microns in diameter, respectively.

[3]Criteria for definite chronic bronchitis required symptoms of cough or sputum on most days for at least 3 months/year, for 2 years or more. Criteria for definite asthma required a history of wheezing and a physician's diagnosis of asthma. Asthma self-reporting was validated with information from medical charts.

individual pollutants, exposure groupings (for example, mean concentrations or exceedance frequencies), and time frames.

Abbey et al. (1993b) reported on the 10-year incidence (1977-1987) of chronic respiratory disease in relation to long-term ambient concentrations of air pollutants (TSPs), ozone, and sulfur dioxide (SO_2). Symptom incidence was determined for 1977-1987 by questionnaire (NHLBI). Confounding variables included in the analysis were education, sex, possible symptoms in 1977, and years worked with a smoker. The mortality results in the SDAs are summarized in a later section on air-pollution mortality findings. For TSPs, exposure was grouped into several magnitudes (average hours exposed to TSP at over 60, 100, 150, and 200 $\mu g/m^3$). Self-reported respiratory symptoms, as noted above, were grouped into asthma, chronic bronchitis, and AOD (any of asthma, chronic bronchitis, and emphysema). The outcome of the study noted increases in the incidence of definite symptoms of AOD and chronic bronchitis with hours exposed to TSP at over 100, 150, and 200 $\mu g/m^3$ and asthma above of 150 and 200 $\mu g/m^3$ (AOD, RR 1.36, 95% CI 1.11-1.66 for 1,000 hours above 200 µg/m3 TSP; chronic bronchitis, RR 1.33, 95% CI 1.07-1.65 for 1,000 hours above 200 µg/m3; and asthma, RR 1.74, 95% CI 1.11-2.72 for 1,000 hours above 200 $\mu g/m^3$).

In the same report, mean concentration and average annual exceedance frequencies of 100, 120, 150, and 200 parts per billion (ppb) were not associated with new cases of any respiratory outcomes, although a possible association between ozone and exceedances of 100 ppb and new cases of asthma (point estimate RR 1.40, 95% CI 0.99-2.34) was noted for 500 hours of average annual increment. An elevated risk in men (not women) was associated with ozone and exceedances of 100 ppb and new cases of asthma (point estimate RR 1.95, 95% CI 1.0-3.94) for 500 hours of annual increment. Because of multicollinearity, the analyses were unable to show whether TSP or ozone was more strongly associated with new cases of asthma (ozone and TSP correlation 0.74). There was no association between SO_2 and respiratory symptoms; however, the average ambient concentrations were low. There also was no association between nitrogen dioxide (NO_2) and each of the respiratory outcomes (Abbey et al. 1993a).

Another report by Abbey et al. (1993c) analyzed the 10-year incidence (1977-1987) of chronic respiratory disease associated with long-term ambient concentrations of sulfate (SO_4) particles. The 10-year cumulative exposure to SO_4 particles was determined for each participant in 1977-1987. Multivariate analysis was conducted for AOD, chronic bronchitis, and asthma for new cases of disease, persistent prevalence (that is, symptoms in both 1977 and 1987), and change in severity of symptoms (from 1977 to 1987). The 10-year mean ambient concentration of SO_4 particles was strongly associated with the development of definite asthma (RR 2.87, 95% CI 1.03-7.55 per increment of 7 $\mu g/m^3$) but not with AOD and chronic bronchitis. Working with a smoker and having AOD before the age of 16 years were strongly associated with asthma.

Finally, Abbey et al. (1995) examined respiratory outcomes in a subset of the cohort (n = 1,868) in relation to estimated long-term ambient concentrations of $PM_{2.5}$ and other air pollutants. Exposure to $PM_{2.5}$ was estimated with regression of site- and season-specific regression equations from paired $PM_{2.5}$ and visibility observations (1979-1986) and applied to visibility data at nine airports in California. The subset of the cohort was selected on the basis of having lived at least 80% of months (1966-1986) close to the airports. Long-term means of each subject's estimated monthly $PM_{2.5}$ mean concentrations and exceedance frequencies were cumulated over 1966-1977 according to ZIP code by monthly residence. A 45$\mu g/m^3$ increase in mean $PM_{2.5}$ exposure was associated with a greater risk of incident chronic bronchitis (RR 1.81,

95% CI 0.98 to 3.25). (When a larger subset of the cohort with less stringent residency criteria is included, this association is stronger, $p < 0.05$.) There was no association with onset of asthma and AOD for $PM_{2.5}$ (means or exceedance frequencies). Mean $PM_{2.5}$ was associated with a change in severity score for AOD, chronic bronchitis, and asthma. Meaningful regression coefficients applied for AOD at all levels of $PM_{2.5}$, for chronic bronchitis at $PM_{2.5}$ levels above 20 $\mu g/m^3$, and for asthma at levels above 40 $\mu g/m^3$.

Cross-Sectional or Case-Control Studies of Air Pollution

While the majority of epidemiologic studies of morbidity and mortality associated with community air pollution are time series (ecologic) design, the committee focused on cross-sectional or case-control studies of air pollution. The time series studies examine daily mortality or morbidity, while the focus for the committee is on long-term health effects.

A population-based study in France examined the relationship between SO_2 concentration and asthma (Baldi et al. 1999). A random sample of adults 25-59 years old who resided for at least 3 years during 1974-1976 in 24 areas of seven French towns were selected. Air pollution was measured over the same 3 year period by pollution-monitoring stations (subjects lived within 500 meters of a station). There was an ecologic correlation between mean annual regional SO_2 concentration and the prevalence of asthma ($r = 0.45$, $p = 0.01$), defined as responding affirmatively to the question "Have you ever had asthma?" In individual-level, cross-sectional analysis, higher mean annual SO_2 was associated with a greater risk of self-reported asthma (OR 1.24 for each 50 ug/m^3 increment, 95% CI 1.08-1.44), when age, educational attainment, and smoking history were controlled for. Geographic clustering of data was taken into account by using random effects. Limitations include the cross-sectional design and the use of self-reported asthma; strengths include the population-based sampling and direct air-pollution monitoring.

Karakatsani et al. (2003) conducted a nested case-control study of Greeks enrolled in a population-based cohort study, the European Prospective Study into Cancer and Nutrition. Residents of greater Athens completed a questionnaire, which was used to recruit 168 participants who reported a history of COPD, chronic bronchitis, emphysema, or respiratory symptoms (including chronic productive cough for 3 months per year for 2 years). The same number of age- and sex-matched controls without respiratory conditions or symptoms was selected. A thoracic-disease specialist visited, interviewed, and measured with spirometry each subject ($n = 84$) at home to confirm the diagnosis of COPD. Air pollution was ascertained retrospectively on the basis of average long-term concentrations of black smoke and NO_2 recorded at 14 monitoring stations for the decade 1987-1997. Boroughs were classified into quintiles of NO_2 concentration. Residential and employment histories were used to calculate time-weighted averages for each subject. Subjects who resided in rural areas or other cities were assigned to categories based on their presumed pollution exposure. Conditional logistic regression revealed an association between the highest quartile of estimated exposure during the preceding 5 years and the risk of COPD (OR 1.89, 95% CI 0.83-4.31). Exposure during the preceding 20 years was not associated with COPD (OR 1.31, 95% CI 0.52-3.28). Study strengths include the population-based recruitment of cases and controls, the attempt to confirm the diagnosis of COPD with physician examination, the objective exposure assessment, and statistical control for sociodemographic and smoking variables. The study had several limitations: There was a lack of uniform criteria for diagnosing COPD; although exposure was objectively ascertained, the lack of monitoring data on subjects who lived outside greater Athens reduced the accuracy of exposure classification; and the wide confidence intervals, reflecting low precision of the effect estimates, limit interpretation of the data.

In a population-based sample of adults aged 40 years or older, investigators studied the relation between regional SO_2 concentration in the Osaka prefecture in Japan and the prevalence of self-reported chronic bronchitis (Tsunetoshi et al. 1971). Average SO_2 concentrations for a 3-year period before the study began were noted. The researchers found a moderate relationship between chronic-bronchitis prevalence and regional average SO_2 when they controlled for age and smoking (mean prevalence increased 1.94 for each SO_2 increment of 1 mg/100 cm^2 per day). There was no relationship between regional SO_2 and the prevalence of reduced 1-second forced respiratory volume (FEV_1). Limitations include the use of an exposure measurement based on averaging SO_2 over a long time (3 years) before the study and the lack of control for socioeconomic status (SES) or other exposures.

A population-based, cross-sectional study of 18,873 people 20-44 years old evaluated the relationship between regional mean annual NO_2 concentration and asthma prevalence across Italy (De Marco et al. 2002). Mean annual outdoor NO_2 was measured with fixed monitoring stations near the study subjects' residences; concentrations were measured for the period 1996-1999 (surveys took place in 1998-2000). Asthma prevalence was measured with a question asking whether the respondent had had an attack of asthma during the preceding 12 months. Higher ambient NO_2 was associated with a greater risk of asthma attacks, when climate, age, sex, smoking, social class, season, and type of contact (telephone vs mail) were controlled for (OR per standard-deviation increment in NO_2 1.13, 95% CI 0.98-1.32). The confidence interval did not exclude absence of an association. Study strengths include the population-based sampling and objective exposure measurement. A limitation of the study, for the committee in interpreting the data for purposes of its charge, is the use of "asthma attacks" as a study outcome, which probably overrepresents exacerbation of previously established asthma, rather than incident asthma cases; the cross-sectional design; and the lack of information about distance between monitoring stations and subjects' residences.

A population-based study in western Australia compared 255 cases of asthma that required hospitalization with 903 population-based controls (Hunt and Holman 1987). Residential SO_2 was estimated with a validated model based on meteorologic data and industry emissions data. There was no relation between mean residential SO_2 and risk of asthma hospitalization (OR 0.8-1.1). There was also no association between frequent high peak exposure (hours of exposure at over 486 $\mu g/m^3$ per year) and risk of hospitalization. A major limitation for the committee in interpreting the data for purposes of its charge is that asthma hospitalizations could reflect either incident disease or exacerbation of pre-existing disease. In addition, most asthma patients are never hospitalized for the disease, so hospitalization is a poor measure of disease causation.

Air-Pollution Mortality Studies

Mortality studies of respiratory outcomes are, for purposes of this report, often difficult to interpret and inconclusive. One reason is that many mortality studies use composite ICD codes instead of minor groupings or individual codes, which would have greater specificity. A second is that because asthma and chronic bronchitis are rarely fatal, mortality studies tend to be insensitive to any relationship between an environmental or occupational exposure and long-term respiratory effects. Finally, although emphysema is the respiratory effect that is the exception because it can be fatal, most emphysema deaths are related to cigarette-smoking. Further complicating matters, emphysema deaths are often caused by pneumonia or cardiovascular disease, so ascertainment of emphysema deaths is not robust.

Respiratory mortality findings in several large-scale cohorts have been reported: American Cancer Society (ACS) (Pope et al. 1995, 2002), Six-Cities (Dockery et al. 1993), SDAs (Abbey et al. 1999), and Netherlands Cohort Study on Diet and Cancer (Hoek et al. 2002). Those studies, however, examined outcomes that are too broad to draw conclusions from, considering that they group composite ICD codes (for example, 460-519) under the broad labels "cardiopulmonary diseases", "respiratory diseases", and "non-malignant respiratory diseases." A recent analysis of the ACS cohort (Pope et al. 2004) performed somewhat more diagnosis-specific analyses with the same methods as Pope et al. (2002). The RR of "COPD and allied conditions" (ICD codes 490-496) in relation to air-pollution exposure was not increased after adjusting for former and current smoking.

Air Pollution: Other Support Studies

Garshick et al. (2003) studied US male veterans in Massachusetts (n = 2,628) who resided near major roadways; such residence is an indicator of motor vehicle exhaust exposure. Veterans who lived within 50 meters of a major roadway were compared with those who lived more than 400 meters away. By virtue of their age (mean age 60.6 years), the veterans were not likely to be Gulf War veterans. They were drawn from the general population of southeastern Massachusetts, and they had not been treated in a VA medical center in the year before being surveyed. Estimates of individual exposure were based on current residential address (without information on residential history) linked to road type and traffic-count data in a geographic information system. Living near a major roadway appeared to be associated with increased reporting of persistent wheeze (OR 1.31, 95% CI 1.00-1.71), as did living near a major roadway with high traffic volume (over 10,000 vehicles per 24 hours) (OR 1.7, 95% CI 1.2-2.4), compared with living near a roadway with lower traffic volume. Self-reports of physician-diagnosed asthma or COPD (defined as chronic bronchitis or emphysema) were analyzed as confounders and effect modifiers. Associations were adjusted for cigarette-smoking, age, and occupational exposure to dust. The authors noted that limitations of the study include lack of information on duration of residence at each address and information about home exposure to NO_x from cooking or heating. Information is lacking about the health effects of the nonresponders, because the study had a response rate of 58%.

Zhang et al. (1999) studied the effects of air pollution on respiratory health of adults in three Chinese cities. A study of parents of schoolchildren was performed on 4,108 adults who resided in four school districts of three major cities.[4] Questionnaires adapted from the American Thoracic Society (ATS) Epidemiologic Standardization project were used to collect information on health status, occupation, level of education, smoking history, indoor air pollution in the home (coal use and smoking), history of respiratory illnesses, and symptoms. The self-reported symptoms ascertained were cough, phlegm, wheeze, and persistent cough and phlegm (PCP, an indicator of chronic bronchitis). Self-reported respiratory illnesses "ever diagnosed by a physician" were asthma and bronchitis, but the latter could have included acute or chronic bronchitis. Exposure to air pollution was determined on the basis of ambient air pollution data from monitoring stations in each district. Four-year average concentrations of TSP, SO_2, and

[4]A separate report covered findings on schoolchildren, but this young population is not relevant to Gulf War veterans.

NOx were assessed to estimate long-term exposure to outdoor air pollution. The trend for TSP was Lanzhou > Wuhan-urban > Guangzhou > Wuhan-suburban. The differences for SO_2 and NO_x were less pronounced. Crude prevalences of each respiratory symptom in both mothers and fathers were Lanzhou > Wuhan urban + suburban > Guangzhou. The ORs and 95% CIs compared with Guangzhou, were determined with a logistic-regression model, which adjusted for age, years of residence, occupation, education, smoking status, home coal use, and use of ventilation device use (chimney, exhaust hood, and exhaust fan). For both mothers and fathers, the ORs (with Guangzhou as a reference) for each respiratory symptom were Lanzhou > Wuhan urban + suburban. The findings suggest that increased TSP concentration is associated with increased symptoms. The ORs for the only symptom indicative of chronic bronchitis (PCP) ranged from 0.86 to 12.62, and all demonstrated an association except for the ORs of the mothers who lived in Wuhan-suburban. Physician-diagnosed asthma and bronchitis showed inconsistent trends. For bronchitis (acute or chronic), ORs for mothers followed the same trend as respiratory symptoms (Lanzhou OR 9.69, 95% CI 5.50-17.06). In a comparison of urban with suburban Wuhan, only the asthma OR for the father was increased (OR 3.59, 95% CI 1.36-9.49). A limitation of the study is that it did not associate air-pollution concentrations themselves with health outcomes; it only associated residence in some regions with health outcomes. The authors cautioned that nonmeasured between-city factors may have been responsible for the associations.

In an ecologic study in Sweden (Bjornsson et al. 1994), the risk of chronic-bronchitis symptoms was higher in Gotborg than Uppsala (OR 1.2, 95% CI 1.02-1.4). There was no difference in the prevalence of self-reported asthma. Although Gotborg was more polluted, there were also differences in climate and SES that could have accounted for the findings.

An ecologic study evaluated the relation between short-term SO_2 peaks and emergency-department visits for asthma in low income neighborhoods in New York City in 1968-1972 (Goldstein and Weinstein 1986). No association was observed between days of "high" SO_2 (defined according to three threshold values) and days with high numbers of emergency-department visits for asthma. Limitations include the lack of control for confounding factors, such as smoking and sociodemographic characteristics, and the likelihood that emergency-department visits reflected exacerbation of pre-existing asthma rather than incident asthma cases.

Two other studies compared the prevalence of asthma or chronic bronchitis among geographic regions that had different air-pollution magnitudes. The geographic areas probably differ in other important ways, such as sociodemographic characteristics of the inhabitants, smoking prevalence, and allergen exposure. Because there were no specific measurements of air pollution, it is difficult to draw any inferences from the studies (Papageorgiou et al. 1997; Woods et al. 2000). The Woods et al. study was a large population-based cross-sectional survey of people 20-44 years old. Self-reported "air-pollution annoyance" was associated with a greater risk of self-reported physician-diagnosed asthma (OR 1.11, 95% CI 1.09-1.14) and chronic bronchitis symptoms (OR 1.14, 95% CI 1.11-1.17). The self-reported-exposure measure is suspect, however, in that persons who have respiratory disease may be more likely to remember and report perceived air-pollution annoyance.

An ecologic study in Brisbane, Australia, examined the association between weekly smoke density (coefficient of haze) and admissions to the casualty department of the Royal Brisbane Hospital at night (Derrick 1970). There was no noteworthy correlation between smoke density and weekly number of asthma admissions (r = -0.04 to -0.05).

Hastings and Jardine (2002) evaluated the association between measured particulate air pollution and upper respiratory disease rates in soldiers deployed to Bosnia in 1997-1998. The study used a composite upper respiratory disease definition that included upper and lower respiratory tract diseases. No specific information on asthma, chronic bronchitis, or COPD was presented.

Zelikoff et al. (2002) has conducted a review of the toxicology of inhaled wood. Additionally, several studies (for example, Aditama 2000; Kunii et al. 2002; Sastry 2002) have conducted studies of mortality and morbidity (primarily through the examination of lung function) of wood smoke.

Domestic gas-stove use releases NO_2, a potential respiratory irritant, into the indoor environment (Samet et al. 1987). Many epidemiologic studies examining the effects of gas-stove use have focused on healthy members of the adult population (Dow et al. 1999; Jarvis et al. 1996, 1998; Ng et al. 1993; Ostro et al. 1993; Samet et al. 1987; Viegi et al. 1992, 1991). In those studies, the effect of gas stove exposure on the development of respiratory symptoms, including asthma symptoms and pulmonary function impairment has been inconclusive.

Hydrogen Sulfide and Respiratory Diseases

The city of Rotorua, New Zealand, is above a geothermally active area with substantial hydrogen sulfide (H_2S) exposure. About one-fourth of the population of 40,000 is regularly exposed to H_2S over 200 μ/m^3 (143 ppb). A series of studies by Bates et al. investigated morbidity and mortality from the full range of diseases, including respiratory diseases (Bates et al. 1997; Bates et al. 1998, 2002). The impetus for the studies was a 1981 World Health Organization report that recommended research in Rotorua to take advantage of the natural conditions to study the health effects of H_2S.

Bates et al. (1997), using census data, compared deaths in Rotorua with those in the rest of New Zealand (1981-1990). First examining the composite category respiratory diseases (ICD codes 460-519), they found the SMR to be higher in Rotorua (SMR 1.18, 95% CI 1.08-1.29, $p < 0.001$). They also found an elevated SMR for chronic obstructive respiratory disease (CORD), ICD-9 codes 490-496, which include asthma, bronchitis, COPD, and allied conditions (SMR 1.20, 95% CI 1.06-1.35, $p < 0.004$). Rotorua has a higher density of Maori residents than other areas of New Zealand. The authors noted the potential for underreporting of Maori mortality statistics because ethnicity on death certificates is based on funeral directors' impressions.

In a subsequent report, Bates (2002) used hospital-discharge data over a 3-year period (1993-1996) to calculate standardized incidence ratios (SIRs) for respiratory and other diseases (and subgroupings) in Rotorua residents. Exposure was designated as high, medium, and low on the basis of area of residence where H_2S was mapped outdoors with passive sampling. Exposure-response trends were found for diseases of the respiratory system (p for trend was < 0.0001), and for CORD and allied conditions, codes 490-496; p for trend was < 0.0001. The authors had no information on smoking and SES as potential confounders.

In a third report, Bates et al. (1998) used hospital-discharge data over a decade (1981-1990) to calculate SIRs for respiratory and other diseases (and subgroupings) in Rotorua residents. No exposure groups were designated. The SIRs for respiratory diseases (ICD codes 460-519) were not increased (SIR 1.01, 95% CI 0.99-1.04). CORD was not increased. A major limitation of the series of Bates studies for purposes of the present report is the grouping of respiratory diseases without specifying whether they were asthma, bronchitis, COPD, or individual conditions. Additionally, the Bates studies were the only epidemiologic studies of H_2S found by the committee that examined long-term health outcomes. Due to the paucity of literature, the committee did not make a separate conclusion on H_2S.

Occupational Studies

Osterman et al. (1989a) studied a cohort of 145 male silicon carbide production workers in Quebec, Canada. Individual exposures were to respirable dust and to SO_2 at relatively low concentrations (less than 1.5 ppm). Exposures were estimated based on the basis of job-specific measurements and linkage to worker-specific job titles and employment duration. Average duration of employment was 14 years. The estimates included a measure of cumulative exposure, average exposure, and most recent exposure. It is notable that the plant had been closed in the 6 months preceding the study, so the evaluation of outcome probably occurred after an exposure-free interval. Respiratory symptoms were ascertained with a translated version of the ATS respiratory-disease questionnaire. Lung function was also measured and reported separately (Osterman et al. 1989b). Although all symptoms occurred more frequently in current smokers (53.8% of the study population), analyses adjusting for age and current smoking indicated a dose-dependent association between chronic phlegm and both average and cumulative exposure to SO_2. For cumulative SO_2 exposure, the highest exposure (over 3 ppm-years) had OR 11.8, 95% CI 2.58-52.9; moderate exposure (>1.0-3.0) OR 2.94, 95% CI 0.84-10.3; and lowest exposure (>0.25-1.0) OR 1.43, 95% CI 0.42-4.83, with the referent being 0-0.25 ppm-years. The strong SO_2-symptom associations persisted and were almost identical with those obtained from regression models that did not include a dust variable. There was no evidence of a dust-SO_2 interaction. The association was more closely related to exposure concentration rather than to duration. A similar dose-dependent association was observed between SO_2 exposure and chronic wheeze. The associations with respirable dust were generally negative. Because the study measured symptoms only 6 months after cessation of exposure, it is not known whether they were reduced or eliminated after a longer exposure-free period.

In a companion article, Osterman et al. (1989b) performed pulmonary-function testing—FEV_1 and forced vital capacity (FVC)—on the same group of 145 former silicon carbide production workers. The cohort experienced reductions in FEV_1 and FVC values, but they were unrelated to cumulative and average SO_2 exposures. No effects of a dust-SO_2 interaction were seen.

Mortality Studies

Studies of respiratory-system mortality in particular occupations are often difficult to interpret. They tend to examine composite or poorly defined outcomes (for example, "respiratory diseases" as a group of ICD codes) or to provide scanty information about exposure (for example, studies of professional drivers (Borgia et al. 1994; Rafnsson and Gunaarsdottir 1991) and highway workers (Maizlish et al. 1988). Other studies examine occupations that entail exposure to chemicals of uncertain relevance to Gulf War veterans, including studies of urban firefighters (Aronson et al. 1994; Baris et al. 2001; Beaumont et al. 1991; Feuer and Rosenman 1986). Although most mortality studies had negative results, three found higher mortality from emphysema (Maizlish et al. 1988) or from a composite category of nonmalignant respiratory diseases (Aronson et al. 1994; Feuer and Rosenman 1986); the design of the three studies, however, precluded adjustment for the effects of smoking, a major risk factor for death from emphysema. A separate analysis of the ACS prospective study found that emphysema mortality was not meaningfully increased among workers exposed to diesel exhaust, after adjustment for the effects of smoking (Boffetta et al. 1988). A large study of firefighters in 27 states (over 5,700 deaths), which included a mix of urban and rural firefighting jurisdictions, did not find higher mortality from COPD (Burnett et al. 1994).

Support Studies

The effects of occupational exposure to engine exhaust were studied in 116 Copenhagen street-cleaners in comparison with a similar number of cemetery workers (Raaschou-Nielsen et al. 1995). Environmental monitoring confirmed that street cleaners had higher average exposures to air pollutants (except ozone) than did cemetery workers, but similar wages and similar exertion. Cemetery workers were younger and less likely to smoke cigarettes. The study did not indicate whether the symptom questionnaire was sent after an exposure-free interval, but the likelihood is that there was no interval, inasmuch as this was a study of current workers. The study found, after adjustment for age and smoking, that street-cleaners were at higher risk for chronic bronchitis (OR 2.5, 95% CI 1.2-5.1) and asthma (OR 2.3, 95% CI 1.0-5.1). Asthma and chronic bronchitis were defined on the basis of responses to the standard questionnaire by the British Medical Research Council. The average duration of employment was 5-9 years. A limitation of the study is the potential for nonmeasured differences between the two types of workers that could confound the exposure-outcome relationships.

Occupational exposure to diesel-exhaust emissions was associated with increased self-reported symptoms of cough and sputum and with lower pulmonary function in coal miners vs matched controls (Reger et al. 1982). When disparities in various health characteristics between workers in or at diesel-using mines and their matched controls were related to an index of diesel exposure, they showed no noteworthy trends. Although a pattern consistent with early airway disease was shown, factors other than diesel may be responsible inasmuch as exposure duration and concentrations were low.

The respiratory health of 259 workers at five salt mines was evaluated with a questionnaire and spirometry (Gamble and Jones 1983); no direct exposure measurements were available. Comparisons within the study population showed a dose-related association of phlegm and diesel-exhaust exposure, no noteworthy trend for cough and dyspnea, and no association with spirometry was seen.

Residence near a factory that produced plastic-coated wallpaper, which emitted combustion products of paraffin oil, was associated with a 24% increase in asthma prevalence defined by computerized medication-dispensing patterns (95% CI 4%-44%) (Dunn et al. 1995). The factory also emitted azodicarbonamide, which has been associated with occupational asthma.

Investigators evaluated clerical and industrial workers (in four engineering factories) in Brisbane, Australia (Smithurst and Williams 1976). Although cough and phlegm were more common among industrial than clerical workers, there was no specific evaluation of exposure to combustion products. There also was no statistical control for potentially confounding variables, such as SES.

A study of 1,933 men 22-54 years old living in Norway found that self-reported occupational exposure to SO_2 was associated with a greater decline in FEV_1 from initial examination (1965-1970) to followup (1988-1990). Investigators demonstrated a decline in FEV_1 after occupational diesel-exhaust exposure, but the decline normalized after an exposure-free period of 3 days (Ulfvarson et al. 1987).

Several other morbidity studies assessed occupational exposures but were limited by lack of exposure information or other features. One study (Fleming and Charlton 2001) found that transport workers have an increased risk of physician-diagnosed asthma (PR 116, 95% CI 101-131), but no measurements of exposure were available. Occupational exposure to engine exhaust was not associated with adult asthma in a study in Sweden (Toren et al. 1999). Other studies are limited in that they did not provide specific estimates of exposure to combustion products but rather studied exposures to a composite category (for example, vapors, gas, dust, or fumes) (Flodin et al. 1996; Kogevinas et al. 1999; Xu and Christiani 1993; Zock et al. 2001).

Some studies have assessed the effect of forest firefighting on various intermediate measures or indexes of pulmonary function rather than on respiratory diseases themselves. Forest firefighters' exposures might be more relevant to Gulf War veterans' exposures than to urban firefighters' exposures, which include combustion products of synthetic materials (Burgess et al. 1999). Most forest-firefighter studies, however, did not examine effects on lung function after an exposure-free period. An exposure-free period is important for distinguishing between reversible, short-term outcomes and long-term outcomes. In one study that had an exposure-free period of 2.5 months after a fire, firefighters were noted to have decreased indexes of expiratory function (FEV_1, and FEF_{25-75}) (Betchley et al. 1997).

Liu et al. (1992) studied 63 members of the US Department of Agriculture Forest Service hotshot crews in northern Montana before and after the forest-fire season. Crews worked full-time in May-November. Spirometric measures indicated declines in FVC, FEV_1, and FEF_{25-75}, and results of methacholine challenge indicated an increase in airway responsiveness. Findings were independent of smoking. The duration of the exposure-free interval between fire exposure and testing appears to have been at most 2 weeks, so it is difficult to determine whether effects are short-term effects, which may reverse, or long-term effects.

A prospective study of 1,768 urban firefighters in 1970-1976 found no exposure-related decline in pulmonary function. The mean FEV_1 and FVC were not reduced by more than 3% over the 6 years (Musk et al. 1979). A study of retirees from the same urban fire department did not find appreciably reduced respiratory function that was unrelated to smoking (Musk et al. 1982). Urban-firefighter studies, however, are probably less relevant to Gulf War veterans (see above) than are studies of rural firefighters, because of the nature of the materials in urban fires.

Biomass-Fuel Combustion

Several studies evaluated the effects of exposure to products of biomass fuel combustion for heating or cooking, which includes combustion of wood, dung, and agricultural residue. The homes in question often do not have a separate kitchen or a way to vent fumes. The studies assessed exposure by self-reporting of duration of cooking-fuel use and, in some cases, by measurement of air quality at the time of the survey.

Population-based Studies

A study in India used data from the population-based National Family Health Survey (n = 38,595) to examine people 60 years old or older (Mishra 2003). On the basis of survey items about 10 cooking fuels, the author classified cooking-smoke exposure as high (only biomass fuels), medium (a mix of biomass and cleaner fuels, such as kerosene, petroleum gas, biogas, or electricity), and low (only cleaner fuels). Asthma was reported by the head of the household (the respondent) for each member of the household in response to the question "Does anyone [in the household] suffer from asthma?" When sociodemographic factors and smoking history were controlled for, biomass-fuel use was associated with a greater risk of asthma than the use of clean fuels (OR 1.59, 95% CI 1.30-1.94). The risk was also increased for the medium group (mixed fuels) vs clean fuels (OR 1.24, 95% CI 1.04-1.49). The asthma results were stronger for women (OR 1.83, 95% CI 1.32-2.53) than men (OR 1.46, 95% CI 1.14-1.88). The strengths of the study are its population-based design, thorough ascertainment of fuel use, and control for confounding. Limitations include the cross-sectional design and the use of a self-reported definition of asthma that did not require symptoms or a physician diagnosis. No information is available on duration of exposure.

Albalak et al. (1999) studied all 241 adults in two rural Bolivian villages. The villages were similar, except that one used indoor cooking and the other outdoor cooking. They were given a Spanish translation of the British Medical Research Council questionnaire for chronic bronchitis. Measured kitchen PM_{10} was substantially higher in the indoor-cooking village; total daily integrated PM_{10} exposure based on a time-budget analysis was also much higher. The outdoor-cooking village had a lower risk of chronic bronchitis, after adjustment for age, sex, and exclusion of smokers (OR 0.4, 95% CI 0.2-0.8). The villages were similar in a variety of socioeconomic indicators. The validation of exposure with direct ambient-air monitoring (specifically PM_{10}) is a strength of the study. Although duration of residence was not reported, air monitoring was carried out over a 10-month period, and a case of chronic bronchitis was identified by uninterrupted cough for at least 3 months over 2 years.

Other Biomass Studies

A case-control study from Mexico City recruited 127 women who had chronic bronchitis or chronic airway obstruction (FEV_1 less than 75% predicted) from a tertiary referral hospital (Perez-Padilla et al. 1996). They had reported a range of 2.5-25 years of cooking with a woodstove. There were four different groups: people who had tuberculosis, interstitial lung disease, or ear nose and throat (ENT) conditions (sinusitis, otitis media, or deviated nasal septum) and healthy visitors of hospitalized patients with no respiratory symptoms or pulmonary function impairment. The primary exposure was to wood smoke while cooking. The selection of controls that had tuberculosis or interstitial lung disease is suspect because such subjects may differ from persons who have chronic airway disease in a variety of important ways. In analyses that used the other control groups, wood-smoke exposure was associated with a greater risk of chronic bronchitis without chronic airway obstruction than in ENT controls (OR 3.6, 95% CI 1.7-8) or healthy visitor controls (OR 8.1, 95% CI 3.4-14). The analysis controlled for age, cigarette-smoking, region of origin, income, education, and place of residence. Wood-smoke exposure was not associated with the risk of chronic airway obstruction without chronic bronchitis. Wood-smoke exposure was associated with a greater risk of chronic airway obstruction plus chronic bronchitis compared with ENT controls (OR 5.2, 95% CI 1.9-15) and healthy controls (OR 15, 95% CI 4-55). Cumulative lifetime exposure (the product of average hours per day of exposure and years of exposure) was also linearly related to a greater risk of chronic bronchitis only than in the ENT or visitor controls. Findings in the tuberculosis and interstitial-lung-disease control groups are difficult to interpret, because these conditions could be related to wood-smoke exposure; alternatively, the conditions, because they are severe diseases, might reduce the likelihood of cooking and consequent exposure. In addition, wood-smoke exposure could be a cause of the ENT conditions and result in a bias toward the null value in the analyses. The small sample resulted in imprecise estimates with wide confidence intervals.

A study in the hill region of Nepal evaluated 1,375 people (Pandey 1984). They reported exposure to domestic smoke produced by burning firewood, straw, and other biomass fuels, and their homes were likely to have been poorly ventilated. The cross-sectional prevalence of chronic bronchitis increased with hours spent near the fireplace. In women, chronic bronchitis was observed among smokers, ex-smokers, and never smokers. In men, it was observed in all groups except nonsmokers. However, the study did not control for SES.

Quereshi (1994) randomly selected two villages in Kashmir. In Gujjar, inhabitants live in single-room hutments and burn firewood in a mud hearth for cooking and heating. In Wahidpora, living conditions are better; kerosene stoves, gas stoves, and electric heaters are more commonly used. The SES was lower in Gujjar, and the prevalence of cigarette-smoking was also lower. The prevalence of chronic bronchitis was higher in Gujjar (10.1%) than in Wahidpora (5.1%). Among Gujjar residents, the prevalence of chronic bronchitis increased with average hours spent near the fireplace (no statistical testing was performed). In a pooled analysis of both villages, the prevalence of chronic bronchitis among women but not men varied with hours spent near the fireplace. A major limitation of the study is the lack of control for confounding variables, such as cigarette-smoking and SES, both within and between villages.

A case-control study in Saudi Arabia recruited 50 people who had COPD defined by airflow obstruction with pulmonary-function testing and 71 healthy controls (Dossing et al. 1994). Exposure to indoor fire during childhood was associated with a greater risk of COPD among women (96% of COPD cases vs 29% of controls) and men (78% vs 39%) ($p < 0.01$ and $p < 0.05$, respectively). Among women, the likelihood of long-term exposure (to indoor fire over 20 years) was higher in the COPD group than in controls (67% vs 5%) ($p < 0.01$). A serious limitation of the study is the lack of control for smoking, age, SES, and other factors.

A case-control study in Bogotá, Columbia, recruited 104 people who had obstructive airways disease (defined with pulmonary-function testing among pulmonary outpatients and medical-ward patients that showed below 70% of predicted FEV_1/FVC and FEV_1) and 104 age-matched controls (surgical or gynecology inpatients or general-medicine outpatients) in three community hospitals (Dennis et al. 1996a, 1996b). Cases and controls averaged more than 15 years of wood use, usually beginning in childhood or adolescence. Use of wood as a cooking fuel was associated with a greater risk of obstructive airways disease (OR 3.92, 95% CI 1.7 to 9.1), when smoking, passive smoke exposure, age, hospital, and gasoline use were controlled for. A study strength is the use of pulmonary-function testing to define cases. Limitations include the lack of control for SES and the limited evaluation of wood-smoke exposure in multivariate analysis (for example, no exposure-response relationship was examined). In addition, the recruitment process in a variety of inpatient and outpatient settings did not clearly result in controls that were comparable with cases.

Investigators examined the use of planchas (wood-burning chimney stoves) compared with open wood fires by 340 women in the rural highlands of Guatemala (Bruce et al. 1998). Although cough and phlegm production were less common among those using planchas, the risk of chronic bronchitis was similar (OR 0.57, 95% CI 0.22-1.46) after adjustment for age. The risk was increased after further adjustment for other indicators of SES (OR 0.72, 95% CI 0.26-1.98). The investigators noted that use of planchas was related to other indicators of higher SES, such as radio ownership, spousal employment in business and trade, and cement or tile floors (as opposed to dirt floors). The authors commented on the potential for strong confounding in studies that use fuel type as an exposure measure.

A population-based study in India evaluated 3,608 nonsmoking women in their homes in villages of Chandigarh in northern India (Behera and Jindal 1991). Cooking with a chulla—which uses dung, crop residues, and agricultural wastes—was associated with a higher prevalence of chronic bronchitis than using a kerosene stove, liquefied petroleum gas, or mixed fuel (2.9% vs 1.3%, 2.5%, and 1.2%, respectively; $p < 0.05$). There was no statistical difference in the prevalence of asthma, but there were very few cases. A major limitation of the study is the lack of control for confounding factors apart from sex and smoking, such as SES.

Investigators in Finland conducted a mail-based survey of Finnish university students to examine the effect of wood-stove heating during childhood (age 0-6 years) on the development of asthma and allergic conditions in young adulthood (age 18-25 years) (Kilpelainen et al. 2001). There was no association between wood-stove exposure during childhood and ever having a self-reported physician diagnosis of asthma (OR 0.99, 95% CI 0.65-1.53) or other atopic conditions when sex, SES, parental atopy, number of older siblings, residential environment at the age of 0-6 years (farm, nonfarm rural, and urban), passive smoking during childhood, furred pets in the home during childhood, and history of day care were controlled for. Study limitations include the cross-sectional survey design and the lack of control for cigarette-smoking.

Additional studies have linked biomass-smoke exposure to impaired pulmonary function with spirometry (Pandey et al. 1985; Peters et al. 1999) and symptom questionnaire (Behera 1997), to increased bronchial hyperresponsiveness with methacholine bronchoprovocation (Jindal et al. 1996), and to increased mortality and morbidity (Smith 2000).

The committee excluded some reports because they contained no specific information about asthma, chronic bronchitis, or COPD (Amoli 1998; Perez-Padilla et al. 2001). Another study was excluded because the statistical analysis could not be clearly interpreted (Golshan et al. 2002): a population-based study in Isfahan, Iran, examined the relation between cooking-fuel use and self-reported respiratory conditions, but the multivariate analysis could not be clearly interpreted, in that both wood and kerosene fuel were included in the same analysis and the referent group was not clearly defined.

Conclusions

Asthma

The series of related studies of Seventh-Day Adventists comprise the only high quality study of asthma incidence related to outdoor air pollution in adults. The studies found that new cases of asthma were associated with combustion-product exposure in air pollutants (Abbey et al. 1993b, 1993c, 1995)The study of Gulf War veterans of Cowan et al. (2002), which used an objective exposure-measurement method, found an association between oil-well fire smoke and asthma in Gulf War veterans, but it could not distinguish between new cases arising after the war and exacerbation of pre-existing conditions. Although the other key Gulf War study based on the Iowa cohort (Lange et al. 2002), which had the advantage of avoiding the potential selection bias of the Cowan et al. study, found no relationship between exposure and asthma, its definition of asthma was inadequate. The study of Mishra (2003) also supports an association between biomass combustion and prevalent asthma. Other studies of biomass-fuel combustion and outdoor air pollution support a relationship between combustion exposure and asthma (Baldi et al. 1999; Garshick et al. 2003; Raaschou-Nielsen et al. 1995) (Table 5.4).

The committee concludes, from its assessment of the epidemiologic literature, that there is limited/suggestive evidence of an association between exposure to combustion products and incident asthma.

TABLE 5.4 Key Studies of Asthma

Reference	Type of Study and Population	Exposure Determination	Health Outcome and How Measured	Results	Adjusted OR (95% CI or p)	Limitations
Abbey et al. 1993b,c	Prospective cohort, n = 3,914, 1977-1987	TSP, ozone, sulfates Exceedance frequencies expressed as average. hours exceeding TSP thresholds of 60, 75, 100, 150, 175, 200 μg/m^3	AOD, asthma, chronic bronchitis incidence via symptom questionnaire	TSP and asthma	TSP > 200 μg/m^3 associated with new cases asthma (RR 1.74, CI 1.11-2.72) with increase in average annual exceedance frequency of 1,000 hr/yr; TSP>150 μg/m^3 associated with new cases of asthma (RR 1.23, $p<0.05$) with increase in average annual exceedance frequency of 1,000 hr/yr	Symptom questionnaire, varying specificity in measures of exposure
Abbey et al. 1993a	Prospective cohort, n = 3,914, 1977-1987	Sulfates (10-yr mean ambient concentrations)	Same as above	10-yr mean ambient concentrations of SO_4 associated only with asthma	Asthma RR 2.87, CI 1.03-7.55 per increment of 7 μg/m^3	Same as above
Cowan et al. 2002	Case-control study, 873 cases of asthma vs 2,464 controls US DOD registry, Army personnel only	Exposure modeling via troop positions and air-monitoring data; cumulative exposure and number of days at high concentrations (defined as ≥65 μg/m^3)	Physician-diagnosed asthma 3-6 years after war	Asthma associated with both estimates of exposure, dose-response	Cumulative exposure: OR 1.24 (CI 1.00-1.55) for intermediate exposure, 1.40 (CI 1.11-1.75) for high exposure No. days at high concentrations: OR 1.22 (CI 0.99-1.51) for 1-5 days, 1.41 (CI 1.12-1.77) for 6-30 days	Self-selected population, pre-exposure asthma status unknown, active-duty military (Army only)
Mishra 2003	Population-based National Family	Self-reported exposure to cooking smoke from biomass	Affirmative response to question "Does	Asthma associated with biomass-fuel	OR 1.59, CI 1.30-1.94 for biomass vs clean fuel	Prevalent cases, limited nature of

Reference	Type of Study and Population	Exposure Determination	Health Outcome and How Measured	Results	Adjusted OR (95% CI or p)	Limitations
	Health Survey (n=38,595), adults 60 years old or older	fuels, cleaner fuels, or mix	anyone [in the household] suffer from asthma?"	use	OR 1.24, CI 1.04-1.49 for mixed fuel vs clean fuel	question

NOTE: AOD=airway obstructive disease; CI=confidence interval; DOD=Department of Defense; OR=odds ratio; RR=relative risk; TSP=total suspended particles.

Chronic Bronchitis

Chronic bronchitis is defined by symptoms of chronic cough and sputum production. A major prospective study of outdoor air pollution with more than a decade of exposure (Abbey et al. 1993b, 1995) and a cross-sectional study of biomass-fuel combustion (Albalak et al. 1999) revealed associations between long-term exposure to combustion products and chronic bronchitis (Table 5.5). Supporting findings were reported by five other studies (Dennis et al. 1996b; Garshick et al. 2003; Osterman et al. 1989a; Perez-Padilla et al. 1996; Raaschou-Nielsen et al. 1995). The study of Gulf War veterans in Iowa of Lange (2002) showed no relationship between exposure to oil-well fires and chronic bronchitis, but the standard epidemiologic definition of chronic bronchitis was not used, so acute and chronic bronchitis could not be distinguished. Although the studies reviewed by the committee indicate a probable relationship between long-term (over 1 year) exposure to combustion products and chronic bronchitis, a key unresolved issue is whether shorter-term exposures (less than 1 year) can cause the condition. The committee found inadequate published data that address the effect of shorter-term combustion-product exposures (less than 1 year) on the risk of developing chronic bronchitis.

A related issue is the exposure-free period after combustion-product exposure. Will chronic bronchitis remit after exposure cessation? If so, how long does it take for symptoms to remit? Only one of the studies in this chapter examined people after an exposure-free period. Osterman et al. (1989a) examined silicon carbide workers with SO_2 and dust exposure 6 months after cessation of exposure. They found strong symptom-SO_2 associations after adjusting for the effects of dust exposure. The study suggests that chronic-bronchitis symptoms can persist for at least 6 months after cessation of combustion-product exposure, but there are no data from this study or others to indicate whether chronic-bronchitis symptoms might abate thereafter. It is instructive to examine the influence of smoking on the natural history of chronic bronchitis. Smoking is the dominant risk factor for chronic bronchitis. It is well known that chronic bronchitis, when defined as mucous hypersecretion, usually remits after smoking cessation (Fletcher 1976; Kanner et al. 1999; Willemse et al. 2004). In the Lung Health Study, most of the people who had COPD (defined by airway obstruction) and chronic cough had resolution of the cough by a year after sustained smoking cessation (Kanner et al. 1999). At 5-year followup, remission of symptoms persisted among the sustained quitters. Similarly, Fletcher (1976) showed that the most people who had chronic bronchitis had resolution of their symptoms after smoking cessation.

TABLE 5.5 Key Studies of Chronic Bronchitis

Reference	Type of Study and Population	Exposure Determination	Health Outcome and How Measured	Results	Adjusted OR (95% CI or p)	Limitations
Abbey et al. 1993b,c	Prospective cohort n=3,310, 1977-1987	TSP, ozone, sulfates Exceedance frequencies were expressed as average. hours exceeding TSP thresholds of 60, 75, 100, 150, 200 μg/m^3	AOD, asthma, chronic bronchitis incidence via symptom questionnaire	TSP and AOD, chronic bronchitis	TSP > 200 μg/m^3 associated with new cases AOD (RR 1.36, CI 1.11-1.66), chronic bronchitis (RR 1.33, CI 1.07-1.65) with increase in average annual exceedance frequency of 1000 hr/yr	Symptom questionnaire, varying specificity in measures of exposure
Abbey et al. 1995	Prospective cohort n=1,631, 1987	$PM_{2.5}$ exposure estimated by regression of site, season-specific regression equations from paired $PM_{2.5}$-visibility observations (1979-1986) and visibility data at nine airports throughout California; long-term averages of each subject's estimated monthly $PM_{2.5}$ mean concentrations and exceedance frequencies cumulated 1966-1977 according to ZIP code by monthly residence	Same as above	Onset of AOD and chronic bronchitis related to $PM_{2.5}$ exposure, onset of asthma not noteworthy for increasing cutoffs of $PM_{2.5}$, increased magnitudes of regression coefficients of AOD significant at all cutoffs, chronic bronchitis significant >20 μg/m^3	Onset of chronic bronchitis RR 1.81 (0.98-3.25) per 45-μg/m^3 increase in mean concentration	Same as above
Albalak 1999	Two villages in Bolivia (n = 241), one with outdoor kitchens, other with indoor kitchens	PM_{10} for kitchen and total daily integrated	Chronic bronchitis via British Medical Research Council questionnaire	Outdoor-kitchen village associated with lower risk of chronic bronchitis than indoor-kitchen village	OR 0.4 (95% CI 0.2-0.8) with adjustment for age and sex and excluding smokers	

NOTE: AOD=airway obstructive disease; CI=confidence interval; DOD=Department of Defense; OR=odds ratio; PM=particulate matter; RR= relative risk; TSP=total suspended particles.

Consequently, even if it could be shown that long-term exposure to combustion products caused chronic bronchitis, it might be expected to remit after exposure cessation without long-term health consequences. The committee found inadequate published data to evaluate the natural history of chronic bronchitis after cessation of exposure to combustion products.

The committee concludes, from its assessment of the epidemiologic literature, that there is inadequate/insufficient evidence of an association between short-term exposure (less than 1 year) to combustion products and chronic bronchitis.

Emphysema

Emphysema is a pathologic process involving air-space enlargement distal to the terminal bronchioles accompanied by destruction of the bronchiolar walls. Its major risk factor is cigarette-smoking. The ACS prospective study found that emphysema mortality was not considerably increased among workers exposed to diesel exhaust after adjustment for the effects of smoking (Boffetta et al. 1988). A study of veterans exposed to oil-well fires did not find a relationship with emphysema (Smith et al. 2002). Other studies that included emphysema in the analysis were methodologically inadequate.

The committee concludes, from its assessment of the epidemiologic literature, that there is inadequate/insufficient evidence of an association between exposure to combustion products and the development of emphysema.

Chronic Obstructive Pulmonary Disease (COPD)

The committee did not identify any high-quality studies that evaluated the effect of exposure to combustion products on the risk of COPD, as defined by objective evidence of irreversible airflow obstruction with spirometry, for example, GOLD criteria (Pauwels et al. 2001). The study of Karakatsani (2003) used a clinical definition of COPD, but the 95% CI for FEV1 percent predicted among COPD cases ranged from 86 to 95%, which did not include values less than 80% of the predicted value. That range indicates that most subjects would not meet the GOLD criteria for airway obstruction, which require an FEV1 of less than 80% of predicted values (Pauwels et al. 2001). Several studies of biomass-smoke exposure used measures of airflow obstruction but had methodologic limitations that precluded clear conclusions about the connection between combustion exposure and COPD (Dennis et al. 1996a, 1996b; Dossing et al. 1994; Perez-Padilla et al. 1996).

The committee concludes, from its assessment of the epidemiologic literature, that there is inadequate/insufficient evidence of an association between exposure to combustion products and the development of COPD as defined by irreversible airflow obstruction.

Although some toxicologic studies do provide mechanistic insight as to how inhaled combustion products might act to bring about symptoms associated with asthma or COPD (for example, reviewed in Barnes 1995; Ichinose et al. 1998; MacNee and Donaldson 2003; Takano et al. 1998), the published toxicologic literature has a number of shortcomings that diminish its usefulness for extrapolation to either the human exposure scenario in general or the Gulf War experience specifically. Most controlled-exposure studies either are of short duration, fail to examine long-term residual effects, or use compromised animal models. In addition, the endpoints selected for examination in those studies cannot be specifically linked to the pathogenesis of any particular respiratory disease.

REFERENCES

Abbey DE, Colome SD, Mills PK, Burchette R, Beeson WL, Tian Y. 1993a. Chronic disease associated with long-term concentrations of nitrogen dioxide. *Journal of Exposure Analysis and Environmental Epidemiology* 3(2):181-202.

Abbey DE, Nishino N, McDonnell WF, Burchette RJ, Knutsen SF, Beeson WL, Yang JX. 1999. Long-term inhalable particles and other air pollutants related to mortality in nonsmokers. *American Journal of Respiratory and Critical Care Medicine* 159(2):373-382.

Abbey DE, Ostro BE, Petersen F, Burchette RJ. 1995. Chronic respiratory symptoms associated with estimated long-term ambient concentrations of fine particulates less than 2.5 microns in aerodynamic diameter (PM2.5) and other air pollutants. *Journal of Exposure Analysis and Environmental Epidemiology* 5(2):137-159.

Abbey DE, Petersen F, Mills PK, Beeson WL. 1993b. Long-term ambient concentrations of total suspended particulates, ozone, and sulfur dioxide and respiratory symptoms in a nonsmoking population. *Archives of Environmental Health* 48(1):33-46.

Abbey DE, Petersen FF, Mills PK, Kittle L. 1993c. Chronic respiratory disease associated with long-term ambient concentrations of sulfates and other air pollutants. *Journal of Exposure Analysis and Environmental Epidemiology* 3(Suppl 1):99-115.

Aditama TY. 2000. Impact of haze from forest fire to respiratory health: Indonesian experience. *Respirology* 5(2):169-174.

Al-Khalaf B. 1998. Pilot study: The onset of asthma among the Kuwaiti population during the burning of oil wells after the Gulf War. *Environment International* 24(1-2):221-225.

Albalak R, Frisancho AR, Keeler GJ. 1999. Domestic biomass fuel combustion and chronic bronchitis in two rural Bolivian villages. *Thorax* 54(11):1004-1008.

Amoli K. 1998. Bronchopulmonary disease in Iranian housewives chronically exposed to indoor smoke. *European Respiratory Journal* 11(3):659-663.

Aronson KJ, Tomlinson GA, Smith L. 1994. Mortality among fire fighters in metropolitan Toronto. *American Journal of Industrial Medicine* 26(1):89-101.

Baldi I, Tessier JF, Kauffmann F, Jacqmin-Gadda H, Nejjari C, Salamon R. 1999. Prevalence of asthma and mean levels of air pollution: Results from the French PAARC survey. *European Respiratory Journal* 14(1):132-138.

Balmes J, Becklake M, Blanc P, Henneberger P, Kreiss K, Mapp C, Milton D, Schwartz D, Toren K, Viegi G. 2003. American Thoracic Society Statement: Occupational contribution to the burden of airway disease. *American Journal of Respiratory and Critical Care Medicine* 167(5):787-797.

Baris D, Garrity TJ, Telles JL, Heineman EF, Olshan A, Zahm SH. 2001. Cohort mortality study of Philadelphia firefighters. *American Journal of Industrial Medicine* 39(5):463-476.

Barnes PJ. 1995. Air pollution and asthma: Molecular mechanisms. *Molecular Medicine Today* 1(3):149-155.

Bates MN, Garrett N, Graham B, Read D. 1997. Air pollution and mortality in the Rotorua geothermal area. *Australian and New Zealand Journal of Public Health* 21(6):581-586.

Bates MN, Garrett N, Graham B, Read D. 1998. Cancer incidence, morbidity and geothermal air pollution in Rotorua, New Zealand. *International Journal of Epidemiology* 27(1):10-14.

Bates MN, Garrett N, Shoemack P. 2002. Investigation of health effects of hydrogen sulfide from a geothermal source. *Archives of Environmental Health* 57(5):405-411.

Beaumont JJ, Chu GS, Jones JR, Schenker MB, Singleton JA, Piantanida LG, Reiterman M. 1991. An epidemiologic study of cancer and other causes of mortality in San Francisco firefighters. *American Journal of Industrial Medicine* 19(3):357-372.

Behera D, Jindal SK. 1991. Respiratory symptoms in Indian women using domestic cooking fuels. *Chest* 100(2):385-388.

Behera D. 1997. An analysis of effect of common domestic fuels on respiratory function. *Indian Journal of Chest Diseases & Allied Sciences* 39(4):235-243.

Betchley C, Koenig JQ, van Belle G, Checkoway H, Reinhardt T. 1997. Pulmonary function and respiratory symptoms in forest firefighters. *American Journal of Industrial Medicine* 31(5):503-509.

Bjornsson E, Plaschke P, Norrman E, Janson C, Lundback B, Rosenhall A, Lindholm N, Rosenhall L, Berglund E, Boman G. 1994. Symptoms related to asthma and chronic bronchitis in three areas of Sweden. *European Respiratory Journal* 7(12):2146-2153.

Boffetta P, Stellman SD, Garfinkel L. 1988. Diesel exhaust exposure and mortality among males in the American Cancer Society prospective study. *American Journal of Industrial Medicine* 14(4):403-415.

Borgia P, Forastiere F, Rapiti E, Rizzelli R, Magliola ME, Perucci CA, Axelson O. 1994 . Mortality among taxi drivers in Rome: A cohort study. *American Journal of Industrial Medicine* 25(4):507-517.

Bruce N, Neufeld L, Boy E, West C. 1998. Indoor biofuel air pollution and respiratory health: The role of confounding factors among women in highland Guatemala. *International Journal of Epidemiology* 27(3):454-458.

Burgess JL, Brodkin CA, Daniell WE, Pappas GP, Keifer MC, Stover BD, Edland SD, Barnhart S. 1999. Longitudinal decline in measured firefighter single-breath diffusing capacity of carbon monoxide values. A respiratory surveillance dilemma. *American Journal of Respiratory and Critical Care Medicine* 159(1):119-124.

Burnett CA, Halperin WE, Lalich NR, Sestito JP. 1994. Mortality among fire fighters: A 27 state survey. *American Journal of Industrial Medicine* 26(6):831-833.

Christie D, Robinson K, Gordon I, Webley C, Bisby J. 1987. Current mortality in the Australian petroleum industry: The healthy-worker effect and the influence of life-style factors. *Medical Journal of Australia* 147(5):222, 224-225.

Coombe MD, Drysdale SF. 1993. Assessment of the effects of atmospheric oil pollution in post war Kuwait. *Journal of the Royal Army Medical Corps* 139(3):95-97.

Cowan DN, Lange JL, Heller J, Kirkpatrick J, DeBakey S. 2002. A case-control study of asthma among U.S. Army Gulf War veterans and modeled exposure to oil well fire smoke. *Military Medicine* 167(9):777-782.

Dagg TG, Satin KP, Bailey WJ, Wong O, Harmon LL, Swencicki RE. 1992. An updated cause specific mortality study of petroleum refinery workers. *British Journal of Industrial Medicine* 49(3):203-212.

De Marco R, Poli A, Ferrari M, Accordini S, Giammanco G, Bugiani M, Villani S, Ponzio M, Bono R, Carrozzi L, Cavallini R, Cazzoletti L, Dallari R, Ginesu F, Lauriola P, Mandrioli P, Perfetti L, Pignato S, Pirina P, Struzzo P. 2002. The impact of climate and traffic-related NO2 on the prevalence of asthma and allergic rhinitis in Italy. *Clinical and Experimental Allergy* 32(10):1405-1412.

Dennis RJ, Maldonado D, Norman S, Baena E, Castano H, Martinez G, Velez JR. 1996a. Wood smoke exposure and risk for obstructive airways disease among women. *Chest* 109(3 Suppl):55S-56S.

Dennis RJ, Maldonado D, Norman S, Baena E, Castano H, Martinez G, Velez JR. 1996b. Wood smoke exposure and risk for obstructive airways disease among women. *Chest* 109(1):115-119.

Derrick EH. 1970. A comparison between the density of smoke in the Brisbane air and the prevalence of asthma. *Medical Journal of Australia* 2(15):670-675.

Dockery DW, Pope CA 3rd, Xu X, Spengler JD, Ware JH, Fay ME, Ferris BG Jr, Speizer FE. 1993. An association between air pollution and mortality in six U.S. cities. *New England Journal of Medicine* 329(24):1753-1759.

Dossing M, Khan J, al-Rabiah F. 1994. Risk factors for chronic obstructive lung disease in Saudi Arabia. *Respiratory Medicine* 88(7):519-522.

Dow L, Phelps L, Fowler L, Waters K, Coggon D, Holgate ST. 1999. Respiratory symptoms in older people and use of domestic gas appliances. *Thorax* 54(12):1104-1106.

Draxler R, McQueen J, Stunder B. 1994. An evaluation of air pollutants exposures due to the 1991 Kuwait oil fires using a Langrangian Model. *Atmospheric Environment* 28:2197-2210.

Dunn CE, Woodhouse J, Bhopal RS, Acquilla SD. 1995. Asthma and factory emissions in northern England: Addressing public concern by combining geographical and epidemiological methods. *Journal of Epidemiology and Community Health* 49(4):395-400.

Eisner MD, Yelin EH, Katz PP, Earnest G, Blanc PD. 2002. Exposure to indoor combustion and adult asthma outcomes: Environmental tobacco smoke, gas stoves, and woodsmoke. *Thorax* 57(11):973-978.

Feuer E, Rosenman K. 1986. Mortality in police and firefighters in New Jersey. *American Journal of Industrial Medicine* 9(6):517-527.

Fleming DM, Charlton JR. 2001. The prevalence of asthma and heart disease in transport workers: A practice-based study. *British Journal of General Practice* 51(469):638-643.

Fletcher CM. 1976. *The Natural History of Chronic Bronchitis and Emphysema: An Eight-year Study of Early Chronic Obstructive Lung Disease in Working Men in London.* Oxford: Oxford University Press.

Flodin U, Ziegler J, Jonsson P, Axelson O. 1996. Bronchial asthma and air pollution at workplaces. *Scandinavian Journal of Work, Environment & Health* 22(6):451-456.

Gamble JF, Jones WG. 1983. Respiratory effects of diesel exhaust in salt miners. *American Review of Respiratory Disease* 128(3):389-394.

Garshick E, Laden F, Hart JE, Caron A. 2003. Residence near a major road and respiratory symptoms in U.S. Veterans. *Epidemiology* 14(6):728-736.

Goldstein IF, Weinstein AL. 1986. Air pollution and asthma: Effects of exposures to short-term sulfur dioxide peaks. *Environmental Research* 40(2):332-345.

Golshan M, Faghihi M, Marandi MM. 2002. Indoor women jobs and pulmonary risks in rural areas of Isfahan, Iran, 2000. *Respiratory Medicine* 96(6):382-388.

Gray GC, Smith TC, Kang HK, Knoke JD. 2000. Are Gulf War veterans suffering war-related illnesses? Federal and civilian hospitalizations examined, June 1991 to December 1994. *American Journal of Epidemiology* 151(1):63-71.

Hanis NM, Shallenberger LG, Donaleski DL, Sales EA. 1985. A retrospective mortality study of workers in three major U.S. refineries and chemical plants. Part 1: Comparisons with U.S. population. *Journal of Occupational Medicine* 27(4):283-292.

Hastings DL, Jardine S. 2002. The relationship between air particulate levels and upper respiratory disease in soldiers deployed to Bosnia (1997-1998). *Military Medicine* 167(4):296-303.

Hoek G, Brunekreef B, Goldbohm S, Fischer P, Van den Brandt PA. 2002. Association between mortality and indicators of traffic-related air pollution in the Netherlands: A cohort study. *Lancet* 360(9341):1203-1209.

Hong CY, Ng TP, Wong ML, Koh KTC, Goh LG, Ling SL. 1994. Lifestyle and behavioural risk factors associated with asthma morbidity in adults. *Quarterly Journal of Medicine* 87(10):639-645.

Hunt TB, Holman CD. 1987. Asthma hospitalisation in relation to sulphur dioxide atmospheric contamination in the Kwinana industrial area of Western Australia. *Community Health Studies* 11(3):197-201.

Ichinose T, Takano H, Miyabara Y, Sagai M. 1998. Long-term exposure to diesel exhaust enhances antigen-induced eosinophilic inflammation and epithelial damage in the murine airway. *Toxicological Sciences* 44(1):70-79.

Jarvis D, Chinn S, Luczynska C, Burney P. 1996. Association of respiratory symptoms and lung function in young adults with use of domestic gas appliances. *Lancet* 347(8999):426-431.

Jarvis D, Chinn S, Sterne J, Luczynska C, Burney P. 1998. The association of respiratory symptoms and lung function with the use of gas for cooking. European Community Respiratory Health Survey. *European Respiratory Journal* 11(3):651-658.

Jindal SK, Gupta D, D'Souza GA, Kalra S. 1996. Bronchial responsiveness of non-smoking women exposed to environmental tobacco smoke or biomass fuel combustion. *Indian Journal of Medical Research* 104:359-364.

Kanner RE, Connett JE, Williams DE, Buist AS. 1999. Effects of randomized assignment to a smoking cessation intervention and changes in smoking habits on respiratory symptoms in smokers with early chronic obstructive pulmonary disease: The Lung Health Study. *The American Journal of Medicine* 106(4):410-416.

Kaplan SD. 1986. Update of a mortality study of workers in petroleum refineries. *Journal of Occupational Medicine* 28(7):514-516.

Karakatsani A, Andreadaki S, Katsouyanni K, Dimitroulis I, Trichopoulos D, Benetou V, Trichopoulou A. 2003. Air pollution in relation to manifestations of chronic pulmonary disease: A nested case-control study in Athens, Greece. *European Journal of Epidemiology* 18(1):45-53.

Kilpelainen M, Koskenvuo M, Helenius H, Terho E. 2001. Wood stove heating, asthma and allergies. *Respiratory Medicine* 95(11):911-916.

Kogevinas M, Anto JM, Sunyer J, Tobias A, Kromhout H, Burney P, Chinn S, Luczynska C, Jarvis D, Lai E, Abramson M, Kutin J, Vermeire P, Van Bastelaer F, Magnussen H, Nowak D, Wichmann HE, Heinrich J, Wjst M, Gialson T, Gislason D, Prichard J, Allwright S, MacLeod D, Bugiani M, Bucca C, Romano C, De Marco lo Cascio R, Campello C, Marinoni A, Cerveri I, Casali L, Crane J, D'Souza W, Pearce N, Barry D, Town I, Gulsvik A, Omenaas E, Bakke P, Soriano J, Roca J, Muniozguren N, Gonzalez JR, Capelastegui A, Martinez-Moratalla J, Almar E, Perez JM, Oereira A, Sanchez J, Quiros J , Huerta I, Boman G, Janson C, Bjornsson E, Rosenhall L, Norrman E, Lundback B, Lindholm N, Plaschke P, Burr M, Layzqll J, Hall R, Harrison B, Stark J, Buist S, Vollmer W, Osborne M. 1999. Occupational asthma in Europe and other industrialised areas: A population-based study. *Lancet* 353(9166):1750-1754.

Kunii O, Kanagawa S, Yajima I, Hisamatsu Y, Yamamura S, Amagai T, Ismail IT. 2002. The 1997 haze disaster in Indonesia: its air quality and health effects. *Archives of Environmental Health* 57(1):16-22.

Lange JL, Schwartz DA, Doebbeling BN, Heller JM, Thorne PS. 2002. Exposures to the Kuwait oil fires and their association with asthma and bronchitis among gulf war veterans. *Environmental Health Perspectives* 110(11):1141-1146.

Liu D, Tager IB, Balmes JR, Harrison RJ. 1992. The effect of smoke inhalation on lung function and airway responsiveness in wildland fire fighters. *American Review of Respiratory Disease* 146(6):1469-1473.

MacNee W, Donaldson K. 2003. Mechanism of lung injury caused by PM10 and ultrafine particles with special reference to COPD. *European Respiratory Journal - Supplement* 40:47s-51s.

Maizlish N, Beaumont J, Singleton J. 1988. Mortality among California highway workers. *American Journal of Industrial Medicine* 13(3):363-379.

Makker HK, Ayres JG. 1999. Work-related asthma in an aircraft engine mechanic. *Respiratory Medicine* 93(1):69-70.

McQueen J, Draxler R. 1994. Evaluation of model back trajectories of the Kuwait oil fires smoke plume using digital satellite data. *Atmospheric Environment* 28:2159-2174.

Meyer JD, Holt DL, Chen Y, Cherry NM, McDonald JC. 2001. SWORD '99: Surveillance of work-related and occupational respiratory disease in the UK. *Occupational Medicine* 51(3):204-208.

Mishra V. 2003. Effect of indoor air pollution from biomass combustion on prevalence of asthma in the elderly. *Environmental Health Perspectives* 111(1):71-78.

Musk A, Smith T, Peters J, McLaughlin E. 1979. Pulmonary function in firefighters: Acute changes in ventilatory capacity and their correlates. *British Journal of Industrial Medicine* 36(1):29-34.

Musk AW, Peters JM, Bernstein L, Rubin C, Monroe CB. 1982. Pulmonary function in firefighters: A six-year follow-up in the Boston Fire Department. *American Journal of Industrial Medicine* 3(1):3-9.

Ng TP, Hui KP, Tan WC. 1993. Respiratory symptoms and lung function effects of domestic exposure to tobacco smoke and cooking by gas in non-smoking women in Singapore. *Journal of Epidemiology and Community Health* 47(6):454-458.

Osterman JW, Greaves IA, Smith TJ, Hammond SK, Robins JM, Theriault G. 1989a. Respiratory symptoms associated with low level sulphur dioxide exposure in silicon carbide production workers. *British Journal of Industrial Medicine* 46(9):629-635.

Osterman JW, Greaves IA, Smith TJ, Hammond SK, Robins JM, Theriault G. 1989b. Work related decrement in pulmonary function in silicon carbide production workers. *British Journal of Industrial Medicine* 46(10):708-716.

Ostro BD, Lipsett MJ, Mann JK, Krupnick A, Harrington W. 1993. Air pollution and respiratory morbidity among adults in southern California. *American Journal of Epidemiology* 137(7):691-700.

Pandey MR. 1984. Domestic smoke pollution and chronic bronchitis in a rural community of the Hill Region of Nepal. *Thorax* 39(5):337-339.

Pandey MR, Regmi HN, Neupane RP, Gautam A, Bhandari DP. 1985. Domestic smoke pollution and respiratory function in rural Nepal. *Tokai Journal of Experimental and Clinical Medicine* 10(4):471-481.

Papageorgiou N, Gaga M, Marossis C, Reppas Chr, Avarlis P, Kyriakou M, Tsipra S, Zeibecoglou K, Tracopoulos G. 1997. Prevalence of asthma and asthma-like symptoms in Athens, Greece. *Respiratory Medicine* 91(2):83-88.

Pauwels RA, Buist AS, Calverley PM, Jenkins CR, Hurd SS. 2001. Global strategy for the diagnosis, management, and prevention of chronic obstructive pulmonary disease. NHLBI/WHO Global Initiative for Chronic Obstructive Lung Disease (GOLD) Workshop summary. *American Journal of Respiratory and Critical Care Medicine* 163(5):1256-1276.

Perez-Padilla R, Regalado J, Vedal S, Pare P, Chapela R, Sansores R, Selman M. 1996. Exposure to biomass smoke and chronic airway disease in Mexican women. A case-control study. *American Journal of Respiratory and Critical Care Medicine* 154(3 Pt 1):701-706.

Perez-Padilla R, Perez-Guzman C, Baez-Saldana R, Torres-Cruz A. 2001. Cooking with biomass stoves and tuberculosis: A case control study. *International Journal of Tuberculosis and Lung Disease* 5(5):441-447.

Peters EJ, Esin RA, Immananagha KK, Siziya S, Osim EE. 1999. Lung function status of some Nigerian men and women chronically exposed to fish drying using burning firewood. *Central African Journal of Medicine* 45(5):119-124.

Petruccelli BP, Goldenbaum M, Scott B, Lachiver R, Kanjarpane D, Elliott E, Francis M, McDiarmid MA, Deeter D. 1999. Health effects of the 1991 Kuwait oil fires: A survey of US army troops. *Journal of Occupational and Environmental Medicine* 41(6):433-439.

Pope CA 3rd, Burnett RT, Thun MJ, Calle EE, Krewski D, Ito K, Thurston GD. 2002. Lung cancer, cardiopulmonary mortality, and long-term exposure to fine particulate air pollution. *Journal of the American Medical Association* 287(9):1132-1141.

Pope CA 3rd, Burnett RT, Thurston GD, Thun MJ, Calle EE, Krewski D, Godleski JJ. 2004. Cardiovascular mortality and long-term exposure to particulate air pollution: Epidemiological evidence of general pathophysiological pathways of disease. *Circulation* 109(1):71-77.

Pope CA 3rd, Thun MJ, Namboodiri MM, Dockery DW, Evans JS, Speizer FE, Heath CW Jr. 1995. Particulate air pollution as a predictor of mortality in a prospective study of U.S. adults. *American Journal of Respiratory and Critical Care Medicine* 151(3 Pt 1):669-674.

Proctor SP, Heeren T, White RF, Wolfe J, Borgos MS, Davis JD, Pepper L, Clapp R, Sutker PB, Vasterling JJ, Ozonoff D. 1998 . Health status of Persian Gulf War veterans: Self-reported symptoms, environmental exposures and the effect of stress. *International Journal of Epidemiology* 27(6):1000-1010.

Qureshi KA. 1994. Domestic smoke pollution and prevalence of chronic bronchitis/asthma in a rural area of Kashmir. *Indian Journal of Chest Diseases & Allied Sciences* 36(2):61-72.

Raaschou-Nielsen O, Nielsen ML, Gehl J. 1995. Traffic-related air pollution: Exposure and health effects in Copenhagen street cleaners and cemetery workers. *Archives of Environmental Health* 50(3):207-213.

Rafnsson V, Gunaarsdottir H. 1991. Mortality among professional drivers. *Scandinavian Journal of Work, Environment & Health* 17(5):312-317.

Reger R, Hancock J, Hankinson J, Hearl F, Merchant J. 1982. Coal miners exposed to diesel exhaust emissions. *Annals of Occupational Hygiene* 26(1-4):799-815.

Reijula K, Haahtela T, Klaukka T, Rantanen J . 1996. Incidence of occupational asthma and persistent asthma in young adults has increased in Finland. *Chest* 110(1):58-61.

Rodriguez de la Vega A, Rojas BO, Batule BM, Sparis GP. 1981. Environmental factors related to bronchial asthma evolution with special reference to kerosene. *Revista Cubana de Medicina* 20(6):605-613.

Rodriguez de la Vega A, Casaco A, Garcia M, Noa M, Carvajal D, Arruzazabala L, Gonzales R. 1990. Kerosene-induced asthma. *Annals of Allergy* 64(4):362-363.

Rushton L, Alderson MR. 1981. An epidemiological survey of eight oil refineries in Britain. *British Journal of Industrial Medicine* 38(3):225-234.

Samet JM, Marbury MC, Spengler JD. 1987. Health effects and sources of indoor air pollution. Part I. *The American Review of Respiratory Disease* 136(6):1486-1508.

Sastry N. 2002. Forest fires, air pollution, and mortality in southeast Asia. *Demography* 39(1):1-23.

Skyberg K, Ronneberg A, Kamoy JI, Dale K, Borgersen A. 1986. Pulmonary fibrosis in cable plant workers exposed to mist and vapor of petroleum distillates. *Environmental Research* 40(2):261-273.

Skyberg K, Ronneberg A, Christensen CC, Naess-Andresen CF, Borgersen A, Refsum HE. 1992. Lung function and radiographic signs of pulmonary fibrosis in oil exposed workers in a cable manufacturing company: A follow up study. *British Journal of Industrial Medicine* 49(5):309-315.

Smith KR. 2000. Inaugural article: national burden of disease in India from indoor air pollution. *Proceedings of the National Academy of Sciences of the United States of America* 97(24):13286-13293.

Smith TC, Heller JM, Hooper TI, Gackstetter GD, Gray GC. 2002. Are Gulf War veterans experiencing illness due to exposure to smoke from Kuwaiti oil well fires? Examination of Department of Defense hospitalization data. *American Journal of Epidemiology* 155(10):908-917.

Smithurst BA, Williams GM. 1976. A study of chronic bronchitis in Brisbane in two groups of workers: The effects of cigarette smoking, pollution and industrial exposure on the disease. *Public Health* 90(4):149-156.

Takano H, Ichinose T, Miyabara Y, Shibuya T, Lim HB, Yoshikawa T, Sagai M. 1998. Inhalation of diesel exhaust enhances allergen-related eosinophil recruitment and airway hyperresponsiveness in mice. *Toxicology and Applied Pharmacology* 150(2):328-337.

Todd GR, Buick B. 2000. Asthma due to kerosene exposure: Three case reports. *International Journal of Occupational Medicine and Environmental Health* 13(1):23-25.

Toren K, Balder B, Brisman J, Lindholm N, Lowhagen O, Palmqvist M, Tunsater A. 1999. The risk of asthma in relation to occupational exposures: A case-control study from a Swedish city. *European Respiratory Journal* 13(3):496-501.

Tsai SP, Dowd CM, Cowles SR, Ross CE. 1992. A prospective study of morbidity patterns in a petroleum refinery and chemical plant. *British Journal of Industrial Medicine* 49(7):516-522.

Tsunetoshi Y, Shimizu T, Takahashi H, Ichinosawa A, Ueda M. 1971. Epidemiological study of chronic bronchitis with special reference to effect of air pollution. *Internationales Archiv fur Arbeitsmedizin* 29(1):1-27.

Ulfvarson U, Alexandersson R, Aringer L, Svensson E, Hedenstierna G, Hogstedt C, Holmberg B, Rosen G, Sorsa M. 1987. Effects of exposure to vehicle exhaust on health. *Scandinavian Journal of Work, Environment & Health* 13(6):505-512.

Viegi G, Paoletti P, Carrozzi L, Vellutini M, Ballerin L, Biavati P, Nardini G, Di Pede F, Sapigni T, Lebowitz MD, Giuntini C. 1991. Effects of home environment on respiratory symptoms and lung function in a general population sample in north Italy. *The European Respiratory Journal* 4(5):580-586.

Viegi G, Carrozzi L, Paoletti P, Vellutini M, DiViggiano E, Baldacci S, Modena P, Pedreschi M, Mammini U, Di Pede C. 1992. Effects of the home environment on respiratory symptoms of a general population sample in middle Italy. *Archives of Environmental Health* 47(1):64-70.

Willemse BW, Postma DS, Timens W, ten Hacken NH. 2004. The impact of smoking cessation on respiratory symptoms, lung function, airway hyperresponsiveness and inflammation. *The European Respiratory Journal* 23(3):464-476.

Wong O, Harris F, Rosamilia K, Raabe GK. 2001a. An updated mortality study of workers at a petroleum refinery in Beaumont, Texas, 1945 to 1996. *Journal of Occupational and Environmental Medicine* 43(4):384-401.

Wong O, Harris F, Rosamilia K, Raabe GK. 2001b. Updated mortality study of workers at a petroleum refinery in Torrance, California, 1959 to 1997. *Journal of Occupational and Environmental Medicine* 43(12):1089-1102.

Woods RK, Burton DL, Wharton C, McKenzie GH, Walters EH, Comino EJ, Abramson MJ. 2000. Asthma is more prevalent in rural New South Wales than metropolitan Victoria, Australia. *Respirology* 5(3):257-263.

Xu X, Christiani DC. 1993. Occupational exposures and physician-diagnosed asthma. *Chest* 104(5):1364-1370.

Zelikoff JT, Chen LC, Cohen MD, Schlesinger RB. 2002. The toxicology of inhaled woodsmoke. *Journal of Toxicology and Environmental Health. Part B, Critical Reviews* 5(3):269-282.

Zhang J, Qian Z, Kong L, Zhou L, Yan L, Chapman RS. 1999. Effects of air pollution on respiratory health of adults in three Chinese cities. *Archives of Environmental Health* 54(6):373-381.

Zock JP, Sunyer J, Kogevinas M, Kromhout H, Burney P, Anto JM. 2001. Occupation, chronic bronchitis, and lung function in young adults. An international study. *American Journal of Respiratory and Critical Care Medicine* 163(7):1572-1577.

6

CARDIOVASCULAR DISEASE

Cardiovascular diseases are the leading cause of death in the United States. Morbidity (other than hypertension) and death from cardiovascular disease occur after the age of 50. Death is due to coronary heart disease or cerebrovascular disease. Factors that contribute to increased risk of those diseases can be assumed to contribute either to chronic risk or to acute triggering of an event. Although dividing putative risk factors between chronic and acute effects is somewhat artificial, it is useful for the present review. If exposures that occurred in the Gulf War play a role in the onset of cardiovascular disorders, it is necessary to postulate that the exposures contribute to chronic processes, such as atherosclerosis. Those chronic processes are complex and multifactorial, eventually occur to some extent in nearly all adults, and are believed to begin in adolescence. There are many established risk factors for cardiovascular diseases, including smoking, male sex, diabetes, hypertension, family history, and blood lipid concentrations. Determining that a relatively brief exposure to combustion products in the Persian Gulf is associated with occurrence or acceleration of atherosclerotic cardiovascular disease—and results in increased incidence of disease years later—is a substantial challenge. Determining that such an effect occurs after an exposure-free period is even more difficult.

The vascular biology of ischemic heart disease and the effect of combustion products on the cardiovascular system are rapidly evolving subjects of scientific inquiry. Much additional information that will inform the toxicologic and epidemiologic database can be expected in the next 2-10 years.

As previously noted, the committee's inclusion criteria require specificity of outcome, methodologic rigor, and some exposure information. Studies that meet the committee's inclusion criteria are referred to as primary studies; ecologic and toxicologic studies, studies of self-reported exposure or multiple exposures, and studies of intermediate[1] outcomes or with lack of specificity about outcomes, such as a broad range of International Classification of Diseases (ICD) codes, are considered support studies. For relevance to Gulf War veterans, the committee focused on long-term cardiovascular effects that persist after exposure ceases (see Chapter 2).

[1] Intermediate outcomes are indexes of altered functioning consistent with later development of a diagnosis (for example, reduced lung volume and increased cytokine concentrations) but without predictive validity.

FUELS AND CARDIOVASCULAR DISEASE

Several studies (Huang 1986; Pollini et al. 1986, 1989; Van Peenen et al. 1985) have been conducted in the petroleum industry to identify and assess potential cardiovascular risk factors. However, the studies did not look specifically at whether exposure to petroleum products or fuels was associated with an increased risk of cardiovascular disease. Instead, they attempted to identify behavioral risk factors and potential screening tools that could form the basis of behavior-modification programs and health risk assessments among petroleum industry-workers.

In contrast, cohort mortality studies of petroleum-refinery workers (such as Christie et al. 1987; Dagg et al. 1992; Hanis et al. 1985; Kaplan 1986; Rushton and Alderson 1981; Tsai et al. 1992; Wong et al. 2001a, 2001b) have examined mortality due to cardiovascular and cerebrovascular diseases. The researches typically used job titles to assess exposure and this can lead to misclassification of exposures. The studies found no increased risk of cardiovascular or cerebrovascular diseases among petroleum-industry workers compared with the general population. In fact, in many studies, mortality was lower than expected. For example, in Wong et al. (2001b), ischemic heart disease had a standard mortality ratio (SMR) of 0.88, 95% confidence interval (CI) 0.77-0.99; chronic endocardial disease and other myocardial insufficiencies had an SMR of 0.08, 95% CI 0.00-0.46; and all other heart disease had an SMR of 0.64, 95% CI 0.43-0.92. As discussed previously, the "healthy-worker effect" probably contributed to those findings.

The committee is unable to draw a conclusion of association given the lack of studies that specifically examined the relationship between exposure to fuels and cardiovascular diseases and the large confounding role of hypertension, high blood pressure, smoking, diet and exercise—which are not often controlled for in cohort mortality studies—in the etiology of those diseases.

COMBUSTION PRODUCTS AND CARDIOVASCULAR DISEASE

The literature on combustion product exposure and cardiovascular disease is large and complex and the there have been recent publications that provide background for this burgeoning area of research (for example, Brook et al. 2004). However, a substantial portion of the literature concerns occupational cohorts in specific occupations (for example, vehicle drivers and tunnel workers) whose exposure is of uncertain relevance to the exposures in the Persian Gulf; such studies are nonetheless considered in this review. Another, larger group of studies, regarding acute exposure to particulate air pollution and cardiovascular events (morbidity and mortality), were not considered relevant to this review; these studies, typically time-series or case-crossover analyses, provide information on events that occurred within days of exposure and so are not relevant to Gulf War exposure and onset of cardiovascular effects long after return from the Gulf War. One useful background reference would be the recently published statement on air pollution and cardiovascular diseases from the American Heart Association.

A common difficulty in assessing the literature for this review is the lack of specificity of diagnoses reported in published articles. For example many articles treat “cardiopulmonary mortality” as one outcome. That provides some information on effects, but it is difficult to translate such a highly heterogeneous outcome into specific diagnoses to support conclusions on specific health outcomes.

This section covers the effect of exposure to combustion products on long-term cardiovascular outcomes, including ischemic heart disease, myocardial infarction, and cerebrovascular disease. It is divided into studies of Gulf War veterans, air-pollution studies, and occupational studies. Each subsection begins with primary studies that had strong methods and exposure information, and then takes up support studies that are not as methodologically robust. If the support studies' findings are consistent with those of the primary studies, they add weight to the primary evidence.

Gulf War Veteran Studies

In February 1991, retreating Iraqi forces set fire to more than 600 oil wells. Fires burned over a 10-month period, until November 1991, exposing thousands of US troops to combustion products. The two studies summarized below (Smith et al. 2002; Proctor et al, 1998) were the only well-designed Gulf War studies that examined cardiovascular effects expressly in relation to combustion-product exposure. The study of Smith et al (2002), the stronger of the two studies by virtue of its objectively documented exposures did not find a relationship; that finding is consistent with several studies of Gulf War veterans that are not reported here because they did not examine specific exposures in relation to symptoms. Another study (Kang et al. 2000), a large and representative, population-based study of 15,000 Gulf War veterans, did not find greater self-reporting of coronary heart disease among Gulf War veterans than among controls Similarly, mortality studies of Gulf War veterans have not found excess cardiovascular disease deaths.

Smith et al. (2002) examined hospitalization patterns of all active-duty personnel who were deployed to the Gulf War in 1991-1999 (n = 405,142) and who were in the Persian Gulf during the oil-well fires. For each active-duty veteran (hospitalized and nonhospitalized alike), the study assigned an oil-smoke exposure by using National Oceanic and Atmospheric Administration modeling (Draxler et al. 1994; McQueen and Draxler 1994). Six exposure categories were created on the basis of average daily exposure and duration of exposure. The largest category of exposure to particulate matter (137,000 personnel) was 1-260 $\mu g/m^3$ for 1-25 days; this was similar in dose but of much shorter duration than the exposure of those in the American Cancer Society (ACS) cohort (see below and Chapter 5). The study examined hospitalizations in relation to exposure. Hospitalizations were for any cause, for major diagnoses in International Classification of Diseases, 9th Edition-Clinical Modification, and for nine specific diagnoses potentially related to oil-well fires.[2] A subject who had been hospitalized with one of the specific diagnoses before the war was excluded from further analysis. The study examined only hospitalizations in Department of Defence (DOD) hospitals because of the availability of data. It found decreased risk of ischemic heart disease among exposed than among nonexposed veterans (relative risk [RR] 0.82, 95% CI 0.68-0.99). One limitation of the study is that hospitalizations were captured only for DOD hospitals, which care for active-duty personnel or veterans with medical benefits. The authors pointed out, however that rates of service attrition were comparable across all exposure categories, including absence of exposure to smoke from oil-well fires.

Proctor et al. (1998) examined self-reported exposures in relation to the symptom experience of two cohorts of Gulf War veterans from Massachusetts (Ft. Devens) and New

---

[2]Asthma; ischemic heart disease; emphysema, acute bronchitis, chronic bronchitis, bronchitis not specified as acute or chronic; malignant neoplasms of the respiratory and intrathoracic organs; malignant neoplasms of the oral pharynx, nasopharynx, and hypopharynx; and pneumoconiosis due to silica or silicates, pneumoconiosis due to inorganic dust, and unspecified pneumoconiosis; pneumopathy due to inhalation of the other dust; respiratory conditions due to chemical fumes and vapors; and other diseases of the respiratory system.

Orleans. The study's nearly 300 subjects made up a stratified random sample of 2,949 troops from Ft. Devens and 928 troops from New Orleans, both including active-duty, reserve, and National Guard troops. The response rate was 58-85% of those participating in an earlier study who could be contacted and located. The control group (n = 50) was Gulf-era veterans deployed to Germany. Subjects were given symptom checklists (covering the previous 30 days), exposure questionnaires, and a neuropsychologic test battery; were interviewed about combat exposure; and underwent diagnostic interviews for posttraumatic stress disorder (PTSD). Each of the 52 symptoms on the symptom checklist was assigned by four independent judges to one of nine body systems, including one for "cardiac symptoms", defined as irregular heartbeats (or "heart flutters"), chest pain, or racing heart. The exposure questionnaire, given only to Gulf War-deployed subjects, contained eight items, four of which were related to combustion products: "smoke from burning oil wells", "vehicle exhaust", "smoke from tent heaters", "smoke from burning human waste". In the Gulf War-deployed cohort, multiple regression adjusting for age, sex, education, and PTSD diagnosis was used to determine symptom-exposure relationships. Self-reported exposure to smoke from oil-well fires had no noteworthy associations, however, vehicle exhaust ($p = 0.026$), smoke from burning human waste ($p = 0.001$), and smoke from tent heaters ($p < 0.001$) were associated with cardiac symptoms. But in a second set of multiple regression-analyses with exposures entered as independent variables, vehicle exhaust and smoke from burning human waste were no longer associated with those symptoms. The findings reported above were essentially unchanged when subjects who met criteria for PTSD were removed from analyses. The study limitations were self-reported symptoms and exposures, moderate to low response rate, and lack of representativeness of the entire Gulf War cohort.

Air-Pollution Studies

Respiratory mortality findings have been reported from several large, longitudinal cohorts with long-term exposures, usually more than 5 years—ACS (Pope et al. 1995), Six-Cities (Dockery et al. 1993), Netherlands Cohort Study on Diet and Cancer (Hoek et al. 2002), and Seventh-Day Adventists (SDAs) (Abbey et al. 1999). All but the SDA study relied on a broad mortality category—cardiopulmonary. Two further analyses, however, provided greater specificity regarding mortality in the ACS and Six-Cities cohorts.

For the ACS cohort, Pope et al. (2004) undertook a more diagnosis-specific analysis with the same methods as their previous report (Pope et al. 2002). The analysis expanded on earlier findings, including 7-16 years of followup of people enrolled in 1982. Exposures to particulate matter were assigned to each participant on the basis of his or her ZIP code at the time of enrollment. For cardiovascular-disease mortality as a composite category, the study found increased RR of 1.12 (95% CI 1.08-1.15) per increase of 10 $\mu g/m^3$ in $PM_{2.5}$.[3] Within that category, deaths from ischemic heart disease (ICD-9 codes 410-414) were increased (RR 1.18, 95% CI 1.14-1.23) even after adjustment for smoking. Deaths from dysrhythmias, heart failure, and cardiac arrest (ICD-9 codes 420-429) were also increased (RR 1.13, 95% CI 1.05-1.21).

A reanalysis of the Six-Cities cohort by Krewski et al. (2003) found that cardiovascular mortality—instead of the less-specific "cardiopulmonary" mortality—was increased (RR 1.41, 95% CI 1.13-1.76 per increase of 18.6 $\mu g/m^3$ in $PM_{2.5}$). The vast majority of cardiovascular mortality was from ischemic heart disease. Nevertheless, although the Six-Cities and ACS findings have been robust to intense scrutiny and reanalysis, the exposure-assessment scheme is

[3] $PM_{2.5}$ is a notation for particulate matter less 2.5 μg in diameter.

still far from definitive. The Netherlands Cohort Study on Diet and Cancer (Hoek et al. 2002), focusing on motor-vehicle exhaust as a source of air pollution, reported on one composite category covering over 50 ICD codes—cardiopulmonary mortality (most of which was from ischemic heart disease). The study had an improved assessment of exposure compared with the prior cohort studies. It found that living for up to 8 years near a major road had an RR of 1.95 (95% CI 1.09-3.51) for cardiopulmonary mortality (codes 400-440 or 460-519). It did not report on more-specific mortality categories, but most cardiopulmonary mortality was from ischemic heart disease.

The city of Rotorua, New Zealand, is above a geothermally active area with substantial hydrogen sulfide (H_2S) exposures. About one-fourth of the population of 40,000 is regularly exposed to H_2S exceeding 200 $\mu g/m^3$ (143 ppb). A series of studies by Bates and co-workers investigated morbidity and mortality from the full range of diseases, including respiratory diseases (Bates et al. 1997, 1998, 2002). The mortality study (Bates et al. 1997), using census data, compared deaths in Rotorua with those in the rest of New Zealand (1981-1990). It found higher SMRs for hypertensive disease (codes 401-405: SMR 1.61, 95% CI 1.24-2.05, $p < 0.001$) but lower SMR for ischemic heart disease (codes 410-414: SMR 0.95, 95% CI 0.89-1.01, $p < 0.10$) and other heart disease (codes 420-429: SMR 0.70, 95% CI 0.58-0.84, $p < 0.001$). The authors interpreted those findings as canceling one another, owing to differences in coding: the rest of New Zealand, unlike Rotorua, is more likely to classify heart disease as "other heart disease" rather than the more-specific hypertensive disease.

Bates et al. (2002) later used hospital-discharge data over a 3-year period (1993-1996) to calculate standardized incidence ratios (SIRs) for respiratory and other diseases (and subgroupings) for Rotorua residents. Exposures were assigned as high, medium, and low, on the basis of mapping of H_2S with passive sampling in residential census-area units of 1,000-3,000 people. Exposure-response trends were found for circulatory-system diseases (ICD codes 390-459: p for trend = 0.0001); for ischemic heart disease (codes 410-414: p for trend < 0.02), cerebrovascular disease (codes 430-438: p for trend = 0.01), and diseases of arteries, arterioles, and capillaries (codes 440-448, p for trend = 0.002). The authors had no information on smoking and socioeconomic status (SES) as potential confounders and no information on residential histories or daily variations for work or study. The limited exposure-assessment information makes it difficult to interpret a dose-response relationship for cardiovascular disease.

In a third study, Bates et al. (1998) used hospital-discharge data over a decade (1981-1990) to calculate SIRs for cardiovascular disease (and subgroupings) for Rotorua residents. In contrast with the other incidence study (Bates et al. 2002), no exposure categories were assigned. The SIRs were slightly increased for cardiovascular disease (codes 390-459: SIR 1.05, 95% CI 1.02-1.07, $p = 0.001$). But the overall figure masked a variety of lower risks of some minor disease groupings, and higher risks of others. Lower risks were those of diseases of pulmonary circulation (codes 415-417: SIR 0.72, 95% CI 0.54-0.93, $p = 0.01$) and cerebrovascular disease (codes 430-438: SIR 0.85, 95% CI 0.79-0.91, $p < 0.001$). Greater risks were those of hypertensive disease (codes 401-405: SIR 1.15, 95% CI 1.00-1.32, $p = 0.05$), other heart disease (codes 420-429: SIR 1.06, 95% CI 1.00-1.13, $p = 0.04$), and diseases of arteries, arterioles, and capillaries (codes 440-448: SIR 1.17, 95% CI 1.07-1.28; $p = 0.001$). The Bates studies were the only epidemiologic studies of H_2S found by the committee that examined long-term health outcomes. Due to the paucity of literature, the committee did not make a separate conclusion on H_2S.

Occupational Studies

Gustavsson et al. (2001) conducted a case-control study of myocardial infarction among men and women (45-70 years old) in Stockholm, Sweden. Strict diagnostic criteria and a population-based design were used to identify the first, nonfatal myocardial infarction. A detailed occupational history was obtained with a questionnaire, which was followed by a sophisticated job-exposure matrix to provide quantitative exposure intensity of motor-vehicle exhaust as assessed with carbon monoxide (CO) and other combustion products as assessed with respirable particles. Exposures were expressed in terms of highest intensity during at least 1 year of work and cumulative exposure. Exposures were presumably higher in earlier decades, and time in occupation contributed to the cumulative-exposure estimate. Information on potential confounders (age, sex, smoking, hypertension, obesity, and diabetes), was obtained and incorporated into the analysis. It is not clear whether SES was used in the analysis, considering that referents were somewhat more likely to be of higher SES (25% of referents vs 19% of cases) and cases were substantially more likely to be manual workers (34% of cases vs 25% of referents). Fairly consistent effects were observed for combustion products, and there was evidence of a dose-response relationship. Myocardial infarction was, after adjustment, increased in the combustion-product group with high intensity during at least 1 year of occupational exposure (RR 2.11, 95% CI 1.23-3.60) and with intermediate intensity (RR 1.42, 95% CI 1.05-1.92). The analysis of the exposure-response trend generated an RR of 1.24, 95% CI 1.07-1.51. An exposure-response trend was also found for the other exposure category, cumulative exposure (in milligrams of respirable particles per cubic meter per year). The group with high cumulative exposure to combustion products had RR 1.35, 95% CI 1.02-1.79, and the group with intermediate cumulative exposure had RR 1.22, 95% CI 0.91-1.64. For the motor-vehicle exhaust group (which included many of the same subjects as the combustion-products group), myocardial infarction was not increased with high exposure (after adjustment), but was increased with intermediate exposure (RR 1.32, 95% CI 1.01-1.73). The trend analysis for the motor-vehicle exhaust group was not noteworthy. Examples of high combustion-product exposure referred to exposures at the threshold limit value. Examples of occupations with high combustion-product exposure were ship engine room crew, firefighters, engineers and technicians in energy production, chimney sweeps, and blacksmiths.

Mortality was studied in a subset of the large ACS cohort to assess occupational exposure to diesel exhaust (Boffetta et al. 1988). The study, initiated in 1984, enrolled 1.2 million people. The focus was on men (40-79 years old) and used a crude job-exposure matrix (based on 2-digit standard industrial classification codes) to determine exposure to diesel exhaust. Men with and without exposure to diesel exhaust were compared. Exposure was not associated with an increased risk of ischemic heart disease (RR 0.98) on the basis of 398 deaths, but there was an increased risk of cerebrovascular disease (codes 430-438: RR 1.61, $p < 0.05$) on the basis of 62 deaths, and of "arteriosclerosis" a minor ICD category (code 440: RR 3.12, $p < 0.05$) on the basis of 10 deaths. However, mortality attributed on death certificates to arteriosclerosis is nonspecific and thus difficult to interpret.

Alfredsson et al. (1993) performed an incidence and mortality study of myocardial infarction among bus drivers in Sweden over a 15-year period. It relied on two population-based registries—one of first acute myocardial-infarction hospitalizations and another of all deaths. Registries were linked to census records of occupation. Comparing male bus drivers with people in other occupations, the study found a higher incidence of myocardial infarction in bus drivers (RR 1.4, 95% CI 1.1-1.8, adjusted for age, calendar year, county, and SES); the effect appeared to decline in retirement. The cohort-mortality study found a small excess of myocardial-infarction deaths and ischemic-heart-disease deaths in bus drivers (RR 1.1, 95% CI 1.0-1.3) with adjustment for age and county but not for smoking or SES. However, the increased mortality risk was unlikely to have been due to smoking inasmuch as lung-cancer mortality was not increased in those workers.

A cohort-mortality study compared 5,529 tunnel (high exhaust) and bridge (low exhaust) workers to the rest of the NYC during 1952-1981 (Stern et al. 1988). Although the focus of the study was on CO, there is no evidence that it was not a study of all combustion products. There was a substantial excess of deaths from atherosclerotic heart disease (ICD-9 codes 410-414). Bridge workers had an SMR for atherosclerotic heart disease of 0.85, and tunnel workers 1.35 (90% CI 1.09-1.68, $p < 0.05$); the effect was much larger in tunnel workers who had more than 10 years on the job. Risk differences between tunnel and bridge workers decreased after separation from employment. No exposure assessment was conducted other than some representative CO monitoring. There was no control for confounders (SES, smoking, and so on), but the lack of excess lung-cancer or emphysema deaths and the identical smoking rates in tunnel and bridge workers suggest that the effect is unlikely to be related to smoking. Bridge and tunnel workers are drawn from the same applicant pool, so SES differences are less likely.

A mortality study in a cohort of Montreal bus drivers (Paradis et al. 1989) found an excess of death from circulatory system diseases (codes 390-458: SMR 122; 95% CI 105-140) and ischemic heart disease (codes 410-414: SMR 120, 95% CI 102-141) in bus drivers with less than 30 years of exposure. Deaths from circulatory system disease and ischemic heart disease were not increased, however, among those with more than 30 years of employment (SMRs 99 and 95, respectively) and there were no increased risks in those employed more than 5 years (circulatory disease SMR 109, 95% CI 99-119; ischemic heart disease SMR 106; 95% CI 95-118). The findings do not preclude a small effect, but there was no control for important confounders such as smoking.

Rushton et al. (1983) studied mortality in a cohort of bus maintenance workers in London was. When they compared those workers with the male population of England and Wales, they found a deficit of ischemic heart disease. However, there was no control for SES, smoking, or other confounders.

Several similar occupational mortality studies were difficult to interpret owing to lack of exposure data or lack of control for confounders (Borgia et al. 1994; Hansen 1989; Maizlish et al. 1988; Michaels and Zoloth 1991; Stern et al. 1981) or lack of control groups (Herbert et al. 2000).

Eight mortality studies were conducted in urban firefighters (Aronson et al. 1994; Beaumont et al. 1991; Burnett et al. 1994; Demers et al. 1992; Deschamps et al. 1995; Feuer and Rosenman 1986; Heyer et al. 1990; Musk et al. 1978) there was one cohort study of coronary heart disease incidence (Glueck et al. 1996), and one study of ischemic heart disease incidence among firefighters nested in a cohort study (Dibbs et al. 1982). Those studies share several features and collectively do not inform the committee's evaluation of the relationship between combustion-product exposure in the Persian Gulf and cardiovascular disease, for the following reasons: all studies were of urban firefighters whose exposures are of uncertain relevance to fossil-fuel combustion-product exposure during the Gulf War; firefighters are typically screened for health problems, and those with health problems often leave the line of work earlier, so such studies are especially susceptible to the healthy-worker effect, which can strongly bias observed relationships, especially in the case of cardiovascular disease (Murray et al. 1979), making the negative associations observed in the majority of the studies impossible to interpret; and firefighters probably differ from people in other occupations with regard to several potentially confounding factors that may influence the incidence of cardiovascular disease. Only the Dibbs et al. study, nested within the Normative Aging Study, has the capability to adjust for potential confounding factors, although the analysis is unclear as to whether the authors have done so.

There is relatively consistent epidemiologic evidence of the relation between ischemic heart disease (including myocardial infarction) and long-term exposure to fossil-fuel combustion products, including motor-vehicle exhaust and combustion-derived fine particulate matter. Several well-designed primary studies support an association (Dockery et al. 1993; Gustavsson et al. 2001; Hoek et al. 2002; Pope et al. 2004), as do several support studies (Alfredsson et al. 1993; Bates et al. 1997; Stern et al. 1988). However, the increased risk is small in absolute terms, and there is no adequate epidemiologic evidence to support the role of relatively short exposures (similar to that experienced in the Gulf War), followed by an exposure-free period, and then development of ischemic heart disease events. The committee recognizes that scientific inquiry in this subject is rapidly evolving, and that more definitive information may be available in the next several years.

The committee concludes, from its assessment of the epidemiologic literature, that there is inadequate/insufficient evidence to determine whether an association exists between short-term exposure (less than 2 years) to combustion products and the development of ischemic heart disease after an exposure-free period of months to years.

REFERENCES

Abbey DE, Nishino N, McDonnell WF, Burchette RJ, Knutsen SF, Beeson WL, Yang JX. 1999. Long-term inhalable particles and other air pollutants related to mortality in nonsmokers. *American Journal of Respiratory and Critical Care Medicine* 159(2):373-382.

Alfredsson L, Hammar N, Hogstedt C. 1993. Incidence of myocardial infarction and mortality from specific causes among bus drivers in Sweden. *International Journal of Epidemiology* 22(1):57-61.

Aronson KJ, Tomlinson GA, Smith L. 1994. Mortality among fire fighters in metropolitan Toronto. *American Journal of Industrial Medicine* 26(1):89-101.

Bates MN, Garrett N, Graham B, Read D. 1997. Air pollution and mortality in the Rotorua geothermal area. *Australian and New Zealand Journal of Public Health* 21(6):581-586.

Bates MN, Garrett N, Graham B, Read D. 1998. Cancer incidence, morbidity and geothermal air pollution in Rotorua, New Zealand. *International Journal of Epidemiology* 27(1):10-14.

Bates MN, Garrett N, Shoemack P. 2002. Investigation of health effects of hydrogen sulfide from a geothermal source. *Archives of Environmental Health* 57(5):405-411.

Beaumont JJ, Chu GS, Jones JR, Schenker MB, Singleton JA, Piantanida LG, Reiterman M. 1991. An epidemiologic study of cancer and other causes of mortality in San Francisco firefighters. *American Journal of Industrial Medicine* 19(3):357-372.

Boffetta P, Stellman SD, Garfinkel L. 1988. Diesel exhaust exposure and mortality among males in the American Cancer Society prospective study. *American Journal of Industrial Medicine* 14(4):403-415.

Borgia P, Forastiere F, Rapiti E, Rizzelli R, Magliola ME, Perucci CA, Axelson O. 1994. Mortality among taxi drivers in Rome: A cohort study. *American Journal of Industrial Medicine* 25(4):507-517.

Brook RD, Franklin B, Cascio W, Hong Y, Howard G, Lipsett M, Luepker R, Mittleman M, Samet J, Smith SC Jr, Tager I. 2004. Air pollution and cardiovascular disease: a statement for healthcare professionals from the Expert Panel on Population and Prevention Science of the American Heart Association. *Circulation* 109(21):2655-2671.

Burnett CA, Halperin WE, Lalich NR, Sestito JP. 1994. Mortality among fire fighters: A 27 state survey. *American Journal of Industrial Medicine* 26(6):831-833.

Christie D, Robinson K, Gordon I, Webley C, Bisby J. 1987. Current mortality in the Australian petroleum industry: The healthy-worker effect and the influence of life-style factors. *Medical Journal of Australia* 147(5):222, 224-225.

Dagg TG, Satin KP, Bailey WJ, Wong O, Harmon LL, Swencicki RE. 1992. An updated cause specific mortality study of petroleum refinery workers. *British Journal of Industrial Medicine* 49(3):203-212.

Demers PA, Heyer NJ, Rosenstock L. 1992. Mortality among firefighters from three northwestern United States cities. *British Journal of Industrial Medicine* 49(9):664-670.

Deschamps S, Momas I, Festy B. 1995. Mortality amongst Paris fire-fighters. *European Journal of Epidemiology* 11(6):643-646.

Dibbs E, Thomas HE Jr, Weiss ST, Sparrow D. 1982. Fire fighting and coronary heart disease. *Circulation* 65(5):943-946.

Dockery DW, Pope CA 3rd, Xu X, Spengler JD, Ware JH, Fay ME, Ferris BG Jr, Speizer FE. 1993. An association between air pollution and mortality in six U.S. cities. *New England Journal of Medicine* 329(24):1753-1759.

Draxler R, McQueen J, Stunder B. 1994. An evaluation of air pollutants exposures due to the 1991 Kuwait oil fires using a Langrangian Model. *Atmospheric Environment* 28:2197-2210.

Feuer E, Rosenman K. 1986. Mortality in police and firefighters in New Jersey. *American Journal of Industrial Medicine* 9(6):517-527.

Glueck C, Kelley W, Wang P, Gartside P, Black D, Tracy T. 1996. Risk factors for coronary heart disease among firefighters in Cincinnati. *American Journal of Industrial Medicine* 30(3):331-340.

Gustavsson P, Plato N, Hallqvist J, Hogstedt C, Lewne M, Reuterwall C, Scheele P. 2001 . A population-based case-referent study of myocardial infarction and occupational exposure to motor exhaust, other combustion products, organic solvents, lead, and dynamite. *Epidemiology* 12(2):222-228.

Hanis NM, Shallenberger LG, Donaleski DL, Sales EA. 1985. A retrospective mortality study of workers in three major U.S. refineries and chemical plants. Part 1: Comparisons with U.S. population. *Journal of Occupational Medicine* 27(4):283-292.

Hansen ES. 1989. Mortality of auto mechanics. A ten year follow-up. *Scandinavian Journal of Work, Environment & Health* 15(1):43-46.

Herbert R, Schechter C, Smith DA, Phillips R, Diamond J, Carroll S, Weiner J, Dahms TE, Landrigan PJ. 2000. Occupational coronary heart disease among bridge and tunnel officers. *Archives of Environmental Health* 55(3):152-163.

Heyer N, Weiss NS, Demers P, Rosenstock L. 1990. Cohort mortality study of Seattle fire fighters: 1945-1983. *American Journal of Industrial Medicine* 17(4):493-504.

Hoek G, Brunekreef B, Goldbohm S, Fischer P, Van den Brandt PA. 2002. Association between mortality and indicators of traffic-related air pollution in the Netherlands: A cohort study. *Lancet* 360(9341):1203-1209.

Huang YY. 1986. Prevalence and unawareness of hypertension in the petrochemical industrial population in China. *Preventive Medicine* 15(6):643-651.

Kang HK, Mahan CM, Lee KY, Magee CA, Murphy FM. 2000. Illnesses among United States veterans of the Gulf War: A population-based survey of 30,000 veterans. *Journal of Occupational and Environmental Medicine* 42(5):491-501.

Kaplan SD. 1986. Update of a mortality study of workers in petroleum refineries. *Journal of Occupational Medicine* 28(7):514-516.

Krewski D, Burnett RT, Goldberg MS, Hoover BK, Siemiatycki J, Jerrett M, Abrahamowicz M, White WH. 2003. Overview of the reanalysis of the Harvard Six Cities Study and American Cancer Society Study of Particulate Air Pollution and Mortality. *Journal of Toxicology and Environmental Health. Part A* 66(16-19):1507-1551.

Maizlish N, Beaumont J, Singleton J. 1988. Mortality among California highway workers. *American Journal of Industrial Medicine* 13(3):363-379.

McQueen J, Draxler R. 1994. Evaluation of model back trajectories of the Kuwait oil fires smoke plume using digital satellite data. *Atmospheric Environment* 28:2159-2174.

Michaels D, Zoloth SR. 1991. Mortality among urban bus drivers. *International Journal of Epidemiology* 20(2):399-404.

Murray FJ, Schwetz BA, Nitschke KD, Crawford AA, Quast JF, Staples RE. 1979. Embryotoxicity of inhaled sulfuric acid aerosol in mice and rabbits. *Journal of Environmental Science and Health. Part C: Environmental Health Sciences* 13(3):251-266.

Musk AW, Monson RR, Peters JM, Peters RK. 1978. Mortality among Boston firefighters, 1915--1975. *British Journal of Industrial Medicine* 35(2):104-108.

Paradis G, Theriault G, Tremblay C. 1989. Mortality in a historical cohort of bus drivers. *International Journal of Epidemiology* 18(2):397-402.

Pollini G, Maugeri U, Jedrychowski W, Bernardo A, Flak E, Jedrychowska I. 1989. Coronary heart disease risk score and ECG abnormalities in apparently healthy workers from petrochemical industry. The Pavia Study. *Giornale Italiano di Medicina del Lavoro* 11(6):273-278.

Pollini G, Maugeri U, Tringali S, Jedrychowski W, Flak E. 1986. Prevalence of hypertension and cardiovascular risk factors in workers of petrochemical industry. The Pavia Study. *Giornale Italiano di Medicina del Lavoro* 8(3-4):89-108.

Pope CA 3rd, Burnett RT, Thun MJ, Calle EE, Krewski D, Ito K, Thurston GD. 2002. Lung cancer, cardiopulmonary mortality, and long-term exposure to fine particulate air pollution. *Journal of the American Medical Association* 287(9):1132-1141.

Pope CA 3rd, Burnett RT, Thurston GD, Thun MJ, Calle EE, Krewski D, Godleski JJ. 2004. Cardiovascular mortality and long-term exposure to particulate air pollution: Epidemiological evidence of general pathophysiological pathways of disease. *Circulation* 109(1):71-77.

Pope CA 3rd, Thun MJ, Namboodiri MM, Dockery DW, Evans JS, Speizer FE, Heath CW Jr. 1995. Particulate air pollution as a predictor of mortality in a prospective study of U.S. adults. *American Journal of Respiratory and Critical Care Medicine* 151(3 Pt 1):669-674.

Proctor SP, Heeren T, White RF, Wolfe J, Borgos MS, Davis JD, Pepper L, Clapp R, Sutker PB, Vasterling JJ, Ozonoff D. 1998 . Health status of Persian Gulf War veterans: Self-reported symptoms, environmental exposures and the effect of stress. *International Journal of Epidemiology* 27(6):1000-1010.

Rushton L, Alderson MR. 1981. An epidemiological survey of eight oil refineries in Britain. *British Journal of Industrial Medicine* 38(3):225-234.

Rushton L, Alderson MR, Nagarajah CR. 1983. Epidemiological survey of maintenance workers in London Transport Executive bus garages and Chiswick Works. *British Journal of Industrial Medicine* 40(3):340-345.

Smith TC, Heller JM, Hooper TI, Gackstetter GD, Gray GC. 2002. Are Gulf War veterans experiencing illness due to exposure to smoke from Kuwaiti oil well fires? Examination of Department of Defense hospitalization data. *American Journal of Epidemiology* 155(10):908-917.

Stern FB, Halperin WE, Hornung RW, Ringenburg VL, McCammon CS. 1988. Heart disease mortality among bridge and tunnel officers exposed to carbon monoxide. *American Journal of Epidemiology* 128(6):1276-1288.

Stern FB, Lemen RA, Curtis RA. 1981. Exposure of motor vehicle examiners to carbon monoxide: A historical prospective mortality study. *Archives of Environmental Health* 36(2):59-65.

Tsai SP, Dowd CM, Cowles SR, Ross CE. 1992. A prospective study of morbidity patterns in a petroleum refinery and chemical plant. *British Journal of Industrial Medicine* 49(7):516-522.

Van Peenen PF, Blanchard AG, Wolkonsky PM. 1985. Cardiovascular risk factors in employees of a petrochemical company. *Journal of Occupational Medicine* 27(3):217-219.

Wong O, Harris F, Rosamilia K, Raabe GK. 2001a. An updated mortality study of workers at a petroleum refinery in Beaumont, Texas, 1945 to 1996. *Journal of Occupational and Environmental Medicine* 43(4):384-401.

Wong O, Harris F, Rosamilia K, Raabe GK. 2001b. Updated mortality study of workers at a petroleum refinery in Torrance, California, 1959 to 1997. *Journal of Occupational and Environmental Medicine* 43(12):1089-1102.

7

REPRODUCTIVE AND DEVELOPMENTAL OUTCOMES

This chapter examines reproductive and developmental outcomes of exposure to fuel and combustion products. The outcomes of interest include infertility, preterm birth and low-birth rate, as well as birth defects and childhood cancers.

In previous reports, Institute of Medicine committees focused primarily on exposures that occurred in men and women before conception. Preconception exposure was considered the most relevant to the Gulf War veterans' experience. Those committees assumed that pregnancies during Gulf War deployment would have been rare that pregnant women would have been immediately evacuated. A newly published study (Araneta et al. 2004), however, indicates that there were many more pregnancies than previously reported and that pregnancies were typically ascertained 2-6 weeks after conception. Thus, it is likely that most pregnant women would have been evacuated during the first 6-12 weeks of pregnancy; that inference led the present committee to expand its search of the epidemiologic literature to include reproductive outcomes, with relevant environmental exposures, during the first trimester of pregnancy.

STUDIES OF BIRTH DEFECTS IN GULF WAR VETERANS

Several studies investigated reproductive effects of service in the Gulf War. Most were of birth defects, and none analyzed whether effects were related to specific biologic or chemical compounds. Early studies did not find any adverse effects, but more recent ones have reported excess cardiac birth defects and other adverse reproductive outcomes in offspring of men and women who served in the Gulf War.

Early studies of Gulf War veterans failed to identify an excess of birth defects in offspring of deployed vs nondeployed veterans. A small study of two Mississippi National Guard units deployed to the Gulf War (n = 282) found no excess rate of birth defects in National Guard members' children compared with rates expected on the basis of surveillance systems and previous surveys (Penman et al. 1996). A much larger study of all live births in military hospitals (n = 75,000) in 1991-1993, included a comparison population of births to nondeployed personnel. The risk of birth defects was the same in children of Gulf War personnel as in the control population (Cowan et al. 1997). The study was limited to military hospitals and thereby excluded persons not being cared for in those hospitals (for example, members of the National Guard, reservists, and those who left the military over the course of the study). National Guard and reserve troops, as noted earlier, constituted a relatively high percentage of US troops deployed to the Gulf War. Anecdotal reports of an excess of Goldenhar syndrome, a rare congenital anomaly that affects the development of facial structures, prompted another study of birth defects. The syndrome is not specifically coded in the reporting of birth defects, so the authors reviewed medical records of birth-defect categories that would have subsumed the Goldenhar syndrome. Too few cases of the syndrome were found to support definitive conclusions (Araneta et al. 1997).

A large, population-based Department of Veterans Affairs study of 15,000 US Gulf War veterans vs 15,000 non-deployed veterans found that both male and female veterans self-reported higher rates of birth defects among liveborn infants, including "moderate to severe" defects (odds ratios [ORs] 1.8-2.8). The defects were grouped into broad categories; the largest (n = 151) was described as "isolated anomaly". Male veterans self-reported a higher rate of miscarriage among their partners (OR 1.62, 95% confidence interval [CI] 1.32-1.99) than did controls. Concerned about reporting bias, the investigators suggested that those observations be confirmed by a review of medical records (Kang et al. 2001).

A population-based study in several states captured births in all hospitals, both military and civilian, and matched birth certificates with military records during the period 1989-1993 (Araneta et al. 2003). The study measured the prevalence of birth defects among infants of Gulf War veterans and non-deployed veterans in states that conducted active case ascertainment of birth defects. Military record of 684,645 Gulf War veterans and 1,587,102 non-deployed veterans were electronically linked with 2,314,908 birth certificates from Arizona, Hawaii, Iowa, and selected counties of Arkansas, Califonia, and Georgia; 11,961 Gulf War veterans' infants and 33,052 non-deployed veterans' infants were identified. Of those, 450 infants had mothers who served in the Gulf War and 3966 had non-deployed veteran mothers. After examining 48 specific categories of birth defects, the study found a greater prevalence of three defects—tricuspid valve insufficiency (relative risk [RR] 2.7, 95% CI 1.1-6.6), aortic valve stenosis (RR 6.0, 95% CI 1.2-31.0), and renal agenesis (RR 2.4, 95% CI 0.7-8.3)—in infants conceived after the war by Gulf War-deployed men in comparison with non-Gulf War-deployed men. Aortic valve stenosis and renal agenesis had higher RRs among infants conceived after the war by Gulf War veteran men than among infants conceived before the war. The study also found a greater prevalence of hypospadias in male infants (RR 6.3, 95% CI 1.5-26.3) conceived during or after the war and born to female Gulf War veterans (in comparison with non-Gulf War-deployed females). The study was not designed to determine whether the excess risk was caused by environmental agents, and it should be interpreted as an exploratory study that investigated 48 categories of birth defects.

A recently published population-based UK study probed the prevalence of birth defects and fetal deaths in all UK Gulf War veterans and Gulf War-era controls (that is, veterans who were not deployed to the gulf war)—a total of 105,735 veterans—studied with a validated postal questionnaire (Doyle et al. 2004). The study period covered conception after the Gulf War and before November 1997. Male Gulf War veterans reported a higher risk of miscarriages in their partners than the comparison cohort (OR 1.4, 95% CI 1.3-1.5). They also reported a higher proportion of offspring with any type of malformation (OR 1.5, 95% CI 1.3-1.7). Examination by type of malformation revealed some evidence of an increased risk of malformation but it was weakened when the analyses were restricted to clinically confirmed conditions. Female veterans did not report an excess of miscarriage, and stillbirths and malformations were too few to be usefully analyzed.

Five reproductive outcomes (livebirth, stillbirth, spontaneous abortion, ectopic pregnancy, and induced abortion) were analyzed among female veterans during or after the Gulf War compared to nondeployed female veterans (Araneta et al. 2004). A postal survey was sent to every woman identified by the Department of Defense as having a pregnancy-related admission to a military hospital from August 2, 1990 to May 31, 1992. The responses were validated with medical records; it was observed that female veterans with post-Gulf War conceptions (n = 292) were at increased risk for spontaneous abortion (OR 2.92, 95% CI 1.9-4.6) and ectopic pregnancy (OR 7.70, 95% CI 3.0-19.8) compared with nondeployed female veterans (n = 427). No difference was found between pregnancies of Gulf War-deployed women and those of non-Gulf War-deployed women.

FUELS AND REPRODUCTIVE AND DEVELOPMENTAL OUTCOMES

In reviewing the literature on paternal and maternal exposure to fuels, the committee found several studies on adverse reproductive outcomes, including infertility, spontaneous abortion, childhood leukemia, neuroblastoma, and Prader-Willi syndrome—which may result from genetic alterations in either sperm or egg. The studies related to each of those outcomes are discussed below (Table 7.1).

TABLE 7.1 Selected Epidemiologic Studies—Reproductive Outcomes and Exposure to Fuel

Reference	Population	Exposed Cases	Estimated Relative Risk
Acute nonlymphocytic leukemia			
Case-Control Study			
Buckley et al. 1989	Paternal exposure to petroleum products		
	None	93	1.0
	1–1,000 days duration	32	1.4 (0.8–2.5)
	> 1,000 days duration	53	2.4 (1.3–4.1)
	Before conception	NA	2.0 (p < 0.05)
	During gestation	NA	2.8 (p < 0.05)
Leukemia			
Case-Control study			
Shu et al. 1988	Maternal occupational exposure during pregnancy		
	Gasoline	38	1.6 (0.8–3.1)
	Diesel oil	16	1.4 (0.6–3.3)
	Kerosene	16	1.4 (0.6–3.1)
	Maternal occupational exposure during pregnancy by histopathologic cell type		
	Gasoline		
	ANLL	13	2.1 (1.1–4.3)
	ALL	21	1.7 (1.0–3.0)
	Kerosene		
	ANLL	6	2.3 (0.9–6.3)
	ALL	9	1.5 (0.6–3.4)

Reference	Population	Exposed Cases	Estimated Relative Risk
Neuroblastoma			
Case-Control Studies			
De Roos et al. 2001	Maternal occupational exposure		
	Nonvolatile hydrocarbons, self-reported exposure	26	1.2 (0.7–2.2)
	Nonvolatile hydrocarbons, industrial hygienist reviewed exposure	12	1.1 (0.5–2.5)
	Diesel fuel, self-reported exposure	12	1.3 (0.5–3.1)
	Diesel fuel, industrial hygienist reviewed exposure	3	0.9 (0.2–4.4)
	Gasoline, self-reported exposure	14	1.6 (0.6–3.8)
	Gasoline, industrial hygienist reviewed exposure	3	0.8 (0.2–4.2)
	Paternal occupational exposure		
	Nonvolatile hydrocarbons, self-reported exposure	130	1.3 (0.9–1.9)
	Nonvolatile hydrocarbons, industrial hygienist reviewed exposure	91	1.5 (1.0–2.2)
	Diesel fuel, self-reported exposure	72	1.2 (0.8–1.9)
	Diesel fuel, industrial hygienist reviewed exposure	42	1.5 (0.8–2.6)
	Kerosene, self-reported exposure	26	1.1 (0.6–2.0)
	Kerosene, industrial hygienist reviewed exposure	16	1.0 (0.5–2.2)
	Gasoline, self-reported exposure	77	0.8 (0.5–1.2)
	Gasoline, industrial hygienist reviewed exposure	45	0.8 (0.5–1.3)
	Adjusted for frequently co-occurring hydrocarbons and paints for paternal exposure to diesel fuel	NA	2.0 (1.0–4.3)
Kerr et al. 2000	Maternal exposure to petroleum	23	3.0 (1.5–6.1)
	Paternal exposure to petroleum	53	1.8 (1.1–2.8)
Prader-Willi syndrome			
Case-Control Study			
Cassidy et al. 1989	Paternal occupational exposure to hydrocarbons	24	0.72 (0.28–1.81)

Infertility

Infertility is the inability to conceive after at least 12 months of unprotected intercourse (Rowe et al. 1993). It has been estimated that 10-15% of couples of reproductive age experience some form of infertility (Speroff et al. 1999). There are numerous risk factors for infertility including: advanced age, obesity in women, previous reproductive experiences, genetic factors, and such diseases as chlamydial infection in women and epididymitis in men (Templeton 2000). No studies of infertility in women and exposure to fuels met the committee's inclusion criteria (see Chapter 2) but the committee found one study on semen characteristics.

In men, semen samples can be collected and used to assess sperm production, structure, and function as measures of the effect of exposure on the male reproductive system. A prospective study was conducted to evaluate the effects of mixed, low-level exposure to complex mixtures on reproductive potential in men (Lemasters et al. 1999). The study included 50 men working on aircraft maintenance at an Air Force installation and eight nonexposed men at the same facility.

Semen quality was assessed at baseline, before entry into the exposed job, and at periods of 15 and 30 weeks post-baseline, during which the men were occupationally exposed to solvents or jet fuels (primarily JP4). Although those two periods were chosen to allow for two complete cycles of spermatogenesis, the distal regions of the epididymis contain sperm of different ages.

At baseline (before entry into the workplace) semen was collected but there was no exposure monitoring. For 15 and 30 weeks of occupational exposure, semen assays and exposure assessment—with industrial-hygiene monitoring and breath sampling—were conducted for the exposed group, and only semen assays were requested for the nonexposed office workers.

Overall, for most sperm measures, the mean values remained within normal range throughout the 30 weeks of exposure. The findings by cycle for all exposed subjects were compared with reference values, and all semen measures at all cycles were found to be similar to reference limits except for percent motile,[1] which was consistently lower. The eight nonexposed subjects had sperm measures similar to the exposed group, and their percent motile was also lower at baseline than the reference. Thus, the findings indicate that exposure to jet fuel did not have an apparent effect on semen quality of aircraft-maintenance personnel. Two possible explanations for the findings are that the mixtures are not associated with spermatotoxic effects at low concentrations and that the exposure measured at one point may be inadequate for characterizing the true absorbed dose.

The strengths of the study were that analyses were adjusted for potential confounders, including alcohol, smoking, and caffeine. Limitations of the study include the appreciable differences in age among the men in the different job groups and the low statistical power.

Spontaneous Abortion

The most common cause of spontaneous abortion is a genetic abnormality of the embryo. Risk factors for spontaneous abortion include age, maternal illness, cigarette-smoking, alcohol use, use of some medications, and a previous spontaneous abortion. The risk of pregnancy loss is known to increase with maternal age, especially after the age of 30 or 35 years; and is also high in women under the age of 18 years. In a woman who has had one spontaneous abortion, the probability of a second is estimated to be 13-26%; and the probability of another increases with successive spontaneous abortions (Smith and Suess 1998). Several maternal occupational exposures have been associated with the risk of spontaneous abortion, including exposure to ethylene oxide, antineoplastic agents, and possibly anesthetic gases.

Spontaneous abortion was studied in women living near oil fields in the Amazon basin of Ecuador (San Sebastián et al. 2002). The water in the rivers and streams of that area is contaminated with oils and is used for drinking, cooking, and bathing. Women living in several communities downstream of oil fields ($n = 365$) were compared with women living upstream and farther from the fields ($n = 283$). The concentration of total petroleum hydrocarbons in drinking water were 0.02 to 2.88 ppm in exposed communities. After adjustment for confounders, women in exposed communities were more likely to report pregnancies ending in spontaneous abortion (OR 2.47, 95% CI 1.61-3.79, $p < 0.01$). The multivariate analysis adjusted for age at interview, age at pregnancy, pregnancy order, year of pregnancy, and socioeconomic status (SES).

---

[1] Percent motile depends on time from ejaculation until sample analysis.

Limitations of the study include the assignment of the same exposure status, based on drinking-water measurements, to every woman in a given study area, and the potential for recall bias.

Childhood Cancers

The committee considered any health effect in the child of a veteran as a reproductive effect even if the manifestation was cancer. Childhood cancer is defined by the American Cancer Society as cancer diagnosed between birth and the age of 14 years. The causes of most childhood cancers are not well known, especially with regard to potential environmental risk factors. Some of the suggested risk factors are genetics, advanced maternal age, birthweight of more than 4000 g, prenatal viral exposure, and prenatal radiation exposure (Ross and Swensen 2000).

Developments in treatment and supportive care for some types of cancer have enabled 75% of afflicted children to survive 5 years or more, and mortality from all childhood cancers combined has declined by 50% since 1973. Although childhood cancer is rare, it is still the leading cause of death from disease in children up to 14 years old (ACS 1999).

Leukemia

Leukemia is the most common cancer in children and accounts for almost one-third of all cases of childhood cancer. Acute lymphocytic leukemia (ALL) is the most common leukemia in children, accounting for nearly 75% of all leukemia cases (ACS 2002b). Slightly more prevalent among white children and among boys, ALL generally occurs in early childhood, particularly at the age of 2-3 years. The 5-year survival rate of children who have ALL has increased to nearly 80%, primarily because of advances in treatment (ACS 2002b).

Most of the remaining childhood leukemia cases are categorized as acute myeloid leukemia (AML), which occurs most commonly in the first 2 years of life and less commonly among older children. Developments in treatment have improved the survival rate of children who have AML, who have 5-year survival rate of about 40% (ACS 2002b).

Prenatal exposure to radiation is known to be associated with the development of ALL (IARC 2000). Some genetic disorders—such as Li-Fraumeni syndrome, Down syndrome, and Klinefelter syndrome—also are associated with ALL, and chemotherapeutic agents are associated with secondary leukemia later in childhood or in adulthood.

A population-based case-control study of 204 children under the age of 18 years who had acute nonlymphocytic leukemia (ANLL) or AML examined occupational exposures of parents (Buckley et al. 1989). The cases were age-matched to population controls, and all the mothers were interviewed, as were the fathers if available. During the interviews, information was collected on demographics, occupational histories and exposures, household exposures, lifestyle factors, reproductive and medical histories, complications of delivery, and congenital abnormalities of the child and first-degree relatives. For each exposure, the nature of the exposure, duration, frequency, and timing in relation to the index pregnancy was asked of each parent. All exposures and related information were self-reported. During the interviews, the parents were asked to report occupational exposures to 52 agents, including petroleum products. Among fathers who had been exposed to petroleum products for more than 1,000 days, the OR for ANLL was 2.4 (95% CI 1.3-4.1; p trend = 0.002) for exposure at any time before, during, or after the birth. The point estimate of the risk decreased to 2.0 for paternal exposure only before conception.

A population-based case-control study of 309 children who had leukemia and 618 healthy population controls in urban Shanghai, China, was conducted (Shu et al. 1988). Controls were randomly selected from the Shanghai general population and matched on sex and age. Information on parental lifestyle, radiation exposure, medication use, birth characteristics, and parental occupation was collected through in-person interviews. Maternal and paternal occupations during pregnancy included working in the chemical industry or a related occupation, working in agriculture or metal refining and processing, being a physician or pharmacist, and working in pharmacy manufacturing. Paternal occupation during pregnancy had no influence on the occurrence of leukemia. There were increased adjusted ORs for maternal exposure to gasoline (OR 1.6, 95% CI 0.8-3.1), diesel oil (OR 1.4, 95% CI 0.6-3.3), and kerosene (OR 1.4, 95% CI 0.6-3.1). Risk by leukemia type showed an association between maternal gasoline exposure and ANLL (OR 2.1, 95% CI 1.1-4.3) and ALL (OR 1.7, 95% CI 1.0-3.0) and between exposure to kerosene and ANLL (OR 2.3, 95% CI 0.9-6.3) and ALL (OR 1.5, 95% CI 0.6-3.4). According to the authors, limitations of the study include recall bias (cases were diagnosed over a 12-year period, whereas controls were healthy children selected in 1985-1986) and interviewer bias (trained interviewers could not be blinded to case-control status). Furthermore, the control-selection procedures might have resulted in bias in the favoring of children from large residential areas. Finally, multiple comparisons in the study and lack of validation for parental x-ray, drug, or occupational exposure indicate the need for cautious interpretation.

Four additional studies examined the relationship between parental occupation and childhood leukemia (Gold et al. 1982; Hakulinen et al. 1976; Lowengart et al. 1987; van Steensel-Moll et al. 1985). They were limited by their inability to validate employment history and their lack of details on specific assessment of exposure as in the study by Shu et al. above (1988). The broad exposure group "hydrocarbon related" included many diverse occupations with exposures to chemicals in addition to hydrocarbons, therefore, it is difficult to draw conclusions on exposure to fuels. Three of those studies did not find increased risks of leukemia related to hydrocarbon- or petroleum-product-exposed parental occupations, either before or during pregnancy. The study of van Steensel-Moll (1985) found that maternal exposure to paint, petroleum products, and unspecified chemicals during pregnancy was related to childhood leukemia (RR 2.4, 95% CI 1.2-4.6). No particular periods of pregnancy were specified.

Central Nervous System Cancer

Central nervous system (CNS) cancers include malignant brain and spinal-cord tumors. Brain tumors are the second-most common group of cancers in children, accounting for about 20% of all childhood cancers. Common types of childhood brain tumors are astrocytomas (tumors originating in the brain cells), primitive neuroectodermal tumors (PNETs, tumors that develop from primitive stem cells), and germ-cell tumors. Neuroblastoma, a type of CNS tumor derived from embryonic neural crest cells, is a common form of cancer in children and accounts for 7-10% of all childhood cancers (ACS 2002a).

The etiology of childhood brain cancer appears to be multifactorial; there is no clear primary cause. Such genetic syndromes as Li-Fraumeni syndrome and von Recklinghausen disease are known to be associated with a modest fraction of these tumors. One well-established risk factor for the development of brain tumors is exposure to ionizing radiation, which can occur during the treatment of other cancers. Other factors—such as exposure to nitrates, aspartame, and electromagnetic fields—have been studied, but no conclusive evidence clearly implicates them as causal factors. More than 50% of children with brain tumors (all types combined) survive over 5 years (ACS 2002a).

To study the effects of parental occupational exposure on the incidence of neuroblastoma among children, De Roos et al. (2001) conducted a case-control study of 538 incident cases of neuroblastoma in children under the age of 19 years who had a new and confirmed diagnosis of neuroblastoma and registered at 139 participating hospitals in the US and Canada. Cases were age-matched to controls 1:1 recruited with random-digit dialing. Telephone interviews were conducted with all the mothers, and fathers if available, to obtain information on demographic characteristics, occupational histories, and exposures to specific chemicals. For each job held during the 2-year period before a child's date of birth, the mother and father were asked specifically about 65 chemicals, including the category of "nonvolatile hydrocarbons" and such specific agents as petroleum products, oils and lubricants, cutting oil, diesel fuel, kerosene, and lubricating oil or grease. All self-reported exposures were reviewed by an industrial hygienist in an attempt to reduce the number of incorrect reports of exposures.

Maternal exposure to most chemicals was not associated with neuroblastoma; however, paternal exposure to some hydrocarbons was associated with increased incidence of neuroblastoma. The OR for neuroblastoma related to self-reported paternal exposure to diesel fuels was 1.2 (CI 0.8-1.9), to kerosene 1.1 (CI 0.6-2.0), and to gasoline 0.8 (CI 0.5-1.2). The analyses were rerun using an industrial hygiene review to assign exposure; the OR for diesel fuel was 1.5 (CI 0.8-2.6), for kerosene 1.0 (CI 0.5-2.2), and for gasoline 0.8 (CI 0.5-1.3); adjustment did not indicate increased risk.

The authors noted that they were unable to explore effects of maternal and paternal exposure before conception or during pregnancy separately because exposures overlapped during those periods. The large number of chemicals considered and the retrospective assessment of exposure limit the strength of this study. Overall, the study found weak support for an association between paternal exposure to diesel fuel and neuroblastoma and no support for an association between maternal exposures to any of the chemicals and neuroblastoma.

In another case-control study, interviews were conducted with the mothers and fathers of 183 children 0-14 years old who had neuroblastoma and resided in New York state (excluding New York City) and with the parents of 372 controls selected from the New York state live-birth certificate registry and matched to cases on year of birth (Kerr et al. 2000). Occupational histories and exposure information on 25 specific physical and chemical compounds were collected for both parents. Information was collected on parental occupation during the entire pregnancy with the index child. Mothers reported both their own and the fathers' occupational histories. An increased risk of neuroblastoma was associated with maternal and paternal exposure to petroleum (OR 3.0, 95% CI 1.5-6.1 and OR 1.8, 95% CI 1.1-2.8, respectively). According to the authors, limitations of the study include possible misclassification of job and exposure, the increased likelihood of chance findings due to the large numbers of multiple comparisons, potential interviewer bias because interviewers were not blinded to the disease status of the index child of the mother being interviewed, and collection of exposure information on both parents from mothers.

A case-control study of occupational exposures of parents with children who had astrocytoma (n = 155) or PNET (n = 166) was conducted (Bunin et al. 1994). Cases were compared with matched control children who were identified with random-digit dialing. Kerosene was the only exposure of relevance to this committee, but the study explored an array of occupational and lifestyle exposures. The study found that maternal exposure to kerosene during pregnancy was associated with an increased risk of astrocytoma (OR 8.9, 95% CI 1.1-71.1, $p = 0.04$). No specific information on the nature of the exposure was provided, and the study carries the potential for recall bias.

Prader-Willi Syndrome

Prader-Willi syndrome (PWS) is a neurogenetic disorder generally associated with an abnormality of chromosome 15. About 60-75% (Akefeldt et al. 1995) of patients with PWS have a cytogenetically visible deletion in the q11-q13 region of paternal chromosome 15. Because PWS is highly associated with the loss of paternally derived genetic material, some have speculated that environmental factors may lead to PWS in men's offspring (Magenis 1988; Strakowski and Butler 1987).

The incidence of PWS is 1 in 12,000 affecting both sexes and various races equally. Children with PWS are often characterized as short and having mental retardation or learning disabilities, incomplete sexual development, behavior problems, low muscle tone, and an urge to eat constantly, which often leads to obesity (PWSA 2004).

Akefeldt et al (1995) conducted a case-control study of 15 PWS patients and 13 controls to assess the relationship between PWS and parental exposures to hydrocarbons, including gasoline. The PWS patients were referred by pediatric outpatient departments. The controls were children referred for obesity that had mental retardation but did not fulfill all the diagnostic criteria for PWS. The study did not include a "normal" control group. Both parents of each child completed a questionnaire about their exposure to environmental and occupational agents (for example, gasoline, petrochemicals, and pesticides). Seven of the 15 PWS fathers reported exposure to gasoline ($p = 0.01$) compared with none in the control group. The fathers reported that they had been exposed for 5-17 years (mean, 9 years) before the children's conceptions. Among the seven PWS children whose fathers had been exposed to gasoline, five had molecular genetic deletions. Four of the eight PWS children, whose fathers were not exposed to gasoline also had chromosomal deletions. One PWS mother and two control group mothers reported exposure to gasoline. The results of the study indicate that only gasoline, not hydrocarbons in general, is implicated in the etiology of PWS. However, the authors note that the small number of cases makes it difficult to obtain significant values. Given the difficulty in correctly recalling details about exposure, especially the duration of exposure, the possibility of errors cannot be excluded.

An earlier study found an association between PWS and paternal occupational hydrocarbon exposure at or about time of conception (Strakowski and Butler 1987). The study included 652 PWS patients identified from the National Prader-Willi Syndrome Association. To obtain controls with a genetic disease in which paternal environmental exposure was an unlikely causative factor, the authors chose fragile X syndrome ($n = 66$) and Down syndrome ($n = 268$). The average age of the fathers was 32 years, no different from the national average. Occupations were classified into 23 categories; 12 categories involved considerable occupational exposure to hydrocarbons, and five to lead. The percentage of fathers with unknown occupations was similar in the PWS group (7.1%) and in the controls (7.5%), and they were excluded from statistical calculations. Paternal occupational hydrocarbon exposure in the PWS group (20.8%) was greater than that in the controls (12.0%), (p-value < 0.001).

Although the Akefeldt et al. and Strakowski and Butler studies found associations between PWS and paternal hydrocarbon or gasoline exposure, neither study collected information on potential confounders, such as paternal drug use, radiation exposure, or smoking history. However, despite the lack of control for potential confounders, the consistent associations found in both studies, the presence of paternal chromosomal deletions in 60-75% of PWS patients, and studies showing associations between chromosomal aberrations and occupational exposure to gasoline (Carere et al. 1998; Khalil 1995; Santos-Mello and Cavalcante 1992) suggest that it is biologically reasonable that paternal exposure to hydrocarbons, such as gasoline, is a possible mechanism for paternally derived PWS. Studies have also shown that in nearly all cases involving an interstitial chromosomal deletion in PWS patients (Ledbetter and Cassidy 1988), parental chromosomes have been normal; thus the deletion in PWS patients might be a de novo event.

To explore the hypothesis that hydrocarbon exposure was associated with the chromosomal abnormality in PWS, Cassidy et al. (1989) conducted a study to determine whether there was a difference in the prevalence of occupational exposure to hydrocarbons at the time of conception between fathers of PWS children who have a 15q chromosomal deletion and fathers of PWS children who do not have such a deletion. Using job classification, they assigned exposure to hydrocarbons. Of the 53 fathers of children with 15q deletions, 24 (45%) were engaged in potentially hydrocarbon-exposed occupations compared with 15 (54%) of the 28 fathers of children with apparently normal chromosomes (OR 0.72, 95% CI 0.28-1.81). Although there were no differences in exposure history on the basis of the presence of 15q deletions, the authors recognize that they were unable to determine whether submicroscopic deletions may be present in the children without apparent chromosome abnormalities. They suggest that research on smaller, less visible microdeletions is needed to understand the relationship between hydrocarbon exposure and PWS.

Conclusion

Overall, it is difficult to reach conclusions on the epidemiologic studies of adverse reproductive outcomes and exposure to fuels. Assessment of findings is limited by the small number of studies available on each health outcome, the possibility of recall bias, and the lack of specificity of exposure to the agents of concern in this report.

The committee concludes, from its assessment of the epidemiologic literature, that there is inadequate/insufficient evidence to determine whether an association exists between exposure to fuels and adverse reproductive or developmental outcomes, including infertility, spontaneous abortion, childhood leukemia, central nervous system tumors, neuroblastoma, and Prader-Willi syndrome.

COMBUSTION PRODUCTS AND REPRODUCTIVE AND DEVELOPMENTAL OUTCOMES

This section covers the following outcomes that have been addressed in epidemiologic research in relation to combustion-product exposures: preterm birth, low birthweight (LBW), very low birthweight (VLBW), intrauterine growth retardation (IUGR), birth defects, and childhood cancers.

Adverse Pregnancy Outcomes

The committee sought information on whether maternal or paternal exposure to combustion products before conception or maternal exposure during the first 3 months (first trimester) of gestation affected pregnancy outcomes. A number of adverse outcomes of pregnancy have been studied for possible associations with exposure to combustion products in air pollution. Most studies examined adverse effects on live births including preterm birth, IUGR, and LBW, which have a pronounced influence on infant morbidity and mortality (Pschirrer and Monga 2000). In the studies covered in this chapter, IUGR and LBW were usually analyzed in relation to full-term births. Other studies examined stillbirths or birth defects. The studies reviewed in this section, conducted largely in heavily polluted cities worldwide, examined associations between adverse pregnancy outcomes and combustion products.

Preterm Births

Preterm birth (<37 weeks) is the second leading cause of infant mortality in the United States (MMWR 1999) and a major cause of infant morbidity. Known environmental risk factors include maternal cigarette-smoking and alcohol dependence; other risk factors are a history of preterm birth, maternal race, and multiple gestation (Pschirrer and Monga 2000). Most preterm births in the United States do not result in LBW (Ritz et al. 2000). At least seven studies, in different continents, have explored the effects of air pollution on preterm births (Table 7.2).

The effects of air pollution on preterm births were studied in a cohort of nearly 100,000 births in Los Angeles in 1989-1993 (Ritz et al. 2000). The exposure, based on collections at 17 air quality monitoring stations, was of averaged pollutant measures over distinct periods such as 1, 2, 4, 6, 8, 12, and 26 weeks before birth, and the entire pregnancy period. The authors also calculated average exposures in the first and second month of pregnancy. Pollutants of interest were carbon monoxide (CO), nitrogen dioxide (NO_2), ozone (O_3), and PM_{10} (particulate matter 10 μg in diameter). About 9% of infants in the sample were born preterm. For $PM_{10,}$ a 50-$\mu g/m^3$ increase in concentration over the first month of pregnancy was associated with a 16% increase in the rate of preterm births (RR 1.16, 95% CI 1.06-1.26). For CO, a 3-ppm increase over the first month of pregnancy was associated with a 4% increase in the rate of preterm births (RR 1.04, 95% CI 1.01-1.09). This study was well designed, with analyses controlling for several known risk factors for preterm birth, including age, race, education, parity, access to prenatal care, and previous low-birthweight or preterm births. The authors adjusted for maternal smoking but reported that the adjustment was incomplete.

TABLE 7.2 Preterm Birth and Combustion-Product Exposure

Reference	Population	Pollutants Measured and Exposure Period	Adjusted OR (95% CI or p) by Period and Pollutant	Adjustments	Limitations
Ritz et al. 2000	97,518 live births, Los Angeles, CA 1989-1993	PM_{10}, CO, NO_2, O_3 Month 1 Final 6 weeks	PM_{10} per 50-µg increase Month 1: RR 1.09, 95% CI 0.99-1.20 6 weeks before birth: RR 1.20, 95% CI 1.09-1.33 CO Month 1: RR 1.04, 95% CI 0.99-1.09 6 weeks before birth: RR 1.12, 95% CI 1.08-1.7 NO_2, O_3 Nonsignificant	Maternal age, race, education, parity, access to prenatal care, previous low-weight or preterm births; season of birth or conception	Inadequate adjustment for maternal smoking
Bobak 2000	108,173 live births, Czech Republic 1991	SO_2, TSP, NO_x Trimesters 1-3	SO_2 per 50-µg increase: Trimester 1: OR 1.27, 95% CI 1.16-1.39 Trimester 2: OR 1.25, 95% CI 1.14-1.38 Trimester 3: OR 1.24, 95% CI 1.13-1.36 TSP per 50-µg increase Trimester 1: OR 1.18, 95% CI 1.05-1.31 Trimester 2: OR 1.11, 95% CI 0.97-1.26 Trimester 3: OR 1.12, 95% CI 0.97-1.28 NOx per 50-µg increase Trimester 1: OR 1.10, 95% CI 1.00-1.21 Trimester 2: OR 1.08, 95% CI 0.98 -1.19 Trimester 3: OR 1.11, 95% CI 1.00-1.23	Sex of child; parity, maternal age group, education, marital status, nationality; month of birth	No adjustment for maternal smoking

Reference	Population	Pollutants Measured and Exposure Period	Adjusted OR (95% CI or p) by Period and Pollutant	Adjustments	Limitations
Liu et al. 2003	229,085 live births, Vancouver, Canada 1986-1998	SO_2, NO_2, CO, ozone Month 1 Last month	SO_2 per 5-ppb increase Month 1: OR 0.95, 95% CI 0.88-1.03 Last month: OR 1.09, 95% CI 1.01-1.19 NO_2 Month 1: OR 1.01, 95% CI 0.94-1.07 Last month: OR 1.08, 95% CI 0.99-1.17 CO per 1-ppm increase: Month 1: OR 0.95, 95% CI 0.89-1.01 Last month: OR 1.08, 95% CI 1.01-1.15 O_3 Month 1: OR 0.98, 95% CI 0.89-1.03 Last month: OR 0.93, 95% CI 0.86-1.00	Maternal age, parity; infant sex, birth weight; birth season	No adjustment for maternal smoking
Wihelm & Ritz 2003	Case-Control Los Angeles, CA 1994-1996	Distance-weighted traffic density (DWTD) Only third trimester specified	DWTD highest quintile Preterm RR 1.08, 95% CI 1.01-1.15	Infant sex; maternal age, race or ethnicity, education; birth season; year of analysis; SES, among other covariates	Could not adjust for active and passive smoking and diet; these are related to SES, which was included in models

Bobak (2000) studied all singleton live births registered in 1991 by the Czech Republic (n = 108,173). The effects of maternal exposure to sulfur dioxide (SO_2), total suspended particulates (TSP), and nitrous oxides (NO_x) were investigated. Daily measurements taken with air monitors in the district of each infant's birth were collected by trimester. After controlling for sex of the child, parity, maternal age group, education, marital status, nationality, and month of birth, a slightly increased OR of premature birth was found for a 50-$\mu g/m^3$ increase in mean concentration of each pollutant. For exposure during the first trimester, SO_2 had an OR of 1.27 (95% CI 1.16-1.39); TSP had an OR of 1.18 (95% CI 1.05-1.31), and NO_x an OR of 1.10 (95% CI 1.00-1.21). Associations with pollutants in the second and third trimester were similar to those found in the first trimester. The study did not adjust for maternal smoking, which is an important risk factor for preterm birth.

Liu et al (2003) studied the relationship between ambient air pollution and preterm birth, LBW, and IUGR among singleton live births in Vancouver, Canada. Ambient exposure to SO_2, NO_2, CO, and O_3 were linked with data obtained from the live-birth database maintained by Statistics Canada. Maternal residence during pregnancy was used to explore exposure during several periods throughout pregnancy: the first, second, and third months of pregnancy and the last and next-to-last months of pregnancy. In addition, exposure during the three trimesters was calculated. They found increased adjusted ORs for preterm birth and SO_2 (OR 1.09, 95% CI 1.01-1.19) and CO (1.08, 95% CI 1.01-1.15) during the last month of pregnancy but not during the first month. The association between preterm birth and SO_2 and CO remained after adjustment for other copollutants. Although the data are not presented, the authors note that they did not find associations between PM_{10} and any of the outcomes. However, they had only 5 years of available data on PM_{10} because there were a small number of births during that period. Overall, the study was of high quality, but a potential limitation is the lack of control for maternal smoking, a risk factor for preterm birth.

A case-control study of preterm and LBW babies in relation to traffic density in Los Angeles County in 1994-1996 was conducted (Wilhelm and Ritz 2003). For each subject, the authors assigned an annual average exposure by using a model of the distance-weighted traffic density and the location of the subject's residence. The traffic density was the same in each trimester. However, the effect was strongest for the last trimester. The magnitude of the preterm-birth effect was small, but there was an increase in preterm births, with an RR of 1.08 (95% CI 1.01-1.51) for the highest quintile of exposure. There was an increased risk of full-term LBW, but no exposure-response relationship was found. In these analyses, the authors adjusted for infant sex, maternal age, maternal race or ethnicity, maternal education, birth season, year of analysis, and other covariates but could not adjust for such potential covariates as active and passive smoking. Because maternal smoking is related to SES indicators, which were included in the models, smoking was probably at least partially accounted for in the multivariate analyses.

Xu et al. (1995) conducted a prospective cohort study of 25,370 pregnant women in Beijing, China, in 1988. Beijing has high ambient mean concentrations of SO_2 (102 $\mu g/m^3$) and TSP (375 $\mu g/m^3$). Air-monitoring data on TSP and SO_2 concentrations were collected, and their effect on preterm births was studied with a time-series analysis of lagged moving averages. After adjustment for several confounders—including season, maternal age, and residential area—increased risks of preterm birth with increased TSP and SO_2 exposure were found. Although the study was well designed, it explored only acute effects of pollutant exposure up to 7 days before delivery.

A case-control study of VLBW (<1500 grams at birth) was conducted in the state of Georgia (Rogers et al. 2000). VLBW babies were largely preterm, so the study was unable to examine the effects of air pollutants on fetal growth independently of the preterm effects. Comparison of 143 mothers of VLBW babies with 202 mothers of babies that weighed more than 2,500 g on the basis of birth records (1986-1988) and face-to-face interviews showed a dose-response relationship between VLBW and increasing maternal exposure to SO_2 and TSP. Complex environmental-transport modeling was performed, and exposure at the birth home and annual average TSP and SO_2 concentrations were estimated for each subject. Although associations were found between the risk of having a VLBW babies and exposures to SO_2 and TSP above the 95th percentile, the study was unable to differentiate between exposures throughout pregnancy and those in the first trimester.

An ecologic design was used to compare Teplice, a highly polluted district in the Czech Republic (where high-sulfur coal is combusted, with Prachatice, a less polluted one (Sram et al. 1996). Teplice's SO_2 and TSP concentrations in winter 1993, for example, were comparable with those in the infamous London fog of 1952. The authors found a higher prevalence of preterm births (6.2% vs 3.4%, $p < 0.01$) in Teplice, but they were not able to adjust for covariates. It was noted that preterm birth was highly related to maternal smoking status.

In summary, the well-designed study of Ritz et al. (2000) found evidence of a relationship between preterm birth and combustion-product exposure. Its analysis controlled for several known risk factors for preterm birth (such as maternal age, race, education, and access to prenatal care). Several other studies reviewed by the committee provide supportive evidence of a relationship (Bobak 2000; Liu et al. 2003; Wilhelm and Ritz 2003).

The committee concludes, from its assessment of the epidemiologic literature, that there is limited/suggestive evidence of an association between combustion-product exposure during pregnancy and preterm birth, but the data provided inadequate/insufficient evidence of an association between combustion-product exposure at specific periods during pregnancy (for example, first trimester) and preterm birth.

Low Birthweight and Intrauterine Growth Retardation

LBW (birthweight <2500 g) affects 5-8% of pregnancies in the United States (Ventura et al. 1998). Retarded fetal growth (IUGR) refers to birthweight falling below the 10th percentile of national standards. Its known risk factors include infant sex and race, maternal weight gain, cigarette-smoking, and alcohol consumption. LBW can be the result of either preterm birth or retarded fetal growth in a preterm or full-term birth. LBW is a measure of retarded fetal growth if a study's analysis adjusts for gestational age or is restricted to full-term births. Most studies evaluated in this section examined full-term births for LBW and IUGR and excluded preterm births (Table 7.3).

TABLE 7.3 Low Birthweight or Intrauterine Growth Retardation and Combustion-Product Exposure

Reference	Population	Pollutant Measured and Exposure Period	Adjusted OR (95% CI or p) by Period and Pollutant	Adjustments	Limitations
Dejmek et al. 1999	Czech Republic 1994-1996	$PM_{2.5}$ (low, <27 μg/m^3; medium, 27 μg/m^3 to <37 μg/m^3; high, ≥37 μg/m^3) PM_{10} (low, <40 μg/m^3; medium, 40 μg/m^3 to <50 μg/m^3; high, ≥50 μg/m^3) Each month of gestation	IUGR: $PM_{2.5}$ Month 1, medium level: OR 1.26, 95% CI 0.81-1.95 Month 1, high level: OR 2.11, 95% CI 1.20-3.70 Other pregnancy months nonsignificant PM_{10} Month 1, medium level: OR 1.62, 95% CI 1.07-2.50 Month 1, high level: OR 2.64, 95% CI 1.48-4.71 Other pregnancy months nonsignificant	Year, season, smoking, maternal height, prepregnancy weight, completed high school	
Dejmek et al. 2000 (same population as Dejmek et al 1999)	Czech Republic 1994-1998	PAH, PM_{10}	IUGR: PAH (Teplice) Month 1, medium level: OR 1.59 95% CI 1.06-2.39 Month 1, high level: OR 2.15, 95% CI 1.27-3.63 PM_{10} (Teplice): Month 1, medium level: OR 1.44 95% CI 1.03-2.02 Month 1, high level: OR 2.14 95% CI 1.42-3.23	Year, season, smoking, maternal height, prepregnancy weight, completed high school	

Reference	Population	Pollutant Measured and Exposure Period	Adjusted OR (95% CI or p) by Period and Pollutant	Adjustments	Limitations
Support Studies					
Bobak 2000	126,752 live births, Czech Republic 1991	SO_2, TSP, NO_2 Trimesters 1-3	LBW: SO_2 per 50-µg increase Trimester 1: OR 1.01, 95% CI 0.88-1.17 Trimester 2: OR 0.95, 95% CI 0.82-1.10 Trimester 3: OR 0.97, 95% CI 0.85-1.10 TSP per 50-µg increase Trimester 1: OR 1.13, 95% CI 0.93-1.38 Trimester 2: OR 1.14, 95% CI 0.92-1.40 Trimester 3: OR 1.14, 95% CI 0.93-1.38 No association between pollutants and IUGR	Gestational age; sex of child, parity; maternal age group, education, marital status, nationality; month of birth	No adjustment for maternal smoking
Lee et al. 2003	388,105 live births, South Korea 1996-1998	CO, PM_{10} Trimesters 1-3 Months 1-5 Months 6-10	LBW: CO Trimester 1: OR 1.04, 95% CI 1.01-1.07 Trimester 2: OR 1.04, 95% CI 1.00-1.06 Trimester 3: OR 0.96, 95% CI 0.93-0.99 Months 1-5: OR 1.06, 95% CI 0.98-1.14 Months 6-10: OR 0.88, 95% CI 0.79-0.99 PM_{10} Trimester 1: OR 1.03, 95% CI 1.00-1.07 Trimester 2:OR 1.04, 95% CI 1.00-1.08 Trimester 3: OR 1.00, 95% 0.95-1.04 Months 1-5: OR 1.04, 95% CI 1.01-1.08 Months 6-10: OR 0.94, 95% CI 0.85-1.05	Date, gestational age, infant sex, maternal age, parental education	No adjustment for maternal smoking

Reference	Population	Pollutant Measured and Exposure Period	Adjusted OR (95% CI or p) by Period and Pollutant	Adjustments	Limitations
Liu et al. 2003	229,095 live births, Vancouver, Canada 1986-1998	SO_2, NO_2, CO, Ozone Month 1 Last Month	IUGR: SO_2 per 5-ppb increase: Month 1: OR 1.07, 95% CI 1.01-1.13 NO_2 per 10-ppb increase: Month 1: OR 1.05, 95% CI 1.01-1.11 CO per 1-ppm increase: Month 1: OR 1.06, 95% CI 1.01-1.10 O_3: Month 1: OR 0.99, 95% CI 0.93-1.04	Maternal age, parity, infant sex, gestational age or birthweight, month of birth	
Maisonet et al. 2001	89,557 live births, northeastern United States 1994-1996	CO, PM_{10}, SO_2 Trimesters 1-3	LBW: CO per 1-ppm increase Trimester 1: OR 1.08, 95% CI 0.91-128 Trimester 2: OR 1.14, 95% CI 0.83-1.58 Trimester 3: OR 1.31, 95% CI 1.06-1.62 SO_2 per 10-ppm increase Trimester 1: OR 0.98, 95% CI 0.93-1.03 Trimester 2: OR 1.01, 95% CI 0.93-1.10 Trimester 3: OR 1.01, 95% CI 0.86-1.20 PM_{10} per 10-$\mu g/m^3$ increase Trimester 1: OR 0.93, 95% CI 0.85-1.00 Trimester 2: OR0.93, 95% CI 0.85-1.02 Trimester 3: OR0.96, 95% CI 0.88-1.06	Gestational age; alcohol, smoking; maternal education, age, race or ethnicity, marital status, weight gain, previous terminations; infant sex; season; gestational age, and so on.	

Reference	Population	Pollutant Measured and Exposure Period	Adjusted OR (95% CI or p) by Period and Pollutant	Adjustments	Limitations
Wang et al. 1997	74,671 live births, China 1988-1991	SO_2, TSP Trimesters 1-3	LBW: SO_2 per 100-μg/m^3 increase Trimesters 1, 2 NS after adjusting for trimester 3 Trimester 3: OR 1.11 95% CI 1.06-1.16 TSP per 100-μg/m^3 increase Trimesters 1, 2 NS after adjusting for Trimester 3 Trimester 3: OR 1.10 95% CI 1.05-1.14	Gestational age, residence, year of birth, maternal age, and infant sex.	No adjustment for maternal smoking, but few women in China during study period smoked, so smoking unlikely to be important confounder
Ritz & Yu 1999	125,573 live births, Los Angeles 1989-1993	CO Trimester 3	LBW: CO: 2.2 to <5 ppm OR 1.04, 95% CI 0.96-1.13 ≥ 5 ppm OR 1.22, 95% CI 1.03-1.44	Gestational age; female child; maternal race, education, age; no prenatal care; and so on	Did not examine trimesters 1-2

Two studies of full-term births were published in the Czech Republic (Dejmek et al. 1999, 2000). One of the primary sources of particles in those populations is coal combustion. The first study was of all live singleton births in the heavily polluted district of Teplice, Czech Republic, covering the period 1994-1996 (Dejmek et al. 1999), and the second study covered the years 1994-1998 (Dejmek et al. 2000). The first study examined the effects of PM_{10} exposure during each month of pregnancy. Of the 1,943 enrolled women who gave birth to full-term singleton infants (at 37-43 weeks of gestation), nearly 10% delivered a child who had IUGR. The study also collected information from questionnaires and medical records in addition to vital statistics and environmental monitoring. After adjustment for relevant confounders—including maternal smoking, year, and season—there were associations between IUGR and PM_{10} and $PM_{2.5}$ exposure during the first month of pregnancy. In particular, the OR for medium exposure to PM_{10} was 1.62 (95% CI 1.07-2.50) and for high exposure 2.64 (95% CI 1.48-4.71); for $PM_{2.5}$, the OR for medium exposure was 1.26 (95% CI 0.81-1.95) and for high exposure 2.11 (95% CI 1.20-3.70). ORs for exposures during the other 8 months of pregnancy were mostly close to 1.0. The study was well designed and statistically powerful, controlling for relevant risk factors and assessing first-trimester exposure separately from exposure in other periods.

Another study (Dejmek et al. 2000) examined whether exposure to polycyclic aromatic hydrocarbons (PAHs), usually bound to fine particles, was associated with IUGR in full-term births. The study included a comparison district (Prachatice) with lower pollution. This study was not an independent dataset from the earlier Dejmek et al. study discussed above. It expanded the period of study to 4 years and was designed to explore associations with components of the particles. In multivariate models that adjusted for confounders, higher PAH concentrations during the first month of gestation increased the risk of IUGR and the adjusted ORs were 1.59 (95% CI 1.06-2.39) for medium exposure and 2.15 (95% CI 1.27-3.63) for high exposure. The authors concluded that the risk of delivering a growth-retarded infant increased with the concentration of fine particles and PAHs in the first month of gestation.

Bobak (2000) conducted a study of all singleton live births registered in 1991 by the Czech Republic (n = 126,752 singleton live births). The study linked Czech national birth-register data with area-based measures of air pollution in 67 districts where at least one pollutant was measured (n = 108,173). Maternal exposures to outdoor SO_2, TSP, and NO_2 in each trimester of pregnancy were studied in relation to LBW, IUGR (<10th percentile of birthweight for gestational age and sex) and prematurity (results were given in the previous section). After adjustment for sex of infant, education, parity, age, marital status of mother, and month of birth, LBW was associated with SO_2 and TSP (OR 1.2, 95% CI 1.11-1.30 and 1.15, 95% CI 1.07-1.24, respectively, for a 50-$\mu g/m^3$ increase in mean SO_2 and TSP concentrations in first trimester). When gestational age was also adjusted for, the relationship with SO_2 was substantially weaker, but the TSP relationship remained strong although the confidence interval widened and included the null value. Prematurity was also associated with SO_2, TSP, and NO_2 concentrations during the first trimester (as described in the previous section). Associations in the second and third trimesters were similar to those found in the first trimester; this was expected because there were correlations between pollutants across trimesters. One potential limitation of the study is the lack of control for maternal smoking, a risk factor for LBW.

A study explored the relationship between LBW and exposure to air pollution in South Korea during different gestational phases (Lee et al. 2003). Birthweight was extracted from birth certificates for all full-term singletons born at 37-44 weeks gestational weeks (n = 388,105). Air pollution monitoring data were used to assign exposure during each trimester and each month of pregnancy. After adjustment for sex, birth order, maternal age, parental education level, and gestational age, first-trimester CO and PM_{10} exposure increased LBW risk (OR 1.04, 95% CI 1.01-1.07 and OR 1.03, 95% CI 1.00-1.07, respectively), as did second-trimester exposure to PM_{10}, SO_2, and NO_2, for which ORs were generally between 1.03 and 1.06 with narrow confidence intervals reflecting the large sample size. There were positive (small) dose-response relationships between LBW and CO during the first trimester and LBW and PM_{10} and SO_2 during the second trimester. Point estimates of effect in the third trimester ranged between 0.96 and 1.00. In the monthly analyses, the risk of LBW were higher for CO exposure in months 2-5 and for PM_{10} in months 2-4 than in later months. For SO_2 and NO_2, exposure in months 3-5 was associated with LBW. Further analyses, dividing exposure into the first 5 months and the last months also suggested that earlier exposure was associated with LBW. Exposure during the first 5 months was associated with LBW even if air pollution was low during the last 5 months. A potential limitation is the lack of control for maternal smoking, a risk factor for LBW. Overall, the study found evidence of an association between LBW and early-pregnancy exposure, primarily during the first 5 months.

Liu et al. (2003), as noted in the previous section, explored the relationship between ambient air pollution and preterm birth, LBW, and IUGR among singleton live births in Vancouver, Canada. IUGR was studied only in full-term births. The authors found an increased adjusted OR for LBW and maternal exposure to SO_2 during the first month of pregnancy (OR 1.11, 95% CI 1.01-1.22 per 5-ppb increase). The LBW-SO_2 association persisted even after adjustment for the other pollutants. IUGR was also associated with exposure to NO_2, SO_2, CO during the first month of pregnancy but not during the last month. IUGR was associated with SO_2 and CO exposure during the first trimester. Overall, the study was of high quality. One potential limitation is the lack of control for maternal smoking, a risk factor for adverse pregnancy outcomes.

A study examined the relationship between ambient air pollution in six northeastern US cities and full-term LBW among 89,557 singleton live births (Maisonet et al. 2001). Average exposure during each trimester was estimated for each study subject on the basis of maternal residence from the birth certificate. In the multivariate analyses, an association was found between LBW and third-trimester CO (adjusted OR 1.31 per 1-ppm increase, 95% CI 1.06-1.62). The models adjusted for maternal smoking during pregnancy, alcohol consumption, maternal education, maternal age, maternal race or ethnicity, marital status, weight gain during pregnancy, previous terminations, infant sex, season of birth, prenatal care, gestational age, and other pollutants. No associations were found between LBW and first- or second-trimester CO exposure or between LBW and exposure to PM_{10} in any trimester. Second-trimester SO_2 exposure was not associated with LBW when it was used as a continuous variable; there were some associations when second-trimester SO_2 exposure was entered into the models in quintiles. This high-quality study was well designed and statistically powerful. It controlled for relevant risk factors and assessed first-trimester exposure separately from other periods, but found consistent associations only with third-trimester CO exposure. The ORs between LBW and first-trimester exposure to the three pollutants were consistently less than 1.0.

A community-based study of all pregnant women in four residential areas of Beijing, China, was conducted (Wang et al. 1997). First-parity single live full-term births (n = 74,671) were studied in relation to average TSP and SO_2 exposure at various times throughout pregnancy, means during each trimester, and lagged moving averages in weeks before birth. After adjustment, third-trimester exposure to TSP and SO_2 was most strongly associated with

LBW: ORs increased by a factor of 1.11 for each 100-μg/m^3 increase in SO_2 (95% CI 1.06-1.16) and 1.10 (95% CI 1.05-1.14) for TSP. The other exposure variables, TSP and SO_2 at other times, had little predictive value after adjustment for third-trimester exposure. Most analyses adjusted for gestational age, residence, year of birth, maternal age, and infant sex. Small negative associations between LBW and first- and second-trimester exposure suggested lower risk with higher exposure. Although maternal smoking was not adjusted for, the authors note that few women in China during the study period smoked. Residential exposure to combustion products from burning fuel or cooking are other potentially important confounders which were not adjusted for in this study.

Another study examined the effect of ambient CO on LBW among full-term infants in southern California (Ritz and Yu 1999). It limited exposure assessments to the third trimester because there was evidence that smoking-related effects are mediated by hypoxia during the last trimester. Although not directly informative on first-trimester exposures, the study supports associations between LBW and third trimester exposure. For CO exposure at more than 5.5 ppm, there was a 22% increase in LBW (OR 1.22, 95% CI 1.03-1.44).

Some published studies (for example, Bobak and Leon 1999; Sram et al. 1996; Vassilev et al. 2001a, 2001b) were cross-sectional or ecologic studies and did not differentiate between early-pregnancy exposure (first trimester) and exposure throughout pregnancy. One study (Perera et al. 2003) was only of third-trimester PAH exposure, and another (Wilhelm and Ritz 2003), although well designed, studied traffic patterns in relation to LBW but did not distinguish between first-trimester exposure and exposure throughout pregnancy.

It is not now possible to identify critical periods of gestation during which exposure is associated with increased risks of LBW and IUGR. The data among studies are not consistent: some studies found associations between LBW and early-pregnancy exposure to specific pollutants (for example, Dejmek et al. 1999), between LBW and late-pregnancy exposures to specific pollutants (for example, Maisonet et al. 2001; Ritz and Yu 1999; Wang et al. 1997), or between LBW and exposure to specific pollutants during both early and late pregnancy (for example, Dejmek et al. 2000); others failed to find associations between LBW or IUGR and either early or late exposure to specific pollutants (for example, Bobak 2000; Maisonet et al. 2001). Identifying a specific period of vulnerability is especially difficult because ambient exposures at different times are correlated, and most studies did not adjust for exposure at different points in pregnancy. One study (Lee et al. 2003) attempted to do that and found the most consistent associations with exposures during the first 5 months (that is, the first and second trimesters), a period that overlaps with but is longer than the period of Gulf War exposure. In conclusion, there is inadequate evidence to conclude that early-pregnancy exposure alone, independently of middle- and late-pregnancy exposure to air pollutants, is associated with full-term LBW and IUGR. Although the evidence on exposure during any time during pregnancy and adverse pregnancy end points is accumulating, further studies are needed to determine the relevant exposure time. Studies adjusting for exposure at different times during gestation would be especially informative.

The two studies conducted in the Czech Republic (Dejmek et al. 1999, 2000) were well designed studies and found evidence of a relationship between LBW or IUGR and combustion-product exposure. Their analyses controlled for several known risk factors, including maternal smoking. Several other studies reviewed by the committee provide supportive evidence of a relationship (Bobak 2000; Lee et al. 2003; Liu et al. 2003; Maisonet et al. 2001; Ritz and Yu 1999; Wang et al. 1997) but most were unable to adjust for maternal smoking.

The committee concludes, from its assessment of the epidemiologic literature, that there is limited/suggestive evidence of an association between combustion product exposure during pregnancy and low birthweight or intrauterine growth retardation, but the data provided inadequate/insufficient evidence of an association between combustion-product exposure at specific periods during pregnancy (for example, the first trimester) and low birthweight and intrauterine growth retardation.

Birth Defects

The association between maternal exposure to air pollutants and the risk of birth defects in southern California was studied during 1987-1993 (Ritz et al. 2002). With a population-based, case-control method, average monthly exposure was assigned to birth-defect cases and control pregnancies (n = 10,649) on the basis of ambient-air monitoring data related to maternal residence during gestation. Dose-response relationships were found between cardiac defects and increasing exposure to CO and O_3 during the second month of gestation. In the case of CO, the risk of ventricular septal defect was increased (ORs per quartile of exposure 1.62-2.95). In the case of O_3, the risk of aortic artery and valve defects, pulmonary artery and valve anomalies, and conotruncal defects was similarly increased.

Three studies examined the association between paternal employment as a firefighter and the risk of cardiac birth defects. A case-control study considered 20 birth defect groups in 22,192 live births in British Columbia (Olshan et al. 1990). After adjustment for paternal age and race and maternal age, increased ORs were reported for paternal firefighting and ventricular septal defects (OR 2.7, 95% CI 1.02-7.18) and atrial septal defects (OR 5.91, 95% CI 1.60-21.83), compared with all other occupations. Increased ORs for both types of cardiac defects were also observed when firemen were compared with policemen. The second comparison group was selected to reduce potential confounding due to lifestyle factors and SES. Because the study relied on limited occupational information from birth registers, it was not possible to identify whether the firefighter fathers were urban or rural. However, the investigators tested whether there was any relationship between the year of a child's birth and paternal employment as firefighter, hypothesizing that the risk of birth defects might have increased with increasing use of synthetic materials over the study period of 1952-1973. The findings suggest that paternal employment as a firefighter increases a child's risk of being born with a ventricular or atrial septal defect. No specific information was available about duration of paternal firefighting and potential confounding factors beyond paternal age and race and maternal age.

A cohort study of 836 infants of firefighters in Sweden was conducted (Kallen and Pradat 1992). There was no increased risk of cardiac defects (RR 0.93, 95% CI 0.38-1.92). Ventricular and atrial septal defects were examined separately, but no increased risk was found among infants fathered by firemen. The cohort, however, was relatively small and thus of limited statistical power.

In a study of maternal or paternal exposure, Bates et al. (1997) studied all types of birth defects (ICD codes 40-759) in the offspring of parents living in Rotorua, New Zealand, a city with high geothermal exposure to hydrogen sulfide. No excess birth defects were reported in comparison with residents in the rest of New Zealand. The Bates studies were the only epidemiologic studies of H_2S found by the committee that examined long-term health outcomes. Due to the paucity of literature, the committee did not make a separate conclusion on H_2S.

The committee concludes, from its assessment of the epidemiologic literature, that there is inadequate/insufficient evidence of an association between maternal and paternal combustion product exposure prior to conception or maternal exposure during early pregnancy and specific birth defects, including cardiac effects.

Childhood Cancers

Several childhood cancers have been investigated in relation to combustion-product exposure before birth (that is, before or during gestation): brain cancer, leukemia, and neuroblastoma. Each of those can arise from embryonic cells or poorly differentiated cells. Most studies of childhood cancer used case-control designs and examined cancer in relation to parental exposure.

A California statewide, population-based cancer registry was used to identify cancers diagnosed in children who were less than 5 years old in 1988-1997 (Reynolds et al. 2004). The 4,369 cases were matched to 8,730 controls by birth date and sex. A mother's residential address at the time of her child's birth was used to calculate traffic density. For all cancer sites combined, the OR for the highest traffic-density exposure category compared with the lowest was 0.87 (95% CI 0.75-1.0). For all sites combined and for leukemia, the ORs were also below 1.0. For CNS tumors, the OR was 1.22 (CI 0.87-1.70). The authors found no increase in risk of cancer or leukemia among offspring of mothers living in high traffic density areas.

Raaschou-Nielsen et al. (2001) studied 1,989 children in the Danish Cancer Registry who had leukemia, CNS tumors, or malignant lymphoma diagnosed during 1968-1991 and 5,506 randomly selected control children from the entire childhood population. Residential histories of cases and controls were traced from 9 months before birth until the time of diagnosis. Traffic patterns and concentrations of benzene and NO_2 were calculated for the relevant period, and exposures to air pollution during pregnancy and during childhood were calculated separately. The risks of leukemia, CNS tumors, and all selected cancers combined were not linked to benzene or NO_2, but the risk of lymphomas (specifically Hodgkin's disease) increased by 25% (p for trend = 0.06) and 51% (p for trend = 0.05) with a doubling of the concentration of benzene and NO_2, respectively during pregnancy. The authors note that traffic-related air pollution at the residence does not appear to be associated with leukemias, CNS tumors, or NHL in children. The Hodgkin's disease finding was of borderline significance in univariate models and may be a chance finding or due to multiple testing.

Results from the United Kingdom Childhood Cancer Study were analyzed (McKinney et al. 2003). Eligible cases were children who had a diagnosed malignant disease (including childhood leukemia, ALL, and brain cancer) or specified benign tumor. Cases were 0-14 years while a resident in England, Scotland, or Wales. Controls were randomly selected from the same family-health services in England and Wales and health boards in Scotland. There were 3,838 cases and 7,629 controls. Parents were interviewed to obtain an occupational history. Job titles and associated industries were coded according to the Standard Occupational Classification and Standard Industrial Classification of Economic Activities, respectively. The authors created 31 occupational groups by combining job titles considered to entail the same specific exposures. Timing of parental occupational exposure was also taken into account. When examining fathers occupationally exposed to combustion products at periconception, the authors found small increased risks for childhood leukemia and ALL. (Owing to substantial overlap between three occupational groups with "exhaust fumes" exposure, parents with some jobs may have been exposed to more than one of the agents and therefore included in more than one of the analyses.)

For ALL, paternal exposure to exhaust fumes at periconception had an OR of 1.26 (95% CI 1.02-1.56); exposure to inhaled particulate hydrocarbons, 1.41 (95% CI 1.11-1.79); and driving, 1.26 (95% CI 1.00-1.59). For leukemia, the ORs for paternal exposures were 1.33 (95% CI 1.09-1.61), 1.48 (95% CI 1.19-1.84), and 1.36 (95% CI 1.10-1.68), respectively. For CNS tumors, the ORs for paternal exposure to exhaust fumes and inhaled particulate hydrocarbons at periconception were 1.08 and 1.13, respectively, but the 95% CI included the null. For ALL, maternal exposure to exhaust fumes had an OR of 1.68 (95% CI 0.76-3.74); exposure to inhaled particulate hydrocarbons, 2.26 (95% CI 0.79-6.45); and driving, 1.74 (95% CI 0.63-4.85); but the 95% CIs included the null. The major limitations of this study are the nonspecific assessment of exposure based on occupation and the inability to account for other confounding exposures in the occupational groups. In addition, the creation of 31 occupational groups led to multiple comparisons and raised caution in interpreting the results. The strengths of the study include its size and population-based design.

Vianna et al. (1984) conducted a case-control study of acute leukemia and neuroblastoma. Trained interviewers questioned the mother of each patient and control. Several control groups were used, including children chosen from birth certificates and matched to cases on several risk factors. The neuroblastoma cases were also used as a control group to explore whether the quality of information obtained from parents of children with leukemia and the parents of controls without a malignancy might differ, assuming that neuroblastoma did not share the risk factors of interest with leukemia. Exposure to aromatic hydrocarbons from gasoline exhaust was defined as working full-time in a specified occupation for at least a year before the birth of the child. The authors did not find an association between exposure to aromatic hydrocarbons and increased risk of neuroblastoma, but did report a higher risk of leukemia in patients whose fathers worked in high-exposure occupations ($p = 0.007$). The primary study limitation is reliance on occupational groups to assign measures of exposure to combustion products. However, that limitation would most likely bias results toward the null.

The relationship between parental occupation and leukemia and brain tumors in children was explored (Gold et al. 1982). A nonspecific measure of exposure to combustion products was used (motor-vehicle-related and including driver, motor-vehicle mechanic, service-station attendant, and railroad worker and engineer). There was an increased risk of leukemia in children whose fathers had vehicle-related occupations ($p < 0.05$). No association was observed for brain cancer and vehicle-related occupations. The study is limited by the concurrent exposures to multiple agents in the fathers' occupations.

Cordier et al. (1997) conducted a population-based, case-control study of childhood brain tumors (251 cases and 601 controls) in three European centers. A Job-Exposure Matrix (JEM) was used to estimate parental occupational exposure to PAHs during the 5-year period before birth. Paternal occupation described as motor-vehicle-related had an OR of 1.6 (95% CI 1.0-2.8). The subset of cases with primitive neuroectodermal tumors had an OR of 2.7 (95% CI 1.1-6.6). They also described increased risks, although no dose-response relationship, with paternal exposure specifically to PAHs; the OR for medium exposure 1.8 (95% CI 1.2-2.6), and the OR for high exposure was 1.3 (95% CI 0.8-2.0). Maternal occupation was not associated with increased risk. The study limitations include the use of maternal recall to measure maternal and paternal occupations and the nonspecificity of jobs categorized as PAH-exposed.

No association was found between childhood nervous system tumors and occupational groups broadly defined as hydrocarbon-related (Johnson et al. 1987). Another study (Hakulinen et al. 1976) found similar results in demonstrating no association between brain tumors, leukemia, and lymphoma and paternal occupations described nonspecifically as hydrocarbon-related.

A case-control study of childhood leukemia and parental occupation did not find an increased risk with occupational exposure to exhaust gases (van Steensel-Moll et al. 1985), and another study (Zack et al. 1980) found no association between leukemia or lymphoma and paternal occupation as a motor-vehicle mechanic or service-station attendant. A study examining neuroblastoma and numerous paternal occupations, including firefighter and motor-vehicle operator, also found no increased risk (Olshan et al. 1999).

All the studies were limited by their inability to validate employment history. They also lacked details on specific assessment of exposure to combustion products. The broad exposure groups included many diverse occupations with exposure to other chemicals in addition to combustion products. In addition, the studies should be viewed cautiously because many of them conducted multiple comparisons. They are best used to generate hypotheses that require more precise assessment of exposure to combustion products.

The committee concludes, from its assessment of the epidemiologic literature, that there is inadequate/insufficient evidence of an association between parental combustion product exposure and all childhood cancers studied, including acute lymphocytic leukemia, leukemia, neuroblastoma, and brain cancer.

REFERENCES

ACS (American Cancer Society). 1999. *Childhood Cancer - General Statement.* [Online]. Available: http://www.cancer.org/downloads/CRI/Childhood%20Cancer%20-%20General%20Statement%20_PDF_.pdf [accessed February 21, 2002].

ACS. 2002a. *ACS: Brain and Spinal Cord Tumors in Children.* [Online]. Available: http://www.cancer.org/downloads/CRI/Brain%20and%20Spinal%20Cord%20Tumors%20in%20Children%20_PDF_.pdf [accessed February 21, 2002].

ACS. 2002b. *Childhood Leukemia.* [Online]. Available: http://www.cancer.org/downloads/CRI/Childhood%20Leukemia%20_PDF_.pdf [accessed February 21, 2002].

Akefeldt A, Anvret M, Grandell U, Nordlinder R, Gillberg C. 1995. Parental exposure to hydrocarbons in Prader-Willi syndrome. *Developmental Medicine and Child Neurology* 37(12):1101-1109.

Araneta MR, Kamens DR, Zau AC, Gastanaga VM, Schlangen KM, Hiliopoulos KM, Gray GC. 2004. Conception and pregnancy during the Persian Gulf War: The risk to women veterans. *Annals of Epidemiology* 14(2):109-116.

Araneta MR, Moore CA, Olney RS, Edmonds LD, Karcher JA, McDonough C, Hiliopoulos KM, Schlangen KM, Gray GC. 1997. Goldenhar syndrome among infants born in military hospitals to Gulf War veterans. *Teratology* 56(4):244-251.

Araneta MR, Schlangen KM, Edmonds LD, Destiche DA, Merz RD, Hobbs CA, Flood TJ, Harris JA, Krishnamurti D, Gray GC. 2003. Prevalence of birth defects among infants of Gulf War veterans in Arkansas, Arizona, California, Georgia, Hawaii, and Iowa, 1989-1993. *Birth Defects Research Part A: Clinical and Molecular Teratology* 67(4):246-260.

Bates MN, Garrett N, Graham B, Read D. 1997. Air pollution and mortality in the Rotorua geothermal area. *Australian and New Zealand Journal of Public Health* 21(6):581-586.

Bobak M, Leon DA. 1999. Pregnancy outcomes and outdoor air pollution: An ecological study in districts of the Czech Republic 1986-8. *Occupational and Environmental Medicine* 56(8):539-543.

Bobak M. 2000. Outdoor air pollution, low birth weight, and prematurity. *Environmental Health Perspectives* 108(2):173-176.

Buckley JD, Robison LL, Swotinsky R, Garabrant DH, LeBeau M, Manchester P, Nesbit ME, Odom L, Peters JM, Woods WG. 1989. Occupational exposures of parents of children with acute nonlymphocytic leukemia: A report from the Childrens Cancer Study Group. *Cancer Research* 49(14):4030-4037.

Bunin GR, Buckley JD, Boesel CP, Rorke LB, Meadows AT. 1994. Risk factors for astrocytic glioma and primitive neuroectodermal tumor of the brain in young children: A report from the Children's Cancer Group. *Cancer Epidemiology, Biomarkers & Prevention* 3(3):197-204.

Carere A, Antoccia A, Cimini D, Crebelli R, Degrassi F, Leopardi P, Marcon F, Sgura A, Tanzarella C, Zijno A. 1998. Genetic effects of petroleum fuels: II. Analysis of chromosome loss and hyperploidy in peripheral lymphocytes of gasoline station attendants. *Environmental and Molecular Mutagenesis* 32(2):130-138.

Cassidy SB, Gainey AJ, Butler MG. 1989. Occupational hydrocarbon exposure among fathers of Prader-Willi syndrome patients with and without deletions of 15q. *American Journal of Human Genetics* 44(6):806-810.

Cordier S, Lefeuvre B, Filippini G, Peris-Bonet R, Farinotti M, Lovicu G, Mandereau L. 1997. Parental occupation, occupational exposure to solvents and polycyclic aromatic hydrocarbons and risk of childhood brain tumors (Italy, France, Spain). *Cancer Causes & Control* 8(5):688-697.

Cowan DN, DeFraites RF, Gray GC, Goldenbaum MB, Wishik SM. 1997. The risk of birth defects among children of Persian Gulf War veterans. *New England Journal of Medicine* 336(23):1650-1656.

De Roos AJ, Olshan AF, Teschke K, Poole C, Savitz DA, Blatt J, Bondy ML, Pollock BH. 2001. Parental occupational exposures to chemicals and incidence of neuroblastoma in offspring. *American Journal of Epidemiology* 154(2):106-114.

Dejmek J, Selevan SG, Benes I, Solansky I, Sram RJ. 1999. Fetal growth and maternal exposure to particulate matter during pregnancy. *Environmental Health Perspectives* 107(6):475-480.

Dejmek J, Solansky I, Benes I, Lenicek J, Sram RJ. 2000. The impact of polycyclic aromatic hydrocarbons and fine particles on pregnancy outcome. *Environmental Health Perspectives* 108(12):1159-1164.

Doyle P, Maconochie N, Davies G, Maconochie I, Pelerin M, Prior S, Lewis S. 2004. Miscarriage, stillbirth and congenital malformation in the offspring of UK veterans of the first Gulf war. *International Journal of Epidemiology* 33(1):74-86.

Gold EB, Diener MD, Szklo M. 1982. Parental occupations and cancer in children—a case-control study and review of the methodologic issues. *Journal of Occupational Medicine* 24(8):578-584.

Hakulinen T, Salonen T, Teppo L. 1976. Cancer in the offspring of fathers in hydrocarbon-related occupations. *British Journal of Preventive and Social Medicine* 30(2):138-140.

IARC (International Agency for Research on Cancer). 2000. *Ionizing Radiation, Part 1: X- and Gamma (g)-Radiation, and Neutrons.* 75. Lyon, France: IARC.

Johnson CC, Annegers JF, Frankowski RF, Spitz MR, Buffler PA. 1987. Childhood nervous system tumors—an evaluation of the association with paternal occupational exposure to hydrocarbons. *American Journal of Epidemiology* 126(4):605-613.

Kallen B, Pradat P. 1992. Re: "Birth defects among offspring of firemen". *American Journal of Epidemiology* 135(11):1318-1320.

Kang H, Magee C, Mahan C, Lee K, Murphy F, Jackson L, Matanoski G. 2001. Pregnancy outcomes among U.S. Gulf War veterans: A population-based survey of 30,000 veterans. *Annals of Epidemiology* 11(7):504-511.

Kerr MA, Nasca PC, Mundt KA, Michalek AM, Baptiste MS, Mahoney MC. 2000. Parental occupational exposures and risk of neuroblastoma: A case-control study (United States). *Cancer Causes and Control* 11(7):635-643.

Khalil AM. 1995. Chromosome aberrations in blood lymphocytes from petroleum refinery workers. *Archives of Environmental Contamination and Toxicology* 28(2):236-239.

Ledbetter DH, Cassidy SB. 1988. Etiology of Prader-Willi Syndrome. In: Caldwell ML, Taylor FL, eds. *Prader-Willi Syndrome: Selected Research and Management Issues.* New York: Springer; as cited in Cassidy et al. 1989.

Lee BE, Ha EH, Park HS, Kim YJ, Hong YC, Kim H, Lee JT. 2003. Exposure to air pollution during different gestational phases contributes to risks of low birth weight. *Human Reproduction* 18(3):638-643.

Lemasters GK, Olsen DM, Yiin JH, Lockey JE, Shukla R, Selevan SG, Schrader SM, Toth GP, Evenson DP, Huszar GB. 1999. Male reproductive effects of solvent and fuel exposure during aircraft maintenance. *Reproductive Toxicology* 13(3):155-166.

Liu S, Krewski D, Shi Y, Chen Y, Burnett RT. 2003. Association between gaseous ambient air pollutants and adverse pregnancy outcomes in Vancouver, Canada. *Environmental Health Perspectives* 111(14):1773-1778.

Lowengart RA, Peters JM, Cicioni C, Buckley J, Bernstein L, Preston-Martin S, Rappaport E. 1987. Childhood leukemia and parents' occupational and home exposures. *Journal of the National Cancer Institute* 79(1):39-46.

Magenis RE. 1988. On the origin of chromosome anomaly. *American Journal of Human Genetics* 42(4):529-533.

Maisonet M, Bush TJ, Correa A, Jaakkola JJ. 2001. Relation between ambient air pollution and low birth weight in the Northeastern United States. *Environmental Health Perspectives* 109(Suppl 3):351-356.

McKinney PA, Fear NT, Stockton D, UK Childhood Cancer Study Investigators. 2003. Parental occupation at periconception: Findings from the United Kingdom Childhood Cancer Study. *Occupational and Environmental Medicine* 60(12):901-909.

MMWR (Morbidity and Mortality Weekly Report). 1999. Preterm singleton births—United States, 1989-1996. *Morbidity and Mortality Weekly Report* 48(9):185-189.

Olshan AF, De Roos AJ, Teschke K, Neglia JP, Stram DO, Pollock BH, Castleberry RP. 1999. Neuroblastoma and parental occupation. *Cancer Causes and Control* 10(6):539-549.

Olshan AF, Teschke K, Baird PA. 1990. Birth defects among offspring of firemen. *American Journal of Epidemiology* 131(2):312-321.

Penman AD, Tarver RS, Currier MM. 1996. No evidence of increase in birth defects and health problems among children born to Persian Gulf War Veterans in Mississippi. *Military Medicine* 161(1):1-6.

Perera FP, Rauh V, Tsai WY, Kinney P, Camann D, Barr D, Bernert T, Garfinkel R, Tu YH, Diaz D, Dietrich J, Whyatt RM. 2003. Effects of transplacental exposure to environmental pollutants on birth outcomes in a multiethnic population. *Envirnomental Health Perspectives* 111(2):201-205.

Pschirrer ER, Monga M. 2000. Risk factors for preterm labor. *Clinical Obstetrics and Gynecology* 43(4):727-734.

PWSA (Prader-Willi Syndrome Association). 2004. *Basic Facts About the Prader-Willi Syndrome.* [Online]. Available: http://www.pwsausa.org/ [accessed September 13, 2004].

Raaschou-Nielsen O, Hertel O, Thomsen BL, Olsen JH. 2001. Air pollution from traffic at the residence of children with cancer. *American Journal of Epidemiology* 153(5):433-443.

Reynolds P, Von Behren J, Gunier RB, Goldberg DE, Hertz A. 2004. Residential exposure to traffic in California and childhood cancer. *Epidemiology* 15(1):6-12.

Ritz B, Yu F. 1999. The effect of ambient carbon monoxide on low birth weight among children born in Southern California between 1989 and 1993. *Environmental Health Perspectives* 107(1):17-25.

Ritz B, Yu F, Chapa G, Fruin S. 2000. Effect of air pollution on preterm birth among children born in Southern California between 1989 and 1993. *Epidemiology* 11(5):502-511.

Ritz B, Yu F, Fruin S, Chapa G, Shaw GM, Harris JA. 2002. Ambient air pollution and risk of birth defects in Southern California. *American Journal of Epidemiology* 155(1):17-25.

Rogers JF, Thompson SJ, Addy CL, McKeown RE, Cowen DJ, Decoufle P. 2000. Association of very low birth weight with exposures to environmental sulfur dioxide and total suspended particulates. *American Journal of Epidemiology* 151(6):602-613.

Ross JA, Swensen AR. 2000. Prenatal epidemiology of pediatric tumors. *Current Oncology Reports* 2(3):234-241.

Rowe PJ, Comhaire FH, Hargreave TB, Mellows HJ. 1993. *WHO Manual for the Standardized Investigation and Diagnosis of the Infertile Couple*. New York: Cambridge University Press.

San Sebastián M, Armstrong B, Stephens C. 2002. Outcomes of pregnancy among women living in the proximity of oil fields in the Amazon basin of Ecuador. *International Journal of Occupational and Environmental Health* 8(4):312-319.

Santos-Mello R, Cavalcante B. 1992. Cytogenetic studies on gas station attendants. *Mutation Research* 280(4):285-290.

Shu XO, Gao YT, Brinton LA, Linet MS, Tu JT, Zheng W, Fraumeni JF Jr. 1988. A population-based case-control study of childhood leukemia in Shanghai. *Cancer* 62(3):635-644.

Smith Ma, Suess JA. 1998. Obstetric complications during pregnancy. In: Taylor RB, ed. *Family Medicine: Principles and Practice*. 5th ed. New York: Springer. Pp. 106-121.

Speroff L, Glass RH, Kase NG. 1999. *Clinical Gynecologic Endocrinology and Infertility*. Philadelphia: Lippincott Williams & Wilkins.

Sram RJ, Benes I, Binkova B, Dejmek J, Horstman D, Kotesovec F, Otto D, Perreault SD, Rubes J, Selevan SG, Skalik I, Stevens RK, Lewtas J. 1996. Teplice Program - The impact of air pollution on human health. *Environmental Health Perspectives* 104(suppl. 4):699-714.

Strakowski SM, Butler MG. 1987. Paternal hydrocarbon exposure in Prader-Willi syndrome. *Lancet* 2(8573):1458.

Templeton A. 2000. Infertility and the establishment of pregnancy—overview. *British Medical Bulletin* 56(3):577-587.

van Steensel-Moll HA, Valkenburg HA, van Zanen GE. 1985. Childhood leukemia and parental occupation. A register-based case-control study. *American Journal of Epidemiology* 121(2):216-224.

Vassilev ZP, Robson MG, Klotz JB. 2001a. Outdoor exposure to airborne polycyclic organic matter and adverse reproductive outcomes: A pilot study. *American Journal of Industrial Medicine* 40(3):255-262.

Vassilev ZP, Robson MG, Klotz JB. 2001b. Associations of polycyclic organic matter in outdoor air with decreased birth weight: A pilot cross-sectional analysis. *Journal of Toxicology and Environmental Health. Part A* 64(8):595-605.

Ventura SJ, Martin JA, Curtin SC, Mathews TJ. 1998. *Report of final natality statistics, 1996. Monthly vital statistics report.* Hyattsville, MD: National Center for Health Statistics: Provisional statistics from the National Center for Health Statistics; as cited in Lee et al. 2003.

Vianna NJ, Kovasznay B, Polan A, Ju C. 1984. Infant leukemia and paternal exposure to motor vehicle exhaust fumes. *Journal of Occupational Medicine* 26(9):679-682.

Wang X, Ding H, Ryan L, Xu X. 1997. Association between air pollution and low birth weight: A community-based study. *Environmental Health Perspectives* 105(5):514-520.

Wilhelm M, Ritz B. 2003. Residential proximity to traffic and adverse birth outcomes in Los Angeles County, California, 1994-1996. *Environmental Health Perspectives* 111(2):207-216.

Xu X, Ding H, Wang X. 1995. Acute effects of total suspended particles and sulfur dioxides on preterm delivery: A community-based cohort study. *Archives of Environmental Health* 50(6):407-415.

Zack M, Cannon S, Loyd D, Heath CW Jr, Falletta JM, Jones B, Housworth J, Crowley S. 1980. Cancer in children of parents exposed to hydrocarbon-related industries and occupations. *American Journal of Epidemiology* 111(3):329-336.

8

OTHER HEALTH OUTCOMES

This chapter will review the epidemiologic literature on possible associations between exposure to fuels and combustion products and a variety of health outcomes: posttraumatic stress disorder, neurologic outcomes, multiple chemical sensitivity, dermatologic outcomes, and sarcoidosis. The outcomes discussed in this chapter do not necessarily have a large literature base, but they are reviewed here because there might be veterans who have an interest in them.

NEUROLOGIC OUTCOMES

The committee reviewed the epidemiologic literature on neurologic effects of exposure to fuels and combustion products, focusing on studies that examined long-term effects. Most studies were of occupational exposure.

The committee selected for detailed evaluation only the studies that met its inclusion criteria, which are listed below and discussed in Chapter 2. The first three criteria apply uniformly across all study outcomes; the fourth is reserved for outcomes that are reversible, that is, gradually abating over days or months after cessation of exposure.

- Methodologic rigor. The report of the study had to be a published in a peer-reviewed journal and had to include details of methodology; the study had to include a control or reference group, had to have the statistical power to detect effects, and had to include reasonable adjustment for confounders. Case studies and case series were generally excluded from the committee's consideration.
- Identification of class or agent. The study had to identify fuels or combustion products relevant to the committee's charge (for example, fuels might include gasoline, kerosene, diesel and jet fuel). If agents were not identified, the study may have been included if it was a study of an occupation that entailed a fuel or combustion-product exposure similar to presumed veterans' exposures in the Persian Gulf.
- Specificity of outcome. The study had to specify a distinct outcome rather than a nonspecific group of health outcomes. Lack of specificity occurs primarily in mortality studies that examine all-cause mortality (such as deaths from all nervous system diseases) as opposed to cause-specific mortality (such as deaths from Parkinson's disease). All-cause mortality studies were excluded unless they analyzed specific health outcomes separately.

- Exposure-free period for reversible neurologic effects. To be relevant to Gulf War veterans, the study had to examine long-term rather than short-term effects. Some neurologic outcomes can be determined only after an exposure-free period of weeks or months before evaluation of study subjects. The committee required an exposure-free period period specifically for effects that might be reversible (such as headache, light-headedness, poor coordination, and difficulty in concentrating), but not for irreversible effects (such as neurologic disease and peripheral neuropathy). The rationale for this criterion is described below.

The committee evaluated long-term effects because they are most relevant to the veterans' situation: exposure to fuels and combustion products during the Gulf War but symptoms that persist for years after the exposure. Long-term or very high exposure to fuels produce well-known short-term effects, including headache, light-headedness, poor coordination, difficulty in concentrating, tremors, myoclonus, and seizures (ATSDR 1995). The short-term effects are reversible and do not persist beyond hours or days after cessation of exposure. Long-term effects are often less well studied than short-term effects.

Occupational or other epidemiologic studies of neurologic effects often do not permit distinction between short-term effects (hours or weeks) and long-term effects (months or years), because many studies examine workers who have both past and current exposure. Consequently, if a study finds a neurologic effect (for instance, headache or fatigue), it is difficult to determine whether the effect will persist after cessation of the exposure unless an exposure-free period of weeks or months has passed before the effect is measured. Many of the available studies were not designed to determine whether an effect was a long-term or a short-term effect.

The challenge of distinguishing long-term and short-term effects is greater in the case of neurobehavioral effects than neurologic diseases for reasons related to onset, reversibility, and availability of objective testing. Neurobehavioral effects (such as symptoms of memory loss and fatigue) can be short-term effects, long-term effects, or both; they can appear within hours of exposure or later; and they can persist or disappear after cessation of exposure. Neurobehavioral effects cannot usually be verified with pathologic or biochemical tests, although objective and validated neurobehavioral tests of memory, attention, and other functions can be used in addition to symptom reporting (IOM 2003). Conversely, neurologic diseases are generally believed to be irreversible after a confirmed diagnosis and are associated with abnormal results of pathology or biochemistry tests. Thus, in evaluating the body of evidence, the committee required that there had been an exposure-free period of weeks or months before testing for a potentially reversible effect. For studies of peripheral neuropathy and neurologic diseases, the committee did not require an exposure-free period, because these effects are almost always long-lasting (although some degree of recovery or lack of progression is possible).

Fuels

This section covers fuel exposure and two neurologic effects: peripheral neuropathy and neurobehavioral effects. Some studies of neurologic effects, whether of those particular outcomes or others, were excluded by the committee for lack of methodologic rigor, nonspecific outcomes (Christie et al. 1987; Dagg et al. 1992; Hanis et al. 1985; Miller et al. 1986; Tsai et al. 1992; Wen et al. 1984), or lack of an exposure-free period in the case of reversible outcomes (Hakkola et al. 1997; Kilburn and Warshaw 1995; Kumar et al. 1988; Odkvist et al. 1987; Struwe et al. 1983).

Peripheral Neuropathy

The committee defined peripheral neuropathy as requiring a diagnosis with a thorough neurologic examination confirmed by quantitative laboratory testing, preferably using nerve-conduction studies and electromyography. Because peripheral neuropathy is often irreversible, the committee did not require a study to meet its criterion for an exposure-free period. Nevertheless, if the study reported *other* outcomes that were reversible (such as, symptoms or neurobehavioral effects), those findings were not evaluated in the absence of an exposure-free period.

Knave et al. (1976, 1978) studied peripheral neuropathy through symptom reporting, neurologic examination, and nerve-conduction studies among 29 aircraft-factory workers. Other neurologic symptoms or outcomes were not considered by the committee, because of the lack of an exposure-free interval period. The 1976 study had two jet-fuel exposure groups: heavily and less heavily exposed. No internal controls that lacked a history of exposure were included, but external controls in four other industries were used as the comparison group. The jet fuel was a mixture of gasoline and kerosene that included the aromatic hydrocarbons benzene, toluene, xylene, and trimethylbenzene. Neurologists evaluated symptoms of polyneuropathy: pain, temperature, touch, discriminative sensitivity, joint kinesthesia, and paresis. Symptoms of "restless legs" (62% vs 19%), pain (31% vs 13%) and paresthesias (77% vs 25%) were more frequent in the heavily exposed group than in the less heavily exposed group. Symptoms of polyneuropathy were more prevalent in the heavily than in the less heavily exposed (pain 30% vs 6%; temperature 69% vs 43%; discriminative sensitivity 15% vs 6%). No other symptoms were increased in the heavily exposed group. Remarkably, 19% of the less heavily exposed compared and none of the heavily exposed had diminished reflexes.

If the neuropathy symptoms are grouped, the heavily exposed workers had a higher frequency of those symptoms than did the less heavily exposed. The less heavily exposed had a higher frequency of symptoms than did four external control groups. An age-stratified analysis was attempted but the samples were too small. For most vibration-sensation measurements and conduction velocities, differences from one external control group were not noteworthy, except that there was a marked difference in hand-vibration threshold between the less heavily exposed group and one control group.

In the 1978 study, the same exposed jet-fuel workers were compared with internal controls that had no jet-fuel exposure (matched for age, employment duration, and education) (Knave et al. 1978). The electroneurographic studies included conduction velocities and action potentials of four major peripheral nerves. The results were conflicting because, although the exposed group displayed lower nerve action potentials in the sural nerve, the nonexposed group displayed slower ulnar and median conduction velocities. The differences were statistically significant. There were higher peripheral vibration thresholds in the exposed group, but differences were nonsignificant.

The overall results of those two studies indicated that although symptomatic differences are related to exposure, there were no objective measures to support a relationship between jet-fuel exposure and neuropathy. The limitations of the studies include small samples and the lack of an internal nonexposed group of controls.

The committee concludes, from its assessment of the epidemiologic literature, that there is inadequate/insufficient evidence to determine whether an association exists between exposure to fuels and peripheral neuropathy.

Neurobehavioral Effects

A team of Australian researchers (Maruff et al. 1998) studied neurologic and cognitive abnormalities in young adults engaged in chronic petrol-sniffing, a form of substance abuse relatively common in tribal groups, including aborigines. The study was of 33 current sniffers (over 6 months), 30 ex-sniffers (abstained for at least 6 months), and 34 nonsniffers in two remote aboriginal communities. Petrol-sniffing involves inhaling petrol directly from a 375-mL soft-drink can whose top has been removed and whose contents have been replaced with about 200 mL of leaded petrol. Petrol-sniffing induces euphoria, relaxation, and slurred speech. A total of 112 men were recruited for the study, but subjects were excluded if they had a history of any hospitalization for acute toxic encephalopathy from petrol-sniffing. Current petrol sniffers were required to abstain from sniffing for at least 12 hours before testing because acute effects of petrol-sniffing can last up to 6 hours. Exposure was based on blood lead and hydrocarbon concentrations and a semistructured interview (with medical-record comparison).

Neurobehavioral outcomes were measured with neurologic examination and 10 neurobehavioral tests in the Cambridge Neuropsychological Test Automated Battery. Conventional neuropsychologic tests of attention, memory, and learning were not suitable, because subjects were in remote communities where English was not the primary language. The Cambridge test battery is considered appropriate for cross-cultural use with an indigenous group for whom English is not the primary language.

Subjects were recruited with the aid of local community health workers, and paid research assistants were recruited from the same communities. On entry into the study, all subjects were interviewed about petrol-sniffing behavior, history of alcohol and other drug use, school attendance, and employment. Petrol-sniffing history was verified with three different methods: local community health-clinic records, assessment by local community health worker, and assessment by research assistants who spoke the same language. Current sniffers, ex-sniffers, and nonsniffers were similar in age (20 years), education, alcohol use, and cannabis use. The only significant difference among the three groups was that nonsniffers were more likely to be in full-time school or employment. Ex-sniffers had abstained for an average of 2.4 years. Current sniffers and ex-sniffers were similar in age at which petrol-sniffing began, number of 375-mL cans per week, years of sniffing (6.2-7.5 years). Current sniffers and ex-sniffers met or had met, respectively, Diagnostic and Statistical Manual of Mental Disorders-IV criteria for inhalant abuse. Current sniffers had significantly increased blood lead (in log micromoles per liter) compared with ex-sniffers and nonsniffers. Lead concentrations in gasoline in Australia are 0.4 and 0.8 g/L.

The physician who conducted the neurologic examination and the neuropsychologist who performed the cognitive-test battery were blinded to subjects' petrol-sniffing status. Ex-sniffers (the group with an exposure-free period of at least 6 months) displayed higher rates of abnormal tandem gait and bilateral palmomental reflexes than did nonsniffers. Ex-sniffers also displayed cognitive deficits in two areas of the test battery: visual-recognition memory and pattern-location paired-associates learning. Current sniffers had the highest rates of abnormal neurologic signs and cognitive deficits. Blood lead and length of time of sniffing correlated significantly with the magnitude of both neurologic and cognitive deficits, whereas blood hydrocarbon concentrations did not. Hydrocarbons or their metabolites, however, are quickly cleared from the blood and then excreted or stored in lipid-rich tissues.

Although hydrocarbons cannot be excluded as a contributor, lead is the most likely component of jet fuels that produces the observed long-term effects. The study found a correlation between blood lead and neurobehavioral outcomes and a lack of correlation between blood toluene or benzene and outcomes. Chronic lead exposure, accumulated over a lifetime, has been found within the last several years to be associated with cognitive deficits in adults (Muldoon et al. 1996; Payton et al. 1998). In the petrol-sniffers study by Maruff et al. (1998), relatively high tetraethyl lead exposure occurred, as indicated by the blood lead concentrations of 1.08 and 1.58 μmol/L in ex-sniffers and current sniffers, respectively. Those concentrations are likely to be much higher and of much longer duration than the ones possibly sustained by Gulf War veterans. No published studies of Gulf War veterans assayed for bone or blood lead, most likely because environmental lead concentrations during the Gulf War did not implicate lead as a health concern. The US Army Environmental Hygiene Agency, which collected more than 4,000 samples in its comprehensive air-monitoring program during the Gulf War's oil-well fires, found ambient lead (mean concentration 0.675 $\mu g/m^3$) which were orders of magnitude below US occupational standards and below the concentrations found in ambient air in most US cities (Rostker, 2000). Tent heaters were another possible source of lead exposure of US troops, but heaters typically burned kerosene and jet diesel fuel, neither of which contains lead as an additive. Lead is an additive only to gasoline. A study of tent-heater emissions with kerosene and jet fuels found lead in ambient air to be negligible, less than 0.1 ppm (Zhou and Cheng 2000).

Several population-based Gulf War studies found a relationship between veterans' self-reported fuel exposure and their self-reported neuropsychologic or cognitive symptoms or nonspecific symptoms (Iowa Persian Gulf Study Group 1997; Kang et al. 2000; Spencer et al. 2001; Suadicani et al. 1999; Unwin et al. 1999). However, because of recall bias, the committee considered them as providing weak evidence of a relationship (Boyd et al. 2003).

In conclusion, the study by Maruff et al. (1998) was well designed, but the neurobehavioral effects that it found among former petrol-sniffers are most likely related to lead in petrol rather than to petrol itself. The studies from the Gulf War provide weak evidence of a relationship between fuel exposure and neurobehavioral effects.

The committee concludes, from its assessment of the epidemiologic literature, that there is inadequate/insufficient evidence to determine whether an association exists between exposure to fuels and neurobehavioral effects.

Combustion Products

To identify long-term neurologic effects of combustion products, the committee evaluated numerous epidemiologic studies, virtually all of which covered three general types of neurologic effects: posttraumatic stress disorder (PTSD), neurobehavioral effects (assessed with symptom reporting or performance on validated neurobehavioral tests or batteries), and some neurologic diseases.

Several studies were selected for detailed evaluation because they met the committee's inclusion criteria for neurologic effects (described above). Studies were excluded for lack of methodologic rigor, nonspecific outcomes, or, most commonly, lack of an exposure-free period in the case of reversible outcomes (Arnold et al. 1985; Camerino et al. 1993; Hakkola et al. 1996, 1997; Sram et al. 1996; Strauss et al. 1992). The remainder of this section reviews the studies that met the committee's inclusion criteria.

Posttraumatic Stress Disorder

PTSD is a commonly studied neurologic effect in firefighters, one of the occupations of interest to this committee. It is a highly disabling anxiety disorder that affects 3-4% of the US population (US DHHS 1999), and that can occur after exposure to an extreme traumatic event, such as death or the threat of death. Its hallmark symptoms are frequent replaying of the traumatic event, avoidance of stimuli associated with the trauma, numbing of general responsiveness, and increased arousal. PTSD qualifies as a long-term, rather than a short-term, effect because of its persistence: it persists more than 12 months in about half the cases (APA 1994). Numerous studies have found increased rates of PTSD diagnosis or symptoms after exposure to such catastrophic events as war, terrorism, sexual or physical abuse, natural disasters, and serious injury (Kessler 2000). Trauma appears to have a dose-response relationship with PTSD: the greater the intensity or frequency of traumatic exposure, the greater the likelihood of developing PTSD or other serious mental-health outcomes (Kang et al. 2003). In many, especially Vietnam veterans, PTSD has lasted for years or decades (Bremner et al. 1996).

Studies of firefighters in at least three countries met the committee's criteria for inclusion. Overall, the prevalence of PTSD symptoms across firefighter samples was 15-40%. A study in Kuwait that used the Impact of Events Scale (IES) found the prevalence of PTSD symptoms in firefighters to be 18.5% (al-Naser and Everly 1999). A study in Germany of 402 firefighters engaged in different work functions found the prevalence of PTSD symptoms to be 18.2% (Wagner et al. 1998). A study comparing Canadian and US firefighters that used the IES found a similar prevalence of PTSD symptoms: 17 and 22%, respectively (Corneil et al. 1999). Although not explicitly a study of PTSD, another US study of firefighters found that 33-41% reported significant distress on the General Health Questionnaire and other measures of psychologic well-being (Boxer and Wild 1993). In a related study, firefighters reported that the most stressful aspect of their job was catastrophic injury to themselves or others (Beaton et al. 1998). None of the studies cited above used diagnostic interviews. Symptom scales are generally for screening purposes, so they probably overestimate the prevalence of a PTSD diagnosis, which can be determined only with an interview.

Firefighters are exposed to both traumatic events and combustion products. Although PTSD in firefighters theoretically might be a toxic effect of exposure to combustion products, no studies of firefighters have examined PTSD as such an effect. The most plausible explanation is that PTSD is an emotional and physiologic response to the psychologic trauma of fighting fires. First, many studies have documented that trauma is a nonspecific cause of PTSD in numerous highly exposed populations (Kessler 2000). Second, the prevalence of PTSD symptoms in firefighters is well within the range found in other occupational groups that have high trauma exposure. Police and other rescue workers (Asukai et al. 2002; Weiss et al. 1995) and Vietnam and Gulf War veterans (Kang et al. 2003; Kulka et al. 1990) experience rates of PTSD symptoms comparable with those of firefighters. Third, no other occupational groups exposed to combustion products have been studied for PTSD as an outcome measure. Taken together, the evidence suggests that PTSD symptoms in firefighters are a response to traumatic events rather than toxic effects of combustion-product exposure.

Few Gulf War studies examined whether self-reported combustion-product exposure was related to PTSD as an outcome measure, and none found a relationship (Proctor et al. 1998; Unwin et al. 1999). None of the studies with objectively measured oil-well fire smoke examined PTSD as an outcome measure. In studies that did not include combustion products as an exposure, PTSD symptoms or diagnoses were more likely in Gulf War veterans with combat exposure or injury (Baker et al. 1997; Kang et al. 2003; Labbate et al. 1998; Wolfe et al. 1998), in women (Wolfe et al. 1993), in veterans who had been exposed to missile attack (Perconte et al. 1993), and in those with grave-registration duties (Sutker et al. 1994). The prevalence of PTSD increases with increasing combat exposure (Kang et al. 2003).

The committee concludes, from its assessment of the epidemiologic literature, that there is inadequate/insufficient evidence to determine whether an association exists between exposure to combustion products and posttraumatic stress disorder as a toxicologic effect.

Neurobehavioral Effects

Choi (1983) studied delayed neurologic sequelae in 65 of 2,360 victims of acute carbon monoxide intoxication (549 of whom were admitted to a South Korea hospital) in 1976-1981. The intoxication occurred at home, where coal, the main domestic fuel, is used for cooking and heating (under the floor). Symptoms most frequently appeared 15-30 days after exposure. Signs and symptoms were noted, and computed-tomographic (CT) scans were performed. The vast majority of the 65 had been unconscious for up to a day. The most common symptoms of delayed neurologic sequelae included "mental deterioration", urinary or fecal incontinence, gait disturbance, and mutism. The most common signs were masked face, Glabella sign, and grasp reflex. CT scans performed on 17 of the 65 subjects revealed five with low density of both basal ganglia, two with decreased density of white matter in the cerebral cortex, and the rest normal. About 75% of patients recovered within a year.

Kilburn (1999) studied the effects of diesel exhaust in 10 railroad workers and six electricians. The author did not indicate how the workers were selected except to say that their selection was "not random". The railroad workers were either train crewmen or diesel-engine repairmen. They continued to be exposed to diesel exhaust, so findings could be confounded by continuing exposure. The electricians, however, were examined 9 months after having been exposed to diesel exhaust in an underground tunnel for 7-18 months. The author investigated symptoms, including the Profile of Mood States, and used 26 neurobehavioral tests. The results were compared with those in general population controls who had no chemical exposure and whose names were drawn from voter-registration rolls. The two groups of workers were found to be impaired in all neurobehavioral functions. The results were not stratified according to past vs continuing exposure, and no environmental-exposure monitoring was conducted. The results of the study are difficult to interpret primarily because the study sample was small and included people whose selection was nonrandom and who had continuing exposure.

Several Gulf War studies included analysis of combustion-product exposure and neurobehavioral effects. They found positive relationships between self-reported exposure and self-reported neuropsychologic, cognitive, or mood symptoms or multiple unexplained symptoms (Iowa Persian Gulf Study Group 1997; Kang et al. 2000; Proctor et al. 1998; Spencer et al. 2001; Unwin et al. 1999; White et al. 2001; Wolfe et al. 2002). Because combustion-product exposure in those studies was self-reported and not confirmed by independent exposure assessment, the committee deemed the studies to provide weak evidence of an effect.

The two studies with objectively measured combustion-product exposure are methodologically weak. The Choi study (1983) was a case series without a control group. The Kilburn study (1999) had serious limitations, especially in subject selection. Those studies, taken together with Gulf War studies, all of which had self-reported exposure, provide only weak evidence of a relationship.

The committee concludes, from its assessment of the epidemiologic literature, that there is inadequate/insufficient evidence to determine whether an association exists between exposure to combustion products and neurobehavioral effects.

Neurologic Diseases

Rotorua, New Zealand, is above a geothermally active area with substantial hydrogen sulfide (H_2S) exposure. About one-fourth of the population of 40,000 is regularly exposed to H_2S at over 200 μg/m^3 (143 ppb). A series of studies by Bates et al. investigated morbidity and mortality from peripheral nervous system (ONS)and central nervous system (CNS) diseases (Bates et al. 1997, 1998, 2002). The impetus for the studies was a 1981 World Health Organization report which recommended research expressly in Rotorua to take advantage of the natural conditions to study the health effects of H_2S.

Using census data, Bates et al. (1997) compared deaths in Rotorua with deaths in the rest of New Zealand (1981-1990). First examining diseases of the nervous system and sense organs as a whole (International Classification of Diseases [ICD] codes 320-398), they found the standardized mortality ratio (SMR) to be nonsignificant (SMR 1.07; 95% confidence interval [CI] 0.82-1.36). They also found nonsignificant SMRs for groupings of nervous-system diseases with more than four deaths: inflammatory diseases of the CNS (ICD codes 320-326), hereditary and degenerative diseases of the CNS (ICD codes 330-337), other disorders of the CNS (ICD 340-349), and disorders of the PNS (ICD codes 350-359). Although the study concluded that there were no indications of excess mortality, the authors noted that they were unable to adjust for ethnicity differences. Rotorua has a higher density of Maori residents than do other areas of New Zealand. The authors noted the potential for underreporting of Maori mortality statistics because ethnicity on death certificates is based on funeral directors' impressions.

In a second study, Bates et al. (1998) used hospital-discharge data over a decade (1981-1990) to calculate standardized incidence ratios (SIRs) for neurologic, respiratory, and cardiovascular diseases (and subgroupings) for Rotorua residents. No exposure groups were assigned. Significant findings were found for diseases of the nervous system and sense organs (SIR 1.11, 95% CI 1.07-1.15), and for these nervous-system disease subgroupings: other disorders of the CNS (ICD codes 340-349, SIR 1.22, 95% CI 1.11-1.33), disorders of the PNS (ICD codes 350-359, SIR 1.35, 95% CI 1.21-1.51), and disorders of the eye and adnexa (ICD codes 360-379, SIR 1.12, 95% CI 1.05-1.19). In addition, the following individual discharge diagnoses were statistically significant: migraine (ICD code 346, SIR 1.40, 95% CI 1.12-1.72), other conditions of the brain (ICD code 348, SIR 2.5, 95% CI 1.89-3.26), mononeuritis of the upper limb and mononeuritis multiplex (code 354, SIR 1.47, 95% CI 1.29-1.67), mononeuritis of the lower limb (ICD code 355, SIR 2.06, 95% CI 1.46-2.81), cataract (ICD code 366, SIR 1.26, 95% CI 1.14-1.38), disorders of the conjunctiva (ICD code 372, SIR 2.09, 95% CI 1.66-2.59), disorders of the orbit (ICD code 376, SIR 1.69, 95% CI 1.12-2.44).

In a separate report, Bates et al. (2002) studied exposure to H_2S in relation to hospital-discharge data (1993-1996). Exposures were continuing and so might be excluded from consideration, but the committee does not require an exposure-free period for studies of peripheral and nervous system diseases inasmuch as that they are most likely irreversible (as opposed to, for example, to neurobehavioral symptoms). Exposures were assigned as high, , and low on the basis of area of residence where H_2S was mapped with passive sampling. Exposure-response trends were found for diseases of the nervous system and sense organs (p for trend <0.0001) as a whole. Significant exposure-response trends were also found for some neurologic-disease subgroupings: other disorders of the CNS (ICD codes 340-349: p for trend <0.0001) and disorders of the PNS (ICD codes 350-359: p for trend = 0.027), disorders of the eye and adnexa (ICD codes 360-379: p for trend <0.0001) and disorders of the ear and mastoid process (ICD codes 380-389: p for trend <0.0001). In each of those cases, the SIRs for high exposure ranged from 2.0 to 2.68. SIRs for medium and low exposure were smaller but also significant. The major limitation of this study is the method of exposure assessment, which was based on residential location at the time of diagnosis. The authors acknowledge that such residential exposure assignment neglected to take into account residential histories or individual variation regarding daily mobility for work or study. They noted that subjects with low-exposure assignment based on residence probably work in the main business district of Rotorua, which is in a high-exposure area. Thus, there is a potential for exposure misclassification. Additionally, the Bates studies were the only epidemiologic studies of H_2S found by the committee that examined long-term health outcomes. Due to the paucity of literature, the committee did not make a separate conclusion on H_2S.

Norman et al. (1983) performed a case-control study to determine risk factors for multiple sclerosis (ICD code 340), one of the diseases included in the Bates et al. nervous-system subgroupings (ICD codes 340-349). They studied 4,371 case-control pairs of World War II and Korea veterans to determine whether climatic factors, including air pollution, or latitude influenced risk. Air pollution was measured according to mean annual days of exposure to smog. Although air pollution and other factors were found to significantly influence the risk of multiple sclerosis when analyzed separately, their effects were found to be nonsignificant after adjustment for latitude.

In summary, the three studies of H_2S exposure of Bates et al. were evaluated, as was a separate study of multiple sclerosis. However, the committee excluded overbroad ICD codes and nonspecific health outcomes and focused on individual neurologic diseases or subgroupings of nervous-system diseases. Of the three studies of Bates et al., only one examined nervous-system subgroupings in relation to exposure. It found exposure-response relationships with nervous-system subgroupings in a hospital-discharge survey (Bates et al. 2002). The limitation of that study was assignment of exposure (residence only) and potential for exposure misclassification. The case-control study of Norman et al. (1983) did not find a relationship between combustion product exposure and multiple sclerosis, which was one of the ICD codes covered by Bates et al. No other studies of nervous-system subgroupings or the individual diseases met the committee's criteria for inclusion.

The committee concludes, from its assessment of the epidemiologic literature, that there is inadequate/insufficient evidence of an association between exposure to combustion products and nervous-system disease subgroupings or individual nervous-system diseases.

MULTIPLE CHEMICAL SENSITIVITY

Multiple chemical sensitivity (MCS), also known as idiopathic environmental intolerance; it is a controversial, highly disabling set of symptoms evoked by low-level chemical exposures. MCS is not formally recognized as a diagnosis in the 10th revision of ICD. Major medical associations question the existence of MCS as a unique clinical entity (AAAAI 1999; AMA 1992; American College of Physicians 1989). In the absence of an established diagnosis, epidemiologists and other researchers have developed case definitions by using a combination of self-reported symptoms. Therefore, the committee evaluated the evidence of a relationship between relevant exposures during the Gulf War and case definitions of MCS.

Case definitions of MCS specify an array of symptoms (for example, fatigue, cognitive impairment, respiratory inflammation, and headache) elicited by exposure to relatively low levels of chemicals that have diverse structures and mechanisms of action (Cullen 1987; Simon et al. 1993). Symptomatic persons often report the belief that their symptoms are caused or later triggered by pesticides, fuels, combustion products, perfumes, and other chemical agents (Caress et al. 2002; Fiedler and Kipen 2001). Numerous studies of people who met an epidemiologic definition of MCS, including Gulf War veterans (Black et al. 1999), reported inability to work and significantly reduced quality of life (Fiedler et al. 1996; Jason et al. 2000).

Background: Epidemiology of MCS Symptoms in Veteran and Civilian Populations

The epidemiology of MCS has been examined in seven large or population-based studies of Gulf War veterans and in three population-based studies of US civilians. The Gulf War studies found that the prevalence of MCS—according to various case definitions based on symptom self-reporting—ranged from 2 to 6%. Each study found the prevalence in Gulf War veterans to be significantly higher than that in nondeployed veterans (Proctor 2000). The prevalence in Gulf War veterans is similar to that found in the general US population (Table 8.1).

TABLE 8.1 Prevalence of MCS Symptoms in Gulf War and US Population-Based Samples

Gulf War Sample	MCS Symptoms or Related Condition	Prevalence in Gulf War-Deployed vs Nondeployed Veterans
Reid et al. 2001, n = 3,531 UK Gulf War veterans	MCS[a]	1.3% vs 0.2-0.3% in two non-Gulf War-deployed groups
Reid et al. 2002, n = 3,531 UK Gulf War veterans	Sensitivity to at least one of 11 Gulf War chemicals	27.7% vs 12.7-14.2% in two non-Gulf War-deployed groups
Black et al. 2000, n = 3,695 Gulf War veterans	MCS/IEI[b]	5.4% vs 2.6%
Goss Gilroy 1998, n = 3,113 Gulf War veterans	MCS symptoms[c]	2.8% vs 0.5%
Gray et al. 2002, n = 11,868 Gulf War veterans	Self-reported physician-diagnosed MCS	1.6% vs 0.4%
Proctor et al. 2001, n = 180 Gulf War veterans	Presumptive MCS[d]	2.9% vs 0%
Fukuda et al. 1998, n = 3,723 Gulf War veterans	Chemical sensitivity[e]	5.0% vs 2.0%

US Population-Based Sample	Condition	Prevalence
Kreutzer et al. 1999, n = 4,046	Self-reported doctor-diagnosed illness ("environmental illness" or MCS)	6.3% doctor-diagnosed illness; 11.9% reported sensitivity to more than one type of chemical
Meggs et al. 1996, n = 1,027	Chemical sensitivity[f]	4.1%
Caress et al. 2002, n = 1,579	Self-reported physician-diagnosed MCS or self-reported a hypersensitivity[g]	3.1% doctor-diagnosed MCS, 12.6% hypersensitivity

[a] Criteria of Simon et al. 1993.
[b] Operational case definition based on expert consensus and review of literature.
[c] Positive responses to two sets of eight systemic symptoms produced by normal or routine exposures to at least two substances (set by a panel of physician experts in allergy, immunology, occupational health, environmental health, clinical epidemiology, and psychiatry).
[d] Cullen criteria (1987).
[e] Single item on symptom questionnaire.
[f] Reported becoming sick after smelling chemical odors almost daily.
[g] Affirmative response to question "Compared to others, do you have an unusual sensitivity to common chemical products?"

Hypotheses About MCS Etiology

The etiology of MCS is unknown, but it has been hypothesized to involve CNS sensitization of mesolimbic pathways after exposure to chemicals or biologic stressors (Graveling et al. 1999). Studies of similar symptom clusters (for example, fibromyalgia and chronic fatigue syndrome, CFS) implicate a multifactorial process of exposure to biologic stressors followed by sensory amplification, reduced hypothalamic-pituitary function, lability of the autonomic nervous system, and psychosocial factors (Clauw 2001). Several researchers believe that the initial step in onset of MCS symptoms requires high exposure and/or repeated fluctuating moderate exposure, after which symptoms can be triggered by lower exposure (Bell et al. 2001; Clauw 2001). Animal studies have shown that the amygdala is vulnerable to sensitization, in which repeated exposure to a specific agent leads to increased response at doses lower than those normally expected to yield a response (Graveling et al. 1999). Altered hypothalamic-pituitary functioning has been identified in rodents sensitized to a chemical (Sorg et al. 1996, 1998, 2001).

Evaluation of the Evidence: Inclusion Criteria

For the purposes of this report, the committee evaluated studies of MCS in populations exposed to fuels or combustion products. The committee's inclusion criteria required methodologic rigor, including criteria for a case definition, and a reasonably representative sample. Another inclusion criterion is the evaluation of subjects after an exposure-free period (free of the fuel or combustion product) to ensure the identification of long-term, rather than short-term, effects.

Nine studies met the committee's inclusion criteria: six of Gulf War veterans and three of occupational or general populations. Although two of the nine studies had verified exposure, most had self-reported exposure and self-reported health outcomes via questionnaire. Studies varied in methods, samples of veterans, definitions of exposure (for example, causal exposure vs trigger) and case definitions of MCS. One of the studies was quite small (for example, Davidoff et al. 1998), did not select matched controls, and suffers from recall bias. The studies described below were of fuels, combustion products, or both.

Gulf War Studies

One Gulf War study had an experimental design that used controlled exposure to fuels in already symptomatic veterans (Fiedler et al. 2004); it was published after the committee's cutoff date for inclusion in this volume. The remaining studies had cross-sectional designs. Most studies did not ask about first onset of symptoms. The only study of first onset is an occupational study by Davidoff (1998), which is reviewed in the next section.

Using exposure surveys rather than controlled exposure, Fiedler et al. (2000) investigated biologic, psychologic, and social factors that contributed to ill health in 58 veterans who had CFS. A subgroup of 19 veterans met criteria for both CFS and MCS symptoms, but the results were not stratified for this comorbid group. Another group that met criteria only for MCS was excluded because it had only four subjects. The 58 ill veterans were compared with 45 healthy veterans. Investigators found that ill veterans were significantly more likely to report becoming ill in the Gulf War from smoke from tent heaters, burning human waste, oil-well fires, vehicle exhaust, and two other exposures (pesticides and anti-nerve-gas pills) but not from debris from Scuds or antitank shells. The total environmental-exposure score was significantly higher in the ill veterans than in the healthy veterans. Ill veterans were also more likely to report traumatic events related to combat, such as reporting that they might have killed someone or that they sat with someone dying of battle wounds. The limitations of this study include issues related to study design, including self-reported exposure and symptoms, and the potential for recall bias.

A large, population-based study of Iowa veterans (n = 3,965) found self-reported prevalence of MCS symptoms at 5.4% in deployed veterans vs 2.6% in nondeployed veterans, with an odds ratio (OR) of 1.92, 95% CI 1.22-3.04 (Black et al. 2000). The criteria for MCS symptoms were set by a panel of physicians who had with expertise in allergy, immunology, occupational health, environmental health, clinical epidemiology, and psychiatry. Although the study did not ask about Gulf War exposures that might have initially caused symptoms, it did ask about 10 potential triggers that exacerbate symptoms, including "smog", "vehicle exhaust", and "organic chemicals, solvents, glues, paint, and fuel". Three of the exposures were more likely to act as triggers in Gulf War deployed than nondeployed (smog: OR 3.39, 95% CI 1.67-6.86; vehicle exhaust: OR 2.10, 95% CI 1.34-3.30; solvents: OR 1.80, 95% CI 1.21-2.68).

Reid et al. (2001) examined associations between MCS symptoms and self-reported exposure in a large, population-based random sample of the entire UK force of 53,000 Gulf War deployed veterans. A postal survey was conducted in 1997-1998, and cases of MCS were defined by the symptom-based criteria established by Simon et al. (1993). Those criteria require symptoms that lasted at least 3 months in at least three organ systems, including the CNS, and sensitivity to four or more substances from a list of numerous potential irritants (for example, smoke or engine exhaust, personal hygiene products, cleaning products, pesticides, treated water, fabrics or dyes, floor coverings, office products, asphalt or tar, fuels, solvents or glues, paints or adhesives, formaldehyde, etc.). The prevalence of MCS was 1.3% in Gulf War veterans, a rate significantly greater than that in two non deployed control groups. Potential exposures were to a list of more than 17 items on a standard Gulf War exposure questionnaire, six of which were relevant to the committee: "diesel or petrochemical fumes", "exhaust from heaters", "smoke from oil fires", "burning rubbish/feces", "diesel on skin", and "Scud missile explosion". The exposures were the same as in Unwin et al. (1999), as was the response rate, 65.1%. Reid et al. (2001) found that in Gulf War-deployed veterans MCS was associated with "exhaust from heaters" (OR 2.8, 95% CI 1.1-7.5), "smoke from oil fires" (OR 4.6, 95% CI 1.6-13.3), and "burning rubbish/feces" (OR 5.8, 95% CI 2.0-16.7). MCS was also associated with numerous other Gulf War exposures, particularly to pesticides, but nonsignificantly with exposure to "diesel or petrochemical fumes" (OR 2.2, 95% CI 0.8-5.9). Exposure to personal pesticides and pesticides on clothing carried increased ORs of 10-12.

In a later paper on the same cohort, Reid et al. (2002) provided more information about veterans' chemical sensitivities based on a questionnaire developed by Kipen et al. (1995). Reid et al. found that nearly 30% of their entire sample of Gulf War veterans reported that at least one of 11 common triggering agents brought about symptoms after deployment (vs before deployment). The list of triggering agents was distinct from the list of Gulf War exposures used in their 2001 publication. Smog, vehicle exhaust or fumes, and "organic chemicals, solvents, glues, paint, or fuel" were significantly more likely to be triggers for Gulf War veterans than for a nondeployed Gulf War-era control group. ORs were 2.6, 95% CI 2.1-3.2 for smog; 60.1, 95% CI 27.4-132.1 for vehicle exhaust; and 19.6, 95% CI 11.0-34.6 for organic chemicals, solvents, glues, paint, or fuel.

Bell et al. (1998) compared rates of self-perceived chemical intolerance in random samples of deployed and nondeployed Gulf War veterans at the Tucson Veterans Affairs Medical Center. The study also asked about perceived exposure to chemical agents during the Gulf War. A 15-minute telephone interview collected data on the veterans' self-perceptions of their health (at the time of the interview, 6 months before, and just before entering and after leaving military service) and self-reports of the diagnosis of PTSD and of intolerance to chemical odors of 17 substances: five items on a previously validated screening index (pesticide, paint, car exhaust, perfume, and new carpet) and 12 items suggested by veterans. Self-reports regarding 12 exposures in the Gulf War were also solicited, three of which were relevant: "smoke from oil-well fires", "diesel exhaust", and "raw fuels". None of those three exposures was found to be associated with being an ill (n = 14) vs a healthy (n = 10) Gulf War veteran. An ill veteran was defined as one who had poor health after service vs before service. The researchers considered the findings preliminary.

Miller and Prihoda (1999) recruited a group of 72 Persian Gulf War veterans through advertisements in MCS patient-group newsletters and word of mouth. No attempt was made to identify individual veterans who met the criteria for MCS, but the sample of veterans obtained had symptoms and symptom-severity scores that were comparable with those of MCS patients who were included in the same study. Veterans were asked to report exposures that they thought had led to their symptoms. Of the Gulf War veterans, 26% reported that "oil fumes" exposure during the Gulf War initiated their illness. However, this study is limited by the self-selected nature of the veteran sample and was not constructed to test hypotheses of causality.

MCS Studies in Non-Gulf War Veteran Populations

Davidoff et al. (1998) studied a cohort of day laborers exposed to gasoline vapors while excavating a new subway tunnel. The laborers inadvertently dug into soil that was contaminated with gasoline from a storage tank belonging to a gasoline station that had closed 30 years earlier. Two months after workers first noticed the odor of gasoline, the digging operation was closed down when investigators found benzene at 60 ppm. No air measurements of gasoline were taken, because pumps malfunctioned, but the authors reported that those workers' symptoms of headache, throat irritation, eye irritation, and cough were consistent with gasoline at 150 and 500 ppm. Study participants were given medical examinations and laboratory studies around the time of the closure and were interviewed by telephone 10-13 months afterward. Study resources were limited, so the authors could not identify a matched control sample of similar workers. Instead, the day laborers were matched to a sample of 20 people from a previous study who had MCS (Davidoff and Keyl 1996) and 24 people from a general population sample (recruited via random-number table from a telephone phone directory).

The authors point out that the cohort of day laborers was unique in several respects: none had complained of MCS when contact with gasoline was made; all subjects were men of low socioeconomic status (SES), and the cohort was viewed as "naive" because none were members of a support group, were being seen by clinical ecologists, or identified themselves as having MCS.

Some 10-13 months after closure of tunnel operations, the authors interviewed by telephone 30 workers randomly drawn from the original group of workers. Of those 30, 17 reported three or more chemical sensitivities that predated the tunnel operation, three reported no new or intensified sensitivities, and 10 reported three or more new or intensified chemical sensitivities. Of the 10 workers in the latter group, eight (or 26.7% of the 30 workers) had MCS, according to the 1987 Cullen criteria (1987). None of the 10 had a distinct profile on the first physical examination at the time of tunnel closure. None of the 10 reported disability 10-13 months later; all were either employed or seeking employment. The symptom cluster was precipitated by extremely high concentrations of gasoline vapors. Finally, it should be noted that 17 of the 30 workers reported three or more sensitivities that predated the tunnel operations, and ten others who had MCS reported either new or intensified sensitivities. The limitations of this study acknowledged by the authors are the small sample, less than optimally matched control groups, and potential for recall bias.

Caress et al. performed a two-phase population-based survey of 1,579 people living in the Atlanta, Georgia, metropolitan area. The investigators sought to examine prevalence, causation and exacerbation of MCS symptoms (Caress and Steinemann 2003; Caress et al. 2002). Nearly 13% of the sample reported "an unusual sensitivity to common chemical products", and 3.1% of the sample reported being diagnosed by a medical doctor with "MCS or environmental illness". The subjects who reported sensitivities were asked a series of further questions. About 13% of them reported a loss of employment caused by their sensitivities. The most common symptoms were headache, burning eyes, asthma or asthma-like symptoms, nausea or stomach upset, and inability to concentrate. Responding to the question "What produces your symptoms?", 72.5% identified car exhaust. Other common triggers were perfume, cleaners, pesticides, and tobacco smoke. When asked "Do you know or suspect the following as the original cause?", nearly 16% selected "petroleum"[1] (Table 8.2), but more than one-third of hypersensitive respondents were not sure of the cause. A small fraction of respondents who had hypersensitivity reported a history of prior emotional problems, but nearly 38% said that they developed emotional problems after the emergence of physical symptoms.

[1] The other major causes were pesticides (27.5%), solvents and (27.5%), and building materials (17.4%).

TABLE 8.2 Common Triggers and Original Causes Reported by People with Chemical Sensitivity (n = 235) Population-Based Sample

"What triggers a reaction?"	**%**		
Perfume	81.2		
Cleaners	88.4		
Fresh ink	26.1		
Appliances	10.1		
Pesticides	81.2		
Chlorine/H_2O	39.1		
Tobacco smoke	82.6		
New carpet	53.6		
Furniture	39.1		
Salon/barber	60.9		
Public parks	52.2		
Car exhaust	72.5		
"Do you know or suspect the following as the original cause?"	**% Yes**	**% No**	**% Maybe**
Pesticides	27.5	34.8	33.3
Solvents	27.5	30.4	37.7
Building materials	17.4	43.5	34.8
Petroleum	15.9	43.5	36.2

SOURCES: Caress et al. 2002; Caress and Steinemann 2003.

In summary, one key study that incorporated objective exposure measurement found a relationship between symptoms of MCS and fuel exposure. That study was of first-onset MCS symptoms in an occupational population unknowingly exposed to fuel vapors. In that study, Davidoff et al. (1998) found that 26.7% of their day-laborer sample met symptom-based criteria for MCS after several months of exposure to fuel while digging a subway tunnel. The strength of that study is that many of the workers had never complained of MCS or identified themselves as having MCS. The study was limited by the small sample and lack of a matched control group of workers, although the authors compared findings with two other control groups. Because of the limitations noted above and described in the text, the study does not meet the committee's criteria for a primary study that would support an association. Although several studies of Gulf War veteran or civilian samples also found an association, they were limited by self-reported exposure and possibility of recall bias.

The committee concludes, from its assessment of the epidemiologic literature, that there is inadequate/insufficient evidence of an association between exposure to fuels and combustion products and symptoms consistent with an epidemiologic definition of MCS.

DERMATOLOGIC OUTCOMES

Dermatologic or skin effects associated with exposure to fuels or combustion products have predominantly been studied in toxicologic and controlled clinical studies (Chapter 3). Most studies assessed the effects of acute exposure and its immediate outcomes. Only a handful of epidemiologic studies, mostly cross-sectional, examined the relationship between exposure and long-term dermatologic effects; each one examined some form of dermatitis, and they are discussed below.

Dermatitis is inflammation of the skin as evidenced by signs of scaling, crusting, redness, and swelling. Several studies reviewed in this section (Table 8.3) looked for relationships between dermatitis and occupational exposure.

Wolf et al. (1994) evaluated the use and reliability of specially tailored trays used in patch testing for differentiating between allergic and irritant contact dermatitis among Israeli soldiers who developed hand dermatitis from contact with oils and fuels. Forty-one soldiers in an infantry, armored, and artillery division who had dermatitis were compared with 64 controls not occupationally exposed to oils and fuels. All patients underwent a history and physical examination, and patch testing with the special supplementary tray that included gun oil, hydraulic oil, automotive lubricant oil, white spirit, and gasoline. Seven of the 41 soldiers (17%) had one or more positive tests with the supplementary tray, although none of the controls did. The patch testing was conducted in a blind manner.

In a later study, Wolf et al. (1996) included more soldiers who had occupational dermatitis (n = 111), more persons in the control group (n = 73), and a second control group of 20 soldiers in the same division who had extensive exposure to oils and fuels but no dermatitis. The authors found that 28% of the soldiers who had occupational dermatitis had one or more positive skin reactions to the supplementary tray, whereas none of those in either control group had such reactions. The authors concluded that allergic contact dermatitis does occur, but the study did not provide any details of the patch-test dilutions in five of the patients, nor was there any mention of specific results at 48 hours and 96 hours. Although the study provides some indication that exposure to oils, fuels, and white spirits can result in allergic contact dermatitis, no data were provided about whether the dermatitis cleared after cessation of exposure. In addition, the reading of results of patch tests is subjective.

TABLE 8.3 Dermatitis and Fuel Exposure

Reference	Type of Study and Population	Exposure Determination	Health Outcome and How Measured	Results	Adjusted OR (95% CI or p)	Limitations
Wolf et al. 1996	111 soldiers with dermatitis vs 73 in control group	Controlled exposures to gasoline and other oils via patch testing with supplementary tray of fuel and oil	Dermatitis	28% of soldiers with dermatitis showed 1 or more positive reactions to supplementary tray; 0% of controls tested positive		No details on patch-test dilutions; no information on results in 48 and 96 hrs. Reading of results subjective; no information on whether dermatitis cleared after exposure
Jia et al. 2002	30 sewing-machine workers vs 30 age-matched workers in spinning mill in China	Gasoline used as solvent	Dermatitis assessed with questionnaire and skin testing for lipids		Dermatitis, OR 5.0 ($p < 0.001$); hyperkeratosis, OR 3.3 ($p < 0.05$); dryness, OR 3.0 ($p < 0.001$); onychosis, OR 11.25 ($p < 0.001$); stratum corneum lipids significantly lower in exposed group ($p < 0.05$)	
Jee et al. 1985	79 ball-bearing factory workers vs 263 zipper-manufacturing workers in Taiwan	Kerosene used as solvent in ball-bearing factory	Dermatitis classified by dermatologist	84% exposed to kerosene (either heavily or lightly) had dermatitis vs 1% of unexposed; among those heavily exposed, 91% had dermatitis, as did 78% of those lightly exposed		Not clear whether dermatologists blinded to exposure status
Venn et al. 2001	9,844 adults and children in Jimma, Ethiopia	Mixed exposure to kerosene, gasoline, or	Questionnaire and allergen skin testing in		Self-reported eczema in preceding year (OR 2.82,	Cannot distinguish between direct skin

Reference	Type of Study and Population	Exposure Determination	Health Outcome and How Measured	Results	Adjusted OR (95% CI or p)	Limitations
		electricity and biomass fuel vs only biomass fuel in home heating	subset of 2,372 adults and children		95% CI 1.61-4.96); kerosene use in preceding year significantly associated with eczema (OR 3.20, 95% CI 1.62-6.32); higher rates of skin sensitization to *D. pteronyssinus* or mixed threshings among those with mixed fuel exposure vs biomass only (OR 1.78, 95% CI 1.06-2.97)	exposure to fuel vs inhalation exposure to combustion products

Jia et al. (2002) studied the dermatologic effects of gasoline exposure among 52 female sewing machine workers in a cross-sectional study in China. The women were exposed daily (7 hours a day) to 500 mL of gasoline in cleaning and applying transfers or decals to the machines. The workplace was ventilated, and the concentration of gasoline in the air was below the maximum allowed, 300 mg/m^3. The women were matched by age with female workers of similar SES from a spinning mill (n = 52). Of the 52 exposed and nonexposed workers, 30 were sampled and interviewed about their occupational history, frequency of hand-washing during the day, and use of skin-care products. Skin samples were collected from the back of their hands to determine stratum corneum lipid concentrations (ceramide, fatty acid, and cholesterol) because these lipids were hypothesized to have been dissolved by the fuel exposure. The results showed that prevalences of hyperkeratosis, dryness, onychosis, and dermatitis were increased among the exposed compared with the non-exposed. The prevalence ratios were 3.33 ($p < 0.05$) for hyperkeratosis; 3.00 ($p < 0.001$) for dryness; 11.25 ($p < 0.001$) for onychosis; and 5.00 ($p < 0.001$) for dermatitis. The authors reported that most workers developed dermatitis within 1 month of starting to use gasoline and that all workers had been exposed for at least a year. Stratum corneum lipid concentrations were significantly lower in the exposed group. The authors did not report whether the skin and nail changes continued after exposure ceased.

Another cross-sectional study (Jee et al. 1985) examined the prevalence of dermatitis and exposure to kerosene among ball-bearing factory workers in Taiwan. Kerosene is used as a degreasing agent in the factory. Seventy-nine female workers who were identified as being exposed were compared with 263 workers employed at a zipper-manufacturing company. The groups had similar age distributions, educational backgrounds, and income levels. Safety personnel at the ball-bearing plant classified the 79 workers into two groups on the basis of exposure. Those classified as heavily exposed to kerosene (n = 34) had direct contact for about 5 hours/day and wore gloves without inner gloves for about 3 hours/day. Those considered lightly exposed (n = 45) did not wear gloves during the day.

Two dermatologists examined the hands and forearms of the heavily and lightly exposed and the nonexposed. They found that 84% of those exposed to kerosene (either heavily or lightly) had dermatitis compared with only 1% of the nonexposed. Among those heavily exposed, 91% had dermatitis; among those lightly exposed 78%. Dermatitis was classified as erythema (65% in both groups), eczema (15% in both groups), or defatting (4% in both groups), but the data were not stratified by type of dermatitis. Patch testing via the standard trays of the National Taiwan University Hospital and the American Academy of Dermatology was performed on five of 12 exposed workers who had severe eczema, and four of the five tested negative. The role and effects of other exposures in the factory (such as to antirust oil) cannot be ruled out. No information was provided on whether the dermatologists were blinded to the exposure status of each worker.

Venn et al. (2001) studied nearly 10,000 adults and children living in Jimma, a city in Ethiopia, to explore the risk of allergy in relation to increased use of cleaner fuels (kerosene, gas, and electricity) in the home. The city is in the midst of a transformation from biomass fuel, which is burned in open fires in poorly-ventilated homes, to cleaner fuels for heating and cooking. The study was prompted by clinicians' observation of increasing rates of asthma and allergies. The city has no major industry, has light traffic levels, and is otherwise not polluted. The study collected symptom and lifestyle questionnaire data and results of allergen skin testing on a subset of 2,372 adults and children. It compared subjects who used a mix of cleaner fuels and biomass to a group that used only biomass fuel. After adjusting for age, sex, and SES, the study found higher rates of skin sensitization to *D. pteronyssinus* or mixed threshings among those with the combination exposure (OR 1.78, 95% CI 1.06-2.97) than among those who used only biomass. It also found increases in self-reported eczema in the preceding year (OR 2.82, 95% CI 1.61-4.96). More specifically, it found that kerosene use, but not gas or electricity use, was significantly associated with eczema (OR 3.20, 95% CI 1.62-6.32). Findings were similar to those in an earlier publication of the same investigators when they compared location of residence (urban site of Jimma with several nearby rural sites) as a proxy for type of heating-fuel use (Yemaneberhan et al. 1997). One study limitation is that pollutant concentrations in the home were not measured. The authors concluded that an increased risk of allergy is associated with the use of cleaner fuels, but their findings could not distinguish the contribution of direct contact with the cleaner fuels or of indoor air pollution from combustion products.

In a cross-sectional study of male farmers in Iowa (n = 382) and the wives of farmers (n = 256), risk factors for farm-related dermatitis were examined (Park et al. 2001). The men and women were identified through the Iowa Farm Family Health and Hazard Survey that inquires about the prevalence of health conditions and injuries among farmers. A followup survey asked about demographics, farm characteristics, work practices, health-related behaviors, skin problems, and exposure to specific chemicals or substances. Nationally representative samples of US male farmers and wives of farmers who identified themselves as farmers and had completed an occupational-health supplement regarding problems with their skin were found through the National Health Interview Survey. A significantly higher risk of dermatitis was seen among farmers' wives who reported being exposed to petroleum products (OR 2.51, 95% CI 1.05-6.05), than those who did not report that exposure. However, no increase was seen among the male farmers (OR 0.39, 95% CI 0.09-1.76). Specific petroleum products or exposures were not delineated, and the study is further limited by the relatively low response rate (39%), which may imply selection bias. No data on length of exposure were provided.

Brender et al. (2003) studied the prevalence of rashes in 214 black people living near a former creosote wood-treatment facility contaminated with polycyclic aromatic hydrocarbons (PAHs). Increased PAHs were found in soil and in groundwater and led to classification of the site on the US Environmental Protection Agency's National Priorities List. In comparison with residents of a nearby community largely of blacks, those living near the wood-treatment facility had higher rates of rashes (relative risk 5.7, 95% CI 3.0-10.9). Most of the rashes were not documented by a physician or an interviewer. The prevalence of rashes was significantly higher among members of the community exposed to higher soil concentrations of anthracene (over 1,000 μg/kg). Anthracene is a solid PAH and is used in wood preservatives.

Rashes are frequently reported by Gulf War veterans, but only one study of Gulf War veterans searched for relationships between dermatitis and self-reported exposure during the Gulf War (Proctor et al. 1998). No exposure to combustion products or fuels or any other self-reported exposure was related to dermatitis, defined as rashes, eczema, or skin allergies.

Many fuels (for example, gasoline and kerosene) are generally acknowledged skin irritants, as indicated by the studies discussed above. Irritant contact dermatitis is evident soon after exposure but usually disappears soon after removal of the irritant. There are few epidemiologic studies, however, of exposure to fuels and irritant and allergic contact dermatitis.

The committee concludes, from its assessment of the epidemiologic literature, that there is inadequate/insufficient evidence to determine whether an association exists between exposure to fuels and combustion products and chronic irritant and allergic contact dermatitis after cessation of exposure.

SARCOIDOSIS

Sarcoidosis is an inflammatory disorder that features accumulation of T lymphocytes and mononuclear phagocytes. The lungs are most frequently affected and undergo inflammatory changes, fibrosis, and other abnormalities; but skin, eyes, and lymph nodes may also be affected. Its etiology is unknown, but it is thought to be triggered by a hypersensitive response to exogenous or endogenous antigens. The prevalence of sarcoidosis in the United States is 10-40 per 100,000. Its frequency is higher in nonwhite and women, but it is also common in whites and men in the United States and throughout the world. Three epidemiologic studies examined the relationship between occupational or residential exposure to fires and sarcoidosis (Table 8.4).

Kajdasz et al. (2001) conducted a case-control study of 44 people who had sarcoidosis. The study was designed to determine whether rural exposure, including the use of residential fireplaces and wood stoves, is related to onset. Cases were recruited from the Medical University of South Carolina Ambulatory Care System and were compared with controls (age-, race-, and sex-matched) recruited through random-digit dialing. A total of 49 people were recruited, but there is little information on how. Of the 49, 44 met the inclusion/exclusion criteria; one person was excluded because of active treatment for tuberculosis, and four declined to participate. Cases were required to have biopsy-confirmed sarcoidosis or, when the biopsy was inconclusive, clinical signs and symptoms of sarcoidosis combined with radiographic findings. The authors noted that "all diagnoses were confirmed by pulmonologists, dermatologists, or ophthalmologists with prior experience in diagnosing and treating sarcoidosis." Trained interviewers administered a questionnaire, which covered exposure history, including magnitude of exposure, from birth through disease development. The questionnaire also covered employment history, smoking, and other factors. Six exposures were included, including home use of a coal stove, wood stove, or fireplace; use of insecticides (other than for home extermination); use of well or spring water; and living or working on a farm. No other details about the types of exposure were asked for other than frequency of use.

In multivariate models, which controlled for demographic and geographic influences, the use of wood stoves (OR 3.1, 95% CI 1.2-7.9) and fireplaces (OR 5.7, 95% CI 1.8-18.4) was significantly related to the occurrence of sarcoidosis, and the use of coal stoves and insecticides/herbicides was not. Exposure-response relationships between number of times used per week as an ordinal variable and the risk of sarcoidosis were evaluated. Wood-stove use had an adjusted OR of 1.4, 95% CI 1.1-1.8, and fireplace use an adjusted OR of 1.8, 95% CI 1.3-2.6.

TABLE 8.4 Case-Control Studies of Sarcoidosis and Combustion Product Exposure

Reference, Country	Cases	Controls	Exposure Determination	Exposure	Adjusted OR (95% CI or p)	Comments
Kajdasz et al. 2001	44 patients with sarcoidosis recruited from Medical University of South Carolina ambulatory-care system	88 persons recruited with random-digit dialing, matched for race, sex, age	Questionnaire administered face to face by trained interviewers covering exposures from birth to onset, employment, smoking, and other factors	Use of wood stove: never or none, less than weekly, weekly, several times per week, daily	In multivariable, multiple-risk-factor conditional logistic-regression model with pairwise interaction terms, increasing woodstove use (adjusted OR 1.4, 95% CI 1.1-1.8) and increased fireplace use (adjusted OR 1.8, 95% CI 1.3-2.6)	Dose-response gradient for woodstoves and fireplaces (reported as marginally significant)
Prezant et al. 1999, New York City, US	All New York City firefighters 1985-1998	All EMS health-care workers in fire department 1995-1998	Biopsy-proven sarcoidosis, pulmonary function (FVC, FEV, diffusing capacity for CO), airway hyperreactivity, maximal oxygen consumption	Occupational	25 cases in firefighters (21 new, four prior), one prior case in health-care worker controls; average annual incidence 12.9/100,000 in firefighters (1985-1998) vs 0 in controls (1995-1998); pulmonary function normal in 68% of firefighters with sarcoidosis; all cases remained at work	

Reference, Country	Cases	Controls	Exposure Determination	Exposure	Adjusted OR (95% CI or p)	Comments
Kern et al. 1993, US	46 Providence, RI, firefighters class of 1979	53 firefighters classes of 1974, 1980; 50 police officers classes of 1973-1981	Questionnaire, chest radiographs, neopterin, IL-2, chlamydia serology	Occupational	Four sarcoidosis cases in firefighter index group, no cases in two control groups; serum neopterin significantly increased in 20% of index firefighter cohort, 22% of firefighter controls, 4% of police officers; via logistic regression firefighting found to be only significant determinant of neopterin increase (OR 5.8, 95% CI 1.3-26.9)	

NOTE: CI=confidence interval; CO=carbon monoxide; FEV=forced expiratory volume; FVC=forced vital capacity; OR=odds ratio.

The study had numerous limitations, such as inadequate description of how the cases without biopsy confirmation were diagnosed and the lack of control for employment history (besides farming), recall bias, and lack of measurement of pollutant concentrations. The authors noted that sarcoidosis could be associated with a component of wood-burning or wood-handling, namely contact with smoke, ash, wood particles, or wood molds.

Researchers with the New York City Fire Department (Prezant et al. 1999) studied a cohort of more than 11,000 firefighters to determine incidence, prevalence, and severity of sarcoidosis over a 13-year period (1985-1998). The research grew out of a pulmonary surveillance program that began in 1985. In 1995, the program added a control group of emergency medical service (EMS) prehospital health-care workers (about 2,700). Cases of sarcoidosis were defined by biopsy that showed evidence of noncaseating granulomas. The methods of case ascertainment were the same in the two groups, except for the timeframe: chart reviews of all currently employed to identify those with pre-existing sarcoidosis, referral to a pulmonary specialist of workers who had signs or symptoms of pulmonary disease, routine chest radiography during wellness medical evaluations, review of all disability leave and retirement applications, and disclosure of study goals to health and safety personnel in employee unions. Cases were studied with physiologic measures of flow rates, diffusing capacity for carbon monoxide, lung volumes, airway hyperreactivity, and maximal oxygen consumption.

The overwhelming majority of firefighters (94%) were white men, compared with 44 % of the controls. Nearly 15.9% of the controls were black men and 15.3% were Hispanic men. The program uncovered 25 cases of sarcoidosis in firefighters (1985-1998). Of the 25 cases, 24 were in white firefighters and one case was found in a black firefighter. One pre-existing case was found in the controls. The average annual incidence of sarcoidosis was 12.9 per 100,000 in firefighters and 0% in the controls. The point prevalence in 1998 was 222 per 100,000 in firefighters and 35 per 100,000 in the controls. Pulmonary function was normal in 68% of the firefighter cases, and maximal oxygen consumption was normal in 59%. Firefighter cases showed minimal impairment, and all were working in the fire department. A strength of the study is the systematic screening program, which probably resulted in fairly complete ascertainment of incident cases. Limitations include the lack of specific exposure assessment and of analysis of duration or frequency of exposure to combustion products. There was no control for potential confounders, such as race or familial aggregation of sarcoidosis (for example, if firefighters are more likely than EMS workers to have siblings enter the job). In addition, there is no way to determine the role of combustion products or exposure to other toxicants, allergens, or infectious agents.

Kern et al. (1993) were the first to study the relationship between firefighting and sarcoidosis. The study stemmed from a cluster of three cases among 10 white firefighters who had trained together as apprentices in 1979. Sarcoidosis appeared 6-8 years later. When the cluster came to light, the investigators hypothesized that a factor intrinsic to firefighting, such as recurrent smoke exposure, might act synergistically with an infectious agent. One agent implicated at the time in sarcoidosis was *Chlamydia pneumoniae*. The investigators conducted a case-finding survey with a questionnaire sent to 1,282 active and retired male firefighters and police officers who had worked or were working in Providence, Rhode Island. They later set up a cohort study comparing the class of 1979 firefighters (n = 46) with two control groups: one was the classes of 1974 and 1980 firefighters (n = 53), and the other was of police officers (classes of 1973-1981, n = 50). They had winnowed questionnaire responders down to those still employed as firefighters or police officers, believing that current occupation was a key to interpreting laboratory results. Investigators compared medical history, exposures, chest radiographs, and seromarkers of T-lymphocyte activation; serum neopterin and interleukin-2 receptors, which are surrogate markers of lymphocytic alveolitis, were used because subjects were not willing to undergo bronchoalveolar lavage. Radiographs were read by specialists who were blinded to occupational group.

A total of four sarcoidosis cases were found in the firefighter index group (including the three original cases), and no cases were found in the two control groups. Although the three groups did not differ by *Chlamydia* serology or interleukin-2 concentrations, serum neopterin was significantly increased in 20% of the index firefighter cohort, 22% of the firefighter controls, and 4% of the police officers. By logistic regression, firefighting was found to be the only significant determinant of neopterin increse (OR 5.8, 95% CI 1.3-26.9). The authors concluded that *Chlamydia* was not likely to be related to cases of sarcoidosis, but that firefighting was. They recommended more studies on neopterin and more studies of firefighters. The limitations of the study are the small sample, the low statistical power (sarcoidosis is a relatively rare disease), the lack of a risk estimate for firefighters vs police officers, the lack of exposure assessment for combustion products, and the lack of assessment of coexposures to other chemicals in the workplace.

The committee concludes, from its assessment of the epidemiologic literature, that there is inadequate/insufficient evidence to determine whether an association exists between exposure to combustion products and sarcoidosis.

REFERENCES

AAAAI (American Academy of Allergy, Asthma and Immunology). 1999. Idiopathic environmental intolerances. American Academy of Allergy, Asthma and Immunology (AAAAI) Board of Directors. *Journal of Allergy and Clinical Immunology* 103(1 Pt 1):36-40.

al-Naser F, Everly GS Jr. 1999. Prevalence of posttraumatic stress disorder among Kuwaiti firefighters. *International Journal of Emergency Mental Health* 1(2):99-101.

AMA (American Medical Association). 1992. Clinical ecology. Council on Scientific Affairs, American Medical Association. *JAMA* 268(24):3465-3467.

American College of Physicians. 1989. Clinical ecology. American College of Physicians. *Annals of Internal Medicine* 111(2):168-178.

APA (American Psychiatric Association). 1994. *Diagnostic and Statistical Manual of Mental Disorders: DSM-IV*. 4th ed. Washington, DC: APA.

Arnold IM, Dufresne RM, Alleyne BC, Stuart PJ. 1985. Health implication of occupational exposures to hydrogen sulfide. *Journal of Occupational Medicine* 27(5):373-376.

Asukai N, Kato H, Kawamura N, Kim Y, Yamamoto K, Kishimoto J, Miyake Y, Nishizono-Maher A. 2002. Reliability and validity of the Japanese-language version of the impact of event scale-revised (IES-R-J): Four studies of different traumatic events. *Journal of Nervous and Mental Disease* 190(3):175-182.

ATSDR (Agency for Toxic Substances and Disease Registry). 1995. *Toxicological Profile for Fuel Oils*. Atlanta, GA: US Department of Health and Human Services, Public Health Service, ATSDR.

Baker DG, Mendenhall CL, Simbartl LA, Magan LK, Steinberg JL. 1997. Relationship between posttraumatic stress disorder and self-reported physical symptoms in Persian Gulf War veterans. *Archives of Internal Medicine* 157(18):2076-2078.

Bates MN, Garrett N, Graham B, Read D. 1997. Air pollution and mortality in the Rotorua geothermal area. *Australian and New Zealand Journal of Public Health* 21(6):581-586.

Bates MN, Garrett N, Graham B, Read D. 1998. Cancer incidence, morbidity and geothermal air pollution in Rotorua, New Zealand. *International Journal of Epidemiology* 27(1):10-14.

Bates MN, Garrett N, Shoemack P. 2002. Investigation of health effects of hydrogen sulfide from a geothermal source. *Archives of Environmental Health* 57(5):405-411.

Beaton R, Murphy S, Johnson C, Pike K, Corneil W. 1998. Exposure to duty-related incident stressors in urban firefighters and paramedics. *Journal of Traumatic Stress* 11(4):821-828.

Bell IR, Baldwin CM, Schwartz GE. 1998. Illness from low levels of environmental chemicals: Relevance to chronic fatigue syndrome and fibromyalgia. *American Journal of Medicine* 105(3A):74S-82S.

Bell IR, Baldwin CM, Schwartz GE. 2001. Sensitization studies in chemically intolerant individuals: Implications for individual difference research. *Annals of the New York Academy of Sciences* 933:38-47.

Black DW, Doebbeling BN, Voelker MD, Clarke WR, Woolson RF, Barrett DH, Schwartz DA. 1999. Quality of life and health-services utilization in a population-based sample of military personnel reporting multiple chemical sensitivities. *Journal of Occupational and Environmental Medicine* 41(10):928-933.

Black DW, Doebbeling BN, Voelker MD, Clarke WR, Woolson RF, Barrett DH, Schwartz DA. 2000. Multiple chemical sensitivity syndrome: Symptom prevalence and risk factors in a military population. *Archives of Internal Medicine* 160(8):1169-1176.

Boxer PA, Wild D. 1993. Psychological distress and alcohol use among fire fighters. *Scandinavian Journal of Work, Environment & Health* 19(2):121-125.

Boyd KC, Hallman WK, Wartenberg D, Fiedler N, Brewer NT, Kipen HM. 2003. Reported exposures, stressors, and life events among Gulf War Registry veterans. *Journal of Occupational and Environmental Medicine* 45(12):1247-1256.

Bremner J, Southwick S, Darnell A, Charney D. 1996. Chronic PTSD in Vietnam combat veterans: Course of illness and substance abuse. *The American Journal of Psychiatry* 153(3):369-375.

Brender JD, Pichette JL, Suarez L, Hendricks KA, Holt M. 2003. Health risks of residential exposure to polycyclic aromatic hydrocarbons. *Archives of Environmental Health* 58(2):111-118.

Camerino D, Cassitto MG, Gilioli R. 1993. Prevalence of abnormal neurobehavioral scores in populations exposed to different industrial chemicals. *Environmental Research* 61(2):251-257.

Caress SM, Steinemann AC. 2003. A review of a two-phase population study of multiple chemical sensitivities. *Environmental Health Perspectives* 111(12):1490-1497.

Caress SM, Steinemann AC, Waddick C. 2002. Symptomatology and etiology of multiple chemical sensitivities in the Southeastern United States. *Archives of Environmental Health* 57(5):429-436.

Choi IS. 1983. Delayed neurologic sequelae in carbon monoxide intoxication. *Archives of Neurology* 40(7):433-435.

Christie D, Robinson K, Gordon I, Webley C, Bisby J. 1987. Current mortality in the Australian petroleum industry: The healthy-worker effect and the influence of life-style factors. *Medical Journal of Australia* 147(5):222, 224-225.

Clauw DJ. 2001. Potential mechanisms in chemical intolerance and related conditions. *Annals of the New York Academy of Sciences* 933:235-253.

Corneil W, Beaton R, Murphy S, Johnson C, Pike K. 1999. Exposure to traumatic incidents and prevalence of posttraumatic stress symptomatology in urban firefighters in two countries. *Journal of Occupational Health Psychology* 4(2):131-141.

Cullen MR. 1987. The worker with multiple chemical sensitivities: An overview. *Occupational Medicine* 2(4):665-661.

Dagg TG, Satin KP, Bailey WJ, Wong O, Harmon LL, Swencicki RE. 1992. An updated cause specific mortality study of petroleum refinery workers. *British Journal of Industrial Medicine* 49(3):203-212.

Davidoff AL, Keyl PM. 1996. Symptoms and health status in individuals with multiple chemical sensitivities syndrome from four reported sensitizing exposures and a general population comparison group. *Archives of Environmental Health* 51(3):201-213.

Davidoff AL, Keyl PM, Meggs W. 1998. Development of multiple chemical sensitivities in laborers after acute gasoline fume exposure in an underground tunneling operation. *Archives of Environmental Health* 53(3):183-189.
Fiedler N, Kipen HM. 2001. Controlled exposures to volatile organic compounds in sensitive groups. *Annals of the New York Academy of Sciences* 933:24-37.
Fiedler N, Giardino N, Natelson B, Ottenweller JE, Weisel C, Lioy P, Lehrer P, Ohman-Strickland P, Kelly-McNeil K, Kipen H. 2004. Responses to controlled diesel vapor exposure among chemically sensitive Gulf War veterans. *Psychosomatic Medicine* 66(4):588-598.
Fiedler N, Kipen H, DeLuca J, Kelly-McNeil K, Natelson B. 1996. A controlled comparison of multiple chemical sensitivities and chronic fatigue syndrome. *Psychosomatic Medicine* 58(1):38-49.
Fiedler N, Lange G, Tiersky L, DeLuca J, Policastro T, Kelly-McNeil K, McWilliams R, Korn L, Natelson B. 2000. Stressors, personality traits, and coping of Gulf War veterans with chronic fatigue. *Journal of Psychosomatic Research* 48(6):525-535.
Fukuda K, Nisenbaum R, Stewart G, Thompson WW, Robin L, Washko RM, Noah DL, Barrett DH, Randall B, Herwaldt BL, Mawle AC, Reeves WC. 1998. Chronic multisymptom illness affecting Air Force veterans of the Gulf War. *Journal of the American Medical Association* 280(11):981-988.
Goss Gilroy Inc. 1998. *Health Study of Canadian Forces Personnel Involved in the 1991 Conflict in the Persian Gulf.* Ottawa, Canada: Goss Gilroy Inc. Department of National Defence.
Graveling R, Pilkington A, George J, Butler M, Tannahill S. 1999. A review of multiple chemical sensitivity. *Occupational and Environmental Medicine* 56(2):73-85.
Gray GC, Reed RJ, Kaiser KS, Smith TC, Gastanaga VM. 2002. Self-reported symptoms and medical conditions among 11,868 Gulf War-era veterans: The Seabee Health Study. *American Journal of Epidemiology* 155(11):1033-1044.
Hakkola M, Honkasalo ML, Pulkkinen P. 1996. Neuropsychological symptoms among tanker drivers exposed to gasoline. *Occupational Medicine* 46(2):125-130.
Hakkola M, Honkasalo ML, Pulkkinen P. 1997. Changes in neuropsychological symptoms and moods among tanker drivers exposed to gasoline during a work week. *Occupational Medicine* 47(6):344-348.
Hanis NM, Shallenberger LG, Donaleski DL, Sales EA. 1985. A retrospective mortality study of workers in three major U.S. refineries and chemical plants. Part 1: Comparisons with U.S. population. *Journal of Occupational Medicine* 27(4):283-292.
IOM (Institute of Medicine). 2003. *Gulf War and Health, Volume 2: Insecticides and Solvents.* Washington, DC: The National Academies Press.
Iowa Persian Gulf Study Group. 1997. Self-reported illness and health status among Gulf War veterans. A population-based study. The Iowa Persian Gulf Study Group. *JAMA* 277(3):238-245.
Jason LA, Taylor RR, Kennedy CL. 2000. Chronic fatigue syndrome, fibromyalgia, and multiple chemical sensitivities in a community-based sample of persons with chronic fatigue syndrome-like symptoms. *Psychosomatic Medicine* 62(5):655-663.
Jee SH, Wang JD, Sun CC, Chao YF. 1985. Prevalence of probable kerosene dermatoses among ball-bearing factory workers. *Scandinavian Journal of Work, Environment & Health* 12(1):61-65.
Jia X, Xiao P, Jin X, Shen G, Wang X, Jin T, Nordberg G. 2002. Adverse effects of gasoline on the skin of exposed workers. *Contact Dermatitis* 46(1):44-47.
Kajdasz DK, Lackland DT, Mohr LC, Judson MA. 2001. A current assessment of rurally linked exposures as potential risk factors for sarcoidosis. *Annals of Epidemiology* 11(2):111-117.
Kang HK, Mahan CM, Lee KY, Magee CA, Murphy FM. 2000. Illnesses among United States veterans of the Gulf War: A population-based survey of 30,000 veterans. *Journal of Occupational and Environmental Medicine* 42(5):491-501.
Kang HK, Natelson BH, Mahan CM, Lee KY, Murphy FM. 2003. Post-traumatic stress disorder and chronic fatigue syndrome-like illness among Gulf War veterans: A population-based survey of 30,000 veterans. *American Journal of Epidemiology* 157(2):141-148.

Kern DG, Neill MA, Wrenn DS, Varone JC. 1993. Investigation of a unique time-space cluster of sarcoidosis in firefighters. *American Review of Respiratory Disease* 148(4 Pt 1):974-980.

Kessler RC. 2000. Posttraumatic stress disorder: The burden to the individual and to society. *Journal of Clinical Psychiatry* 61(Suppl 5):4-12.

Kilburn KH. 1999. Neurobehavioral and respiratory findings in jet engine repair workers: A comparison of exposed and unexposed volunteers. *Environmental Research* 80(3):244-252.

Kilburn KH, Warshaw RH. 1995. Neurotoxic effects from residential exposure to chemicals from an oil reprocessing facility and superfund site. *Neurotoxicology and Teratology* 17(2):89-102.

Kipen HM, Hallman W, Kelly-McNeil K, Fiedler N. 1995. Measuring chemical sensitivity prevalence: A questionnaire for population studies. *American Journal of Public Health* 85(4):574-577.

Knave B, Persson HE, Goldberg JM, Westerholm P. 1976. Long-term exposure to jet fuel: An investigation on occupationally exposed workers with special reference to the nervous system. *Scandinavian Journal of Work, Environment & Health* 2(3):152-164.

Knave B, Olson BA, Elofsson S, Gamberale F, Isaksson A, Mindus P, Persson HE, Struwe G, Wennberg A, Westerholm P. 1978. Long-term exposure to jet fuel. II. A cross-sectional epidemiologic investigation on occupationally exposed industrial workers with special reference to the nervous system. *Scandinavian Journal of Work, Environment & Health* 4(1):19-45.

Kreutzer R, Neutra RR, Lashuay N. 1999. Prevalence of people reporting sensitivities to chemicals in a population-based survey. *American Journal of Epidemiology* 150(1):1-12.

Kulka RA, Schlenger WE, Fairbank JA, Hough RL, Jordan BK, Marmar CR, Weiss DS. 1990. *Trauma and the Vietnam War Generation: Report of Findings from the National Vietnam Veterans Readjustment Study.* New York: Brunner/Mazel.

Kumar P, Gupta BN, Pandya KP, Clerk SH. 1988. Behavioral studies in petrol pump workers. *International Archives of Occupational and Environmental Health* 61(1-2):35-38.

Labbate LA, Cardena E, Dimitreva J, Roy M, Engel CC. 1998. Psychiatric syndromes in Persian Gulf War veterans: An association of handling dead bodies with somatoform disorders. *Psychotherapy and Psychosomatics* 67(4-5):275-279.

Maruff P, Burns CB, Tyler P, Currie BJ, Currie J. 1998. Neurological and cognitive abnormalities associated with chronic petrol sniffing. *Brain* 121(Pt 10):1903-1917.

Meggs WJ, Dunn KA, Bloch RM, Goodman PE, Davidoff AL. 1996. Prevalence and nature of allergy and chemical sensitivity in a general population. *Archives of Environmental Health* 51(4):275-282.

Miller BG, Cowie HA, Middleton WG, Seaton A. 1986. Epidemiologic studies of Scottish oil shale workers: III. Causes of death. *American Journal of Industrial Medicine* 9(5):433-446.

Miller CS, Prihoda TJ. 1999. A controlled comparison of symptoms and chemical intolerances reported by Gulf War veterans, implant recipients and persons with multiple chemical sensitivity. *Toxicology and Industrial Health* 15(3-4):386-397.

Muldoon S, Cauley J, Kuller L, Morrow L, Needleman H, Scott J, Hooper F. 1996. Effects of blood lead levels on cognitive function of older women. *Neuroepidemiology* 15(2):62-72.

Norman JE Jr, Kurtzke JF, Beebe GW. 1983. Epidemiology of multiple sclerosis in U.S. veterans: 2. Latitude, climate and the risk of multiple sclerosis. *Journal of Chronic Diseases* 36(8):551-559.

Odkvist LM, Arlinger SD, Edling C, Larsby B, Bergholtz LM. 1987. Audiological and vestibulo-oculomotor findings in workers exposed to solvents and jet fuel. *Scandinavian Audiology* 16(2):75-81.

Park H, Sprince NL, Whitten PS, Burmeister LF, Zwerling C. 2001. Farm-related dermatoses in Iowa male farmers and wives of farmers: A cross-sectional analysis of the Iowa Farm Family Health and Hazard Surveillance Project. *Journal of Occupational and Environmental Medicine* 43(4):364-369.

Payton M, Riggs K, Spiro A3, Weiss S, Hu H. 1998. Relations of bone and blood lead to cognitive function: The VA Normative Aging Study. *Neurotoxicology and Teratology* 20(1):19-27.

Perconte S, Wilson A, Pontius E, Dietrick A, Kirsch C, Sparacino C. 1993. Unit-based intervention for Gulf war soldiers surviving a SCUD missile attack: Program description and preliminary findings. *Journal of Traumatic Stress* 6(2):225-238.

Prezant DJ, Dhala A, Goldstein A, Janus D, Ortiz F, Aldrich TK, Kelly KJ. 1999. The incidence, prevalence, and severity of sarcoidosis in New York City firefighters. *Chest* 116(5):1183-1193.

Proctor SP, Heeren T, White RF, Wolfe J, Borgos MS, Davis JD, Pepper L, Clapp R, Sutker PB, Vasterling JJ, Ozonoff D. 1998. Health status of Persian Gulf War veterans: Self-reported symptoms, environmental exposures and the effect of stress. *International Journal of Epidemiology* 27(6):1000-1010.

Proctor SP, Heaton KJ, White RF, Wolfe J. 2001. Chemical sensitivity and chronic fatigue in Gulf War veterans: A brief report. *Journal of Occupational & Environmental Medicine* 43(3):259-264.

Proctor SP. 2000. Chemical sensitivity and gulf war veterans' illnesses. *Occupational Medicine* 15(3):587-599.

Reid S, Hotopf M, Hull L, Ismail K, Unwin C, Wessely S. 2001. Multiple chemical sensitivity and chronic fatigue syndrome in British Gulf War veterans. *American Journal of Epidemiology* 153(6):604-609.

Reid S, Hotopf M, Hull L, Ismail K, Unwin C, Wessely S. 2002. Reported chemical sensitivities in a health survey of United Kingdom military personnel. *Occupational and Environmental Medicine* 59(3):196-198.

Rostker, B. 2000. *Environmental Exposure Report: Oil Well Fires*. [Online]. Available: http://www.gulflink.osd.mil/owf_ii/ [accessed August 6, 2004].

Simon G, Daniell W, Stockbridge H, Claypoole K, Rosenstock L. 1993. Immunologic, psychological, and neuropsychological factors in multiple chemical sensitivity. A controlled study. *Annals of Internal Medicine* 119(2):97-103.

Sorg BA, Bailie TM, Tschirgi ML, Li N, Wu WR. 2001. Exposure to repeated low-level formaldehyde in rats increases basal corticosterone levels and enhances the corticosterone response to subsequent formaldehyde. *Brain Research* 898(2):314-320.

Sorg BA, Willis JR, Nowatka TC, Ulibarri C, See RE, Westberg HH. 1996. Proposed animal neurosensitization model for multiple chemical sensitivity in studies with formalin. *Toxicology* 111(1-3):135-145.

Sorg BA, Willis JR, See RE, Hopkins B, Westberg HH. 1998. Repeated low-level formaldehyde exposure produces cross-sensitization to cocaine: Possible relevance to chemical sensitivity in humans. *Neuropsychopharmacology* 18(5):385-394.

Spencer PS, McCauley LA, Lapidus JA, Lasarev M, Joos SK, Storzbach D. 2001. Self-reported exposures and their association with unexplained illness in a population-based case-control study of Gulf War veterans. *Journal of Occupational and Environmental Medicine* 43(12):1041-1056.

Sram RJ, Benes I, Binkova B, Dejmek J, Horstman D, Kotesovec F, Otto D, Perreault SD, Rubes J, Selevan SG, Skalik I, Stevens RK, Lewtas J. 1996. Teplice Program - The impact of air pollution on human health. *Environmental Health Perspectives* 104(Suppl 4):699-714.

Strauss P, Orris P, Buckley L. 1992. A health survey of toll booth workers. *American Journal of Industrial Medicine* 22(3):379-384.

Struwe G, Knave B, Mindus P. 1983. Neuropsychiatric symptoms in workers occupationally exposed to jet fuel-a combined epidemiological and casuistic study. *Acta Psychiatrica Scandinavica, Supplementum* 303:55-67.

Suadicani P, Ishoy T, Guldager B, Appleyard M, Gyntelberg F. 1999. Determinants of long-term neuropsychological symptoms: The Danish Gulf War Study. *Danish Medical Bulletin* 46(5):423-427.

Sutker PB, Uddo M, Brailey K, Vasterling JJ, Errera P. 1994. Psychopathology in war-zone deployed and nondeployed Operation Desert Storm troops assigned graves registration duties. *Journal of Abnormal Psychology* 103(2):383-390.

Tsai SP, Dowd CM, Cowles SR, Ross CE. 1992. A prospective study of morbidity patterns in a petroleum refinery and chemical plant. *British Journal of Industrial Medicine* 49(7):516-522.

Unwin C, Blatchley N, Coker W, Ferry S, Hotopf M, Hull L, Ismail K, Palmer I, David A, Wessely S. 1999. Health of UK servicemen who served in Persian Gulf War. *Lancet* 353:169-178.

US DHHS (US Department of Health and Human Services). 1999. *Mental Health: A Report of the Surgeon General*. Rockville, MD: US Department of Health and Human Services, Substance Abuse and Mental Health Services Administration, Center for Mental Health Services, National Institutes of Health, National Institute of Mental Health.

Venn AJ, Yemaneberhan H, Bekele Z, Lewis SA, Parry E, Britton J. 2001. Increased risk of allergy associated with the use of kerosene fuel in the home. *American Journal of Respiratory and Critical Care Medicine* 164(9):1660-1664.

Wagner D, Heinrichs M, Ehlert U. 1998. Prevalence of symptoms of posttraumatic stress disorder in German professional firefighters. *American Journal of Psychiatry* 155(12):1727-1732.

Weiss DS, Marmar CR, Metzler TJ, Ronfeldt HM. 1995. Predicting symptomatic distress in emergency services personnel. *Journal of Consulting and Clinical Psychology* 63(3):361-368.

Wen CP, Tsai SP, Gibson RL, McClellan WA. 1984. Long-term mortality of oil refinery workers. II. Comparison of the experience of active, terminated and retired workers. *Journal of Occupational Medicine* 26(2):118-127.

White RF, Proctor SP, Heeren T, Wolfe J, Krengel M, Vasterling J, Lindem K, Heaton KJ, Sutker P, Ozonoff DM. 2001. Neuropsychological function in Gulf War veterans: Relationships to self-reported toxicant exposures. *American Journal of Industrial Medicine* 40(1):42-54.

Wolf R, Movshowitz M, Brenner S. 1994. Contact dermatitis in Israeli soldiers. *Journal of Toxicology and Environmental Health* 43(1):7-11.

Wolf R, Movshowitz M, Brenner S. 1996. Supplemental tests in the evaluation of occupational hand dermatitis in soldiers. *International Journal of Dermatology* 35(3):173-176.

Wolfe J, Brown P, Kelley J. 1993. Reassessing war stress: Exposure and the Persian Gulf War. *Journal of Social Issues* 49(4):15-31.

Wolfe J, Proctor SP, Davis JD, Borgos MS, Friedman MJ. 1998. Health symptoms reported by Persian Gulf War veterans two years after return. *American Journal of Industrial Medicine* 33(2):104-113.

Wolfe J, Proctor SP, Erickson DJ, Hu H. 2002. Risk factors for multisymptom illness in US Army veterans of the Gulf War. *Journal of Occupational and Environmental Medicine* 44(3):271-281.

Yemaneberhan H, Bekele Z, Venn A, Lewis S, Parry E, Britton J. 1997. Prevalence of wheeze and asthma and relation to atopy in urban and rural Ethiopia. *Lancet* 350(9071):85-90.

Zhou Y, Cheng YS. 2000. Characterization of emissions from kerosene heaters in an unvented tent. *Aerosol Science and Technology* 33(6):510-524.

9

HYDRAZINES AND NITRIC ACID

This chapter discusses the committee's review and evaluation of epidemiologic studies and toxicologic information on persistent human health effects that might have resulted from exposure to hydrazines and nitric acid (HNO_3). This format is a departure from previous chapters in which the number of epidemiologic studies on exposure to fuels and combustion products were too numerous to include all in one chapter.

US military personnel present in the Persian Gulf region during Operation Desert Storm might have been exposed to inhibited red fuming nitric acid (IRFNA) and possibly unsymmetrical dimethylhydrazine (UDMH) if it was used as rocket fuel when they were near disintegrating incoming short-range ballistic missiles, commonly known as Scuds, that dispersed uncombusted fuel, oxidizers, and combustion products (DOD 2001). Somewhat fewer than 100 Scuds were launched by Iraq; about 50 were directed at Kuwait and the remainder came down in or near Israel (DOD 2001). Many of the Scuds broke apart on re-entry, each releasing about 300 lb of residual oxidizer and 100 lb of fuel (DOD 2001). Disintegration would have had to occur less than 3 km above the ground for those chemicals not to have been dissipated by the time they reached the ground (DOD 2000). If the chemicals did reach the ground, they could potentially expose an area of 2-3 km by 100-200 m but would evaporate within a few hours (DOD 2000). The National Research Council (NRC 1998) noted that in the vicinity of a rocket launch, nitric acid would be more likely to be in the form of an aqueous aerosol than a gas. The amount of nitric acid that would result if an ignited launch were aborted would greatly exceed the amount produced if combustion proceeded.

Military personnel in the vicinity of incoming Scuds reported experiencing an array of acute health effects, including burning sensations, tearing eyes, runny noses, nausea, vomiting, dizziness, sleeplessness, headaches, and blurred vision (DOD 2001). After aerial breakup of Scuds, "some cases" required medical treatment or hospitalization, but there were no instances of pulmonary edema (DOD 2000). After direct contact with several Iraqi missiles captured at a storage facility, there were two or three cases of skin burns (DOD 2001). The committee is not aware of other uses of hydrazines or nitric acid during the Gulf War that might have resulted in exposure of US military personnel.

Hydrazines have similar chemical structures but they differ in their production, uses, and adverse health effects (ATSDR 1997). Symmetrical (or 1,2-) dimethylhydrazine will not be considered here, because it is not used as a rocket propellant, as are hydrazine, monomethylhydrazine (MMH), and unsymmetrical (or 1,1-) dimethlyhydrazine. Although Iraq had apparently experimented with UDMH as a rocket fuel, it is more likely that kerosene was the rocket fuel used during the Gulf War (DOD 2001).

Nitric acid, probably in the form of IRFNA, was used as an oxidizer for the propellant in the Scuds (DOD 2000). Metal corrosion is inhibited if a halogen compound, such as hydrogen fluoride or iodine, is added to red fuming nitric acid (RFNA) (DOD 2000). The oxidizer's color and fuming properties result from the high concentration of nitric acid, relative to nitrogen dioxide, in the liquid (EFMA 1997).

The remainder of this chapter contains the committee's evaluation of the scientific literature on adverse, persistent health effects of hydrazines and nitric acid. It begins by reviewing toxicologic information on those chemicals, then reviews human studies related to whether persistent health effects might be associated with exposure to hydrazines and nitric acid, and finally presents the committee's conclusions.

TOXICOLOGY

This section provides an overview of toxicologic information on two chemicals—UDMH and RFNA—that may have been dispersed over Gulf War veterans by disintegrating Scuds. Because toxicologic data on those chemicals are sparse, the findings on similar chemicals are also reviewed. Data on hydrazine and MMH are considered in addition to those on UDMH, and information on nitric acid in general is reviewed with the extremely limited data specifically on RFNA. For each of those sets of chemicals (hydrazines and nitric acids), the following information is presented: uses, physical and chemical properties, exposure limits recommended by national and international government bodies and organizations, toxicokinetic properties, summaries of experimental studies, and any evidence of genetic susceptibility and of interactions between the chemicals in question and other substances.

The committee's approach was to use toxicity data, primarily from experimental animal studies, for background information and as supporting evidence. Therefore, an extensive review of toxicologic studies was not appropriate here. Several organizations—for example, the Agency for Toxic Substances and Disease Registry (ATSDR 1997), the International Agency for Research on Cancer (IARC 1974, 1999a, 1999b, 1999c) the National Institute for Occupational Safety and Health (NIOSH 1976), and the National Research Council (NRC 1996, 1998, 2000)—have conducted reviews of hydrazine- and nitric acid-related compounds. The reader is referred to those sources for more detailed reviews of the toxicologic data on the compounds.

Hydrazines

Hydrazines contain two nitrogen atoms joined by a single covalent bond. Hydrazine, UDMH, and MMH are used as rocket propellants. Hydrazine is also used for such applications as agricultural pesticides and water treatment (IARC 1999b). UDMH is also used for chemical syntheses, as an absorbent for acid gas, and as a plant-growth control agent (NRC 2000). MMH is also used as a chemical intermediate (NRC 2000). Some physical and chemical characteristics of hydrazines are listed in Table 9.1.

TABLE 9.1 Chemical Identity and Selected Physical and Chemical Properties of Hydrazines and Nitric Acid

Properties	Hydrazine	MMH	UDMH	Nitric Acid
Synonyms	Diamine, diamide, anhydrous hydrazine, hydrazine base	Methylhydrazine	1,1-Dimethylhydrazine, dimazine, dimazin	Aqua fortis, azotic acid, hydrogen nitrate, nitryl hydroxide; white fuming nitric acid (WFNA, 97.5% HNO_3), red fuming nitric acid (RFNA, 85% HNO_3), concentrated nitric acid (CNA, 68-70% HNO_3)
CAS registry no.	302-01-2	60-34-4	57-14-7	7697-37-2
Molecular weight	32.05	46.07	60.10	63.01
Chemical formula	N_2H_4	CH_6N_2	$C_2H_8N_2$	HNO_3
Color	Colorless	Colorless	Colorless	Colorless, yellowish, or reddish-brown
Physical state	Liquid	Liquid	Liquid	Liquid
Boiling point	113.5°C	87.5°C	63.9°C	83°C (WFNA) 121°C (CNA)
Melting point	2°C	–52.4°C	–58°C	–42°C (WFNA) –38°C (monohydrate) –18°C (trihydrate)
Solubility	Miscible with water and methyl, ethyl, propyl, and isobutyl alcohols; insoluble in chloroform and diethyl ether	Soluble in hydrocarbons; miscible with water and low-molecular-weight monohydric alcohols	Miscible with water, alcohol, ether, dimethyl formamide, and hydrocarbons	Miscible in water
Vapor pressure	14.1 mm Hg at 25°C	49.63 mm Hg at 25°C	157 mm Hg at 25°C	57 mm Hg at 25°C (WFNA) - 49 mm Hg at 20°C (CNA)
Flash point	37.8°C (closed cup)	–8.33°C	–15°C (closed cup)	Not flammable

Properties	Hydrazine	MMH	UDMH	Nitric Acid
Explosive limits	4.7-100% by volume in air	Not found	2-95% by volume in air	Not found
Disassociation constant	na	na	na	pKa < 0
Conversion factor	1 ppm = 1.31 mg/m^3 1 mg/m^3 = 0.76 ppm	1 ppm = 1.88 mg/m^3 1 mg/m^3 = 0.53 ppm	1 ppm = 2.5 mg/m^3 1 mg/m^3 = 0.41 ppm	1 ppm = 2.6 mg/m^3 1 mg/m^3 = 0.38 ppm

NOTE: CAS=Chemical Abstracts Services; MMH=monomethylhydrazine; UDMH=unsymmetrical dimethylhydrazine; na=not applicable.
SOURCES: ATSDR (1997), EFMA (1997), IARC (1992, 1999b), NRC (1996, 2000).

Exposure limits and carcinogenic classifications have been recommended for hydrazines by such organizations as ACGIH, ATSDR, the US Environmental Protection Agency (EPA), IARC, NRC, and the Occupational Safety and Health Administration (OSHA). Those limits and classifications are summarized in Table 9.2.

Toxicokinetics

Animal studies using inhalation, dermal, and oral exposures have been conducted on the absorption, distribution, metabolism, and excretion of hydrazines. The toxicokinetics of hydrazines appears to differ among animal species (ATSDR 1997), and there are differences in the metabolic pathways of hydrazine, UDMH, and MMH (ATSDR 1997).

Hydrazines are rapidly absorbed into the blood, and they and their metabolites are distributed to various tissues, such as the kidney, liver, lung, muscle, bladder, and pancreas (ATSDR 1997; Kaneo et al. 1984; Pinkerton et al. 1967). Plasma concentrations in male rats given UDMH subcutaneously at 50 mg/kg rapidly decreased after exposure, with a half-life of about 1 hour (Fiala and Kulakis 1981). UDMH was detectable in the blood of dogs within 30 sec of application (at 5-30 mmol/kg) to their shaved chests, but blood concentrations did not start to rise substantially for about 5 minutes (Smith and Clark 1971). Similar results were reported for cutaneous absorption of hydrazine (at 3-15 mmol/kg) (Smith and Clark 1972).

There does not appear to be preferential accumulation in specific tissues. Hydrazines with a free amino group are able to react with endogenous alpha-keto acids, which can produce adverse health effects (ATSDR 1997). Hydrazine undergoes acetylation and can react with cellular molecules in vivo (Kaneo et al. 1984; Llewellyn et al. 1986; Preece et al. 1991). UDMH undergoes demethylation and can react with cellular molecules (Mitz et al. 1962).

Evidence suggests that at least some hydrazines are metabolized by both enzymatic and nonenzymatic pathways (ATSDR 1997; Godoy et al. 1984; Tomasi et al. 1987). The metabolic process may be dose-dependent and saturable (Preece et al. 1992). Three cytochrome P450 isozymes (CYP2E1, CYP2B1, and CYP1A1/2) are involved in metabolism of hydrazine (Delaney and Timbrell 1995; Jenner and Timbrell 1994; Timbrell et al. 1982). Hydrazine has also been shown to be metabolized by another enzymatic pathway (peroxidases) and by a nonenzymatic pathway (a copper-ion-mediated pathway) (Sinha 1987). Hydrazine metabolism produces free radicals and carbonium ion intermediates that may be responsible for adverse health effects (ATSDR 1997). Koizumi et al. (1998) found that metabolism of hydrazine in humans is affected by genotypes of an isozyme of *N*-acetyltransferase, NAT2.

Hydrazines and their metabolites are excreted in urine and in expired air (ATSDR 1997). Llewellyn et al. (1986) reported that unchanged hydrazine, acetyl hydrazine, and diacetylhydrazine were found in the urine of hydrazine-treated animals.

TABLE 9.2 Recommended Exposure Limits for Hydrazines and Nitric Acid

Organization	Chemical	Type of Exposure Limit	Recommended Exposure Limit	Reference
ACGIH	Hydrazine	TLV	0.01 ppm, A3, skin (adopted 1995)	ACGIH 2003
	UDMH	TLV	0.01 ppm, A3, skin (adopted 1995)	ACGIH 2003
	MMH	TLV	0.01 ppm, A3, skin (adopted 1995)	ACGIH 2003
	Nitric acid	TLV	2.0 ppm (adopted 1976)	ACGIH 2003
	Nitric acid	STEL	4.0 ppm	
ATSDR	Hydrazine	MRL	0.004 ppm (intermediate-duration inhalation exposure)	ATSDR 1997
	UDMH	MRL	0.0002 ppm (intermediate-duration inhalation exposure)	
EPA	Hydrazine	Evaluation of carcinogenicity	Probably human carcinogen (group B2)	IRIS 2003
IARC	Hydrazine and UDMH	Evaluation of carcinogenicity	Overall evaluation: possibly carcinogenic in humans (Group 2B); sufficient evidence of carcinogenicity in experimental animals; inadequate evidence in humans	IARC 1999
	Nitric acid (included in review of strong-inorganic-acid mists, in which exposure to sulfuric acid dominated most studies)	Evaluation of carcinogenicity	Overall evaluation: strong-inorganic-acid mists containing sulfuric acid are carcinogenic in humans (group 1); sufficient evidence from occupational exposures	IARC 1992
NIOSH	Hydrazine	REL	0.03 ppm	NIOSH 1997
		IDLH	50 ppm	
	MMH	REL	0.04 ppm	
		IDLH	20 ppm	
	UDMH	REL	0.06 ppm	

Organization	Chemical	Type of Exposure Limit	Recommended Exposure Limit	Reference
		IDLH	15 ppm	
NIOSH	Nitric acid	REL	2.0 ppm	NIOSH 1994
		STEL	4.0 ppm	
		IDLH	25 ppm	
NRC	Hydrazine	SMAC	0.02 ppm (30-day exposure)	NRC 1996 2000
	MMH	AEGL-2	0.11 ppm (8-hr exposure)	
	UDMH		0.38 ppm (8-hr exposure)	
OSHA	Hydrazine	PEL	1.0 ppm	OSHA 1997 (29 CFR 1910.1000)
	UDMH		0.5 ppm	
	Nitric acid		2.0 ppm	OSHA 1972 (29 CFR 1910.93)

NOTE: UDMH=unsymmetrical dimethylhyrazine; MMH=monomethylhydrazine; ACGIH=American Conference of Governmental Industrial Hygienists; TWA=time-weighted average; TLV=threshold limit value (TWA for 8-hr workday and 40-hr workweek); STEL=short-term exposure limit (TWA for 15 min); A3=confirmed animal carcinogen with unknown relevance to humans; skin=potentially large contribution to exposure by cutaneous route; ATSDR=Agency for Toxic Substances and Disease Registry; EPA=US Environmental Protection Agency; IARC=International Agency for Research on Cancer; NIOSH=National Institute for Occupational Safety and Health; OSHA=Occupational Safety and Health Administration; MR= minimal risk level; REL=recommended exposure limit (TWA for 10-hr workday during 40-hr workweek); IDLH=concentration immediately dangerous to life or health; AEGL-2=acute exposure guideline level 2; SMAC=spacecraft maximum allowable concentration; PEL=permissible exposure limit (TWA for 8-hr workday during 40-hr workweek).

Experimental Studies

Experimental studies of the toxicity of hydrazines in humans and laboratory animals are summarized here. This section focuses on studies that examined chronic effects of hydrazines, particularly effects shown to persist after cessation of exposure. Epidemiologic studies assessing the adverse health effects of hydrazines are reviewed later in this chapter. On the basis of experimental data, chronic health effects of concern in relation to hydrazines are cancer and injuries to the respiratory tract, liver, and nervous and reproductive systems.

Respiratory Effects

MacEwen et al. (1970) exposed seven male volunteers (23-44 years old) to MMH at 90 ppm for 10 minutes by inhalation. The group consisted of smokers, former smokers, and nonsmokers. Acute effects included mild to moderate irritation of the nose, throat, and eyes; but there was no excessive lacrimation or coughing. No substantial exposure-related effects as measured with spirometry or clinical chemistry were observed during the 60 days after exposure, except for a 3-5% increase in Heinz body formation at day 7 that declined after 2 weeks.

Rats and mice exposed by inhalation to UDMH at as low as 0.05 ppm for 6 months showed effects on the lungs (hyperplasia) and nasal mucosa (inflammation, hyperplasia, and dysplasia) (Haun et al. 1984; Vernot et al. 1985). Dogs subchronically exposed at 25 ppm UDMH showed lung irritation and damage, but exposure at 5 ppm did not cause those effects (Rinehart et al. 1960). No studies that assessed respiratory effects after cessation of exposure of laboratory animals to hydrazines were found.

Hepatic Effects

Multiple hepatic effects have been observed in laboratory animals exposed to hydrazine and UDMH by inhalation and orally. Hepatotoxic changes (fatty changes, hyperplasia, hemosiderosis, increased serum enzymes, degeneration, and pigmentation of Kupffer cells) were observed in rats, mice, dogs, and monkeys subchronically or chronically exposed by inhalation to hydrazine at 0.25-14 ppm or to UDMH at 0.05-25 ppm (Comstock et al. 1954; Haun 1977; Haun and Kinkead 1973; Haun et al. 1984; House 1964; Rinehart et al. 1960; Vernot et al. 1985; Weatherby and Yard 1955). Oral exposure to hydrazine also caused hepatotoxic effects in rats, mice, and hamsters (Biancifiori 1970; Preece et al. 1992; Wakabayashi et al. 1983; Weatherby and Yard 1955).

Nervous System Effects

The nervous system appears to be a target for hydrazine and UDMH. Hydrazine has been used as a chemotherapeutic agent, and some cancer patients treated with hydrazine orally at 0.2-0.7 mg/kg/day experienced neurologic effects, such as nausea, vomiting, dizziness, excitement, lethargy, and neuritis (ATSDR 1997; Ochoa et al. 1975); the side effects subsided on cessation of treatment. Nervous system effects (such as tremors, vomiting, convulsions, lethargy, and behavioral changes) have been observed in rats, mice, and dogs repeatedly exposed to hydrazine at 1 ppm or UDMH at up to 140 ppm by inhalation and acutely exposed to hydrazine at 3-15 mmol/kg or UDMH at 5-30 mmol/kg) dermally (Haun and Kinkead 1973; Rinehart et al. 1960; Smith and Clark 1971, 1972; Weeks et al. 1963).

Reproductive and Developmental Effects

Keller et al. (1984) conducted a teratogenicity assessment of MMH and UDMH in rats with intraperitoneal administration but reported that developmental toxicity occurred only at doses that were toxic to the dams. Reproductive effects (ovarian and testicular atrophy, endometrial inflammation, endometrial cysts, and aspermatogenesis) were observed in hamsters and mice exposed by inhalation to hydrazine at 1-5 ppm (Vernot et al. 1985) and UDMH at 0.05 ppm (Haun et al. 1984).

Cancer

A number of animal studies have reported increases in the incidence of cancers after exposure to hydrazines (reviewed in ATSDR 1997; IARC 1999b; NRC 1996, 2000). Studies of hamsters exposed to UDMH by subcutaneous injection have had both positive findings (Ernst et al. 1987) and negative findings (Jeong and Kamino 1993). Oral exposures (by gavage or in drinking water) to UDMH or hydrazine (administered as hydrazine sulfate or isonicotinic acid hydrazide), however, have produced increased tumor rates (particularly of respiratory or hepatic tissues) in multiple strains of mice, rats, and hamsters (Bhide et al. 1976; Biancifiori 1970; Biancifiori et al. 1964, 1966; Bosan et al. 1987; Maru and Bhide 1982; Roe et al. 1967; Severi and Biancifiori 1968; Steinhoff and Mohr 1988; Toth 1969).

Inhalation exposure, which would be most relevant to the Gulf War experience, has been less intensively investigated but also produced positive findings. Year-long exposure of rats and hamsters to hydrazine at 0.05, 0.25, 1.0, or 5.0 ppm for 6 hr/day, 5 days/wk followed by at least a year of observation before sacrifice led to dose-dependent increases in the incidence of lesions of the nasal epithelium (Vernot et al. 1985). Mice had slight increases in the incidence of lung adenomas in the high-dose group, but the small groups of dogs (four males and four females per dose level) showed no consistent response (Vernot et al. 1985). Inhalation exposure of rats and mice to UDMH was associated with leukemia and tumors of the lung, nasal passages, bone, pancreas, pituitary, blood vessels, liver, and thyroid (Haun et al. 1984). Chronic inhalation of MMH was not found to be carcinogenic in rats or dogs, but it did produce lung, nasal, and liver tumors in mice and nasal, renal, and adrenal tumors in hamsters (Kinkead et al. 1985).

Genotoxicity

Hydrazine and UDMH have been shown to be genotoxic in both in vivo and in vitro tests (reviewed in ATSDR 1997). Hydrazine and UDMH are alkylating agents and produced DNA damage in in vivo assays but had negative results in in vivo assays of unscheduled DNA synthesis, dominant lethal mutation, and gene mutation. Hydrazine and UDMH had positive results in gene-mutation assays in *Salmonella typhimurium* and *Escherichia coli* with and without activation and in *Photobacterium leiognathi* without activation. Mammalian cell assays had positive results for DNA alkylation, transformation, sister chromatid exchange, and unscheduled DNA synthesis without activation, and for gene mutation with and without activation.

Other Health Outcomes

Amyloidosis of the kidneys was observed in hamsters exposed to hydrazine by inhalation at 0.25 ppm for 6 hr/day, 5 days/wk for 1 year but not in rats, mice, or dogs experiencing the same treatment regimen (Vernot et al. 1985). No renal effects were observed in dogs exposed to UDMH by inhalation at 25 ppm (Rinehart et al. 1960) or in mice given hydrazine orally at 9.5 mg/kg/day (Steinhoff et al. 1990).

Case studies have suggested that exposure to hydrazine or hydrazine derivatives is associated with systemic lupus erythematosus or a similar syndrome (Durant and Harris 1980) (Pereyo 1986), but the data are too sparse to support conclusions about an association. In addition, decreased T helper-cell counts observed in mice given UDMH by injection at 75 mg/kg/day are inconsistent with an autoimmune response (Frazier et al. 1991). In other studies, lymphocyte activity and DNA synthesis were suppressed by in vitro exposure to UMDH, possibly because of effects on interleukin-2 production or intracellular calcium (Bauer et al. 1990; Frazier et al. 1992). Taken together, data from laboratory animal studies fail to provide biologic plausibility of the hydrazine-induced autoimmunity suggested by human case reports.

Hydrazine is a sensitizing agent. Multiple case studies have reported that dermal exposure to solutions containing up to 1% hydrazine causes contact dermatitis (reviewed in ATSDR 1997).

Genetic Susceptibility

Little is known about genetic susceptibility to toxic effects of hydrazines. In laboratory animals, susceptibility to hydrazines varies with species, strain, and age (ATSDR 1997; NRC 2000).

Interactions

No data were found on potential interactions between hydrazines and other chemicals.

Nitric Acid

In addition to its use as an oxidizer in explosives, nitric acid is used as a mineral acid in industrial processes (particularly in metal pickling and electroplating) and is a component in the manufacture of synthetic fertilizers (ACGIH 2003; IARC 1992; Sathiakumar et al. 1997).

Some physical and chemical characteristics of nitric acid are presented in Table 9.1. Naming conventions and several of nitric acid's properties (particularly vapor pressure, melting and boiling points, and color) depend on the proportion of nitrogen dioxide (NO_2) in the nitric acid solution. Reagent grade or "concentrated" nitric acid (CNA) contains about 70% nitric acid. The fuming property is associated with yet more concentrated mixtures, which contain correspondingly less nitrogen dioxide; red fuming nitric acid (RFNA) is about 85% nitric acid, and white fuming nitric acid (WFNA) is about 97.5% nitric acid (ACGIH 2003; EFMA 1997). The designation "inhibited" for the rocket-fuel oxidizers connotes the inclusion of halogen additives (about 1% hydrogen fluoride or iodine) to suppress the corrosive properties of nitric acid on metal equipment (DOD 2000). Nitric acid is not combustible, but it is dangerously reactive with many materials (EPA 1987).

The extreme corrosive potential of this strong acid has long been recognized. As summarized in Table 9.2, ACGIH adopted a TLV of 2 ppm for nitric acid in 1966 on the basis of case reports dating from 1804 and animal studies published in 1954 (Diggle and Gage 1954) (Gray et al. 1954b); this was supplemented by a short-term exposure limit (STEL) of 4 ppm in 1976. NIOSH recommended the same values in 1976, and the Occupational Safety and Health Administration (OSHA) adopted a permissible exposure limit (PEL) for nitric acid of 2 ppm. Authoritative review bodies have drawn their conclusions about nitric acid in large part on the basis of its likely mechanistic similarity to and co-occurrence in occupational mists with other strong inorganic acids (EPA 1987; IARC 1992; NIOSH 1976).

Toxicokinetics

Nitric acid has a corrosive effect upon contact with biological tissues. It produces oxides of nitrogen, particularly nitrogen dioxide, when it spontaneously decomposes or reacts with metals or organic materials (NIOSH 1976). The deposition and toxicity of nitric acid in the respiratory tract is a function of the form of the nitric acid (vapor or aerosol); vapor or small particles penetrate more deeply into the lung. IARC (1992) noted that nitric acid is generally a vapor but that its water solubility when aerosol forms would favor upper airway deposition of larger particles that would have greater potential to alter the pH of mucus in a specific location. More recent investigations suggest that, contrary to expectation, inhaled vapor-phase nitric acid may be converted into or deposited on small particles in the humid atmosphere of the respiratory tract; this would facilitate its transport to and deposition in the deep lung (Chen and Schlesinger 1996). Detailed information on absorption, metabolic processing, tissue-specific distribution, or elimination of nitric acid was not found.

Experimental Studies

Experimental studies that address the toxicity of nitric acid in laboratory animals are summarized here. Epidemiologic studies assessing the adverse health effects of nitric acid are reviewed later. The primary concern of this chapter is effects of nitric acid that might persist after cessation of exposure.

The immediate consequences of contact with nitric acid are severe enough for its acute effects to have led to controlling its occupational use and to additional regulation; therefore, the chronic effects and toxic mechanism of nitric acid have not been extensively investigated with contemporary protocols. On the basis of case reports and experimental data, the chronic health effects of concern for nitric acid are the residual effects of irritation of the eyes, skin, respiratory tract, and gastrointestinal tract; dental erosion; and the possibility that it is carcinogenic.

Residual Effects of Corrosive Action and Irritation

Occupational case reports adequately document the severe and potentially permanent dermal and ocular damage that results from contact with nitric acid, so few animal studies of these effects have been conducted. Dermal contact with concentrated nitric acid can produce burns or severe irritant (acute eczematous) dermatitis, damaging the skin's upper and lower layers within minutes and possibly resulting in permanent scarring and impairment of function (Birmingham 1988). Aside from burns, nitric acid may stain skin yellow to brown because of the conversion of skin proteins to xanthoproteic acid (White 1934). More dilute solutions produce milder irritation and hardening of the epithelium (NIOSH 1976).

Contact of the eye with nitric acid in sufficient amount or concentration can produce corneal opacification; mild injury may resolve, but severe ocular damage may persist as blindness (NIOSH 1976).

Case studies of workers exposed subchronically to vapors of nitric acid have consistently reported erosion of dental enamel, a permanent effect. Most often, however, such exposure occurs in combination with other strong acids, such as sulfuric or hydrochloric acid, which actually may be more potent than nitric acid in this respect (Dettling 1935; Lynch and Bell 1947; tenBruggen Cate 1968).

Similarly, the corrosive effects on the gastrointestinal tract and potentially lethal consequences observed in isolated cases of nitric acid ingestion have obviated the need for experimentation with animals on such outcomes (NIOSH 1976). In any event, this route of exposure would not be pertinent for Gulf War veterans exposed to nitric acid showering down from disintegrating Scud missiles.

Somewhat more toxicologic investigation has been conducted regarding the respiratory consequences of inhaling nitric acid vapors at various concentrations. The report by Diggle and

Gage (1954) of exposure to nitric acid for an unspecified period at 25 ppm (63 mg/m^3) as a no-observed-effect level (NOEL) in rats was first cited by ACGIH when proposing the current TLV of 2 ppm in 1964 and has since served as a primary piece of toxicologic data supporting regulatory levels for nitric acid; the original article, however, provided no detail about the conduct of the assay (NIOSH 1976).

The other long-referenced body of information about the toxicologic effects of inhaling nitric acid (and RFNA in particular) is a series of studies by Gray et al. (1952, 1954a, 1954b). Rats exposed to RFNA (nitrogen dioxide at 9-14 ppm, nitric acid concentration not stated) showed widespread inflammation of the airways, especially of the upper portion, immediately after exposure for 40-96 hours; several weeks later, much of the inflammation had abated, but all lungs examined were reported to have localized areas of "emphysema". The extent and persistence of those effects were not functions of duration of exposure (Gray et al. 1952). Acute 30-minute exposures of male rats to nitrogen dioxide alone, RFNA (8-17% nitrogen dioxide), or WFNA (0.1-0.4% nitrogen dioxide) produced lethal concentrations (LC_{50}s) of 174 ppm, 310 ppm, and 334 ppm, respectively; burns were observed on the animals, but pulmonary edema was the cause of death (Gray et al. 1954b). Those findings have been interpreted as suggesting that the nitrogen dioxide with which nitric acid coexists may be the primary toxic constituent of the vapor mixtures (ACGIH 2003; NIOSH 1976). Chronic exposure of 30 mice, 90 rats, and 10 guinea pigs to RFNA at 4 ppm for 4 hr/day, 5 days/wk for up to 6 months produced no pathologic changes compared with control animals (Gray et al. 1954a).

There have been several studies of nitric acid's effect on isolated animal tissues (Greenberg et al. 1971; Pham-Huu-Chanh et al. 1966; Preziosi and Ciabattoni 1987). Nitric acid has been used to produce animal models of human obstructive airway disease (Greenberg et al. 1971; Mink et al. 1984; Peters and Hyatt 1986; Totten and Moran 1961).

More recently, nitric acid has been one of several components of ambient air pollution investigated in chamber studies. Nitric acid alone was found to penetrate far more deeply into the lung than might have been expected given its anticipated solubility in the mucus of the upper respiratory tract, perhaps as a result of being converted from vapor to particle form (Schlesinger et al. 1994, 1995). Nitric acid also impaired macrophage secretion of superoxide and tumor necosis factor alpha, and this has implications for pulmonary immunocompetence (Schlesinger et al. 1994, 1995) Unlike acid sulfates which can produce hyperreactivity, nitric acid tended to produce hyporeactivity (Schlesinger et al. 1994, 1995).

Cancer

Considerable attention has been addressed to the possibility that nitric acid, like other strong inorganic acids, might contribute to the development of lung or laryngeal cancer in workers exposed to acid mists (IARC 1992). Those acids often occur in combination, and sulfuric acid has been considered the compound most likely to be responsible for any such effect, but they could share a mechanism of toxic action. Soskolne et al. (1989) reviewed the existing information to evaluate whether acids are likely to cause chronic effects, particularly cancer. They focused on the sulfuric acid literature, but asserted that the chronic tissue irritation associated with acid exposure and the perturbations of cellular functioning arising from pH extremes are plausible mechanisms of genotoxic and carcinogenic activity. Swenberg and Beauchamp (1997) concurred that a carcinogenic mechanism of action was feasible but concluded that the evidence from experimental animals neither strongly supports nor refutes the induction of cancer by inorganic acid mists.

Only the experiments of Ballou et al. (1978, 1981) included nitric acid as a test agent; it was used in parallel with hydrochloric acid and sulfuric acid. No significant increases in neoplasia were observed when groups of male rats with short-term inhalation exposure (30 minutes or six 6-hour exposures over 2 weeks) to nitric acid or to other acids were observed over their lifetimes and then compared with untreated and water-vapor-exposed controls.

Genotoxicity

Nitric acid specifically has been subjected to minimal genotoxicity testing that might illuminate any role in respiratory carcinogenesis. ToxNet's Gene-Tox database lists only a virally enhanced cell-transformation assay in Syrian hamster ovary cells with negative results (Heidelberger et al. 1983).

In reviewing nonphysiologic culture conditions that might contribute to positive results of in vitro genotoxicity assays, Scott et al. (1991) concluded that acid pH (but not specifically nitric acid) can produce chromosomal aberrations in a variety of in vitro test systems. Swenberg and Beauchamp (1997) noted that low pH can enhance the occurrence of DNA modifications (by depurination or deamination) that might lead to point mutations and might induce chromosomal aberrations. It is implausible, however, that occupational exposures would cause systemic alterations in pH.

Other Health Outcomes

Soskolne et al. (1989) hypothesized that chronic tissue irritation and extremes of pH associated with acid exposure might foster developmental insults and increase susceptibility to infection. IARC's review of strong inorganic acid mists (1992), however, found no toxicology studies addressing nitric acid's potential to generate reproductive or developmental effects, nor did the present committee's literature search reveal any reproductive-toxicity or immunotoxicity studies.

Genetic Susceptibility

No studies were found that addressed variability in susceptibility to the toxic effects of nitric acid, either between species or among individuals of a given species.

Interactions

The fact that RFNA with a higher concentration of nitrogen dioxide than WFNA (8-17% vs 0.1-0.4%) was found to have a lower LC_{50} (310 ppm vs 334 ppm) (Gray et al. 1954b) has been interpreted as suggesting that nitric acid has a synergistic effect on the primary irritating effect of nitrogen dioxide. Conversely, Mautz et al. (1988) hypothesized that the observed synergy of ozone and nitrogen dioxide is due to their reaction in situ to form nitric acid.

Rats and rabbits have been exposed to various combinations of nitric acid, ozone, and particles intended to simulate actual mixtures of ambient air pollution in California (as opposed to the sulfuric acid combinations that would be representative of air pollution in the eastern United States). Cells recovered from those animals by bronchiolar lavage were used in a variety of bioassays. The findings from chamber studies suggest that nitric acid does contribute to producing features similar to those of human bronchitis and emphysema (Keinman et al. 1995; Mautz et al. 1995; Schlesinger et al. 1995). Beyond the irritating effects of the H+ ion shared with other acids, the nitrate anion itself may have some toxic activity (Schlesinger et al. 1994). Nitric acid appears to be at most mildly synergistic with ozone and particles. The persistence of this set of respiratory effects has not been established.

EPIDEMIOLOGIC STUDIES

The relationship between occupational exposure to chemicals that may have been released from disintegrating Scud missiles (possibly UDMH and RFNA) and the development of long-term, adverse health effects has been examined in several retrospective cohort, case-control, and cross-sectional studies of the general public. Several studies of Gulf War veterans, most of which were cross-sectional and conducted years after the war, did inquire about exposure to scud missile debris. The studies of Gulf War veterans pertaining to possible Scud-related exposures are described below. Similar discussions of occupational studies concerning exposure to hydrazines or to nitric acid and other strong inorganic acids follow with summaries of their most relevant findings.

Gulf War Veteran Studies and Scud Missile Debris Exposure

All the studies of Gulf War veterans and exposure to Scud missile debris reviewed by the committee used questionnaires to identify a broad array of biologic and chemical exposures (usually 10-20 per study) and symptoms (often 25-100 in a checklist format) experienced by the veterans, but few involved any confirmation with clinical examinations or laboratory tests. This sort of study design—involving a host of self-reported symptoms and exposures—has limitations for drawing inferences about symptom-exposure relationships.

About 43% of veterans in the largest, most representative population-based study of US veterans reported exposure to Scud missile debris (Kang et al. 2000), so such exposure during the war was perceived to be common although the Department of Defense (DOD 2001) reported that there were fewer than 50 instances of Scud disintegration that might have exposed US troops.

Several major Gulf War health studies included Scud debris in their lists of exposure options. Some provide evidence of a relationship between self-reported Scud debris exposure and a self-reported health effects; others do not. The studies' key findings with respect to Scud missile debris exposure are summarized below.

Cohorts of Gulf War veterans from Ft. Devens, MA, and New Orleans, LA, have been followed longitudinally and reported on in a series of articles. Surveys were carried out shortly after return in 1991 and at 2-year intervals thereafter: 1992-1993, 1994-1995, and 1996-1997. The survey conducted in 1994-1995 (Proctor et al. 1998) was the first of these to examine symptom-exposure relationships. The study's nearly 300 subjects represented a stratified random sample of 2,949 troops from Ft. Devens and 928 troops from New Orleans, both consisting of active-duty, reserve, and National Guard troops deployed to the Gulf. The response rates for Ft. Devens and New Orleans were 85% and 58%, respectively, of subjects from an earlier study who could be found and contacted again. The control group consisted of 50 veterans deployed to Germany during the Gulf War era (December 1990-August 1991).

Proctor et al. (1998) analyzed the relationships between the subjects' responses to an eight-item exposure questionnaire and a checklist of symptoms experienced during the previous 30 days, adjusted for an index of combat stressors and posttraumatic stress disorder (PTSD) status as determined in a diagnostic interview. Each of the 52 symptoms on the symptom checklist was assigned to one of nine body systems (such as muscoskeletal symptoms) by four independent judges (an occupational-health physician, an environmental-health specialist, an environmental epidemiologist, and a neuropsychologist). Multiple regression adjusted for age, sex, education, combat stress score, and PTSD diagnosis found that "debris from Scuds" was associated with musculoskeletal ($p = 0.017$),[1] neurologic ($p < 0.001$),[2] neuropsychologic ($p = 0.001$),[3] and psychologic[4] symptoms ($p = 0.001$). White et al. (2001) reported on more detailed assessment of neuropsychologic functioning obtained with a neurobehavioral test battery on the same cohort and found no relationship between exposure to Scud debris and poorer performance.

Unwin et al. (1999) mailed questionnaires to population-based random samples of UK veterans deployed to the Gulf War, deployed to Bosnia, or serving but not deployed during the Gulf War era. The self-reported symptoms (within the previous 30 days) and military experiences (including having been within 1 mile of a Scud missile explosion) were contrasted among these groups of respondents. For three clusters of health outcomes of interest—Centers for Disease Control and Prevention (CDC) multi-symptom syndrome, posttraumatic stress reaction, and poor physical functioning—Scud missile debris exposure was uniformly more frequently reported by veterans with each of the sets of symptoms. The estimated Scud missile debris-related risk was higher for those deployed to Bosnia, but for all three symptom clusters the increase was greater than unity only for the Gulf War veterans; numerous other exposures, however, were found to be considerably more strongly associated with these health outcomes.

Reid et al. (2001) studied subgroups of British veterans meeting criteria for chronic fatigue syndrome (CFS)[5] or for multiple chemical sensitivity (MCS) among the respondents to the earlier investigation (Unwin et al. 1999). MCS was increased in the Gulf War sample (frequency 1.3%, 95% CI 1.0-1.7) in comparison with both the Bosnia-deployed (frequency 0.3%, 95% CI 0.1-0.6) and the era veterans (frequency 0.2%, 95% CI 0.1-0.4), whereas the frequency of CFS among the Gulf War veterans (2.1%, 95% CI 1.6-2.6) was increased only in comparison with the veterans deployed to Bosnia (0.7%, 95% CI 0.4-1.2). There was an association between Scud missile debris exposure and CFS in the 76 Gulf War veterans with CFS (OR 2.6, 95% CI 1.5-4.6). The 46 Gulf War veterans with MCS (who included seven of the CFS cases) were not more likely to report Scud debris exposure than the other Gulf War veterans (OR 1.6, 95% CI 0.8-3.0).

Goss Gilroy Inc. (1998) received 6,552 mailed responses from a cohort of almost 10,000 consisting of all Canadian Gulf War veterans and a similar sample of concurrent Canadian forces serving elsewhere. Exposure to Scud missile debris (exploding within 1 km) was one of about 10 exposures lumped into a broader category, created by the authors, termed "psychologic stressors". Other exposures in this category included dead animals; handling prisoners of war (POWs); wearing protective gear other than for training; hearing chemical alarms sounding; having artillery, rockets, mortars, or anything else other than Scud missiles explode in the air 1 km away; witnessing anyone dying; and handling dead bodies. The authors found many relationships between various symptoms and exposure to this category of "psychologic stressors", but the category is so heterogeneous that it would have been difficult to tie any health effect directly to Scud missile debris exposure.

The Danish Gulf War Study secured health information on 686 of the 821 peacekeeping forces sent to the Gulf from August 1990 through 1997 and contrasted it with that on 231

---

[1]Joint pains, backaches, and neckaches or stiffness.
[2]Headaches, numbness in arms or legs, and dizziness.
[3]Difficulties in learning new material, difficulty in concentrating, and confusion.
[4]Inability to fall asleep, frequent periods of feeling depressed, and frequent periods of anxiety or nervousness.
[5]A "case" of CFS was defined using veterans' responses to the study's fatigue scale and the Short Form-36 measure of functional disability. This combination was chosen to approximate the CDC criteria for CFS (Fukuda et al. 1994).

nondeployed military controls (Ishoy et al. 1999b, 2001b). Having been within 2 km of a Scud missile explosion was one of 26 physical, chemical, or biologic exposures investigated for possible association with particular adverse health outcomes. No relationship was found between Scud debris exposure and neuropsychologic symptom clusters (Suadicani et al. 1999), gastrointestinal symptoms (Ishoy et al. 1999a), or male sexual problems (Ishoy et al. 2001a).

Spencer et al. (2001) conducted a nested case-control study of exposure-symptom relationships in cases of unexplained illness (UI) (n = 241) and healthy controls (n = 113) drawn from among 1,119 responders in an earlier mailed survey of Gulf War veterans in Oregon and Washington (Spencer et al. 1998). Investigators used a new case definition for UI (Storzbach et al. 2000) in addition to the more restrictive CDC definition, according to which 115 subjects met the criteria of UI. On the basis of test-retest reliability and other factors, the 144 items on the original exposure questionnaire were winnowed down to 44. Two types of Scud missile debris exposures were among the 44 items retained: "heard Scud alarms" one to five times, six to 30 times, or more than 30 times; and "saw Scud detonate one to five times, six to 30 times, or more than 30 times. Those showed no association with either case definition of UI, whereas a more indirect index of Scud effects (inadequate protection during chemical/Scud alarms) was associated with both case definitions of UI but somewhat more strongly with the CDC definition (OR 3.16, 95% CI 1.28-7.80) than with the more inclusive one (OR 2.39, 95% CI 1.03-5.56). None of those factors was carried into the multivariate logistic modeling analysis.

Fiedler et al. (2000) studied veterans drawn from the DOD registry, comparing 58 subjects who met the case definition of CFS (35 with and 23 without psychiatric comorbidity) with 45 healthy controls. A set of Gulf War exposures (including "Scud debris") derived from the questionnaire developed for the Ft. Devens cohort was used again in this study. As for all the exposure options, more Gulf War veterans with CFS (with or without psychiatric problems) reported environmental exposures, including Scud debris exposure, than did the healthy control veterans ($p < 0.0001$). Unlike most of the other exposure options, Scud debris was not reported to have made the CFS subjects ill at the time of exposure more frequently than the controls.

Using factor analysis on the symptoms reported by 10,423 US Gulf War veterans and 8,960 of their nondeployed contemporaries who responded to a mailed survey (Kang et al. 2000), Kang et al. (2002) identified a new neurologic syndrome associated with Gulf War service characterized by four symptoms: loss of balance or dizziness, speech difficulty, sudden loss of strength, and tremors or shaking. The 277 Gulf War veterans who had all four of those symptoms were categorized as having the syndrome; 6,730 Gulf War veterans who had none of the symptoms were retained as controls. Having been within a mile of a Scud missile explosion was not among the nine exposures that were at least 3 times more commonly reported by the cases than by the controls.

Thus, the results from Gulf War veteran studies regarding Scud missile debris exposure and health effects is mixed, with no consistent pattern emerging.

Occupational Studies of Hydrazine Exposure

The designs, strengths, and weaknesses of the various epidemiology studies related to possible long-terms effects of exposure to hydrazine are summarized in Table 9.3.

Cohort Studies

US Aerospace Cohort

Ritz et al. (1999) conducted a retrospective cohort study of aerospace workers involved in testing the performance of rocket engines using hydrazines (hydrazine, MMH, and UDMH) or other fuels (such as kerosene, liquid oxygen, and beryllium). Because radiation-related activities were also conducted at the facility, those who had ever been monitored for radiation were excluded, leaving 6,107 male subjects employed at the plant for at least 2 years from 1950 to 1980. Death certificates for 1,391 subjects who died in 1960-1994 were obtained from plant pension files or from state vital-statistics offices. Underlying cause of death was abstracted and coded according to ICD-9 by a licensed nosologist. A job-exposure matrix was based on job titles and codes, facility records, manager reports, and an industrial-hygiene review. Monitoring data were not available, but there were inventories of the amount of hydrazines brought into the facility in 1955-1994. Because exposures typically resulted from accidents or unpredictable events, workers were put into presumptive-exposure groups on the basis of their jobs—high, medium, low, and unexposed—reflecting relative likelihood (rather than intensity) of having been exposed to hydrazine. Each person was placed in the highest exposure category in which he had worked for at least 6 months; a second categorization was based on the more stringent criterion of exposure for at least 24 months. In addition, logistic analyses were performed on each of the categorizations to allow for a 0-, 10-, or 15-year lag.

TABLE 9.3 Epidemiologic Studies Related to Exposure to Hydrazines

Reference	Population (Study and Control Group)	Study Design	Health Outcomes Assessed	Agent and Exposure Assessment	Analysis and Adjustment	Comments
US Aerospace Cohort						
Ritz et al. 1999	6,107 male workers employed at least 2 years in 1950-1980 at California rocket-engine testing facility	Retrospective cohort, mortality	Mortality 1960-1994: cancer deaths: lung (ICD-9 162), hematopoietic or lymphopoietic (ICD-9 200-208), bladder or kidney (ICD-9 188, 189), oral cavity-pharynx-larynx-esophagus (ICD-9 140-150, 161), pancreas (ICD-9 157); smoking-related cancers (except lung cancer) (ICD-9 140-150, 157, 161, 188, 189) Emphysema deaths (ICD-9 492)	Hydrazine exposure assessed with job-exposure matrix generated from company records, extensive industrial-hygiene review of facility, and amount of hydrazines used yearly	Internal comparison with about 4,500 nonexposed subjects: conditional logistic regression adjusting for age, pay type, time since hire, or transfer to testing division	Long followup period (average, 29 years) but relatively small number of cancer deaths (404) Smoking histories not available for all subjects, but analysis for "other" smoking-related deaths negative; for 295 subjects with smoking histories, smoking status not related to hydrazine-exposure group Possible confounding exposures: kerosene fuels, chlorine, fluorine, nitric acid, trichloroethylene
Morgenstern and Ritz 2001	Same dataset as Ritz et al. (1999) considered with two other cohorts				Analyses of Ritz et al. (1999) plus external comparison with US white male population	Entire cohort used in external comparisons so dominated by nonexposed and healthy-worker effect that association with hydrazine exposure not evident
UK Hydrazine-Production Cohort						

Reference	Population (Study and Control Group)	Study Design	Health Outcomes Assessed	Agent and Exposure Assessment	Analysis and Adjustment	Comments
Wald et al. 1984	427 men who worked at least 6 months in 1945-1971 at UK hydrazine plant 21 (5%) could not be traced Compared with men of England and Wales for same period (source not specified)	Retrospective cohort, mortality	Mortality through June 1982: cancers deaths: lung	High, moderate, or low exposure to hydrazine assessed from records of area of plant employment and expertise of factory manager	Only observed and expected numbers of deaths stratified by duration of exposure and years since first exposure	Subjects could contribute person-years at risk to multiple exposure categories, depending on which jobs were held; SMRs and confidence intervals can be calculated
Morris et al. 1995	Followup of 406 men in cohort of Wald et al. (1984) Percentage loss to followup not stated. Compared with men of England and Wales for same period (source not specified)	Retrospective cohort, mortality	Mortality through January 1992: cancer deaths: lung, digestive system IHD deaths	Same as for Wald et al. (1984)	SMRs presented stratified by both duration of exposure and years since first exposure	Cohort is quite small, but followup period is substantial Confidence intervals can be calculated

Reference	Population (Study and Control Group)	Study Design	Health Outcomes Assessed	Agent and Exposure Assessment	Analysis and Adjustment	Comments
Italian Power Plant Cohort						
Cammarano et al. 1984	270 men employed at least 6 months in 1960-1969 at thermoelectric power plant in Italy Compared with death rates in Lombardy Cancer Registry.	Retrospective cohort, mortality	Mortality through 1980; lung cancer deaths	Workers exposed to hydrazine solution during loading procedures	Expected values calculated from local cancer registry Results stratified by < or ≥ 10 years of exposure	Only 26 deaths, 15 of them from cancer SMR and 95% CI can be calculated
Cross-Sectional Studies						
King et al. 1969	140 missile-fuel handlers	Cross-sectional review of existing records	Review of reports of annual physicals (1966-1968), including liver, pulmonary, blood, and urine studies; liver biopsies of three subjects with abnormal findings	Known use of hydrazine as missile propellant, no quantification or sampling, considerable coexposure to other haptotoxins but no adjustment	Comparison with clinical standards	Sample of opportunity; no comparison group; no exposure quantification; and possible confounding toxic exposures
Petersen et al. 1970	350-400 people in Danish Air Force who worked with liquid rocket propellants	Cross-sectional	Of 1,193 workers, 46 men had increased SGPT; liver biopsies on 26 of these (six fatty, five uncertain, 15 normal)	UDMH among propellants used	Only biospied person's possible UDMH exposure listed; no systematic analysis	Distribution of subjects with and without UDMH exposure among those with increased SGPT and entire sample not clear
Nomiyama et al. 1998	249 (140 exposed) male employees, 18-60 years old, from five Japanese plants manufacturing hydrazine hydrate	Cross-sectional	Clinical examinations; self-reported symptoms; review of insurance claims at three factories for prevalence of reported conditions	Hydrazine measured in air samples from work breathing zones and urine samples	Rate ratio for exposed vs nonexposed (operational sample size unclear)	Risk estimates expressed as rate ratios of 3-year prevalence from three of five plants for 1992-1994 Uniformity of insurance information questionable

For those with high exposure to hydrazine for a minimum of either 6 or 24 months, lung-cancer mortality was consistently increased irrespective of lag period. Adjusted rate ratios ranged from 1.68 (95% CI 1.12-2.52) for 6 months of exposure and no lag to 2.10 (95% CI 1.36-3.25) for 24 months of exposure with a latent period of at least 15 years. For both the 6-month and 24-month exposure classifications, the relative risks increased with increasing years of latency. For the medium exposure category, the estimates of lung-cancer risk were uniformly somewhat lower for all duration or lag-period combinations. In the analysis by decade of exposure (high exposure for at least 6 months), the highest risk was observed for the period 1960-1969 (RR 2.01, 95% CI 1.21-3.33), when the hydrazines were tested most intensively.

Ritz et al. (1999) invested considerable effort in investigating whether the result for lung-cancer mortality might be attributable to smoking rather than hydrazine exposure. For the 295 workers on whom some information about smoking history was available, no correlation was found between smoking and hydrazine exposure; hydrazine effects in this cohort are unlikely to have been confounded by smoking. Like lung cancer and bladder or kidney cancer, cancers of the upper aerodigestive tract (oral cavity, pharynx, larynx, and esophagus) and of the pancreas are considered to be smoking-related. For those cancer sites, however, risks were not increased by high hydrazine exposure for either more than 6 or 24 months; increases were seen in the medium exposure groups (6 months of exposure: RR 1.69, 95% CI 0.47-6.06; 24 months of exposure: RR1.18, 95% CI 0.26-5.27). For all the smoking-related cancers (other than lung) combined or for emphysema deaths, the risk estimates followed a similar pattern. The lack of increased risk for any of those cancers with high exposure to hydrazine supports the idea that the positive lung-cancer finding was not due to confounding with smoking.

Mortality from hematopoietic or lymphopoietic cancers increased in both medium and high exposure groups, regardless of duration; risk increased slightly, but consistently with lag. With the full 15 years of lag, however, instead of increased risk with duration of exposure, the only increase was for high exposure of at least 6 months (RR 2.83, 95% CI 1.22-6.56). For those cancers, the risk was most markedly increased for the decade 1960-1969 (RR 2.45, 95% CI 0.91-6.58).

Relative risks were also increased for death from bladder or kidney cancer among those with high exposure to hydrazine for at least 6 months (RR 1.65, 95% CI 0.59-4.56) or 24 months (RR 1.80, 95% CI 0.63-5.12) and 15-year lag. No deaths from bladder or kidney cancer were reported among subjects with medium exposure. Mortality, however, is not the best measure of incidence of a cancer that is not highly fatal, as bladder cancer is.

Overall, the investigation was well conducted; it had relatively large numbers of exposed cases, derived exposure duration and latency information on an individual basis, and used a job-exposure matrix to determine probability of exposure to hydrazine. Morgenstern and Ritz (2001) reanalyzed the cohort in this study in comparison with the general US population (in parallel to two other cohorts from the same facility that had potential radiation exposure) and had results virtually identical with those reported here.

UK Hydrazine Production Cohort

A retrospective cohort of 427 male workers at a hydrazine plant in the UK consisted of those who had been employed for at least 6 months in 1945-1971. This population was 95% traceable at the time of the initial followup through 1982 (Wald et al. 1984). Morris et al. (1995) continued the mortality followup of the traceable 406 men through 1992 (an average of 30 years). Exposure to hydrazine was assessed by using the expertise of the factory manager and records indicating where in the plant each subject had been employed. Although no measurements of atmospheric hydrazine had been made, the researchers believed ambient concentrations in the hydrazine-production area of the plant had been 1-10 ppm and near the storage vessels as high as 100 ppm. On the basis of jobs held, each subject was allocated to the groups for which results were presented—high exposure (directly involved in hydrazine production for at least 6 months) or low to moderate exposure. Data on mortality were gathered from the National Health Service records for each employee. Observed incidences were determined by 5-year age groups and compared with expected values derived from men in England and Wales in the same age groups during the same period. Results were presented with and without the constraint of a 10-year latency since first exposure.

For most health outcomes over both followup intervals, the number of expected deaths exceeded the number of observed deaths in the exposed cohort; this implied a healthy-worker effect. The lung was the only cancer site for which observed deaths surpassed the number expected for those working in a high-exposure job for 6 months or more (3 observed vs 2.79 expected); the risk was slightly more increased for those with at least 10 years since first exposure (SMR 1.23, 95% CI 0.25-3.61).

In the low-to-moderate exposure category, cancers of the digestive system were somewhat increased (SMR 1.24, 95% CI 0.57-2.34); no cancers of this type were observed in the high-exposure group. The ICD codes included in this category were not specified, but it is improbable that they correspond to the "upper aerodigestive tract" sites considered by Ritz et al. (1999).

The distribution of ischemic-heart-disease (IHD) deaths suggests that the small increase observed in those who had held a high-exposure job for at least 2 years (SMR 1.08, 95% CI 0.47-2.13) merely represents a random perturbation.

The relatively small number of observed deaths limits the interpretation of the study results. Given that hydrazine exposure was based on jobs listed in employment records, subjects who switched jobs in the company and thus had varied levels of exposure may have diluted the effects of stratification presented by person-years. The methods and interval of followup appear adequate, although Morris et al. (1995) did not report whether more subjects had proved untraceable from 1982 to 1992 in addition to the 5% who were untraceable in the first study.

Italian Power Plant Cohort

Cammarano et al. (1984) conducted a cancer-mortality study among 270 male workers in a thermoelectric power plant in Turbigo (Milan, Italy). The men had worked in the plant for at least 6 months in 1960-1969. on the basis of company registers and census data, all subjects were followed up through 1980. For each of the 26 subjects found to have died during the study period, cause of death was ascertained from the registry of the municipality where the death occurred. Attempts were made to interview next of kin and to trace clinical records where information was lacking or of poor quality. The numbers of expected deaths for various causes were computed from the 1976-1977 Lombardy Cancer Registry for Varese Province, which is within 5 km of Turbig, the small town where most of the workers lived. Analysis of the processes used at the plant indicated that a number of toxic substances in addition to hydrazine were present in the work environment (polycyclic aromatic hydrocarbons (PAHs), asbestos, polychlorinated biphenyls (PCBs), chromium, nickel, and beryllium); the researchers made no assertions about which agent(s) might be responsible for any increase in risk.

The two observed lung-cancer deaths occurred among the workers with 10 years or more of exposure, giving an increased risk estimate with a wide confidence interval (SMR 1.42, 95% CI 0.17-5.12). For all types of cancer, mortality was increased in the entire cohort (SMR 1.98,

95% CI 1.11-3.26), but the excess risk (SMR 2.76) was confined to those with 10 years or more of exposure. Although the results indicate a two-fold to threefold excess risk of cancer overall, the small numbers for each cancer type prevent the identification of any increased risk for a specific site. Furthermore, the effects of exposure to hydrazine cannot be isolated from the effects of the combination of exposures experienced in this work setting, and this limits the study's contribution to the body of evidence on hydrazine as a specific causative agent.

Cross-Sectional Studies

Toxicologic data available since the middle 1950s indicated that hydrazine and UDMH have potential for hepatotoxicity (ATSDR 1997; Choudhary and Hansen 1998; NRC 1996; Shook and Cowart 1957; Wells 1908), so industrial-hygiene programs have included monitoring of liver function in workers exposed to hydrazines, as is evidenced by the studies described below.

Missile-Propellant Handlers at Vandenberg Air Force Base, CA

King et al. (1969) reviewed the records of physical examinations routinely conducted from 1966 through 1968 on 140 asymptomatic people who handled missile fuels (including hydrazine). The liver-function screenings generated the most atypical examination results: 17 people (12%) had increased serum glutamic pyruvic transaminase (SGPT) activity or thymol turbidity, and fatty changes were seen in two of the liver biopsies drawn from the three people with the extreme findings. Little can be concluded from those findings, because reviewed medical records were a sample of opportunity without enhancement by a comparison group, assessment of hydrazine exposure, or adjustment for confounding exposures.

Rocket-Propellant Workers in Danish Air Force

During the early 1960s, routine blood and urine analyses had been performed three or four times a year on 1,193 members of the Danish Air Force, including 350-400 involved in handling liquid rocket propellants (UDMH in particular). In the entire group, 46 men (4%) had one or more instances of increased SGPT; the prevalence of increased SGPT specifically among the propellant workers was not stated. Liver biopsies were performed on the 26 for whom there was not a ready explanation of the SGPT increase and who agreed to the procedure (Petersen et al. 1970). For each of the 26 people, a synopsis of possible exposure to UDMH was given. Six instances of fatty degeneration were found (all in people whose SGPT remained increased at the time of the biopsy) and five additional people had some suggestion of liver damage. All the biopsied subjects appeared to have had some opportunity for UDMH exposure, so an association with liver damage was not obvious in this set. There was no systematic analysis of the relationship between UDMH exposure, SGPT readings, and biopsy findings for the entire sample, so the biopsied subjects constitute a set of case histories. Petersen et al. (1970) expressed interest in whether the hepatic effects would persist after exposure to UDMH ceased, but no report of such a followup study was found.

Japanese Hydrazine Hydrate Workers

Nomiyama et al. (1998) studied workers at five factories in Japan that made hydrazine hydrate (HH) or hydrazine derivatives. After exclusion of 48 subjects who had hepatitis B/C antigens or diabetes, the analysis consisted of 249 males 18-60 years old, of whom 140 had been exposed to hydrazines for 0.5-34 years. A combination of personal air sampling and biologic monitoring (urinary excretion of hydrazine and acetylhydrazine) demonstrated no exposure of the control subjects and an average of 11 ppb in the breathing zones of HH workers. Subjects were given clinical examinations, and they completed questionnaires regarding subjective symptoms, smoking and alcohol and caffeine consumption, and past and present medical history, including exposure to chemical products and medications. Insurance-claim records from 1992 through 1994 from three of the five factories were used to determine prevalence rates of disease. Self-reported symptoms and clinical findings did not differ systematically with exposure. The insurance claims suggested increased risks among HH-exposed workers for viral hepatitis (RR 1.99, 95% CI 1.15-3.43), cirrhosis (RR 2.48, 95% CI 1.51-4.08), thyroid disorders (RR 2.48, 95% CI 1.51-4.08), and cerebrovascular disease other than cerebral infarction (RR 2.26, 95% CI 1.35-3.78). The exposure assessment in this study was well performed. The validity of insurance claims as a proxy for diagnosed diseases, however, limits the interpretation of the findings, because diagnostic criteria would not be expected to be uniform. Presumably, exposure continued during the 3-year period when insurance claims were submitted, so the issue of persistence was not addressed.

Summary

Overall, relatively few epidemiologic studies of exposure to UDMH specifically or hydrazines in general are available. Only a single specific health outcome—lung cancer—was represented in all three cohort mortality studies reviewed by the committee (Cammarano et al. 1984; Morris et al. 1995; Ritz et al. 1999), and they all suggested the possibility of an increase in risk. The analysis of the US cohort by Ritz et al. (1999) demonstrated an association between hydrazine exposure, based on a job-exposure matrix, and risk of lung cancer. Several sources of potential confounding, including sex and radiation exposure, were controlled by study design. Other potentially confounding variables were controlled in multivariate analysis, including age, pay type (a proxy for socioeconomic status), and time since hire or transfer (a proxy for the selective loss of less healthy workers). Although smoking status of most workers was unknown, there was indirect evidence that smoking did not confound the results. There was no association between hydrazine-exposure category and smoking status in a subset of workers who completed a health survey. Moreover, there was no relation between hydrazine-exposure category and the risk of smoking-related nonrespiratory cancers and emphysema. The committee conducted a sensitivity analysis that factored in uncertainties about smoking frequencies in the exposed and nonexposed workers, which gave further assurance that full knowledge of and adjustment for smoking would be unlikely to broaden the reported confidence intervals for lung cancer to include 1.0.

The other two retrospective cohort studies (Cammarano et al. 1984; Morris et al. 1995) of lung cancer were limited by small sample and inadequate study power. In addition, the study of Italian power-plant workers (Cammarano et al. 1984) was limited by its failure to control for coexposure to other carcinogenic substances, including asbestos and PAHs. The lack of internal control subjects and the lack of information on smoking constitute major limitations for both studies. That the confidence interval for lung cancer after high likelihood of exposure to hydrazines as compared with nonexposed internal controls found by Ritz et al. (1999) lies above 1.0 and completely within that of the negative finding in comparison with external control rates (Cammarano et al. 1984) indicates no inconsistency. Consequently, there is inadequate evidence to evaluate the consistency of the association between hydrazine and lung cancer beyond the strong study by Ritz et al. (1999).

Results of experimental studies involving oral and inhalation exposures to hydrazine, UDMH, and MMH show an increased incidence of various types of tumors in animals.

Malignant and benign tumors and preneoplastic changes, have been identified at several sites—including the lung, liver, and nose—in mice, rats, and hamsters exposed to hydrazines; and the available data support a dose-related occurrence of those lesions (Biancifiori 1970; Biancifiori et al. 1964, 1966; Bosan et al. 1987; Kinkead et al. 1985; Mommsen et al. 1982; Roe et al. 1967; Severi and Biancifiori 1968; Steinhoff and Mohr 1988; Toth 1969; Vernot et al. 1985). In vivo and in vitro studies on hydrazines have demonstrated potential mechanisms of carcinogenicity, including mutagenesis, DNA alkylation, and tissue injury (ATSDR 1997). Those mechanisms may be relevant to the carcinogenicity of hydrazines in humans.

The committee concludes, from its assessment of the epidemiologic literature, that there is limited/suggestive evidence of an association between exposure to hydrazines and lung cancer.

The three cohorts reviewed reported somewhat increased mortality from cancer at sites other than the lung (hematopoietic and lymphopoietic, bladder and kidney, digestive tract, and pancreas) and from two noncancer conditions (emphysema and ischemic heart disease). The possibility of nonspecific hepatic effects was raised by three cross-sectional reports, but the studies were largely opportunistic compilations of available information that did not adhere to explicit protocols. The available epidemiologic studies do not provide adequate or consistent evidence of an association between exposure to hydrazines and any of those health outcomes.

The committee concludes, from its assessment of the epidemiologic literature, that there is inadequate/insufficient evidence to determine whether an association exists between exposure to hydrazines and hematopoietic or lymphopoietic cancers, bladder or kidney cancer, digestive tract cancer, pancreatic cancer, mortality from emphysema or ischemic heart disease, or hepatic effects.

Table 9.4 provides the key findings that the committee evaluated in drawing its conclusions of association for exposure to hydrazine.

Occupational Studies of Nitric Acid Exposure

The designs, strengths, and weaknesses of the various epidemiology studies related to possible long-terms effects of exposure to nitric acid are summarized in Table 9.5.

TABLE 9.4 Selected Epidemiologic Studies—Health Outcomes and Exposure to Hydrazines

Reference	Study Population	Exposed Cases	Estimated Relative Risk
Lung Cancer			
Cohort Studies			
Ritz et al. 1999	Male US rocket-engine workers		
	Nonexposed		1.0
	Nonexposed or low exposure, ≥6 months (from Morgenstern and Ritz et al. 2001)	97	
	Medium exposure, ≥6 months		
	No lag	5	0.41 (0.17-1.02)
	10-year lag	4	0.36 (0.13-0.98)
	15-year lag	4	0.42 (0.15-1.16)
	High exposure, ≥6 months		
	No lag	44	1.68 (1.12-2.52)
	10-year lag	42	1.70 (1.13-2.56)
	15-year lag	41	1.93 (1.27-2.93)
	Medium exposure, ≥24 months		
	No lag	7	0.66 (0.31-1.44)
	10- year lag	6	0.65 (0.28-1.49)
	15-year lag	5	0.65 (0.26-1.62)
	High exposure, ≥24 months		
	No lag	36	1.70 (1.11-2.59)
	10-year lag	34	1.76 (1.15-2.71)
	15-year lag	34	2.10 (1.36-3.25)
	Decade of Exposure (high exposure, ≥6 months)		
	1950-1959	NA	0.88 (0.54-1.44)
	1960-1969	NA	2.01 (1.21-3.33)
	1970-1979	NA	1.45 (0.70-3.01)
	1980-1989	NA	0.46 (0.06-3.64)
Morris et al. 1995	Male UK hydrazine-plant workers		
	Any exposure (≥6 months at plant)	8	0.66 (0.29-1.31)[a]
	≥10 years since first exposure	8	0.74 (0.32-1.46)[a]
	Moderate/low exposure	5	0.54 (0.17-1.26)[a]
	≥10 years since first exposure	5	0.60 (0.19-1.40)[a]
	High exposure		
	≥6 months duration	3	1.08 (0.22-3.14)[a]
	≥10 years since first exposure	3	1.23 (0.25-3.61)[a]
	≥2 years duration	1	0.41 (0.01-2.30)[a]
	≥10 years since first exposure	1	0.47 (0.01-2.64)[a]

Reference	Study Population	Exposed Cases	Estimated Relative Risk
Cammarano et al. 1984	Italian power-plant workers		
	All subjects	2	0.87 (0.11-3.15)[b]
	<10 years exposure	0	0
	≥10 years exposure	2	1.42 (0.17-5.12)[b]
Bladder/Kidney Cancer			
Cohort Study			
Ritz et al. 1999	Male US rocket-engine workers		
	Nonexposed		1.0
	Medium exposure, ≥6 months, 15-year lag	0	—
	High exposure, ≥6 months, 15-year lag	7	1.65 (0.59-4.56)
	Medium exposure, ≥24 months, 15-year lag	0	—
	High exposure, ≥24 months, 15-year lag	6	1.80 (0.63-5.12)
Lymphopoietic Cancer			
Cohort Study			
Ritz et al. 1999	Male US rocket-engine workers		
	Nonexposed		1.0
	Nonexposed or low exposure, ≥6 months (from Morgenstern and Ritz et al. 2001)	35	
	Medium exposure, ≥6 months, 15-year lag	5	1.79 (0.65-4.94)
	High exposure, ≥6 months, 15-year lag	11	2.83 (1.22-6.56)
	Medium exposure, ≥24 months, 15-year lag	4	1.32 (0.45-3.90)
	High exposure, ≥24 months, 15-year lag	6	1.42 (0.54-3.72)
	Decade of exposure (high exposure, ≥6 months)		
	1950-1959	NA	0.86 (0.32-2.28)
	1960-1969	NA	2.45 (0.91-6.58)
	1970-1979	NA	0 (0--)[c]
	1980-1989	NA	0.89 (0--)[c]
Oral Cavity, Pharyngeal, Laryngeal, or Esophageal Cancers ("Upper Aerodigestive Tract Cancers")			
Cohort Study			
Ritz et al. 1999	Male US rocket-engine workers		
	Medium exposure, ≥6 months, 15-year lag	3	1.69 (0.47-6.06)
	High exposure, ≥6 months, 15-year lag	3	0.69 (0.19-2.53)
	Medium exposure, ≥24 months, 15-year lag	2	1.18 (0.26-5.27)
	High exposure, ≥24 months, 15-year lag	2	0.57 (0.13-2.61)
Digestive Tract Cancer			
Cohort Study			
Morris et al. 1995	Male UK hydrazine-plant workers		
	Any exposure (≥6 months at plant)	9	0.95 (0.44-1.81)[a]
	≥10 years since first exposure	8	0.95 (0.41-1.87)[a]
	Moderate/low exposure	9	1.24 (0.57-2.34)[a]
	≥10 years since first exposure	8	1.22 (0.53-2.41)[a]
	High exposure	0	0.0

Reference	Study Population	Exposed Cases	Estimated Relative Risk
Pancreatic Cancer			
Cohort Study			
Ritz et al. 1999	Male US rocket-engine workers		
	Nonexposed		1.0
	Medium exposure, ≥6 months, 15-year lag	4	1.95 (0.62-6.12)
	High exposure, ≥6 months, 15-year lag	2	0.48 (0.10-2.25)
	Medium exposure, ≥24 months, 15-year lag	4	2.26 (0.72-7.09)
	High exposure, ≥24 months, 15-year lag	1	0.32 (0.04-2.51)
Smoking-Related Cancers (other than lung; ICD-9 140-150, 157, 161, 188, 189) (presented as evidence that smoking is not confounder)			
Cohort Study			
Ritz et al. 1999	Male US rocket-engine workers		
	Nonexposed		1.0
	Medium exposure, ≥6 months, 15-year lag	7	1.22 (0.54-2.76)
	High exposure, ≥6 months, 15-year lag	12	0.94 (0.47-1.86)
	Medium exposure, ≥24 months, 15-year lag	6	1.17 (0.49-2.79)
	High exposure, ≥24 months, 15-year lag	9	0.90 (0.42-1.92)
Emphysema Deaths (presented as evidence that smoking is not confounder)			
Cohort Study			
Ritz et al. 1999	Male US rocket-engine workers		
	Nonexposed		1.0
	Medium exposure, ≥6 months, 15-year lag	4	2.18 (0.72-6.62)
	High exposure, ≥6 months, 15-year lag	3	0.54 (0.15-1.93)
	Medium exposure, ≥24 months, 15-year lag	3	2.26 (0.64-8.02)
	High exposure, ≥24 months, 15-year lag	3	0.74 (0.21-2.65)
Ischemic Heart Disease			
Cohort Studies			
Morris et al. 1995	Male UK hydrazine-plant workers		
	Any exposure (≥6 months at plant)	26	0.70 (0.46-1.03)[a]
	≥10 years since first exposure	23	0.69 (0.44-1.03)[a]
	Moderate/low exposure	18	0.63 (0.37-1.00)[a]
	≥10 years since first exposure	16	0.62 (0.35-1.01)[a]
	High exposure		
	≥6 months duration	8	0.94 (0.40-1.85)[a]
	≥10 years since first exposure	7	0.92 (0.37-1.90)[a]
	≥2 years duration	8	1.08 (0.47-2.13)[a]
	≥10 years since first exposure	7	1.06 (0.43-2.18)[a]

NOTE: na=not available.

[a] 95% CIs calculated with standard methods from observed and expected numbers presented in original paper.

[b] Risk estimate and 95% CI calculated with standard methods from observed and expected numbers presented in original paper.

[c] Upper limits could not be estimated because of the small numbers of outcome events in the high-exposure category.

TABLE 9.5 Epidemiologic Studies Related to Exposure to Nitric Acid

Reference	Study Populations	Study Design	Health Outcomes Assessed	Agent and Exposure Assessment	Analysis and Adjustment	Comments
Pennsylvania Sheet and Tin Mill Cohort						
Mazumdar et al. 1975	8,465 white male sheet and tin mill workers among 58,828 male steel workers employed in 1953 at seven Allegheny County, Pennsylvania, plants	Prospective cohort mortality	Mortality through 1966 assessed from death certificates: cancer: respiratory, lymphatic/hematopoietic, various heart diseases (if employed ≥5 yr before 1954)	Fumes from acid baths related to work in pickling, coating, or specialty finishing processes	RR calculated from observed deaths in each work area against expected deaths from remainder of total cohort	Small numbers observed and expected preclude calculation of stable CIs for many combinations of jobs and health outcome; ICDs not given
Swedish Metal Pickling Cohort						
Ahlborg et al. 1981	110 men employed at least 1 year at pickling house in 1951-1979	Retrospective cohort	Mortality through 1979: cancer: respiratory tract, laryngeal	Nitric acid component of pickling baths	Expected numbers calculated by sex, calendar year, and age from Swedish Cancer Registry for 1958-1979	This was basically a note reporting a cluster of three laryngeal cancers; smoking not accounted for
US Midwestern Metal Pickling Cohort						
Beaumont et al. 1987	1,165 workers employed at least 6 months in 1940-1965 at one of three midwestern steel-manufacturing facilities in pickling-related job, followed through 1981	Retrospective cohort mortality	Mortality through Oct. 27, 1981: diabetes focus on lung cancer	Nitric acid one of "other acids" used in pickling operations	SMRs for all vs US population; white males working 1950-1954 vs Allegheny County steel workers to control for smoking and other socioeconomic factors	Lung-cancer excess stronger among those exposed to acids other than sulfuric than for those exposed to sulfuric acid only; several approaches taken to show increase not due solely to smoking

Reference	Study Populations	Study Design	Health Outcomes Assessed	Agent and Exposure Assessment	Analysis and Adjustment	Comments
Steenland et al. 1988	Subset of 879 subjects from Beaumont et al. (1987) for whom determinations of ever having had laryngeal cancer could be made	Retrospective cohort	Incidence of laryngeal cancer through early 1986 determined by interviews with living subjects or next of kin, plus medical record reviews; information on smoking also gathered	Nitric acid among acids used in pickling operations	Expected figures calculated from US population data with adjustment for excess smoking in cohort	Significant increase in incidence of laryngeal cancer, but analyses not conducted in detail by three acid categories used in Beaumont et al. (1987)
Steenland and Beaumont 1989	1,156 males in cohort of Beaumont et al. (1987) 14% of those alive in 1981 (162) could not be traced	Retrospective cohort mortality	Mortality through early 1986: lung cancer Information on smoking gathered from subject or next of kin	Nitric acid component of acids used in pickling operations	SMRs calculated from US population from 1940-1978; adjustment for smoking by Axelson technique	Analysis was not stratified by types of acid exposure; control for smoking decreased risk of lung cancer just below significance
Italian Chemical Plant Workers						
Rapiti et al. 1997	125 males ever exposed to acid mixtures among 505 workers at Italian chemical plant any time in 1954-1970	Retrospective cohort	Mortality 1970-1991 with focus on cancer	Scan of medical files containing work histories and annual examinations, as required by 1954 law; nitric and sulfuric acids used in some jobs	SMR (90% CIs) based on regional cause-specific death rates	Vital status determined for 96% of full cohort

Reference	Study Populations	Study Design	Health Outcomes Assessed	Agent and Exposure Assessment	Analysis and Adjustment	Comments
Nitric Acid Production Cohort						
Hilt et al. 1985	287 male production and maintenance workers first employed any time in 1928-1961 at nitric acid production plant and alive 1953, compared with national incidence data	Retrospective cohort	Histologically verified new cancer cases in 1953-1980 in Norwegian Cancer Registry; focus on lung cancers and pleural or peritoneal mesothelioma (plus cancers of unknown origin); also colon, stomach, melanoma	Asbestos exposure dominated exposure to nitric acid; excluded from consideration as key study	SIR with expectations calculated by 5-year age groups for 1953-1980 from Norwegian Cancer Registry; adjusted for smoking	Very significantly increased lung cancer in highly exposed and lightly exposed maintenance workers; nonsignificant O/E=1.6 (3 vs 1.9) for lightly exposed production workers (how many of 190 not stated) for whom nitric acid exposure might be perceptible factor
Hilt 1987	153 men working any time in 1928-1970 at nitric acid production plant and "eligible" for clinical examination 1979-1980 followed through 1985	Prospective cohort	Lung fibrosis and/or pleural plaques, respiratory symptoms	Asbestos exposure dominated exposure to nitric acid; excluded from consideration as key study	Stratification by current, ex-, or never smoker	
Hilt et al. 1991	287 subjects in Hilt et al. (1985) followed through 1988 (8 more years)	Retrospective cohort	Histologically verified new cancer cases in 1953-1988 in Norwegian Cancer Registry; focus on lung cancers and pleural or peritoneal mesothelioma (plus cancers of unknown origin); also colon, stomach, melanoma	Asbestos exposure dominated exposure to nitric acid; excluded from consideration as key study	SIR with expectations calculated by 5-year age groups for 1953-1988 from Norwegian Cancer Registry; adjusted for smoking	O/E for lung cancers among light-exposure group (not subdivided between maintenance and production workers) changed from 2.1 to 1.8 (5 vs 2.4 to 7 vs 4.0), both nonsignificant

Reference	Study Populations	Study Design	Health Outcomes Assessed	Agent and Exposure Assessment	Analysis and Adjustment	Comments
Laryngeal Cancer Case-Control Studies						
Soskolne et al. 1984	50 cases (34 laryngeal) of upper respiratory cancer diagnosed in 1944-1980 in employees of at least 1 year at chemical plant in Louisiana; 175 matched company controls	Case-control	"Upper respiratory" cancer	Work history records used to score occupations in ethanol units for level of exposure to sulfuric acid; occupations outside ethanol units unexposed	ORs; analysis adjusted for alcoholism, tobacco use, and history of ear, nose, or throat disease; controls matched on duration and first year of employment, age, sex, and race	
Soskolne et al. 1992	183 men with histologically confirmed laryngeal cancer diagnosed in 1977-1979 in southern Ontario; 183 matched population controls	Case-control	Laryngeal cancer	Self-reported work histories coded by author for exposure to sulfuric acid	ORs; analysis adjusts for cigarette and alcohol use; controls matched on sex, age, and neighborhood	
Zemla et al. 1987	328 male cases in Upper Silesia located through Institute of Oncology in Poland in 1980-1984; 656 controls without cancer matched on native or immigrant status	Case-control	Laryngeal cancer confirmed histopathologically	Self-reported history of occupational hazards including vapors containing sulfuric, hydrochloric, and nitric acid immigrants assumed to have shorter exposure to industrial pollution.	Unclear how "expected" figures obtained, necessary for chi^2 tests and/or RRs	Nitric acid is assumed component of self-reported exposure; addressed confounding by smoking and alcohol consumption

Reference	Study Populations	Study Design	Health Outcomes Assessed	Agent and Exposure Assessment	Analysis and Adjustment	Comments
Eisen et al. 1994	108 incident cases in cohort of automobile workers exposed to machining fluids at three Michigan plants ≥3yrs before 1985; 540 cohort controls	Nested case-control	Laryngeal cancers detected through 1989	Acid mists (nitric, phosphoric, or sulfuric acid) used in restricted locations at two plants addressed as confounder to machining fluid exposure; exposure based on air sampling, historical records, and plant interviews	OR; used 10-year lags and adjusted for time since hire; controls matched for age, plant, race, and sex	Acid-mist years OR = 0.90 (0.66-1.22) Nitric acid included, but cannot separate its effect from that of other acids
De Stefani et al. 1998	112 incident and histologically confirmed cases from five hospitals in Montevideo from 1993-1995; 509 controls with cancers not related to tobacco or alcohol	Case-control	Laryngeal cancer	Self-reported exposure to strong acid (hydrochloric, nitric, and sulfuric) mists	ORs from unconditional logistic regression adjusted for age, residence, education, income, cigarette smoking, and alcohol consumption	Increased risk for ever exposed (1.6), 1-20 years (1.2), and 21+ years (1.8) of exposure; Nitric acid was included, but cannot separate its effect from other acids
Gustavsson et al. 1998	157 cases of laryngeal cancer among Swedish-born men 40-79 years old living in Stockholm county or five southern counties (388 cases at other three cancer sites); 641 controls matched by region and age group drawn by stratified random sampling of population registers	Case-control	Sought all incident cases from Jan. 1, 1988 to Jan. 31, 1991 of squamous cell carcinoma of "upper gasointestinal tract" (oral cavity, pharynx, larynx, and esophagus reported individually; ICD-9 141, 143, 144, 146, 148, 150, 161); New cases reported weekly from local hospitals or regional cancer registries.	Questionnaire on lifestyle and work history administered by unblinded nurse; likelihood and intensity of 17 factors coded by occupational hygienist from work histories, including "acid mist", PAHs 90% and 85% of identified 605 cases and 756 controls completed	RRs by logistic regression adjusted for age, region, smoking, and alcohol use	Which acids included in "acid mist" category not specified

Reference	Study Populations	Study Design	Health Outcomes Assessed	Agent and Exposure Assessment	Analysis and Adjustment	Comments
Multiple Myeloma Case-Control Study						
Morris et al. 1986	698 cases from four SEER registries from 1977-1981; 1,683 population controls	Case-control	Multiple myeloma	Toxicologist put interviews responses into 20 exposure groups; "acids" (included muriatic, hydrochloric, sulfuric, chromic, nitric, acetic, and other acids)	Mantel-Haenszel ORs adjusted for age, sex, race, and study site	Elevated risk (1.5; 0.8-2.8) for self-respondents, but no risk seen with addition of proxies; Nitric acid was included, but cannot separate its effect from other acids
Bombay Nitric Acid Plant						
Kamat et al. 1984	125 workers chronically exposed to nitric acid fumes	Cross-sectional	Respiratory symptoms (interview), lung function, radiography	Subjects' exposure to nitric acid not estimated, but samples obtained at unidentified times and sites in the plant between 20-40 ppm	No analysis directly relates NO_2 exposure to pulmonary function or radiographic abnormalities	Exposure assessment undefined
Indian Suburban Nitric Acid and Bombay Chemical Plants						
Kolhatkar et al. 1987	113 male workers (70 in nitric acid plant and 43 in urban plant with exposure to nitric acid, plus other acids); 29 nonexposed male workers (15 and 14 from above plants)	Cross-sectional	Respiratory symptoms (interview), lung function, radiography	No measurement of nitric acid or liberated NO_2 fumes; thought to exceed 2-15 ppm ("newer and cleaner" than nitric acid plant in Kamat et al. 1984); no explanation of means of allocation to exposed or nonexposed group	No analysis directly relates NO_2 exposure to pulmonary function or radiographic abnormalities	Exposure assessment undefined

Cohort Studies

Pennsylvania Sheet and Tin Mill Cohorts

Mazumdar et al. (1975) reported on the mortality experience through 1966 of a cohort of 8,465 white men who worked in the sheet and tin mills of seven plants in Allegheny County, Pennsylvania, in 1953 (a subset of a much larger NIOSH cohort of steelworkers). For 1,183 deceased subjects, a licensed nosologist coded underlying causes of death from death certificates according to ICD-7. Exposure to fumes from acid baths (said to contain sulfuric, hydrochloric, or phosphoric acid) was determined through a review of work-history records. Such exposures occurred in the pickling, coating, or specialty finishing processes, which were involved in six of 13 job classifications reported: batch pickling and sheet drying; continuous pickling and electric cleaning; stainless annealing, pickling, and processing; coating; sheet finishing and shipping; and tin finishing and shipping. The study did not specifically identify or evaluate exposure to nitric acid.

Relative risks were calculated from observed deaths in each work area and compared with the number of expected deaths from the remainder of the nonexposed cohort. Job-specific findings were presented for all cancers, with cancers of the respiratory organs or of lymphatic and hematopoietic tissues broken out separately. The incidence of all cancers was notably increased only in workers in stainless annealing, pickling, and processing (6 observed, 2.0 expected; RR 3.32, $p < 0.05$); that one of these cases was a lymphohematopoietic cancer (0.2 expected) and two were respiratory (0.6 expected) suggests increases of both. Cancer of respiratory organs was modestly increased among those who had worked in coating (4 observed, 2.8 expected) or in sheet finishing and shipping (19 observed, 15.6 expected; RR 1.27).

Another cohort of men involved in metal pickling was studied by Ahlborg et al. (1981). One hundred and ten men were employed in a pickling house for at least 1 year in 1951-1979. Nitric acid is a known component of the pickling baths, but no attempts to quantify exposure were made. The incidence of cancers of the respiratory tract and larynx was compared with expected figures as calculated from sex, calendar year, and age for 1958-1979 in the Swedish Cancer Registry. Regardless of a 10-year induction period, there were four observed cases of respiratory tract cancer and three cases of laryngeal cancer. Those are notably higher than the expected figures of 0.66 (0.55 given a 10-year latency) and 0.06 (0.05 given a 10-year latency) respectively. Smoking habits of the subjects were not assessed or accounted for and may confound the results.

US Midwestern Metal Pickling Cohort

Beaumont et al. (1987) retrospectively followed 1,165 workers at three midwestern steel-manufacturing facilities. Subjects were employed for at least 6 months in a pickling-related job from 1940 to 1964. Mortality was followed through 1981 by using vital statistics from the Social Security Administration and Internal Revenue Service. From work-history records, industrial-hygiene and engineering records and surveys, and company personnel expertise, subjects were categorized according to what acids they were exposed to in their metal-pickling jobs: sulfuric acid only, sulfuric and other acids, or other acids only (all members of this category worked at a single factory). Nitric acid was identified as a component of "other acid" exposure (a situation that occurred at only one of the three plants). When the overall cohort was compared with the US population, lung cancer stood out as the only markedly increased cause of death (SMR 1.64, 95% CI 1.14–2.28); the risk of death related to diabetes was also increased (SMR 1.65, 95% CI 0.71–2.26). The lung-cancer increase was extreme for those who had worked only with "other acids"

(SMR 2.24). In an effort to control for smoking and other socioeconomic factors, a comparison was made with Allegheny County steelworkers —the Pennsylvania cohort whose pickling portion was reported on by Mazumdar et al. (1975)—but this required restricting the Midwestern cohort to those employed from 1950 to 1954. Lung cancer mortality was again most increased among those working exclusively with "other acids" (SMR 2.00, 95% CI 1.06–3.78). Although this subset of workers was exposed to acids other than nitric acid (such as hydrochloric, hydrofluoric, and hydrocyanic acids), the findings suggest that sulfuric acid may not be exclusively or primarily responsible for carcinogenic effects observed among those working with strong inorganic acids.

Steenland et al. (1988) examined a subset of 879 subjects from the Midwestern cohort in whom it could be determined whether laryngeal cancer had ever been diagnosed. Beaumont et al. (1987) found two deaths among all the pickling workers; this suggested an increase (SMR 1.93, 95% CI 0.23–6.99) for laryngeal cancer, which has 5-year survival of better than 50%. Steenland et al. (1988) found an additional seven diagnoses of laryngeal cancer (standard incidence ratio [SIR] 2.30; 9 observed cases vs 3.92 expected, with adjustment for smoking). The small number of cases precluded detailed analysis by acid-exposure group and it was not stated whether the 62% sulfuric acid-only, 22% mixed, and 16% "other-acids-only" partition of the full cohort was carried into the subset; but it was reported that four, three, and two of the cases, respectively, were in these categories.

Steenland and Beaumont (1989) followed up mortality in that cohort into 1986 and gathered individual smoking histories from those still living or next of kin. The findings for lung cancer remained increased (SMR 1.55, 95% CI 1.12-2.11), but adjustment for the smoking information dampened the increase (SMR 1.36, 95% CI 0.97-1.84). Results were not presented by the separate acid-exposure groups, so little insight was gained into any effects that might be due to nitric acid or the other nonsulfuric acids used in the pickling jobs.

Italian Chemical Plant Workers

Rapiti et al. (1997) examined occupational risk factors for cancer mortality in a cohort of 505 men employed from 1954 to 1970 in an Italian chemical plant. Vital status through June 1991 was obtained from registry offices. In compliance with a 1954 national law, workers exposed to particular chemicals were examined annually, and the employees' work histories were kept with their medical records. Screening of those files revealed that 125 subjects had been engaged at some point during their employment in the production of acid mixtures that included sulfuric and nitric acids. Compared with regional causes of death, acid exposure was associated with increases stomach cancer (SMR 1.47, 90% CI 0.40-3.80), pancreatic cancer (SMR 1.69, 90% CI 0.09-8.04), lung cancer (SMR 1.62, 90% CI 0.81-2.92), non-Hodgkin's lymphoma (SMR 4.17, 90% CI 0.04-19.7), and leukemia (SMR 1.79, 90% CI 0.09-8.47). The authors discussed the hypothesized association between laryngeal cancer and acid mixtures, but apparently no such deaths were observed in the entire cohort. The exposure circumstances in the plant where nitric acid was used in combination with sulfuric acid are of particular interest, but the small numbers of exposed cases resulted in extremely wide, largely uninformative confidence intervals (even at the 90% level).

Nitric Acid Production Cohort

A cohort of 287 male workers at a nitric acid production plant in Norway was studied by Hilt et al. (1985) through 1980 and followed up by Hilt et al. (1991) through 1988. The subjects were regularly exposed to asbestos in the period 1928-1980, but the researchers focused on workers exposed to asbestos before 1961 who had not died before 1953. The incidence of cancer was calculated on the basis of data from the Norwegian Cancer Registry, which was thought to be comprehensive for cancer diagnosis for the period in question. Exposure to asbestos was assessed through occupational-history records and was the primary exposure of interest for the study. Although the plant workers were engaged in processes related to nitric acid production, no measurements of exposure to this compound were included in the studies. In all likelihood, the increased reported risks of lung cancer and pleural mesothelioma were driven by asbestos exposure. The studies were well-conducted but are of marginal utility for the purposes of this review (and particularly for evaluating respiratory cancers) because the exposure experience of the subjects is dominated by asbestos. The effects of nitric acid exposure were not studied specifically and cannot be inferred.

Case-Control Studies

Laryngeal Cancer

A study of laryngeal cancer performed by Zemla et al. (1987) comprised 328 cases of native and migrant workers in Upper Silesia who were located through the Institute of Oncology in Poland from 1980–1984 and 656 population controls. Self-reported histories of occupational hazards included exposure to vapors containing sulfuric, hydrochloric, and nitric acids. Exposure to acid vapors was associated with an increase in laryngeal cancer among natives (RR 0.57, 95% CI 0.07-2.06), immigrants (RR 4.50, 95% CI 2.06-8.54), and both together (RR 2.0, 95% CI 1.00-3.52). Since the statistics in the table did not appear to correspond with the observed number reported, the committee re-calculated the RR and CI. The numbers indicate that there is a big difference between the natives and the immigrants. However, the study is limited by the use of self-reported and broadly defined exposure-assessment methods.

Eisen et al. (1994) conducted a case-control study of laryngeal cancer among automobile workers exposed to machining fluids in the automobile industry. Qualitative data were also collected on exposure to acid mists (including nitric, phosphoric, and sulfuric acids) in two of the three plants studied. Exposure information was based on self-reports from long-term employees and industrial-hygiene records. Treated as a continuous variable, each year of acid mist exposure was not shown to increase risk of laryngeal cancer (OR 0.90, 95% CI 0.66-1.22).

De Stefani et al. (1998) studied 112 incident and histologically confirmed cases of laryngeal cancer at five hospitals in Montevideo from 1993 to 1995 in comparison with 509 controls with cancers not related to tobacco or alcohol use. Self-reported histories of exposure were gathered by questionnaire and addressed strong inorganic acids (defined as hydrochloric, nitric, or sulfuric acid). Risk of laryngeal cancer was increased with reported exposure to strong acid (OR 1.6, 95% CI 0.9-2.6), and a dose-response relation with years of exposure was suggested: subjects exposed for 1-20 years, OR 1.2, 95% CI 0.6-2.5, and subjects exposed for 20 years, OR 1.8, 95% CI 1.1-3.1. Synergism with heavy smoking (≥36 pack-years) was also demonstrated (OR 11.6, 95% CI 5.5-24.2).

In their case-control study of squamous cell carcinomas of the "upper gastrointestinal tract" diagnosed among Swedish men in 1988-1991, Gustavsson et al. (1998) reported on a set of 157 laryngeal-cancer cases compared with referents from the population registry matched on region and age group. Work histories and other personal information were gathered by nurses in structured in-person interviews. An occupational hygienist abstracted the extent of exposure to 17 occupational factors from the work histories; "acid mist" was one of them, but what specific acids were included was unstated. Exposure to acid mists was found to be associated with an increased risk of laryngeal cancer (OR 1.31, 95% CI 0.41-4.22).

Multiple Myeloma

Morris et al. (1986) performed a case-control study of 698 cases of multiple myeloma from four Surveillance, Epidemiology, and End Results (SEER) registries in 1977-1981 with a population control group of 1,683. Exposure information was self-reported for 68% of the cases and 99% of the controls with family-member proxies providing data for deceased or ill subjects. Exposure to acids (including muriatic, hydrochloric, sulfuric, chromic, nitric, and acetic acids) was associated with an increased risk of multiple myeloma when analysis was limited to self-respondents (OR 1.5, 95% CI 0.8-2.8), but the effect was eliminated when proxy respondents were included (OR 1.0, 95% CI 0.6-1.9).

Non-Cancer Health Outcomes

Cardiovascular Effects

As described above, Mazumdar et al. (1975) followed the mortality of a cohort of Pennsylvania steelworkers employed through 1966. Selected "cardiovascular-renal diseases" were studied in more detail when overall increases were noted among the white workers. Addition of the requirement of having worked for at least 5 years in the plants to the previous criterion of having been employed in 1953 reduced the number of evaluated deaths from those causes to 6,839. The risk of death due to arteriosclerotic heart disease was increased for all the acid-related jobs except coating; the risk posed by batch pickling was especially increased (12 observed, 5.4 expected; RR 2.55, $p < 0.01$). Coating, however, was the only acid-related job category that showed an increased rate of death from hypertensive heart disease (6 observed, 1.1 expected; RR 10.83; $p < 0.01$). For vascular lesions of the central nervous system, sheet finishing (24 observed, 18.3 expected; RR 1.41) and stainless annealing (4 observed, 3.2 expected) showed slight increases.

Respiratory Effects

Three studies evaluated respiratory function among nitric acid plant workers. Kamat et al. (1984) reported increases in dyspnea and cough, chest pain, giddiness, and headaches associated with longer periods of work among 125 men at an Indian nitric acid plant. Kolhatkar et al. (1987) evaluated respiratory symptoms and functions in a study of 113 male workers exposed to nitric acid at two other plants in India and found some chronic restrictive lung changes after long-term occupational exposure. Hilt (1987) documented clinical examinations of 153 men from the cohort of Norwegian nitric acid production workers described above (Hilt et al. 1985, 1991); the subjects were exposed primarily to asbestos, so little can be inferred about the role of nitric acid.

Summary

On the basis of the committee's review of the epidemiologic evidence, no available studies directly examined the association between exposure to nitric acid and long-term human health effects. Most studies were able only to investigate the health effects of nitric acid in combination with other strong inorganic acids, such as sulfuric acid, or other known carcinogens such as asbestos: that is, an independent assessment of nitric acid exposure was impossible because workers were exposed simultaneously to such mixtures. As a result, the health effects associated with exposure to nitric acid alone cannot be assessed.

Given the limitations of the body of evidence described above, it is interesting that what findings there are cluster mostly around respiratory cancers. The cohort studies on sheet and tin mill workers (Mazumdar et al. 1975), steel-pickling workers (Ahlborg et al. 1981; Beaumont et al. 1987), and chemical-plant workers (Rapiti et al. 1997) found an increased risk of lung cancer among those exposed to mixtures of acids. Similarly, several cohort studies (Ahlborg et al. 1981; Eisen et al. 1994; Steenland et al. 1988) and case-control studies (De Stefani et al. 1998; Zemla et al. 1987) indicated an increased risk of laryngeal cancer with exposure to acid mists and strong acid mixtures. Not only could the effects of nitric acid not be separated from those of other agents, but the small samples resulted in relatively small numbers of observed cancers and in inadequate study power.

IARC (1992) included nitric acid in its review of strong inorganic acids for which the conclusion was that strong-inorganic-acid mists containing sulfuric acid are carcinogenic in humans. However, very little is known about the dosimetry of inhaled nitric acid. Nitric acid generally exists in air in the vapor state except in acid fogs. Although the high water solubility and existence in the vapor state suggests that it should undergo substantial removal in the upper respiratory tract, there is some evidence that inhaled vapor-phase nitric acid may be converted into or deposited on small particles in the humid atmosphere of the respiratory tract. That would facilitate its transport to and deposition in the deep lung (Chen and Schlesinger 1996). In contrast, the data supporting a role for sulfuric acid in occupational cancers of the larynx involved exposures to large acid droplets, which would deposit in the upper respiratory tract. Thus, because the form of nitric acid that may have been inhaled by service personnel is not known, an analogy cannot be drawn between the apparent carcinogenic effects of industrial exposures to sulfuric acid and any possible carcinogenic effects of Gulf War exposures to nitric acid.

Furthermore, the underlying mechanism thought to be responsible for the carcinogenicity of strong-inorganic-acid mists would require extensive chronic exposure, which would not be equivalent to a person's being exposed to all of the few Scuds that may have disintegrated over troops during the Gulf War.

The available epidemiologic findings on cancer at other sites and on noncancer health outcomes are largely isolated data points generated in the course of investigating the potential of nitric acid or other strong inorganic acids as respiratory carcinogens.

Several toxicologic and controlled clinical studies have been performed with nitric acid vapors (Abraham et al. 1982; Aris et al. 1993; Beckett et al. 1995; Koenig et al. 1989; Mautz et al. 1995; Schlesinger et al. 1994). Whether those studies involved acute or repeated exposures, however, biologic endpoints were assayed within 24 hours of cessation of exposure. Thus, they do not add compelling information regarding persistent effects of exposure to nitric acid.

The committee concludes, from its assessment of the epidemiologic literature, that there is inadequate/insufficient evidence to determine whether an association exists between exposure to nitric acid and lung, laryngeal, stomach, bladder, colon, pancreatic, or lymphopoietic cancers; melanoma; multiple myeloma; or mortality from cardiovascular diseases.

Table 9.6 provides the key findings reviewed by the committee.

TABLE 9.6 Selected Epidemiologic Studies—Health Outcomes and Exposure to Nitric Acid

Reference	Study Population	Exposed Cases	Estimated Relative Risk
Respiratory Cancer (broken out below where Lung or Larynx was presented separately)			
Cohort Studies			
Mazumdar et al. 1975	Pennsylvania sheet and tin mill cohort (cancer of "respiratory organs", ICD not specified)		
	Jobs with exposure to acid baths (containing sulfuric, hydrochloric, or phosphoric acid)		
	Batch pickling and sheet dryers	0	—
	Continuous pickling and electric cleaning	0	—
	Stainless annealing, pickling, and processing	2	3.33 (0.40-12.03)[b]
	Coating	4	1.43 (0.39-3.66)[b]
	Sheet finishing and shipping	19	1.27 (0.73-1.90)[b]
	Tin finishing and shipping	2	0.56 (0.07-2.01)[b]
Ahlborg et al. 1981	Swedish metal-pickling cohort (respiratory tract cancers, ICD 160-163)		
	No latency	4	6.06 (1.65-15.52)[b]
	>10 years latency	4	7.27 (1.98-18.62)[b]
Beaumont et al. 1987	Midwestern metal-pickling cohort All types of acid exposure	37	1.63 (1.15-2.26)
Lung Cancer			
Cohort Studies			
Steenland and Beaumont 1989	Midwestern metal-pickling cohort (employed 1940-1964)		
	Mortality through 1986 All types acid exposure	41	1.55 (1.12-2.11)
	Adjust for smoking	41	1.36 (0.97-1.84)
Beaumont et al. 1987	Mortality through 1981 All types of acid exposure	35	1.64 (1.14-2.28)[a]
	Sulfuric acid only	19	1.39, $p > 0.05$
	Daily and ≥20 years since first employment	16	1.93, $p < 0.05$
	Sulfuric and other acids	7	1.92, $p > 0.05$
	Other acids only	9	2.24, $p < 0.05$
	Time since first employment		
	0.5-20 years	2	3.26, $p > 0.05$
	≥20 years	7	2.06, $p > 0.05$
	Only those employed 1950-1954)		
	vs US population	9	2.42 (1.11-4.61)
	vs Allegheny County steelworkers	9	2.00 (1.06-3.78)

Reference	Study Population	Exposed Cases	Estimated Relative Risk
Rapiti et al. 1997	Italian chemical-plant workers		
	Exposed to acid mixtures	8	1.62 (0.81-2.92)[c]
Laryngeal Cancer			
Cohort Studies			
Ahlborg et al. 1981	Swedish metal-pickling cohort		
	No latency	3	50.00 (10.32-146.17)[b]
	>10 years latency	3	60.00 (12.38-175.40)[b]
Beaumont et al. 1987	Midwestern metal-pickling cohort		
	Mortality, all acid groups	2	1.93 (0.23-6.99)
Steenland et al. 1988	Incidence, all acid groups (two in "other acids")	9	2.30 (1.05-4.36)[a]
	≤5 years duration (one in "other acids")	3	1.70 (0.35-4.95)[a]
	>5 years duration (one in "other acids")	6	2.76 (1.01-6.02)[a]
Case-Control Studies			
Eisen et al. 1994	Nested case-control in cohort of automobile workers exposed to machining fluids		
	Years exposed to acid mist	na	0.90 (0.66-1.22)
Zemla et al. 1987	Residents of Upper Silesia, Poland		
	Exposed to vapor (including nitric acid)	11	2.00 (1.00-3.52)
	Natives	2	0.57 (0.07-2.06)
	Immigrants	9	4.50 (2.06-8.54)
De Stefani et al. 1998	Residents of Montevideo, Uruguay		
	Exposed to strong acids (including nitric acid)	46	1.6 (0.9-2.6)
	1-20 years	12	1.2 (0.6-2.5)
	≥21 years	34	1.8 (1.1-3.1)
Gustavsson et al. 1998	Swedish men		
	Exposed to acid mist	4	1.31 (0.41-4.22)
Esophageal Cancer			
Case-Control Study			
Parent et al. 2000	Montreal case-control study set		
	All histologic types	15	2.2 (1.2-4.3)
	Exposure to sulfuric acid		
	Nonsubstantial	12	2.0 (1.0-4.0)
	Substantial	3	4.1 (1.0-17.2)
	Squamous cell carcinoma	10	2.8 (1.2-6.1)
	Exposure to sulfuric acid		

Reference	Study Population	Exposed Cases	Estimated Relative Risk
	Nonsubstantial	9	2.2 (1.2-6.3)
	Substantial	1	3.1 (0.3-28.1)
Lymphopoietic Cancer			
Cohort Studies			
Mazumdar et al. 1975	Pennsylvania sheet and tin mill cohort		
	Jobs with exposure to acid baths (containing sulfuric, hydrochloric, or phosphoric acid)		
	Batch pickling and sheet dryers	0	—
	Continuous pickling and electric cleaning	0	—
	Stainless annealing, pickling, and processing	1	5.0 (0.13-27.85)[b]
	Coating	0	—
	Sheet finishing and shipping	0	—
	Tin finishing and shipping	3	3.00 (0.62-8.77)[b]
Rapiti et al. 1997	Italian chemical-plant workers		
	Exposed to acid mixtures	2	1.87 (0.33-5.88)[c]
	Non-Hodgkin's lymphoma	1	4.17 (0.04-19.70)[c]
	Leukemia	1	1.79 (0.09-8.47)[c]
Multiple Myeloma			
Case-Control Study			
Morris et al. 1986	Residents of four US states		
	Self-respondents and proxies	20	1.0 (0.6-1.9)
	Self-respondents only	19	1.5 (0.8-2.8)
Non-Cancer Health Outcomes Arteriosclerotic Heart Disease (Mortality)			
Cohort Study			
Mazumdar et al. 1975	Pennsylvania sheet and tin mill cohort (≥5 years)		
	Jobs with exposure to acid baths (containing sulfuric, hydrochloric, or phosphoric acid)		
	Batch pickling and sheet dryers	12	2.55 (1.15-3.88)[a] ($p<0.01$)
	Continuous pickling and electric cleaning	8 (vs 6.9)	1.17
	Stainless annealing, pickling, and processing	16 (vs 14.0)	1.16
	Coating	12	0.66 (0.35-1.20)[a]
	Sheet finishing and shipping	98	1.07 (0.86-1.29)[a]
	Tin finishing and shipping	26	1.08 (0.69-1.56)[a]

Reference	Study Population	Exposed Cases	Estimated Relative Risk
Hypertensive Heart Disease (Mortality)			
Cohort Study			
Mazumdar et al. 1975	Pennsylvania sheet and tin mill cohort (≥5 years)		
	Jobs with exposure to acid baths (containing sulfuric, hydrochloric, or phosphoric acid)		
	Batch pickling and sheet dryers	0	—
	Continuous pickling and electric cleaning	0	—
	Stainless annealing, pickling, and processing	1 (vs 0.5)	2.0
	Coating	6 (vs 1.1)	10.83 ($p< 0.01$)
	Sheet finishing and shipping	1	0.26 (0.01-1.43)[a]
	Tin finishing and shipping	0	—
Vascular Lesions of CNS (Mortality)			
Cohort Study			
Mazumdar et al. 1975	Pennsylvania sheet and tin mill cohort (≥5 years)		
	Jobs with exposure to acid baths (containing sulfuric, hydrochloric, or phosphoric acid)		
	Batch pickling and sheet dryers	0	—
	Continuous pickling and electric cleaning	0	—
	Stainless annealing, pickling, and processing	4 (vs 3.2)	1.25
	Coating	3	0.75 (0.15-2.19)[b]
	Sheet finishing and shipping	24	1.41 (0.84-1.95)[a]
	Tin finishing and shipping	4	0.74 (0.21-1.97)[a]
Diabetes Mellitus (Mortality)			
Cohort Study			
Beaumont et al. 1987	Midwestern metal-pickling cohort All types of acid exposure	8	1.65 (0.71-3.26)

NOTE: na=not available.
[a] 95% CIs were calculated with standard methods from the observed and expected numbers presented in the original paper.
[b] Risk estimates and 95% CIs were calculated with standard methods from the observed and expected numbers presented in the original paper.
[c] 90% CIs were reported.

REFERENCES

Abraham WM, Kim CS, King MM, Oliver W, Yerger L. 1982. Effects of nitric acid on carbachol reactivity of the airways in normal and allergic sheep. *Archives of Environmental Health* 37(1):36-40; as cited in NRC 1998.

ACGIH (American Conference of Governmental Industrial Hygienists). 2003. *2003 TLVs and BEIs: Threshold Limit Values for Chemical Substances and Physical Agents. Biological Exposure Indices.* Cincinnati, OH: ACGIH.

Ahlborg G Jr, Hogstedt C, Sundell L, Aman CG. 1981. Laryngeal cancer and pickling house vapors. *Scandinavian Journal of Work, Environment and Health* 7(3):239-240.

Aris R, Christian D, Tager I, Ngo L, Finkbeiner WE, Balmes JR. 1993. Effects of nitric acid gas alone or in combination with ozone on healthy volunteers. *American Review of Respiratory Disease* 148(4 Pt 1):965-973; as cited in NRC 2000.

ATSDR (Agency for Toxic Substances and Disease Registry). 1997. *Toxicological Profile for Hydrazines*. Atlanta, GA: US Department of Health and Human Services, Public Health Service, ATSDR.

Ballou JE, Gies RA, Dagle GE, Burton FG, Moss OR. 1978. Late effects of acid inhalation. In: *Pacific Northwest Laboratory Annual Report.* Richland, WA: Pacific Northwest Laboratory. Pp. 6.1-6.2; as cited in Swenberg and Beauchamp 1997.

Ballou JE, Gies RA, Dagle GE, Burton FG, Moss OR. 1981. Late effects of acid inhalation. In: *Pacific Northwest Laboratory Annual Report.* Richland, WA: Pacific Northwest Laboratory. Pp. 223-225; as cited in Swenberg and Beauchamp 1997.

Bauer R, Tarr M, Olsen RG. 1990. Effect of 1,1-dimethylhydrazine on lymphoproliferation and interleukin 2 immunoregulatory function. *Archives of Environmental Contamination and Toxicology* 19(1):148-153.

Beaumont JJ, Leveton J, Knox K, Bloom T, McQuiston T, Young M, Goldsmith R, Steenland NK, Brown DP, Halperin WE. 1987. Lung cancer mortality in workers exposed to sulfuric acid mist and other acid mists. *Journal of the National Cancer Institute* 79(5):911-921.

Beckett WS, Russi MB, Haber AD, Rivkin RM, Sullivan JR, Tameroglu Z, Mohsenin V, Leaderer BP. 1995. Effect of nitrous acid on lung function in asthmatics: A chamber study. *Environmental Health Perspectives* 103(4):372-375.

Bhide SV, D'Souza RA, Sawai MM, Ranadive KJ. 1976. Lung tumour incidence in mice treated with hydrazine sulphate. *International Journal of Cancer* 18(4):530-535.

Biancifiori C. 1970. Hepatomas in CBA/Cb/Se mice and liver lesions in golden hamsters induced by hydrazine sulfate. *Journal of the National Cancer Institute* 44(4):943-953; as cited in ATSDR 1997.

Biancifiori C, Bucciarelli E, Clayson D, Santilli FE. 1964. Induction of hepatomas in CBA/Cd/Se mice by hydrazine sulphate and the lack of effect of croton oil on tumor induction in BALB/c/Cd/Se mice. *British Journal of Cancer* 18:543-550.

Biancifiori C, Giornelli-Santilli FE, Milia U, Severi L. 1966. Pulmonary tumours in rats induced by oral hydrazine sulphate. *Nature* 212(60):414-415.

Birmingham DJ. 1988. Contact dermatitis and related dermatoses associated with petroleum recovery and use. *Occupational Medicine* 3(3):511-523.

Bosan WS, Shank RC, MacEwen JD, Gaworski CL, Newberne PM. 1987. Methylation of DNA guanine during the course of induction of liver cancer in hamsters by hydrazine or dimethylnitrosamine. *Carcinogenesis* 8(3):439-444.

Cammarano G, Crosignani P, Berrino F, Berra G. 1984. Cancer mortality among workers in a thermoelectric power plant. *Scandinavian Journal of Work, Environment & Health* 10(4):259-261.

Chen CC, Schlesinger RB. 1996. Considerations for the respiratory-tract dosimetry of inhaled nitric acid vapor. *Inhalation Toxicology* 8(7):639-654.

Choudhary G, Hansen H. 1998. Human health perspective on environmental exposure to hydrazines: A review. *Chemosphere* 37(5):801-843.

Comstock CC, Lawson LH, Greene EA, Oberst FW. 1954. Inhalation toxicity of hydrazine vapor. *AMA Archives of Industrial Hygiene and Occupational Medicine* 10:416-490; as cited in NRC 1996.

De Stefani E, Boffetta P, Oreggia F, Ronco A, Kogevinas M, Mendilaharsu M. 1998. Occupation and the risk of laryngeal cancer in Uruguay. *American Journal of Industrial Medicine* 33(6):537-542.

Delaney J, Timbrell J. 1995. Role of cytochrome P450 in hydrazine toxicity in isolated hepatocytes in vitro. *Xenobiotica* 25(12):1399-1410.

Dettling J. 1935. Atrophy of the crowns of the teeth of workers engaged in nitriding processes (Odontomalacia nitrosa). *Deutsche Zeitschrift für die Gesamte Gerichtliche Medizin* 25:198; as cited in NIOSH 1976.

Diggle WM, Gage JC. 1954. The toxicity of nitrogen pentoxide. *British Journal of Industrial Medicine* 11:140-144; as cited in NIOSH 1976.

DOD (Department of Defense). 2000. *Information Paper: Inhibited Red Fuming Nitric Acid.* [Online]. Available: http://www.gulflink.osd.mil/irfna/ [accessed August 20, 2003].

DOD. 2001. *Information Paper: Iraq's Scud Ballistic Missiles.* [Online]. Available: http://www.gulflink.osd.mil/scud_info_ii/ [accessed August 20, 2003].

Durant PJ, Harris RA. 1980. Hydrazine and lupus. *New England Journal of Medicine* 303(10):584-585.

EFMA (European Fertilizer Manufacturers Association). 1997. *Guidelines for Transporting Nitric Acid in Tanks*. [Online]. Available: http://www.efma.org/publications/NitricAcid/ [accessed August 20, 2003].

Eisen EA, Tolbert PE, Hallock MF, Monson RR, Smith TJ, Woskie SR. 1994. Mortality studies of machining fluid exposure in the automobile industry III: A case-control study of larynx cancer. *American Journal of Industrial Medicine* 26(2):185-202.

EPA (Environmental Protection Agency). 1987. *Nitric Acid. Chemical Profiles, United States Environmental Protection Agency*. [Online]. Available: http://yosemite.epa.gov/oswer/CeppoEHS.nsf/Profiles/7697-37-2?OpenDocument [accessed August 26, 2003].

Ernst H, Rittinghausen S, Wahnschaffe U, Mohr U. 1987. Induction of malignant peripheral nerve sheath tumors in European hamsters with 1,1-dimethylhydrazine (UDMH). *Cancer Letters* 35(3):313-311.

Fiala E, Kulakis C. 1981. Separation of hydrazine, monomethylhydrazine, 1,1-dimethylhydrazine and 1,2-dimthylhydrazine by high performance liquid chromatography with electrochemical detection. *Journal of Chromatography* 214:229-233; as cited in ATSDR 1997.

Fiedler N, Lange G, Tiersky L, DeLuca J, Policastro T, Kelly-McNeil K, McWilliams R, Korn L, Natelson B. 2000. Stressors, personality traits, and coping of Gulf War veterans with chronic fatigue. *Journal of Psychosomatic Research* 48(6):525-535.

Frazier DE Jr, Tarr MJ, Olsen RG. 1991. The in vitro and in vivo effects of 1,1-dimethylhydrazine (UDMH) on murine lymphocyte subsets and Ia antigen expression. *Immunopharmacology Immunotoxicology* 13(1- 2):25-46.

Frazier DE Jr, Tarr MJ, Olsen RG. 1992. Evaluation of murine lymphocyte membrane potential, intracellular free calcium, and interleukin-2 receptor expression upon exposure to 1,1-dimethylhydrazine. *Toxicology Letters* 61(1):27-37.

Fukuda K, Straus S, Hickie I, Sharpe M, Dobbins J, Komaroff A. 1994. The chronic fatigue syndrome: A comprehensive approach to its definition and study. International Chronic Fatigue Syndrome Study Group. *Annals of Internal Medicine* 121(12):953-959.

Godoy H, Diaz Gomez M, Castro J. 1984. Metabolism and activation of 1,1-dimethylhydrazine and methylhydrazine, two products of N-nitrosodimethylamine reductive biotransformation. In: O'Neill IK, von Borstel RC, Miller CT, Long J, Bartsch H, eds. *N-Nitroso Compounds: Occurrence, Biological Effects and Relevance to Human Cancer*. Vol. 57. Lyons, France: International Agency for Research on Cancer. Pp. 479-484; as cited in IARC 1999b.

Goss Gilroy Inc. 1998. *Health Study of Canadian Forces Personnel Involved in the 1991 Conflict in the Persian Gulf.* Ottawa, Canada: Goss Gilroy Inc., Department of National Defence.

Gray EL, Goldberg SB, Patton FM. 1954a. Toxicity of the oxides of nitrogen: III. Effect of chronic exposure to low concentrations of vapors from red fuming nitric acid. *Archives of Industrial Hygiene and Occupational Medicine* 10:423-425; as cited in NIOSH 1976.

Gray EL, MacNamee JK, Goldberg SB. 1952. Toxicity of NO^2 vapors at very low levels: A preliminary report. *Archives of Industrial Hygiene and Occupational Medicine* 6:20-21; as cited in NIOSH 1976.

Gray EL, Patton FM, Goldberg SB, Kaplan E. 1954b. Toxicity of the oxides of nitrogen: II. Acute inhalation toxicity of nitrogen dioxide, red fuming nitric acid, and white fuming nitric acid. *Archives of Industrial Hygiene and Occupational Medicine* 10:418-422; as cited in NIOSH 1976.

Greenberg SD, Gyorkey F, Jenkins DE, Gyorkey P. 1971. Alveolar epithelial cells following exposure to nitric acid: Electron microscopic study in rats. *Archives of Environmental Health* 22:655-662; as cited in NIOSH 1976.

Gustavsson P, Jakobsson R, Johansson H, Lewin F, Norell S, Rutkvist LE. 1998. Occupational exposures and squamous cell carcinoma of the oral cavity, pharynx, larynx, and oesophagus: A case-control study in Sweden. *Occupational and Environmental Medicine* 55(6):393-400.

Haun CC, Kinkead ER. 1973. *Chronic Inhalation Toxicity of Unsymmetrical Dimethylhydrazine: Oncogenic Effects.* Springfield, VA: Department of Commerce; as cited in ATSDR 1997.

Haun CC. 1977. *Canine Hepatotoxic Response to the Inhalation of 1,1-Demethylhydrazine (UMDH) and 1,1-Dimethylhydrazine with Dimethylnitrosamine (DMNA). AMRL-TR-76-125.* Wright-Patterson Air Force Base, OH: Aerospace Medical Research Laboratory; as cited in ATSDR 1997.

Haun CC, Kinkead ER, Vernot CL. 1984. *Chronic Inhalation Toxicity of Unsymmetrical Dimethlyhydrazine: Oncogenic Effects.* Wright-Patterson Air Force Base, OH: Aerospace Medical Research Laboratory; as cited in ATSDR 1997.

Heidelberger C, Freeman AE, Pienta RJ, Sivak A, Bertram JS, Casto BC, Dunkel VC, Francis MW, Kakunaga T, Little JB, Schechtman LM. 1983. Cell transformation by chemical agents: A review and analysis of the literature. A report of the U.S. Environmental Protection Agency GeneTox Program. *Mutation Research* 114(3):283-385.

Hilt B. 1987. Non-malignant asbestos diseases in workers in an electrochemical plant. *British Journal of Industrial Medicine* 44(9):621-626.

Hilt B, Andersen A, Rosenberg J, Langard S. 1991. Cancer incidence among asbestos-exposed chemical industry workers: An extended observation period. *American Journal of Industrial Medicine* 20(2):261-264.

Hilt B, Langard S, Andersen A, Rosenberg J. 1985. Asbestos exposure, smoking habits, and cancer incidence among production and maintenance workers in an electrochemical plant. *American Journal of Industrial Medicine* 8(6):565-577.

House WB. 1964. *Tolerance Criteria for Continuous Exposure Inhalation Exposure to Toxic Materials. III. Effects on Animals of 90-d Exposure to Hydrazine, Unsymmetrical Dimethylhydrazine (UMDH), Decaborane, and Nitrogen Dioxide. ASD-TR-61-519.* Wright-Patterson Air Force Base, OH: Aerospace Medical Research Laboratory.

IARC (International Agency for Research on Cancer). 1974. *Some Aromatic Amines, Hydrazine and Related Substances, N-Nitroso Compound and Miscellaneous Alkylating Agents.* Lyon, France: IARC.

IARC. 1992. *Occupational Exposures to Mists and Vapours from Strong Inorganic Acids.* 54. Lyon, France: IARC.

IARC. 1999a. *1,1-Dimethylhydrazine.* 71 Pt 3. Lyon, France: IARC.

IARC. 1999b. *Hydrazine.* 71 Pt 3A. Lyon, France: IARC .

IARC. 1999c. *Re-evaluation of some organic chemicals, hydrazine and hydrogen peroxide. Proceedings of the IARC Working Group on the Evaluation of Carcinogenic Risks to Humans. Lyon, France, 17-24 February 1998.* 71 Pt 1. Lyon, France: IARC.

IRIS (Integrated Risk Information System). 2003. *Hydrazine/Hydrazine Sulfate (CASRN 302-01-2)*. [Online]. Available: http://www.epa.gov/iris/subst/0352.htm [accessed February, 2004].

Ishoy T, Andersson AM, Suadicani P, Guldager B, Appleyard M, Gyntelberg F, Skakkebaek NE, The Danish Gulf War Study. 2001a. Major reproductive health characteristics in male Gulf War Veterans. The Danish Gulf War Study. *Danish Medical Bulletin* 48(1):29-32.

Ishoy T, Suadicani P, Andersson A-M, Guldager B, Appleyard M, Skakkebaek NE, Gyntelberg F. 2001b. Prevalence of male sexual problems in the Danish Gulf War Study. *Scandinavian Journal of Sexology: Special Issue* 4(1):43-55.

Ishoy T, Suadicani P, Guldager B, Appleyard M, Gyntelberg F. 1999a. Risk factors for gastrointestinal symptoms. The Danish Gulf War Study. *Danish Medical Bulletin* 46(5):420-423.

Ishoy T, Suadicani P, Guldager B, Appleyard M, Hein HO, Gyntelberg F. 1999b. State of health after deployment in the Persian Gulf. The Danish Gulf War Study. *Danish Medical Bulletin* 46(5):416-419.

Jenner AM, Timbrell JA. 1994. Influence of inducers and inhibitors of cytochrome P450 on the hepatotoxicity of hydrazine in vivo. *Archives of Toxicology* 68(6):349-357.

Jeong JY, Kamino K. 1993. Lack of tumorigenic activity of 1,1-dimethylhydrazine in Syrian golden hamsters treated by subcutaneous injection. *Experimental and Toxicologic Pathology* 45(1):61-63.

Kamat SR, Mahashur AA, Shah SP. 1984. Health study of nitric acid plant workers. *Lung India* 2:84-88.

Kaneo Y, Iguchi S, Kubo H, Iwagiri N, Matsuyama K. 1984. Tissue distribution of hydrazine and its metabolites in rats. *Journal of Pharmacobio-dynamics* 7(8):556-562; as cited in IARC 1999b.

Kang HK, Mahan CM, Lee KY, Magee CA, Murphy FM. 2000. Illnesses among United States veterans of the Gulf War: A population-based survey of 30,000 veterans. *Journal of Occupational and Environmental Medicine* 42(5):491-501.

Kang HK, Mahan CM, Lee KY, Murphy FM, Simmens SJ, Young HA, Levine PH. 2002. Evidence for a deployment-related Gulf War syndrome by factor analysis. *Archives of Environmental Health* 57(1):61-68.

Keinman M, Bhalla DK, Mautz WJ, Osann K, Basbaum C. 1995. *Nitric Acid Toxicity: Potential for Particle and Ozone Interactions*. Irvine, CA: California State Air Resources Board.

Keller WC, Olson CT, Back KC, Gaworski CL. 1984. Teratogenic assessment of three methylated hydrazine derivatives in the rat. *Journal of Toxicology and Environmental Health* 13(1):125-131.

King WH, Byyny RL, Ellerby RA, Williams CR. 1969. Medical evaluation of missile fuel handlers. *Aerospace Medicine* 40(3):315-317.

Kinkead ER, Haun CC, Vernot ER, MacEwen JD. 1985. *A Chronic Inhalation Toxicity Study on Monomethylhydrazine. AFAMRL-TR-85-025*. Wright-Patterson Air Force Base, OH: Aerospace Medical Research Laboratory; as cited in NRC 2000.

Koenig JQ, Covert DS, Pierson WE. 1989. Effects of inhalation of acidic compounds on pulmonary function in allergic adolescent subjects. *Environmental Health Perspectives* 79:173-178.

Koizumi A, Nomiyama T, Tsukada M, Wada Y, Omae K, Tanaka S, Miyauchi H, Imamiya S, Sakurai H. 1998. Evidence on N-acetyltransferase allele-associated metabolism of hydrazine in Japanese workers. *Journal of Occupational and Environmental Medicine* 40(3):217-222.

Kolhatkar VP, Patel MH, Mahashur AA, Rupawate RU, Vaidya PV, Kamat SR. 1987. Comparative study of respiratory changes in nitric acid plant workers. *Journal of the Association of Physicians of India* 35(3):217-219.

Llewellyn BM, Keller WC, Olson CT. 1986. *Urinary Metabolites of Hydrazine in Male Fischer 344 Rats Following Inhalation or Intravenous Exposure. AMRL-TR-86-025*. Wright-Patterson Air Force Base, OH: Aerospace Medical Research Laboratory; as cited in ATSDR 1997.

Lynch JB, Bell J. 1947. Dental erosion in workers exposed to inorganic acid fumes. *British Journal of Industrial Medicine* 4:84-86; as cited in NIOSH 1976.

MacEwen JD, Theodore J, Vernot EH. 1970. *Proceedings of the First Annual Conference on Environmental Toxicology. Human Exposure to EEL Concentrations of Monomethylhydrazine. AMRL-TR-70-102*. Wright-Patterson Air Force Base, OH: Aerospace Medical Research Laboratory; as cited in NRC 2000.

Maru GB, Bhide SV. 1982. Effect of antioxidants and antitoxicants of isoniazid on the formation of lung tumours in mice by isoniazid and hydrazine sulphate. *Cancer Letters* 17(1):75-80.

Mautz WJ, Bhalla DK, Kikkawa Y, Keinman MT, Phalen RF, Rasmussen R, Wong C, Osann K. 1995. *Studies to Determine the Long-Term Effects of Acidic Atmospheres. Final Report to the California Air Resources Board.* Irvine, CA: California State Air Resources Board; as cited in Keinman et al. 1995.

Mautz WJ, Kleinman MT, Phalen RF, Crocker TT. 1988. Effects of exercise exposure on toxic interactions between inhaled oxidant and aldehyde air pollutants. *Journal of Toxicology and Environmental Health* 25(2):165-178.

Mazumdar S, Lerer T, Redmond CK. 1975. Long-term mortality study of steelworkers. IX. Mortality patterns among sheet and tin mill workers. *Journal of Occupational Medicine* 17(12):751-755.

Mink S, Coalson L, Whitley L, Greville H, Jadue C. 1984. Pulmonary function tests in the detection of small airway obstruction in a canine model of bronchiolitis obliterans. *American Review of Respiratory Disease* 130:1125-1133; as cited in Schlesinger et al. 1995.

Mitz MA, Aldrich FL, Vasta BM. 1962. *Study of Intermediary Metabolic Pathways of 1, 1-Dimethylhydrazine (UDMH). AMRL-TDR-62-110.* Wright-Patterson Air Force Base, OH: Aerospace Medical Research Laboratory; as cited in ATSDR 1997.

Mommsen S, Aagaard J, Sell A. 1982. An epidemiological case-control study of bladder cancer in males from a predominantly rural district. *European Journal of Cancer & Clinical Oncology* 18(11):1205-1210.

Morgenstern H, Ritz B. 2001. Effects of radiation and chemical exposures on cancer mortality among Rocketdyne workers: A review of three cohort studies. *Occupational Medicine* 16(2):219-237.

Morris J, Densem JW, Wald NJ, Doll R. 1995. Occupational exposure to hydrazine and subsequent risk of cancer. *Occupational and Environmental Medicine* 52(1):43-45.

Morris PD, Koepsell TD, Daling JR, Taylor JW, Lyon JL, Swanson GM, Child M, Weiss NS. 1986. Toxic substance exposure and multiple myeloma: A case control-study. *Journal of the National Cancer Institute* 76(6):987-994.

NIOSH (The National Institute for Occupational Safety and Health). 1976. *Occupational Exposure to Nitric Acid. Criteria for a Recommended Standard. DHHS (NIOSH) Publication No. 76-141.* [Online]. Available: http://www.cdc.gov/niosh/76-141.html [accessed June 17, 2003].

NIOSH. 1994. *International Chemical Safety Cards*. [Online]. Available: http:www.cdc.gov/niosh/ipcsneng/neng0183.html [accessed February 10, 2004].

NIOSH, DHHS. 1997. *NIOSH Pocket Guide to Chemical Hazards*. Cincinnati, OH: US Department of Health and Human Services, Public Health Service, Centers for Disease Control and Prevention, National Institute for Occupational Safety and Health.

Nomiyama T, Omae K, Tanaka S, Miyauchi H, Koizumi A, Tsukada M, Wada Y, Mogi T, Imamiya S, Sakurai H. 1998. A cross-sectional observation of the effects of hydrazine hydrate on workers' health. *Journal of Occupational Health* 40(3):177-185.

NRC (National Research Council). 1996. Hydrazine. In: NRC. *Spacecraft Maximum Allowable Concentrations for Selected Airborne Contaminants.* Vol. II. Washington, DC: National Academy Press. Pp. 213-234.

NRC. 1998. Appendix F: Acute Toxicity of Nitric Acid. In: *Assessment of Exposure-Response Functions for Rocket-Emission Toxicants.* Washington, DC: National Academy Press. Pp. 197-208.

NRC. 2000. Dimethylhydrazine: Acute exposure guideline levels. In: *Acute Exposure Guideline Levels for Selected Airborne Chemicals.* Washington, DC: National Academy Press. Pp. 155-201.

Ochoa MJ, Wittes R, Krakoff IH. 1975. Trial of hydrazine sulfate (NSC-150014) in patients with cancer. *Cancer Chemotherapy Reports* 59(6):1151-1154.

Parent ME, Siemiatycki J, Fritschi L. 2000. Workplace exposures and oesophageal cancer. *Occupational & Environmental Medicine* 57(5):325-334.

Pereyo N. 1986. Hydrazine derivatives and induction of systemic lupus erythematosus. *Journal of the American Academy of Dermatology* 14(3):514-515.

Peters SG, Hyatt RE. 1986. A canine model of bronchial injury induced by nitric-acid lung mechanisms and morphologic features. *The American Review of Respiratory Disease* 133(6):1049-1054.

Petersen P, Bredahl E, Lauritsen O, Laursen T. 1970. Examination of the liver in personnel working with liquid rocket propellant. *British Journal of Industrial Medicine* 27(2):141-146.

Pham-Huu-Chanh, Maciotta-Lapoujade M, NguyenLuong Thi Ngog Suong, Azum-Gelade M-C. 1966. Study of the immediate effects of aerosol spray of acids on the isolated lungs of guinea pigs. *Agressologie* 7:507-511; as cited in NIOSH 1976.

Pinkerton MK, Hagano EA, Back KC. 1967. *Distribution and Excretion of* ^{14}*C-Monomethylhydrazine. AMRL-TR-67-175*. Wright-Patterson Air Force Base, OH: Aerospace Medical Research Laboratory. Pp.1-17; as cited in NRC 2000.

Preece NE, Ghatineh S, Timbrell JA. 1992. Studies on the disposition and metabolism of hydrazine in rats in vivo. *Human & Experimental Toxicology* 11(2):121-127.

Preece NE, Nicholson JK, Timbrell JA. 1991. Identification of novel hydrazine metabolites by nitrogen-15 NMR. *Biochemical Pharmacology* 41(9):1319-1324.

Preziosi P, Ciabattoni G. 1987. Acid rain effects on arachidonic acid metabolism in perfused and ventilated guinea-pig lung. *Toxicology Letters* 39(1):101-108; as cited in Soskolne et al. 1989.

Proctor SP, Heeren T, White RF, Wolfe J, Borgos MS, Davis JD, Pepper L, Clapp R, Sutker PB, Vasterling JJ, Ozonoff D. 1998. Health status of Persian Gulf War veterans: Self-reported symptoms, environmental exposures and the effect of stress. *International Journal of Epidemiology* 27(6):1000-1010.

Rapiti E, Fantini F, Dell'orco V, Fano V, Blasetti F, Bracci C, Forastiere F, Comba P. 1997. Cancer mortality among chemical workers in an Italian plant. *European Journal of Epidemiology* 13(3):281-285.

Reid S, Hotopf M, Hull L, Ismail K, Unwin C, Wessely S. 2001. Multiple chemical sensitivity and chronic fatigue syndrome in British Gulf War veterans. *American Journal of Epidemiology* 153(6):604-609.

Rinehart WE, Donait E, Green EA. 1960. The sub-acute and chronic toxicity of 1,1-dimethylhydrazine vapor. *American Industrial Hygiene Association Journal* 21:207-210; as cited in ATSDR 1997.

Ritz B, Morgenstern H, Froines J, Moncau J. 1999. Chemical exposures of rocket-engine test-stand personnel and cancer mortality in a cohort of aerospace workers. *Journal of Occupational and Environmental Medicine* 41(10):903-910.

Roe FJ, Grant GA, Millican DM. 1967. Carcinogenicity of hydrazine and 1,1-dimethylhydrazine for mouse lung. *Nature* 216(113):375-376.

Sathiakumar N, Delzell E, Amoateng-Adjepong Y, Larson R, Cole P. 1997. Epidemiologic evidence on the relationship between mists containing sulfuric acid and respiratory tract cancer. *Critical Reviews in Toxicology* 27(3):233-251.

Schlesinger RB, Chen LC, Nadziejko C, Last JA, Pinkerton K. 1995. *Studies to Determine Long-Term Health Effects of Acidic Atmospheres.* Sacramento, CA: California State Air Resources Board, Research Division.

Schlesinger RB, El-Fawal HAN, Zelikoff JT, Gorxzynski JE, McGovern T, Madsiejko CE, Chen LC. 1994. Pulmonary effects of repeated episodic exposures to nitric acid vapor alone and in combination with ozone. *Inhalation Toxicology* 6(1):21-41.

Scott D, Galloway S, Marshall R, Ishidate M Jr, Brusick D, Ashby J, Myhr BC. 1991. Genotoxicity under extreme culture conditions: A report from International Commission for Protection Against Environmental Mutagens and Carcinogens Task Group 9. *Mutation Research* 257(2):147-205.

Severi L, Biancifiori C. 1968. Hepatic carcinogenesis in CBA-Cb-Se mice and Cb-Se rats by isonicotinic acid hydrazide and hydrazine sulfate. *Journal of the National Cancer Institute* 41(2):331-349.

Shook B, Cowart H. 1957. Health hazards associated with unsymmetrical dimethylhydrazine. *Industrial Medicine* 26:333-336; as cited in Petersen et al. 1970.

Sinha BK. 1987. Activation of hydrazine derivatives to free radicals in the perfused rat liver: A spin-trapping study. *Biochimica et Biophysica Acta* 924(2):261-269.

Smith EB, Clark DA. 1971. Absorption of unsymmetrical dimethylhydrazine (UDMH) through canine skin. *Toxicology and Applied Pharmacology* 18(3):649-659.

Smith EB, Clark DA. 1972. Absorption of hydrazine through canine skin. *Toxicology and Applied Pharmacology* 21(2):186-193.

Soskolne CL, Jhangri GS, Siemiatycki J, Lakhani R., Dewar R, Burch JD, Howe GR, Miller AB. 1992. Occupational exposure to sulfuric acid in southern Ontario, Canada, in association with laryngeal cancer. *Scandinavian Journal of Work, Environment and Health* 18(4):225-232.

Soskolne CL, Pagano G, Cipollaro M, Beaumont JJ, Giordano GG. 1989. Epidemiologic and toxicologic evidence for chronic health effects and the underlying biologic mechanisms involved in sub-lethal exposures to acidic pollutants. *Archives of Environmental Health* 44(3):180-191.

Soskolne CL, Zeighami EA, Hanis NM, Kupper LL, Herrmann N, Amsel J, Mausner JS, Stellman JM. 1984. Laryngeal cancer and occupational exposure to sulfuric acid. *American Journal of Epidemiology* 120(3):358-69.

Spencer PS, McCauley LA, Joos SK, Lasarev MR, Schuell T, Bourdette D, Barkhuizen A, Johnston W, Storzbach D, Wynn M, Grewenow R. 1998. U.S. Gulf War Veterans: Service periods in theater, differential exposures, and persistent unexplained illness. Portland Environmental Hazards Research Centre. *Toxicology Letters* 102-103:515-521.

Spencer PS, McCauley LA, Lapidus JA, Lasarev M, Joos SK, Storzbach D. 2001. Self-reported exposures and their association with unexplained illness in a population-based case-control study of Gulf War veterans. *Journal of Occupational and Environmental Medicine* 43(12):1041-1056.

Steenland K, Beaumont J. 1989. Further follow-up and adjustment for smoking in a study of lung cancer and acid mists. *American Journal of Industrial Medicine* 16(4):347-354.

Steenland K, Schnorr T, Beaumont J, Halperin W, Bloom T. 1988. Incidence of laryngeal cancer and exposure to acid mists. *British Journal of Industrial Medicine* 45(11):766-776.

Steinhoff D, Mohr U. 1988. The question of carcinogenic effects of hydrazine. *Experimental Pathology* 33(3):133-143.

Steinhoff D, Mohr U, Schmidt WM. 1990. On the question of the carcinogenic action of hydrazine: Evaluation on the basis of new experimental results. *Experimental Pathology* 39(1):1-9.

Storzbach D, Campbell KA, Binder LM, McCauley L, Anger WK, Rohlman DS, Kovera CA. 2000. Psychological differences between veterans with and without Gulf War unexplained symptoms. *Psychosomatic Medicine* 62(5):726-735.

Suadicani P, Ishoy T, Guldager B, Appleyard M, Gyntelberg F. 1999. Determinants of long-term neuropsychological symptoms: The Danish Gulf War Study. *Danish Medical Bulletin* 46(5):423-427.

Swenberg JA, Beauchamp RO Jr. 1997. A review of the chronic toxicity, carcinogenicity, and possible mechanisms of action of inorganic acid mists in animals. *Critical Reviews in Toxicology* 27(3):253-259.

tenBruggen Cate H. 1968. Dental erosion in industry. *British Journal of Industrial Medicine* 25:249-266; as cited in NIOSH 1976.

Timbrell J, Scales M, Streeter A. 1982. Studies on hydrazine hepatotoxicity: 2. Biochemical findings. *Journal of Toxicology and Environmental Health* 6:955-968.

Tomasi A, Albano E, Botti B, Vannini V. 1987. Detection of free radical intermediates in the oxidative metabolism of carcinogenic hydrazine derivatives. *Toxicologic Pathology* 15(2):178-183.

Toth B. 1969. Lung tumor induction and inhibition of breast adenocarcinomas by hydrazine sulfate in mice. *Journal of the National Cancer Institute* 42(3):469-475.

Totten RS, Moran TJ. 1961. Cortisone and atypical pulmonary "epithelial" hyperplasia: Effects of pretreatment with cortisone on repair of chemically damaged rabbit lungs. *American Journal of Pathology* 38:575-86; as cited in Schlesinger et al. 1995.

Unwin C, Blatchley N, Coker W, Ferry S, Hotopf M, Hull L, Ismail K, Palmer I, David A, Wessely S. 1999. Health of UK servicemen who served in Persian Gulf War. *Lancet* 353:169-178.

Vernot EH, MacEwen JD, Bruner RH, Haun CC, Kinkead ER, Prentice DE, Hall A 3rd, Schmidt RE, Eason RL, Hubbard GB, Young JT. 1985. Long-term inhalation toxicity of hydrazine. *Fundamental and Applied Toxicology* 5(6 Pt 1):1050-1064.

Wakabayashi T, Horiuchi M, Sakaguchi M, Onda H, Misawa K. 1983. Induction of megamitochondria in the mouse and rat livers by hydrazine. *Experimental and Molecular Pathology* 39(2):139-153; as cited in NRC 1996.

Wald N, Boreham J, Doll R, Bonsall J. 1984. Occupational exposure to hydrazine and subsequent risk of cancer. *British Journal of Industrial Medicine* 41(1):31-34.

Weatherby JH, Yard AS. 1955. Observations on the subacute toxicity of hydrazine. *AMA Archives of Industrial Health* 11:413-419; as cited in NRC 1996.

Weeks MH, Maxey GC, Sicks ME, Greene EA. 1963. Vapor toxicity of UDMH in rats and dogs from short exposures. *American Industrial Hygiene Association Journal* 24:137-143; as cited in NRC 2000.

Wells H. 1908. The Pathological Anatomy of Hydrazine Poisoning. *Journal of Experimental Medicine* 10:457-464; as cited in King et al. 1969.

White RF, Proctor SP, Heeren T, Wolfe J, Krengel M, Vasterling J, Lindem K, Heaton KJ, Sutker P, Ozonoff DM. 2001. Neuropsychological function in Gulf War veterans: Relationships to self-reported toxicant exposures. *American Journal of Industrial Medicine* 40(1):42-54.

White R. 1934. Acids, alkalis, and some metallic salts: Burns and ulcerations due to acids. In: *The Dermatergoses or occupational affections of the skin: Giving descriptions of the trade processes, the responsible agents and their actions.* 4. London: HK Lewis and Co. Pp. 122-125; as cited in NIOSH 1976.

Zemla B, Day N, Swiatnicka J, Banasik R. 1987. Larynx cancer risk factors. *Neoplasma* 34(2):223-233.

A

CONCLUSIONS FROM *GULF WAR AND HEALTH VOLUMES 1* AND *2*

Sufficient Evidence of a Causal Relationship

Evidence is sufficient to conclude that there is a causal association between exposure to a specific agent and a specific health outcome in humans. The evidence is supported by experimental data and fulfills the guidelines for sufficient evidence of an association (below). The evidence must be biologically plausible and satisfy several of the guidelines used to assess causality, such as: strength of association, dose–response relationship, consistency of association, and a temporal relationship.

- Benzene and
    - acute leukemia
    - aplastic anemia
- Sarin and a dose-dependent acute cholinergic syndrome that is evident seconds to hours subsequent to sarin exposure and resolves in days to months

Sufficient Evidence of an Association

Evidence is sufficient to conclude that there is a positive association. That is, a consistent positive association has been observed between exposure to a specific agent and a specific health outcome in human studies in which chance and bias, including confounding, could be ruled out with reasonable confidence. For example, several high-quality studies report consistent positive associations, and the studies are sufficiently free of bias, including adequate control for confounding.

- Benzene and adult leukemia
- Solvents and acute leukemia
- Propylene glycol and allergic contact dermatitis
- Pyridostigmine bromide and transient acute cholinergic effects in doses normally used in treatment and for diagnostic purposes
- Anthrax vaccination and transient acute local and systemic effects
- Botulinum toxoid vaccination and transient acute local and systemic effects

Limited/Suggestive Evidence of an Association

Evidence is suggestive of an association between exposure to a specific agent and a specific health outcome, but the body of evidence is limited by the inability to rule out chance and bias, including confounding, with confidence. For example, at least one high-quality study reports a positive association that is sufficiently free of bias, including adequate control for confounding. Other corroborating studies provide support for the association, but they were not sufficiently free of bias, including confounding. Alternatively, several studies of lower quality show consistent positive associations, and the results are probably not due to bias, including confounding.

Cancers

- Tetrachloroethylene and dry-cleaning solvents and
    - bladder cancer
    - kidney cancer
    - organophosphorus insecticides and
    - non-Hodgkin's lymphoma
    - adult leukemia
    - adult leukemia
- Solvents and
    - adult leukemia
    - myelodysplastic syndromes
    - bladder cancer
    - multiple myeloma
- Carbamates and non-Hodgkin's lymphoma
- Benzene and non-Hodgkin's lymphoma

Neurologic Effects

- organophosphorus insecticide exposure with OP poisoning and long-term neurobehavioral effects (that is, abnormal results on neurobehavioral test batteries and symptom findings)
- Solvents and neurobehavioral effects (that is, abnormal results on neurobehavioral test batteries and symptom findings)

Other Health Effects

- Solvents and
    - hepatic steatosis
    - chronic glomerulonephritis
    - reactive airways dysfunction syndrome (RADS) which would be evident with exposure and could persist for months or years
- Insecticides and allergic contact dermatitis
- Sarin at doses sufficient to cause acute cholinergic signs and symptoms and subsequent long-term health effects

Inadequate/Insufficient Evidence to Determine Whether an Association Exists

Evidence is of insufficient quantity, quality, or consistency to permit a conclusion regarding the existence of an association between exposure to a specific agent and a specific health outcome in humans.

Cancers

- Solvents and
    - oral, nasal, or laryngeal cancer
    - stomach, rectal, or pancreatic cancer
    - bone cancer
    - melanoma or nonmelanoma skin cancer
    - ovarian or uterine cancer
    - prostate cancer
- Solvents other than trichloroethylene and cervical cancer
- Solvents other than tetrachloroethylene and dry-cleaning solvents and
    - esophageal cancer
    - bladder cancer
    - lung cancer
- Specific solvents other than benzene and
    - brain and other central nervous system cancers
    - non-Hodgkin's lymphoma
    - acute and adult leukemia
- Solvents other than trichloroethylene and mixtures of benzene, toluene, and xylene and colon cancer
- Benzene and myelodysplastic syndromes
- Insecticides and
    - lung cancer
    - pancreatic cancer
    - soft tissue sarcomas
    - prostate, testicular, or bladder cancers
    - kidney cancers
    - brain and other central nervous system cancers
- Insecticides and solvents
    - Hodgkin's disease
    - hepatobiliary cancers
    - multiple myeloma
- Lindane and solvents and breast cancer
- Parental preconception exposure to insecticides and childhood leukemias, brain and other central nervous system cancers, and non-Hodgkin's lymphoma
- Parental preconception exposure to solvents and neuroblastoma and childhood brain cancers

- Uranium and
  - lymphatic cancer
  - bone cancer

Neurologic Effects

- Insecticides and solvents and
  - peripheral neuropathy
  - Parkinson's disease
  - amyotrophic lateral sclerosis
  - Alzheimer's disease
- Solvents and
  - multiple sclerosis
  - a long-term reduction in color discrimination
  - long-term hearing loss
  - long-term reduction in olfactory function
- Uranium and nervous system disease

Reproductive Effects

- Insecticides and solvents and male or female infertility after cessation of exposure
- Parental preconception exposure to insecticides or solvents and
  - spontaneous abortion or other adverse pregnancy outcomes
  - congenital malformations
- Uranium and reproductive or developmental dysfunction

Other Health Effects

- Insecticides and aplastic anemia
- Solvents other than benzene and aplastic anemia
- Insecticides and solvents and
  - irreversible cardiovascular outcomes
  - persistent respiratory symptoms or impairment after cessation of exposure
- Solvents and
  - cirrhosis
  - alterations in liver function tests after cessation of exposure
  - chronic pancreatitis and other persistent gastrointestinal outcomes
  - the systemic rheumatic diseases: scleroderma, rheumatoid arthritis, undifferentiated connective tissue disorders, and systemic lupus erythematosus
- Exposure to uranium and lung cancer at higher levels of cumulative exposure (>200 mSv or 25 cGy)
- Uranium and
  - nonmalignant respiratory disease
  - gastrointestinal disease
  - immune-mediated disease
  - effects on hematological parameters
  - genotoxic effects
  - cardiovascular effects

  - hepatic disease
  - dermal effects
  - ocular effects
  - musculoskeletal effects
- Pyridostigmine bromide and long-term adverse health effects
- Exposure to sarin at low doses insufficient to cause acute cholinergic signs and symptoms and subsequent long-term adverse health effects
- Anthrax vaccination and long-term adverse health effects
- Botulinum toxoid vaccination and long-term adverse health effects
- Multiple vaccinations and long-term adverse health effects

Limited/Suggestive Evidence of No Association

Evidence is consistent in not showing a positive association between exposure to a specific agent and a specific health outcome after exposure of any magnitude. A conclusion of no association is inevitably limited to the conditions, magnitudes of exposure, and length of observation in the available studies. The possibility of a very small increase in risk after exposure studied cannot be excluded.

- Exposure to uranium and lung cancer at cumulative internal dose levels lower than 200 mSv or 25 cGy
- Uranium and clinically significant renal dysfunction

Consensus Not Reached on Category of Association

- Tetrachloroethylene and dry-cleaning solvents and esophageal cancer
- Trichloroethylene and colon cancer
- Mixtures of benzene, toluene, and xylene and colon cancer
- Tetrachloroethylene and dry-cleaning solvents and lung cancer
- Trichloroethylene and cervical cancer
- Solvents and kidney cancer
- Benzene and solvents and brain and other central nervous system cancers
- Parental preconception exposure to solvents and childhood leukemia
- Organophosphorous insecticide exposure without OP poisoning and long-term neurobehavioral effects (that is, abnormal results on neurobehavioral test batteries and symptom findings)

B

LITERATURE SEARCHES

The information used by the committee was developed through a comprehensive search of the literature. The search used public and commercial databases that cover biologic, medical, toxicologic, chemical, and regulatory information; most of the databases are bibliographic and provide citations to the scientific literature. The references of major review and research articles, books, and reports were also examined.

The specific compounds identified in the literature were divided into three main categories: combustion products, fuels, and hydrazine and nitric acid. The Committee advised staff in identifying appropriate synonyms, Chemical Abstracts Service registry numbers, and additional, related terms. Terms were compared with the controlled vocabularies of the databases to be searched, and database-specific terms were used as search terms. In April 2003 three searches were performed—one for each of the main categories.

The searches were conducted in two major biomedical electronic databases: MEDLINE and EMBASE. MEDLINE, produced by the National Library of Medicine (NLM), indexes 4,600 biomedical journals and contains about 11 million citations. The database covers entries from 1966 to the present. EMBASE, based on the Excerpta Medica database, is produced by Elsevier Science and indexes over 4,000 international journals covering such fields as drug research, toxicology, clinical and experimental human medicine, public health, and occupational health. It covers entries from 1974 to the present. EMBASE has more of an international focus than does MEDLINE. EMBASE contains more than 9 million records and adds about 450,000 records each year. Staff also searched the publication lists of the International Agency for Research on Cancer and the Agency for Toxic Substances and Disease Registry for reference material pertinent to the substances to be examined. In addition, the reference lists of review articles were examined for related citations. Results of searching these various sources were imported into ProCite, a software program designed to store and manage bibliographic data.

This original ProCite database consisted of about 33,000 records. The titles and abstracts of those records were reviewed by staff and committee members, and the citations deemed relevant for the study were copied into a "working" ProCite database, which consisted of about 8,500 records. The working database consisted mostly of epidemiologic studies but also contained case reports, series papers, background documents, and references to pertinent toxicologic sources.

Additional searching in PubMed explored various specific subjects that might be relevant to this study. Literature searches were performed in PubMed for hydrocarbons and for "Gulf War" by using many synonyms and related terms. The combined toxicologic information and environmental-health database called Toxnet and found on the NLM web site was used to search for toxicologic literature related to the three main categories.

C

TYPES OF EPIDEMIOLOGIC STUDIES

This appendix briefly describes the types of studies considered in the body of this report. Some studies enabled the committee to form judgments about the strength of an association between a putative agent and a health outcome and were used as primary studies (for example, cohort and case-control studies); others were not considered useful for that assessment and were considered support studies (for example, cross-sectional studies, case reports, and case series).

EXPERIMENTAL STUDIES IN ANIMALS: ANIMAL MODELS

Studies of laboratory animals and other nonhuman systems are essential for understanding mechanisms of action, biologic plausibility, and possible health effects when experimental research in humans is not ethically or practically possible (Cohrssen and Covello 1989; NRC 1991). Such studies permit a potentially toxic agent to be introduced under conditions controlled by the researcher, such as dose, duration, and route of exposure. Nonhuman studies are also a valuable complement to human studies of genetic susceptibility. Although nonhuman studies often focus on one agent at a time, they more easily enable the study of chemical mixtures and their potential interactions.

Research on health effects of toxic substances includes animal studies that characterize absorption, distribution, metabolism, elimination, and excretion. Animal studies may examine acute (short-term) exposures or chronic (long-term) exposures. They may focus on the mechanism of action (how a toxicant exerts its deleterious effects at the cellular and molecular levels). Mechanism-of-action (or mechanistic) studies encompass a range of laboratory approaches with whole animals and in vitro systems that use tissues or cells from humans or animals. Structure-activity relationships, in which a potential toxicant and a known toxicant are compared with respect to molecular structure and chemical and physical properties, are an important source of hypotheses about mechanisms of action.

In carrying out its charge, the committee used the results of animal and other nonhuman studies in several ways, particularly as markers of health effects that might be important for humans. If an agent, for example, is absorbed and deposited in specific tissues or organs, the committee looked closely for possible abnormalities at those sites in human studies.

One problem with animal studies is the difficulty of finding animal models that permit the study of symptoms rather than disease end points. That is particularly true when one is trying to find an animal model for attributes that we consider peculiar to humans, such as cognition, behavior, and the perception of pain. Many symptoms reported by veterans, such as headache and muscle or joint pain, are difficult to study in standard neurotoxicologic tests in animals (OTA 1990). Another problem is that for some outcomes (for example, cancer and birth defects) animal studies may implicate a chemical as being able to cause such outcomes, but the specific outcome in animals may differ from the outcome in humans. Given the task of this committee, the results of such studies could be considered supportive but not primary evidence of an association with a specific outcome in humans.

EXPERIMENTAL STUDIES IN HUMANS: RANDOMIZED CONTROLLED TRIALS

Experimental studies in humans are the foremost means of establishing causal associations between exposure to an agent and human health outcomes. Experimental studies are used most often in the evaluation of the safety and efficacy of medications, surgical practices, biologic products, vaccines, and preventive interventions. In an experiment, the investigator assigns the agent to be studied and records the outcome. Two key features of experimental studies are prospective design and use of a control group. Randomized controlled trials are considered the gold standard in experimental studies.

In randomized controlled trials, each subject has a known probability of assignment to the test group or the control group, and the various subjects' probabilities are often equal. Large randomized controlled trials are designed to have all possible confounding variables occur with equal frequency in the test and control groups. Blinding—shielding test subjects and controls from knowledge of their assignment—may be another aspect of randomized controlled trials.[1] It is most readily accomplished when subjects in the control group receive a placebo. When both subjects and investigators are unaware of assignment, a study is said to be double-blind. The objective of blinding is to reduce bias introduced by subjects' and investigators' attitudes and expectations for study outcomes.

The value of randomized controlled trials has been so convincingly demonstrated that they are required for ensuring the safety and efficacy of all new medications introduced into the market in the United States. The main drawbacks of randomized controlled trials are their expense, the time needed for completion, and the common practice of systematically excluding many groups of people, which makes results less easy to generalize from.

CONTROLLED EPIDEMIOLOGIC STUDIES (OBSERVATIONAL)

In contrast with randomized controlled trials and other experimental studies in humans, most epidemiologic investigations are "observational". That means simply that the occurrences of exposure to the putative agent and of the particular diseases or outcomes are studied as they arise in the usual course of life and not under the conditions of a planned experiment. However, through various strategies of formal comparative investigations, observational studies in populations are often "controlled". We discuss below the different types of controlled, observational studies considered by the committee.

---

[1]Blinding can also be part of the study design in cohort and case-control studies (see below). Disease outcome and exposure can be determined independently by different groups of researchers, or the exposure assessment in case-control studies can be performed by scientists who are blinded as to the disease status of the subjects.

Cohort Studies

The cohort, or longitudinal, study is an epidemiologic study that follows a defined group, or cohort, over time. It can test hypotheses about whether exposure to a specific agent is related to the development of disease and can examine multiple disease outcomes that may be associated with exposure to a given agent. A cohort study starts with people who are free of the disease in question and classifies them according to whether they have been exposed to the agent of concern. It compares health outcomes in people who have been exposed with outcomes in those who have not. Such a comparison can be used to estimate a risk difference or a relative risk, two statistics that measure association. The risk difference is the rate of a disease in exposed persons minus the rate in nonexposed persons. It represents the absolute number of extra cases of the disease associated with the exposure. The relative risk, or risk ratio, is determined by dividing the rate of the disease in the exposed group by the rate in the nonexposed group. A relative risk greater than 1 suggests a positive association between exposure and disease onset; the higher the relative risk, the stronger the association.

A prospective cohort study selects subjects on the basis of exposure (or lack of it) and follows the cohort to determine the rate at which the disease (or other health outcome) develops. A retrospective (or historical) cohort study differs from a prospective study in terms of temporal direction; the investigator traces backward to classify past exposures in the cohort and then forward to ascertain the rate of disease.

Retrospective cohort studies commonly have been performed in occupational health. They often assess disease-related mortality because of the relative ease of determining vital status of people and the availability of death certificates to determine causes of death. For comparison purposes, cohort studies often use general population mortality (age-, sex-, race-, time-, and cause-specific) because it may be difficult to identify a comparison group of nonexposed workers. The observed number of deaths among workers from a specific cause (such as lung cancer) is compared with the expected number of deaths from that cause. The expected number is calculated by multiplying the annual mortality in the general population by the number of person-years of followup[2] of the workers. The ratio of observed to expected deaths (which by convention is often multiplied by 100) is a standardized mortality ratio (SMR). An SMR greater than 100 generally suggests an increased risk of dying from the specified cause in the exposed group. Many cohort studies refine their measures of health outcomes by using an internal comparison group, which may differ from the cohort in exposure magnitude but otherwise be more similar to the cohort than the general population is.

The major problem in comparing the general population with an occupational cohort is the "healthy-worker effect" (Monson 1990); this effect arises when an employed population of generally healthy people experiences lower mortality than the general population, which consists of both healthy and unhealthy people. The healthy-worker effect is usually due to workers' lower rates of cardiovascular and traumatic deaths. A military population that has a high rate of external traumatic causes of death (such as Gulf War veterans) may be different from many occupational populations. In calculating the SMR, the denominator (expected deaths) is derived from general population figures rather than from an otherwise comparable group of nonexposed workers (which may be unavailable). The "artificially" higher denominator for expected deaths in the general population lowers the SMR, thereby underestimating the strength of an association

[2]*Person-years of followup* refers to the sum of the observation periods for the total number of workers under study. Its purpose is to account for differences in periods of employment of study subjects.

between exposure to the agent and the cause of death. In other words, the healthy-worker effect introduces a bias that diminishes the true disease-exposure relationship.

To counter the influence of the healthy-worker effect, some studies divide the worker population into different groups, on the basis of magnitude of exposure to the agent being studied. Searching for dose-response relationships within the worker population itself is a way of reducing the potential bias introduced by the use of population controls. The problem is that measurements of dose may be imprecise or unavailable, particularly if the exposures occurred decades earlier. Consequently, epidemiologists often rely on job classification as a surrogate of dose. Reliance on job classification introduces the possibility of misclassification bias because the classification may not be a good proxy for the actual exposure or dose. Another problem—not only in determining job classification but especially in determining whether potential confounding exposures (see next paragraph), such as cigarette-smoking by individual workers, are present—is incompleteness of records. Bias introduced by misclassification and confounding can systematically alter study results by diluting or strengthening associations. One major advantage of a cohort study is the ability of the investigator to control the classification of subjects at the beginning of the study. Classification in prospective cohort studies is not influenced by the presence of disease; the disease has yet to occur, and this reduces an important source of potential bias known as selection bias.

A cohort study design also gives the investigator the advantage of measuring and correcting potential confounding. When it is possible to measure a confounding factor,[3] the investigator can apply statistical methods to minimize its influence on the results. Another advantage of a cohort study is that it is possible to calculate absolute rates of disease incidence.[4] A final advantage (especially over cross-sectional studies) is that it may be possible to adjust each subject's followup health status according to his or her baseline health status so that the person acts as his or her own control; this may reduce a source of variation and increase the power to detect effects.

The disadvantages of cohort studies are the high costs associated with a large study population and long periods of followup (especially if the disease is rare), attrition of study subjects, and delay in obtaining results.

Case-Control Studies

The case-control study is useful for testing hypotheses about the relationships between exposure to specific agents and disease. It is especially useful for studying the etiology of rare diseases. When health outcomes are infrequent or rare, longitudinal or cross-sectional studies must be large enough and last long enough to accumulate enough adverse events to support accurate estimation of the risk posed by a particular agent. In case-control studies, subjects (or cases) are selected on the basis of having a disease, and controls are selected on the basis of not having the disease. Cases and controls are then asked about their past exposures to specific agents. Cases and controls might be matched with regard to such characteristics as age, sex, and socioeconomic status to eliminate those characteristics as causes of observed differences in past exposure; alternatively, matching factors can be controlled for in the analysis. The odds of

[3]A confounding factor is a variable that is independently associated with the health outcome and may affect the results of the study because it is distributed differently in the study and control groups.
[4]Incidence is the rate of occurrence of new cases of an illness or disease in a given population during a specified period. Prevalence is the number of cases of an illness or disease existing in a given population at a specific time.

exposure to the agent among the cases are then compared with the odds of exposure among controls. The comparison generates an odds ratio,[5] a statistic that depicts the odds of having a disease among those exposed to the agent of concern relative to the odds among a nonexposed comparison group. An odds ratio greater than 1 indicates a potential association between exposure to the agent and the disease. The greater the odds ratio, the stronger the association. In short, in a case-control study, subjects are selected on the basis of disease presence, and prior exposure is then ascertained.

Case-control studies have the advantages of ease, speed, and relatively low cost. They are also advantageous for their ability to probe multiple exposures or risk factors. However, case-control studies are vulnerable to several types of bias, including recall bias. Other disadvantages are the need to identify representative groups of cases, the need to choose suitable controls, and the need to collect comparable information on exposure of both cases and controls. Those disadvantages might lead to unidentified confounding variables that differentially influence the selection of cases or control subjects or the detection of exposure. Case-control studies are often the first, but not the definitive, approach to testing a hypothesis.

Cross-Sectional Studies

In a cross-sectional study, the population of interest is surveyed at one time. Information about health conditions and exposures to various agents, either present or past, is collected simultaneously. The selection of people to enter the study—in contrast with cohort and case-control studies—is independent of the exposure to the agent under study and independent of disease characteristics. Cross-sectional studies seek to uncover potential associations between exposure to specific agents and development of disease. They may compare disease or symptom rates between groups with and without the exposure to the specific agent or compare exposure to the specific agent between groups with and without the disease. Although cross-sectional studies need not have control groups, studies with control groups are methodologically more sound. Several health studies of Gulf War veterans are controlled cross-sectional surveys that compare a sample of veterans previously deployed to the Gulf War with a sample of veterans who served during the same period but were not deployed to the Gulf War.

Cross-sectional surveys are easier to perform and less expensive to implement than cohort studies. Cross-sectional surveys can identify the prevalence of diseases and exposures in a defined population. They are useful for generating hypotheses. However, they are much less useful for determining cause-effect relationships, because disease and exposure data are collected simultaneously and may be self-reported (Monson 1990). It may also be difficult to determine the temporal sequence of exposure and symptoms or disease.

Case Reports and Case Series

A case report is generally a detailed description of a patient's illness reported by a clinician; the clinician may suspect that the illness is the result of exposure to a specific biologic or chemical agent. Subjects in a case series have the same or a similar disease and experienced identical or similar exposures to a specific agent. Case reports and case series provide information for generating hypotheses about exposure and disease relationships. For Gulf War veterans, registry programs established by the Department of Veterans Affairs and the

[5]An odds ratio is a good estimate of relative risk when the disease under study is rare.

Department of Defense constitute a type of voluntary case series. Any veteran may come forward to receive a clinical examination and a referral for treatment. Because of their documentation of veterans' symptoms and diagnoses, the registries have been valuable in generating hypotheses; but they are not designed for hypothesis-testing or for establishing the prevalence of disease or specific exposures among Gulf War veterans.

The value of case reports and case series is that they can document possible associations between environmental exposures and particular health outcomes. In some situations, they may be useful in suggesting causal relationships if a disease is rare and has a close temporal relationship to an exposure (Kramer and Lane 1992). However, case reports and case series do not have control groups. Because case series are not population-based, many cases caused by an exposure go unreported, and the prevalence of cases may be lower than that in the population at large. Furthermore, the cases may not have been caused by exposure to the specific agent.

Information from Death Certificates

Studies that use mortality data obtained from death certificates tend to be conducted among occupational groups. Death certificates can provide information on occupation, as well as cause of death; occupations listed are used by investigators as surrogates of potential exposures. However, using data from death certificates raises several concerns because an occupation might be listed incorrectly or without actual knowledge of the person's job. That would lead to exposure misclassification and uncertainty regarding the associations reported. In many cases, a biologic or chemical exposure is underestimated if it is based on death-certificate information, and the magnitude of the association under consideration might be overestimated or underestimated. Finally, depending on the disease, studies that use a death-certificate cause of death may underestimate disease prevalence and may misclassify disease outcomes. The information from death certificates, if used by the committee, might provide supportive evidence.

COMMENTS ON THE NATURE OF THE GULF WAR STUDIES

Most studies of Gulf War veterans' health have been cross-sectional and have been conducted years after the war. Few studies included clinical examinations or laboratory tests to verify outcomes. Almost all used questionnaires to identify a broad array of agents to which the veterans may have been exposed (often 10-20 agents per study), and symptoms (often 25-100) appear in a checklist format. Questionnaire studies—using a host of self-reported symptoms and exposures—have limitations for drawing inferences about symptom-exposure relationships. Exposure questionnaires were often general and rarely asked about duration, degree, or frequency of exposure.

Most of the studies were designed to detect the nature and prevalence of veterans' symptoms and illnesses and whether they constituted a new syndrome rather than specifically to assess the effects of exposure to agents of interest to the committee.

Because the studies were generally cross-sectional, they limit opportunities to learn about symptom duration and latency of onset (IOM 2000). They were especially subject to recall bias: veterans who develop symptoms might be more likely than asymptomatic veterans to recall exposures to particular agents

Several approaches were taken to combine reported symptoms with outcome variables. One was to use a statistical method called factor analysis to uncover an underlying structure in reported symptoms (Cherry et al. 2001; Fukuda et al. 1998; Haley and Kurt 1997). A second approach attempted to match symptoms in some way to previously defined syndromes or illnesses (Iowa Persian Gulf Study Group 1997; Nisenbaum et al. 2000; Unwin et al. 1999). In some cases, symptoms were assembled into established syndromes on the basis of criteria devised by the investigators. Other studies did not attempt a synthesis of any sort but searched for associations between exposures to various agents during the Gulf War and individual symptoms.

Another limitation of studies of Gulf War veterans is the problem of multiple comparisons between exposure to numerous agents and health outcomes. When investigators examine a large number of exposure-symptom associations, the chances of reporting a spurious association as statistically significant are increased. Some Gulf War studies took a variety of statistical approaches to adjust for multiple comparisons. However, many did not account for multiple comparisons and reported any association with a p value of 0.05 or less as statistically significant. In some cases, the investigators indicated that they did not adjust for multiple comparisons, because of the exploratory nature of the study and because of their desire to reduce the probability of not finding a true association. Other investigators were more conservative and set a more stringent significance level to reduce the probability of error (Cherry et al. 2001; Haley and Kurt 1997; White et al. 2001).

Many studies noted that exposures to different agents were associated with the health outcomes they measured. Only one study attempted to examine the association between specific agents and specific health outcomes, and it found them to be strongly correlated (Cherry et al. 2001); the interrelationships might reflect information bias and might constitute an important limitation of the study. Thus, although the committee considered the body of evidence on Gulf War veterans, in many instances the studies supported findings rather than providing primary evidence.

REFERENCES

Cherry N, Creed F, Silman A, Dunn G, Baxter D, Smedley J, Taylor S, Macfarlane GJ. 2001. Health and exposures of United Kingdom Gulf war veterans. Part I: The pattern and extent of ill health. *Occupational and Environmental Medicine* 58(5):291-298.

Cohrssen J, Covello V. 1989. *Risk analysis: A Guide to Principles and Methods for Analyzing Health and Environmental Risks.* Washington, DC: Council on Environmental Quality, Executive Office of the President.

Fukuda K, Nisenbaum R, Stewart G, Thompson WW, Robin L, Washko RM, Noah DL, Barrett DH, Randall B, Herwaldt BL, Mawle AC, Reeves WC. 1998. Chronic multisymptom illness affecting Air Force veterans of the Gulf War. *Journal of the American Medical Association* 280(11):981-988.

Haley RW, Kurt TL. 1997. Self-reported exposure to neurotoxic chemical combinations in the Gulf War. A cross-sectional epidemiologic study. *Journal of the American Medical Association* 277(3):231-237.

IOM (Institute of Medicine). 2000. *Gulf War and Health, Volume 1: Depleted Uranium, Sarin, Pyridostigmine Bromide, Vaccines.* Washington, DC: National Academy Press.

Iowa Persian Gulf Study Group. 1997. Self-reported illness and health status among Gulf War veterans. A population-based study. The Iowa Persian Gulf Study Group. *Journal of the American Medical Association* 277(3):238-245.

Kramer M, Lane D. 1992. Causal propositions in clinical research and practice. *Journal of Clinical Epidemiology* 45(6):639-649.

Monson R. 1990. *Occupational Epidemiology.* 2nd edition. Boca Raton, FL: CRC Press, Inc.

Nisenbaum R, Barrett DH, Reyes M, Reeves WC. 2000. Deployment stressors and a chronic multisymptom illness among Gulf War veterans. *Journal of Nervous and Mental Disease* 188(5):259-266.

NRC (National Research Council). 1991. *Animals as Sentinels of Environmental Health Hazards.* Washington, DC: National Academy Press.

OTA (Office of Technology Assessment). 1990. *Neurotoxicity: Identifying and Controlling Poisons of the Nervous System. OTA-BA-436.* Washington, DC: US Government Printing Office.

Unwin C, Blatchley N, Coker W, Ferry S, Hotopf M, Hull L, Ismail K, Palmer I, David A, Wessely S. 1999. Health of UK servicemen who served in Persian Gulf War. *Lancet* 353:169-178.

White RF, Proctor SP, Heeren T, Wolfe J, Krengel M, Vasterling J, Lindem K, Heaton KJ, Sutker P, Ozonoff DM. 2001. Neuropsychological function in Gulf War veterans: Relationships to self-reported toxicant exposures. *American Journal of Industrial Medicine* 40(1):42-54.

D

DESCRIPTIVE TABLES OF CANCER STUDIES

This appendix contains two tables that describe the studies used in Chapter 4 (on cancer). Table D.1 provides information on cohort studies related to exposures to fuels and combustion products, and Table D.2 provides information on case-control studies. The studies are referred to repeatedly in Chapter 4. For each study, the following information is provided: a description of the study population, the number of subjects in the study group, how the type of cancer was determined, how exposure was assessed, what type of analysis was conducted, and which potential confounders were adjusted for.

TABLE D.1 Description of Cohort Studies Related to Exposure to Fuels and Combustion Products

Reference	Population	Study Group	Health-Outcome Assessment	Exposure Assessment	Analysis, Adjustment for Potential Confounders
Imperial Oil Cohort					
Hanis et al. 1979	Mortality experience (1964-1973) of male Imperial Oil workers (at least 1 yr for active workers; at least 5 yrs for inactive workers) in Canada; internal comparison of refinery and non-refinery workers	15,032; 5,731 refinery, 9,301 non-refinery	Vital status followed through provincial registrars, Statistics Canada	Job titles classified as in or outside refinery work	RR; age
Schnatter et al. 1992	Mortality experience (1964-1983) of Imperial Oil workers (at least 1 yr) in Canada; external comparison with Canadian general population	34,597	Vital status followed through Statistics Canada, internal data sources, NDI	Company employment in 11 operating segments and HC exposure assigned by industrial hygienists on basis of detailed work histories	SMR; sex, age, calendar period
Schnatter et al. 1993	Mortality experience (1964-1983) of male Imperial Oil petroleum-marketing and distribution workers (at least 1 yr) in Canada; external comparison with Canadian general population	6,672	Vital status followed through Statistics Canada, internal data sources, NDI	HC exposure frequency assigned by industrial hygienists based on basis of detailed work histories	SMR; sex, age, calendar period
Schnatter et al. 1996	Nested cases of lymphohematopoietic malignancies among Imperial Oil workers (at least 1 yr) in Canada; internal controls selected from males in cohort, matched 4:1 on age and were alive at case date of death	14 leukemia 7 MM 8 NHL	Cause of death on death certificates coded by Statistics Canada	Company employment in 11 operating segments and HC exposure assigned by industrial hygienists on basis of detailed work histories	Mantel-Haenszel OR; age, smoking, family cancer history, frequency of chest x rays
Lewis et al. 2000	Mortality experience (1964-1994) of Imperial Oil workers (at least 1 yr in 1964-1983) in Canada; external comparison with Canadian general population	34,560	Vital status followed through Statistics Canada, internal data sources, NDI	Company employment in 11 operating segments and presumed HC exposure derived from job titles	SMR; sex, age, calendar period

Reference	Population	Study Group	Health-Outcome Assessment	Exposure Assessment	Analysis, Adjustment for Potential Confounders
Lewis et al. 2003	Incidence and mortality experience (1964-1994) of Imperial Oil workers (at least 1 yr, first hire in 1964-1994) in Canada; external comparison with Canadian general population	25,292	Vital status and cancer incidence followed through Statistics Canada, internal data sources, NDI	Similar exposure-group codes developed by industrial hygienist from detailed work histories	SIR, and SMR; sex, age, calendar period
Mobil Oil Cohort					
Raabe et al. 1998	Mortality experience (1946-1987) of Mobil Oil employees (at least 1 yr in 1945-1987) in Beaumont, Texas; external comparison with US general population	7,119	Vital status followed through company records, Pension Benefits Information Inc., SSA, NDI	Company employment; two job categories assigned on basis of job title	SMR; age, sex, race, calendar period
Rosamilia et al. 1999	Cases of lung cancer and controls in cohort of Mobil Oil employees (at least 1 yr in 1946-1987) in Beaumont, Texas	112 cases, 490 controls	Vital status followed through company records, Pension Benefits Information Inc., SSA, NDI	Four job categories assigned from work-history records	OR (nested case-control); age, race, smoking, prior job assignments
Wong et al. 2001	Mortality experience (1946-1996) of Mobil Oil employees (at least 1 yr in 1945-1996) in Beaumont, Texas; external comparison with US general population	7,543	Vital status followed through company records, Pension Benefits Information Inc., SSA, NDI	Company employment; two job categories assigned on basis of job title	SMR; age, sex, race, calendar period
Texaco Mortality Study					
Divine et al. 1985	Mortality experience (1947-1977) of white male Texaco refinery, petrochemical-plant, and research laboratory workers (at least 5 yrs) in the US; external comparison with US white male population	19,077	Vital status followed through company records, SSA	Company employment	SMR; race, sex

Reference	Population	Study Group	Health-Outcome Assessment	Exposure Assessment	Analysis, Adjustment for Potential Confounders
Divine and Barron 1986	Mortality experience (1947-1977) of white male Texaco refinery, petrochemical-plant, and research-laboratory workers (at least 5 years) in the US; external comparison with US white male population	18,798	Vital status followed through company records, SSA	Company employment; job or process unit determined from work histories	SMR; race, sex
Divine et al. 1999a	Mortality experience (1947-1993) of Texaco refinery, petrochemical plant, and research laboratory workers (at least 5 yrs) in the US; external comparison with US general population	28,480	Vital status followed through company records, SSA, NDI, HCFA	Company employment; job or process unit determined from work histories	SMR; race, sex
Divine et al. 1999b	Mortality experience (1947-1993) of Texaco refinery, petrochemical-plant, and research lab workers (at least 5 yrs) in the US; external comparison with US general population	28,480	Vital status followed through company records, SSA, NDI, HCFA	Company employment; job or process unit determined from work histories	SMR; race, sex
Italian Oil Refinery Cohort					
Bertazzi et al. 1989	Mortality experience (1949-1982) of male workers (ever employed) at refinery near Milan, Italy; external comparison with national and local (Lombardy region) male populations	1,595	Vital status followed through Population Statistics Office	Company employment in 29 occupation units determined from work histories	SMR; age, sex, calendar time
Consonni et al. 1999	Mortality experience (1949-1991) of male workers (ever employed in 1949-1982) at refinery near Milan, Italy; external comparison with local (Lombardy region) male population	1,583	Vital status followed through Population Statistics Office	Company employment in 29 occupation units determined from work histories	SMR; age, sex, calendar time

Reference	Population	Study Group	Health-Outcome Assessment	Exposure Assessment	Analysis, Adjustment for Potential Confounders
ACS Cancer Prevention Study II					
Boffetta et al. 1988	Mortality experience (1982-1984) of male subjects, 40-79 yr old, enrolled in ACS Cancer Prevention Study II	461,981	Follow up through personal contact; death certificates obtained from state health departments	Self-administered questionnaire at baseline assessed current, last, and longest-held occupations, exposure to 12 groups of substances	RR; age, smoking factors, other occupational exposures
Pope et al. 1995	Mortality experience (1982-1998) of subjects, at least 30 yr old with one household resident at least 45 yr old, enrolled in ACS Cancer Prevention Study II	552,138	Follow up through personal contact (through 1988) with death certificates obtained from state health departments; record linkage with NDI (through 1989)	Mean concentrations of sulfate and fine-particle air pollution provided by EPA databases	RR; age, sex, race, cigarette-smoking, exposure to passive cigarette-smoking, BMI, drinks per day of alcohol, education, occupational exposure
Pope et al. 2002	Mortality experience (1982-1998) of subjects, at least 30 yr old with one household resident at least 45 yr old, enrolled in ACS Cancer Prevention Study II	About 500,000 (number of subjects depends on pollution index used)	Follow up through personal contact (through 1988) with death certificates obtained from state health departments; record linkage with NDI (through 1998)	Mean concentrations of air pollution (PM, sulfate, SO_2, NO_2) provided by EPA databases	RR; age, sex, race, smoking, education, marital status, body mass, alcohol consumption, occupational exposure, diet
Other Cohorts					
Abbey et al. 1999	Mortality experience (1977-1992) of nonsmoking, white, Seventh Day Adventist residents of California who had lived at least 10 yr within 5 mi of current residence	6,338	Vital status followed through record linkage with California death-certificate files (1977-1992), NDI (1979-1992), church records	Monthly estimates of ambient concentrations of air pollutants (PM_{10}, SO_2, NO_2) provided by fixed-site monitoring stations maintained by CARB provided	RR; sex, years of education, pack-years of past smoking, alcohol use

Reference	Population	Study Group	Health-Outcome Assessment	Exposure Assessment	Analysis, Adjustment for Potential Confounders
Boffetta et al. 2001	Incidence experience (1971-1989) of occupationally active (1960 and 1970 censuses; excluding farmers) residents of Sweden; internal comparisons made across exposure intensities and probabilities; external comparison to Swedish general population	55,883 total exposed cancer cases	Follow up for incidence through Swedish Cancer Register; vital status tracked through national Register of Causes of Death	Job and industry titles classified for probability and intensity of exposure to diesel-engine emissions	SIR, sex, age, calendar year RR; age, calendar period, geographic region, urban or rural residence
Borgia et al. 1994	Mortality experience (1965-1988) of male taxi drivers (registered in 1950-1975) in Rome, Italy	2,311	Vital status tracked through local registry office or through record linkage with national or regional mortality files	Taxi drivers registered in Rome	SMR; age, calendar period
Chow et al. 1994	Incidence experience (1961-1979) of stomach cancer in occupationally active (1960 census) Swedish men; external comparison with Swedish general population	16,872 cases	Cancer incidence tracked through Swedish Cancer-Environmental Registry which links census data to Swedish Cancer Registry	Occupation and industry codes from census data	SIR; age, sex, region
Chow et al. 1995	Incidence experience (1961-1979) of esophageal cancer in occupationally active (1960 census) Swedish men; external comparison with Swedish general population	2,394 cases	Cancer incidence tracked through Swedish Cancer-Environmental Registry which links census data to Swedish Cancer Registry	Occupation and industry codes from census data	SIR; age, sex, region
Gamble et al. 1996	Nested cases of kidney cancer among Exxon employees of at least 1 mo at three US refineries and chemical plants in 1970-1992; internal controls matched on sex, race, age, date of hire, at-risk status	37 cases, 148 controls	Vital status followed through SSA,NDI	Industrial hygienist constructed JEM from company records and job titles	OR (nested case-control); logistic regression BMI, mean arterial pressure, smoking

Reference	Population	Study Group	Health-Outcome Assessment	Exposure Assessment	Analysis, Adjustment for Potential Confounders
Guberan et al. 1992	Incidence and mortality experience (1949-1986) of lung and gastrointestinal cancer in male professional drivers (1949-1961) in canton of Geneva, Switzerland; external comparison with Geneva male population	6,630	Follow up for incidence through Geneva Cancer Registry; vital status tracked through National Office of Statistics	Subjects had valid (in 1949) or new (1949-1961) licenses issued as drivers of heavy-duty-road goods vehicles, taxis, buses, coaches, professional transports; subjects classified as "more" or "less" exposed to exhaust gases	SIR, SMR; age, year
Gustavsson et al. 1990	Incidence (1958-1984) and mortality (1952-1986) experience of male bus garage workers (at least 6 mo in 1945-1970) from five locations in Stockholm, Sweden; external comparisons with Stockholm general population and occupationally active population in Sweden; internal comparisons made for cumulative exposure indices	695	Cancer incidence tracked through Swedish Cancer Registry; mortality ascertained from Statistics Sweden	Industrial hygienist constructed JEM from historical data from garages on numbers and types of diesel engines present, ventilation, job types and duration	SMR; age, sex, cause of death OR; conditional logistic regression, age
Hansen 1993	Mortality experience (1970-1980) of truck drivers (1970 census) in Denmark compared with population of unskilled workers	14,225 truck drivers, 43,024 unskilled laborers	Record linkage with Central Population Register, Death Certificate Register	Truck-driver job title in 1970 census	SMR (expected numbers of deaths in driver group calculated in reference to unskilled group); age, period
Hansen 2000	Nested cases of male breast cancer among Pension Fund members in Denmark in 1970-1989; internal controls matched on age	230 cases	Cancer incidence tracked through Danish Cancer Registry	Job titles obtained from Pension Fund files and Central Person Registry; author assigned exposure to gasoline, combustion products	Conditional logistic regression; birth year, SES

Reference	Population	Study Group	Health-Outcome Assessment	Exposure Assessment	Analysis, Adjustment for Potential Confounders
Hoek et al. 2002	Mortality experience (1986-1994) of a subcohort of males, age 55-69 yr old, in Netherlands Cohort Study on Diet and Cancer	4,492	Vital status followed through Dutch Central Bureau of Genealogy	Self-administered questionnaire at baseline gave location of residence in 1986; exposure to traffic-related air pollution determined through National Air Quality Monitoring Network data	RR; age, sex, education, Quetelet index, occupation, active and passive cigarette-smoking, neighborhood SES score
Huebner et al. 2000	Incidence experience of lymphohematopoietic malignancies among Exxon employees of at least 1 mo at three US refineries and chemical plants in 1970-1992 or US-based employees of at least 1 day in 1979-1982 with all subjects having current, final, or active (1983-1994) employment at Baton Rouge, Louisiana facility; internal controls matched on sex, race, age, date of hire, at-risk status	8,942 59 LH malignancies	Record linkage with the Louisiana tumor registry	Job type obtained from company records	SIR; modified life-table approach stratified by sex, race, age, year of diagnosis
Jarvholm and Silverman 2003	Incidence and mortality experience (1971-1995) of Swedish male construction workers (1971-1993); internal comparisons of truck drivers and heavy-equipment operators within carpenters and electricians; external comparisons to Swedish general population	6,364 truck drivers, 14,364 heavy equipment operators, 119,984 carpenters and electricians	Record linkage with National Cancer Registry and National Death Registry	Job title obtained at initial health examination (1971-1993)	SIR, SMR; age, period, smoking habits
Jarvholm et al. 1997	Incidence experience (1958-1991) of male workers (at least 1 yr) in 26 companies in petroleum industry in Sweden; external comparison with Swedish general population	4,128	Cancer incidence followed through the Swedish Cancer Registry	Employment in refinery operations, distribution, other occupations determined from job titles	SIR (90% CI); sex, age, calendar year

Reference	Population	Study Group	Health-Outcome Assessment	Exposure Assessment	Analysis, Adjustment for Potential Confounders
Kneller et al. 1990	Incidence experience (1980-1984) of stomach cancer in occupationally active (1982 census) residents over 30 yr old in Shanghai, China; internal comparison among census registrants	13,489 cases	Cancer incidence tracked through Shanghai Cancer Registry	Occupation at time of diagnosis or retirement ascertained through interview of patient or next of kin	SIR; age, sex
Krewski et al. 2000	Mortality experience (1974-1991) of participants in Six Cities Study in northeast and midwest US; audit of original study with updated exposure assessment methods	8,111	Annual letters mailed to assess vital status; nonrespondents prompted family follow up and NDI records searches	Air-pollutant measurements from central locations in communities	RR; sex, education, diabetes, hypertension, BMI, smoking history, occupational exposure to dusts or fumes
Lagorio et al., 1994	Mortality experience (1981-1992) of self-employed gas-station attendants (in 1980) in Italy; external comparison with Latium region, Italian general population	2,665	Vital status followed through registries of last municipality of residence with record linkage with National Mortality File (pre-1986) or Regional Death Index	Environmental survey, duration of employment	SMR; age, sex
Lan et al. 2002	Incidence experience (1976-1992) of lung cancer in farmers, 41-75 yr old, in Xuanwei County, China	21,232	Lung-cancer incidence tracked through record searches of six regional hospitals	Interview with standardized questionnaire assessing kitchen practices as surrogates for indoor air pollution	RR; sex, age, family history of lung cancer, chronic bronchitis or emphysema, tuberculosis, other SES and demographic variables

Reference	Population	Study Group	Health-Outcome Assessment	Exposure Assessment	Analysis, Adjustment for Potential Confounders
Larkin et al. 2000	Mortality experience (1959-1976) of railroad workers, 40-64 yr old, with 10-20 yr of experience in 1959	55,395	Vital status tracked through US RBB records	Interstate Commerce Commission job code obtained from US RBB records and classified for diesel exposure	RR; age, calendar year
McLaughlin et al. 1987	Incidence experience (1961-1979) of renal cancer in occupationally active (1960 census) Swedish men; external comparison to Swedish general population	7,405 renal-cell cases 821 renal-pelvis cases	Cancer incidence tracked through Swedish Cancer-Environmental Registry, which links census data to Swedish Cancer Registry	Occupation and industry codes from census data	SIR; age, sex, region
Nafstad et al. 2003	Incidence experience (1972-1998) of lung cancer in males, 40-49 yr old, in Oslo, Norway	16,209	Cancer incidence tracked through Norwegian cancer registry	Estimated average concentrations of air pollutants (SO_2, NO_x) from Norwegian Institute for Air Research records; initial questionnaire established home address	RR; age, education, tobacco-smoke exposure, other pollutant
Nelson et al. 1985, 1987	Mortality experience (1970-1982) of Amoco Oil refinery workers (at least 6 mo, with 1 day in 1970-1980); external comparison with US general population	10,763	Vital status followed through SSA, NDI, company telephone survey	Company employment industrial hygienist assigned three job types and exposure types; frequency on basis of job titles	SMR; age, sex, race

Reference	Population	Study Group	Health-Outcome Assessment	Exposure Assessment	Analysis, Adjustment for Potential Confounders
Poole et al. 1993	Nested cases of kidney cancer and controls from several cohorts of workers in 36 petroleum refineries	102 cases, 408 controls	Author and nosologist confirmed cases from death certificates obtained from each cohort	Industrial hygienists assigned HC exposure types, intensity, and frequency on basis of detailed work histories	RR (nested case-control), conditional logistic regression; control for matching factors: employer and location, age, at-risk status
Rafnsson and Gunnars-dottir 1991	Mortality experience (1951-1988) of professional truck and taxi drivers in Reykjavik, Iceland; external comparison with general male population of Iceland	1,021	Record linkage with National Register, Register of Deceased	Truck and taxi drivers identified through membership rolls of Hreyfill cooperative taxi agency	SMR; age, calendar year
Ritz 1999	Mortality experience (1951-1989) of male uranium-processing plant workers (at least 3 yr, with first hire in 1951-1972) in Ohio; external comparison with US general population; Internal comparison among workers monitored for exposure	3,814	Vital status followed through SSA (pre-1979) NDI (1979-1980)	Exposure matrixes generated by employees, industrial hygienists	SMR, RR (conditional logistic regression); age, calendar year, time since first hired, pay type, radiation dose
Saverin et al. 1999	Mortality experience (1970-1994) of lung cancer in male potash miners (at least 1 yr from 1969-1991) in South Harz Mountains area, Germany; internal comparison within subcohort of subjects who worked underground at least 10 yr, held one job for 80% of their time, had three or fewer underground jobs; external comparison to general male population of Germany	5,536; 3,258 subcohort	Vital status followed through local population registers	Personal and area dust-sampling concentrations were averaged and assigned to work categories of production, maintenance, workshop	RR, age SMR; age

Reference	Population	Study Group	Health-Outcome Assessment	Exposure Assessment	Analysis, Adjustment for Potential Confounders
Soll-Johanning et al. 1998	Incidence experience (1943-1994) of urban bus drivers and tramway employees (1900-1994, alive in 1943) in Copenhagen, Denmark; external comparisons to Copenhagen and Denmark general populations	18,120	Record linkage with Danish Cancer Registry	Urban bus drivers and tramway employees identified through employment records of Copenhagen Traffic Company	SIR; sex, age, calendar period
Soll-Johanning et al. 2003	Nested cases of lung and bladder cancer among urban bus drivers and tramway employees (1900-1994, alive in 1943) in Copenhagen, Denmark; internal comparisons across air pollution index	153 lung, 84 bladder	Record linkage with Danish Cancer Registry	Air-pollution exposure index developed and assigned on basis of bus routes driven	RR; smoking
van Loon et al. 1997	Nested cases of lung cancer among males, 55-69 yr old, in Netherlands Cohort Study on Diet and Cancer (1986-1990); internal comparison with subcohort	524 cases, 1,316 subcohort	Record linkage with national pathology register and all cancer registries in Netherlands	Self-administered questionnaire at baseline gave lifetime occupational history, which was reviewed by occupational hygienist and assigned exposure to PAHs	RR; age, other occupational exposures, smoking, vitamin intake
Vasama-Neuvonen et al. 1999	Nested cases of incident ovarian cancer among occupationally active Finnish women (892,591) in 1971-1995	5,072 cases	Cancer incidence tracked through Finnish Cancer Registry	Job titles from 1970 Census linked with Finnish JEM to establish exposure probability	Poisson regression analysis; birth cohort, follow up period, SES
Wong et al. 1999	Nested cases of leukemia, multiple myeloma, kidney cancer in cohort of 18,135 petroleum-distribution workers in US in 1946-1985; internal controls matched 5:1 on company, age, sex	35 leukemia, 11 MM, 12 kidney	Vitas status followed through SSA, NDI, Death Master File	Cumulative and peak exposure to gasoline assessed through job titles, duration of work	Conditional logistic regression

Reference	Population	Study Group	Health-Outcome Assessment	Exposure Assessment	Analysis, Adjustment for Potential Confounders
Zeegers et al. 2001	Nested cases of bladder cancer among a cohort of men, 55-69 yr old, in Netherlands in 1986-1992; random subcohort selected as controls	532 cases	Record linkage to cancer registries, Dutch national database of pathology reports	Self-administered questionnaire at baseline assessed job histories, exposure to confounders; occupational epidemiologists and industrial hygienists assigned probability of exposure to PAHs, diesel exhaust	Rate ratios, failure-time regression model; cigarette-smoking, age, dietary factors, family history

NOTE: ACS=American Cancer Society; BMI=body-mass index; EPA=Environmental Protection Agency; HC=hydrocarbon; HCFA=Health Care Financing Administration; JEM=job exposure matrix; NDI=National Death Index; OR=odds ratio; PM=particulate matter; RBB=Railroad Retirement Board; RR=relative risk; SES=socioeconomic status; SIR=standardized incidence ratio; SMR=standardized mortality ratio; SSA=Social Security Administration.

TABLE D.2 Description of Case-Control Studies Related to Exposure to Fuels and Combustion Products

Reference	Population	Number of Cases	Number of Controls	Relevant Exposures	Exposure Assessment	Analysis; Adjustment for Potential Confounders
Ahrens et al. 1991	Male laryngeal-cancer cases identified in one hospital in Bremen, Germany, in 1986 with histologic confirmation; nonneoplastic male controls selected from same hospital and matched on age and residence	85 laryngeal	100	Transport and communication, diesel oil, gasoline	In-person interview with standardized questionnaire covering lifetime occupational history with exposure checklist	Unconditional logistic regression; smoking, alcohol consumption, age

Reference	Population	Number of Cases	Number of Controls	Relevant Exposures	Exposure Assessment	Analysis; Adjustment for Potential Confounders
Alguacil et al. 2000	Pancreatic-cancer cases diagnosed at five general hospitals in eastern Spain in 1992-1995; nonneoplastic controls with previous suspicion of pancreatic or biliary cancer selected from same hospitals	185 pancreatic	264	PAHs, diesel-engine exhaust	Interview with standardized questionnaire assessing work in any of 10 activities and specific exposures encountered; industrial hygienists evaluated exposures to 22 agents	Unconditional logistic regression; age, sex, hospital, smoking, alcohol use
Armstrong et al. 2000	Nasopharyngeal cancer cases, 19-74 yr old, among Chinese residents of Selangor and Federal Territory, Malaysia in 1990-1992; cases diagnosed in four area centers with histologic confirmation; healthy population controls selected randomly through multistage area sampling and matched on sex and age	282 nasopharyngeal	282	Motor fuel, oil	In-person interviews assessing detailed occupational histories, residential history, lifestyle and nutritional information; job descriptions, durations, tools, specific agents encountered were included	Multiple logistic regression; smoking, dietary factors
Aronson et al. 1996	Male prostate cancer cases and cancer controls, 35-70 yr old, diagnosed in 19 large Montreal-area hospitals in 1979-1985 and histologically confirmed for one of 19 anatomic cancer sites; age-matched population controls also chosen from electoral lists and with RDD	449 prostatic	2,083 total; 533 population, 1,550 cancer	Diesel-engine emissions, liquid-fuel combustion products, PAHs, Benzo[a]pyrene	In-person interview with segments on work histories (job titles); exposures attributed by team of chemists and industrial hygienists	Unconditional logistic regression; age, family income, Quetelet index, respondent status

Reference	Population	Number of Cases	Number of Controls	Relevant Exposures	Exposure Assessment	Analysis; Adjustment for Potential Confounders
Asal et al. 1988	Cases from 29 hospitals in Oklahoma diagnosed and confirmed in 1981-1984; hospital controls selected from same hospitals and matched on age, sex, race, hospital, date of admission; population controls selected through RDD	315 renal	313 hospital, 336 population	Petroleum refining, distribution	In-person interview assessing occupations, industrial exposures	Logistic regression; weight, age, alcohol consumption, occupations, smoking, snuff use, coffee consumption, kidney stones, hypertension, other medical factors
Barbone et al. 1995	Male lung-cancer cases, 37-93 yr old, diagnosed in 1979-1981 and 1985-1986 in Trieste, Italy, with histologic confirmation; deceased (within 6 mo of cases) male controls selected from registry of Department of Pathology	755 lung	755	Level of air pollution (particle deposition)	Particle deposition measured at fixed-site monitoring stations (deposimeters)	Logistic regression; age, cigarettes/day, occupational carcinogen exposure, social group
Boffetta et al. 2003	Male cases of laryngeal and hypopharyngeal cancer diagnosed in six European centers in 1980-1983 with histologic confirmation; controls selected from census lists, electoral rolls, or population registries and matched for sex and age	1,010 laryngeal and hypopharyngeal	2,176	Railway-transport industry, motor vehicle mechanics	Interview with standardized questionnaire assessing jobs held at least 1 yr; job titles coded	Unconditional logistic regression, age, study area, average tobacco-smoking, average alcohol-drinking

Reference	Population	Number of Cases	Number of Controls	Relevant Exposures	Exposure Assessment	Analysis; Adjustment for Potential Confounders
Brown et al. 1988	White, male laryngeal-cancer cases, 30-79 yr old, diagnosed in 56 hospitals along Gulf Coast of Texas in 1975-1980; controls selected through Texas Department of Health mortality tapes, drivers license records, HCFA-provided Medicare records, and matched on age, vital status, ethnicity, county of residence	183 laryngeal	250	Transportation, driver, diesel and gasoline fumes	Interview (self-reports or proxy) assessing lifetime occupational and residential histories, lifestyle factors, demographic characteristics; industrial hygienist classified job titles for exposure to specific agents	Logistic regression; cigarette smoking, alcohol consumption
Bruske-Hohlfeld et al. 1999	Pooled male lung-cancer cases and controls from two studies in Germany (1988-1993 in Bremen and Frankfurt/Main; 1990-1996 in Nordrhein-Westfalen, Rheinland-Pfalz and Bayern, the Saarland, Thuringen, and Sachen); population controls matched on age, sex, region of residence	3,498 lung	3,541	Professional drivers	In-person interview with standardized questionnaire assessing lifetime occupational history; standardized coding of job titles	Conditional logistic regression; smoking, asbestos exposure

Reference	Population	Number of Cases	Number of Controls	Relevant Exposures	Exposure Assessment	Analysis; Adjustment for Potential Confounders
Bruske-Hohlfeld et al. 2000	Pooled male lung-cancer cases and controls from two studies in Germany (1988-1993 in Bremen and Frankfurt/Main; 1990-1996 in Nordrhein-Westfalen, Rheinland-Pfalz and Bayern, the Saarland, Thuringen, Sachen); population controls matched on age, sex, and region of residence	3,498 lung	3,541	Diesel-engine exhaust, PAHs, Benzo[a]pyrene; transport worker, freight handler	In-person interview with standardized questionnaire assessing lifetime occupational history; specific questions addressed exposure to PAHs; diesel-exhaust exposure derived from job titles; standardized coding of job titles	Conditional logistic regression; smoking, asbestos exposure
Carozza et al. 2000	Glioma cases, age 20 yr old or older, diagnosed in six San Francisco Bay counties in 1991-1994 by Northern California Cancer Center; controls selected through random-digit dialing, matched for age, gender, race	476 glioma	462	Petroleum and gas workers, service-station attendants	In-person interviews with standardized questionnaire assessing detailed lifetime job history	Multiple logistic regression; age, sex, years of education, race
Cole et al. 1972	Lower urinary tract cancer cases, 20-89 yr old, diagnosed and histologically confirmed, among residents of eastern Massachusetts in 18-mo span; controls randomly selected from area resident lists, matched on age, sex	461 lower urinary tract	485	Petroleum-related occupations	In-person interviews collected occupational histories each job listed was assigned occupation titles, levels of occupational exposures	Relative risk; smoking, age

Reference	Population	Number of Cases	Number of Controls	Relevant Exposures	Exposure Assessment	Analysis; Adjustment for Potential Confounders
Costantini et al. 2001	Hematolymphopoietic-cancer cases, 20-74 yr old identified through periodic hospital survey and diagnosed in 12 regions in Italy in 1991-1993 with histologic confirmation; controls randomly selected from municipal demographic files and National Health Services files, matched for age, sex	1,450 NHL 365 HD 652 leukemia	1,779	Transport operators	In-person interview (direct or proxy) with standardized and job-specific questionnaires assessing lifetime occupational history, exposure to specific agents	Mantel-Haenszel OR; age, sex
Dai et al. 1996	Female lung-cancer cases, 30-69 yr old, diagnosed in 1992-1993 in Harbin, China; population controls randomly selected, matched on age, smoking status	120 lung	120	Coal-stove use	In-person interview with standardized questionnaire assessing cooking, heating practices	Unconditional logistic regression; SES and dietary factors, family cancer history
Decoufle and Stanislawczyk 1977	White cancer cases and nonneoplastic controls admitted to Roswell Park Memorial Institute in 1956-1965, comprising 22 cancer sites	25,416 total participants, 6,434 male cancer, 7,515 female cancer		Bus, taxicab, truck drivers; mechanics, repairmen; delivery and route men; locomotive engineers, firemen	Self-reported lifetime occupational histories collected	RR; smoking, age

Reference	Population	Number of Cases	Number of Controls	Relevant Exposures	Exposure Assessment	Analysis; Adjustment for Potential Confounders
Demers et al. 1993	MM cases identified through SEER tumor registries in four geographic areas, under 80 yr old, newly diagnosed in 1977-1981; population controls identified through RDD and population survey of geographic areas	692 MM	1,683	Petroleum, coal refining, manufacturing	Interviews (direct or proxy) with standardized questionnaire to assess occupational history, specific exposure agents; occupations, industries coded according to 1970 US Census	Mantel-Haenszel OR; sex, age, race, study area
De Stefani et al. 1998	Male laryngeal-cancer cases, 30-75 yr old, diagnosed in five hospitals in Montevideo, Uruguay, in 1993-1995; cancer controls selected from same hospitals and timeframe	112 laryngeal	509	Gasoline, diesel exhaust, gasoline exhaust	In-person interview with standardized questionnaire assessing lifetime occupational histories and exposure to specific agents	Unconditional logistic regression; age, residence, education, income, tobacco-smoking and type, alcohol consumption
Dietz et al. 1995	Head- and neck-cancer cases diagnosed at the Department of Otorhinolaryngology at University of Heidelberg, Germany, in 1989-1992; outpatient controls selected from same department and matched on sex, size of residence, age	164 laryngeal 100 oral cavity 105 oropharyngeal or hypopharyngeal	656, 400, 420	Heating, cooking with fossil-fuel stoves	Interview with standardized questionnaire assessing household practices and work conditions	Adjusted ORs; Tobacco, alcohol consumption

Reference	Population	Number of Cases	Number of Controls	Relevant Exposures	Exposure Assessment	Analysis; Adjustment for Potential Confounders
Du et al. 1996	Lung-cancer cases identified from local police registries in Guangzhou, China, in 1985; deceased (unrelated to lung cancer) controls matched on sex, age	849 lung	849	Coal fumes	Next-of-kin interview	Mantel-Haenszel RR; smoking
Dumas et al. 2000	Male cases, controls, 35-70 yr old, diagnosed in 19 large Montreal-area hospitals in 1979-1985 and histologically confirmed for one of 19 cancer sites; frequency-matched by approximate age, population-based controls also chosen from electoral lists, RDD	257 rectal	1,295 cancer, 533 population	Combustion products of soot, coal, wood	In-person interviews with specific question on detail of each job subject had; analyzed and coded by team of chemists and industrial hygienists (about 300 exposures) on semiquantitative scale	Unconditional logistic regression; age, education, respondent status, cigarette-smoking, beer consumption, BMI
Elci et al. 2003	Male laryngeal-cancer cases diagnosed in Oncology Treatment Center of Social Security Agency Okmeydani Hospital in Istanbul, Turkey, in 1979-1984 with histologic confirmation; controls selected from same hospital, timeframe among cases of HD, cancers of skin (nonmelanoma), testis, bone, male breast as well as benign lesions	940 laryngeal	1,519	Diesel exhaust, gasoline exhaust, PAHs	In-person interview with standardized questionnaire assessing lifetime occupational history, tobacco and alcohol use; industrial hygienist performed JEM exposure assignments	Unconditional logistic regression; age, smoking, alcohol consumption

Reference	Population	Number of Cases	Number of Controls	Relevant Exposures	Exposure Assessment	Analysis; Adjustment for Potential Confounders
Farrow et al. 1989	Cases of myelodysplastic syndrome diagnosed at University Hospital of Wales in 1985-1986; outpatient controls selected from same hospitals, timeframe and matched on age and sex	63 myelodysplastic syndrome	63	Petrol, diesel fumes, liquids	In-person interview with standardized questionnaire assessing lifetime occupational history with checklist of 70 specific agents; exposure index based on checklist and duration of particular jobs	Crude OR
Flodin et al. 1987	MM cases, 40-80 yr old, diagnosed in six hospitals in central and southeastern Sweden in 1973-1983 and alive in 1981-1983; controls randomly selected from local population registers	131 MM	431	Engine exhausts	Mailed questionnaire assessing occupational exposures (self-reports)	Mantel-Haenszel OR; age, confounder score
Flodin et al. 1988	Chronic lymphocytic-leukemia cases, 40-80 yr old, diagnosed in five hospitals in central and southeastern Sweden in 1964-1984 and alive in 1981-1983; controls randomly selected from local population registers	111 chronic lymphocytic leukemia	431	Engine exhausts	Mailed questionnaire assessing occupational exposures (self-reports)	Mantel-Haenszel OR; age, confounder score

Reference	Population	Number of Cases	Number of Controls	Relevant Exposures	Exposure Assessment	Analysis; Adjustment for Potential Confounders
Fritschi and Siemiatycki 1996	Male melanoma cases and cancer controls, 35-70 yr old, diagnosed in 19 large Montreal-area hospitals in 1979-1985 and histologically confirmed for one of 19 cancer sites; age-matched population controls also chosen from electoral lists and with RDD	103 melanoma	1,066 total, 533 population, 533 cancer	PAHs, petroleum-related substances	In-person interview with segments on work histories (job titles); exposures attributed by team of chemists and industrial hygienists	Unconditional logistic regression; age, years of schooling, ethnicity
Gerhardsson de Verdier et al. 1992	Colorectal-cancer cases identified through local hospitals and Regional Cancer Registry in Stockholm, Sweden in 1986-1988; cases histologically confirmed and subjects limited to those born in Sweden in 1907-1946 and lived half their lives there; population controls randomly selected from Stockholm County population registry	352 colon 217 rectal	512	Petrol station, automotive repair	Questionnaire administered in person or through mail with followup telephone survey; exposure to list of chemicals or employment in specified occupations determined	Unconditional logistic regression; age, sex, nutritional intake markers, BMI, physical activity, family history of colorectal cancer

Reference	Population	Number of Cases	Number of Controls	Relevant Exposures	Exposure Assessment	Analysis; Adjustment for Potential Confounders
Goldberg et al. 2001	Male cases and controls, 35-70 yr old, diagnosed in 19 large Montreal-area hospitals in 1979-1985 and histologically confirmed for one of 19 cancer sites; frequency-matched by approximate age; population-based controls also chosen from electoral lists and with RDD	497 colon	1,514 cancer, 533 population	Diesel-engine emissions	In-person interviews with specific question on detail of each job subject had; analyzed and coded by team of chemists and industrial hygienists (about 300 exposures) on semiquantitative scale	Unconditional logistic regression; age, respondent status, ethnicity, nonoccupational factors (such as cigarette-smoking, alcohol consumption)
Gustavsson et al. 1998	Oral-cavity, pharyngeal-, laryngeal-, and esophageal-cancer cases among all Swedish men, 40-79 yr old, residing in two regions with reporting from departments of oncology and surgery in 1988-1990; controls randomly selected from population registers and matched on age, region	545	641	PAHs, Welding fumes	Interview with standardized questionnaire assessing lifestyle and environmental factors; occupational hygienist assigned exposure intensity, probability to 17 specific occupational exposures	Unconditional logistic regression; age, region, alcohol consumption, tobacco-smoking

Reference	Population	Number of Cases	Number of Controls	Relevant Exposures	Exposure Assessment	Analysis; Adjustment for Potential Confounders
Gustavsson et al. 2000	Male lung-cancer cases, 40-75 yr old, among stable residents (living outside Sweden no more than 5 yr in 1950-1990) identified through Swedish Cancer Registry in 1985-1990; controls randomly selected from population registers and matched on age, year of inclusion	1,042 lung	2,364	Diesel exhaust, motor exhaust, combustion products (benzo[a]pyrene)	Mailed questionnaire (direct or proxy) established lifetime occupational history; occupational hygienist assigned probability, intensity of exposure to specific agents	Unconditional logistic regression; matching variables, smoking, residential radon level, environmental exposure to NO_2
Hansen et al. 1998	Male lung-cancer cases, born 1897-1966, identified through Danish Cancer Registry in 1970-1989; noncancer controls randomly selected from Central Population Registry and matched on age, sex	28,744 lung	28,744	Lorry, bus drivers; taxi drivers	Record linkage with nationwide pension-fund files	Conditional logistic regression
Hayes et al. 1989	Male lung-cancer cases pooled from three studies in US (Florida in 1976-1979, New Jersey in 1980-1981, Louisiana in 1979-1983)	1,444 lung	1,893	Drivers (truck, heavy equipment, bus, taxi)	Studies reviewed to identify occupations with motor-exhaust exposure	Logistic regression; age, smoking, study area

Reference	Population	Number of Cases	Number of Controls	Relevant Exposures	Exposure Assessment	Analysis; Adjustment for Potential Confounders
Heineman et al. 1992	Male cases of MM diagnosed and reported to Danish Cancer Registry in 1970-1984; controls randomly selected from Danish Central Population Registry and matched on sex, age, year of diagnosis	1,098 MM	4,169	Wholesale tradefuel, oil, gas; gasoline; oil products	Job titles obtained from subjects' most recent tax records; industrial hygienists assigned exposure to 20 major categories, 27 specific substances	Adjusted ORs; age
Howe et al. 1980	Bladder-cancer cases diagnosed in three Canadian provinces in 1974-1976; neighborhood controls matched on age, sex	632 bladder	632	Petroleum industry	In-person interviews assessing lifetime occupational history with 13 a priori suspect industries	Logistic regression, discordant pairs, matching variables
Huebner et al. 1992	Oral- and pharyngeal cancer cases, 18-79 yr old, obtained from population-based cancer registries in five US locations in 1984-1985; controls obtained through RDD, matched on sex, race, age, study area	1,114 oral and pharyngeal	1,268	Petroleum-industry worker, motor vehicle operator, service-station worker	Interview (direct or proxy) with structured questionnaire assessing jobs held at least 6 mo; job titles coded	Multiple logistic regression; smoking, alcohol consumption, study location, age, race

Reference	Population	Number of Cases	Number of Controls	Relevant Exposures	Exposure Assessment	Analysis; Adjustment for Potential Confounders
Iscovich et al. 1987	Bladder-cancer cases admitted to 10 hospital from three counties in Argentina in 1983-1985 with histologic confirmation; hospital controls selected from same hospitals and period (within 3 mo) as cases; neighborhood controls selected from same block as case, matched on sex, age	117 bladder	117 hospital; 117 neighborhood	Work in oil refinery	In-person interview with standardized questionnaire covering lifetime occupational history with exposure checklist (33 agents)	Unconditional logistic regression; age, smoking
Jockel et al. 1992	Lung-cancer cases, age 38-87 yr old, diagnosed in seven hospitals in five cities in Germany with histologic confirmation (recruitment dates not given); hospital controls with diagnosis unrelated to smoking matched on sex, age; population controls randomly selected from residence registries	194 lung	194 hospital, 194 population	SO_2, benzo[a]pyrene, total suspended particles	In-person interview with standardized and supplemental questionnaires assessing residential history; emission index generated from energy-consumption statistics; semiquantitative index combined this with SO_2 emissions, coal use, degree of industrialization	Logistic regression; age, smoking, occupation

Reference	Population	Number of Cases	Number of Controls	Relevant Exposures	Exposure Assessment	Analysis; Adjustment for Potential Confounders
Kadamani et al. 1989	Kidney-cancer cases, 20 yr old or more, diagnosed in 23 hospitals in Oklahoma City and Tulsa in 1981-1983 with histologic confirmation; controls selected through RDD of Oklahoma residents, matched on age, sex	210 kidney	210	Hydrocarbons	In-person interviews assessing occupational histories, lifestyle, demographic factors; likelihood of hydrocarbon exposure assigned by industrial-hygienist review of job titles	Mantel-Haenszel OR; weight, education
Katsouyanni et al. 1991	Female lung-cancer cases diagnosed in seven hospitals in Athens, Greece, in 1987-1989; hospital controls over 35 yr old, admitted within 1 week of case	101 lung	89	Air pollution	Lifetime residential and employment histories were coupled with data from fixed-site monitoring stations according to borough for cumulative exposure index	Multiple logistic regression; age, years of schooling, interviewer
Kauppinen et al. 1995	Deceased pancreatic-cancer cases as of April 1990, 40-74 yr old at diagnosis in 1984-1987; identified cases and controls from Finnish Cancer Registry; controls of similar age, period of diagnoses selected from deceased cases of stomach, colon, or rectal cancer	595 pancreatic	1,622	Engine exhaust; PAHs	Mailed questionnaire to next of kin assessing lifetime work history (job titles); assignment of exposures by industrial hygienist and use of JEM	Unconditional logistic regression; age, sex, tobacco smoking, diabetes mellitus, alcohol consumption

Reference	Population	Number of Cases	Number of Controls	Relevant Exposures	Exposure Assessment	Analysis; Adjustment for Potential Confounders
Kleinerman et al. 2002	Lung-cancer cases, 30-70 yr old, diagnosed in Pingliang and Qingyang, China, in 1994-1998; population controls randomly selected from census lists, matched on age, sex, prefecture	846 lung	1,740	Biomass, coal-fuel use	Direct questions in interview on biomass or coal use for fuel or heating	Unconditional logistic regression; matching variables, color-television ownership, number of cattle, tobacco use
Kogevinas et al. 2003	Pooled bladder-cancer cases, 30-79 yr old, and controls from 11 studies in six European countries in 1976-1996	3,346 bladder	6,840	Petroleum-refining workers, PAHs	Standardized coding of job titles from various studies; JEM applied to assign exposure to specific exposures	Unconditional logistic regression; age, smoking, study center
Lan et al. 2001	Lung-cancer cases diagnosed in Xuan Wei, China, in 1995-1996; controls randomly selected from list of household registrations, matched on sex, age, village, cooking and heating fuel used	97 lung	97	Lifetime-accumulated smoky coal use without ventilation	In-person interview with standardized questionnaire assessing lifestyle factors	Conditional logistic regression, age, sex, pack-years of smoking
Leclerc et al. 1997	Pooled sinonasal-cancer cases and controls from 12 studies in seven countries	930 sinonasal	3,136	Motor-vehicle driver	Standardized coding of job titles from various studies	Logistic regression; age, study
Lindquist et al. 1991	Acute leukemia cases, 15-84 yr old, admitted to five hospitals in Sweden, interviewed in 1980-1983; controls selected from population registry, matched on sex, age	125 acute leukemia	125	Professional drivers	In-person interview with standardized questionnaire assessing occupational, task histories	Discordant pairs; logistic regression

Reference	Population	Number of Cases	Number of Controls	Relevant Exposures	Exposure Assessment	Analysis; Adjustment for Potential Confounders
Magnani et al. 1987	Male cancer cases of five sites, 18-54 yr old, identified from death certificates from three English counties in 1959-1979 (1964 unavailable); deceased controls selected for each case set, matched on age at death, sex, county of residence	244 esophagus 343 pancreas 99 melanoma 147 kidney 432 brain	935 1,315 361 556 1,603	Coal, petroleum-products industry	Occupations listed on death certificates; JEM constructed to assign exposure to 49 agents	Matched ORs; matching variables
Mandel et al. 1995	Renal-cell cancer cases, age 20-79 yr old, from six international sites, diagnosed and confirmed in 1989-1991 with cancer registries or surveillance of clinical and pathology departments; controls selected from population registers, electoral rolls, residential lists, HCFA records, or RDD, depending on site; controls matched on age, exposure	1,732 renal	2,309	Oil refinery industry, gas-station attendants, gasoline, jet fuel, heating oil, kerosene, or diesel fuel	In-person interviews to assess lifetime occupational history, exposure to specific agents	Logistic regression; age, center, BMI, cigarette-smoking
Matos et al. 2000	Male lung-cancer cases identified among residents in four hospitals in Buenos Aires, Argentina, in 1994-1996; hospital controls (unrelated to tobacco use) matched on age, hospital	199 lung	393	Motor-vehicle and truck drivers, railway-transport industry	In-person interview with questionnaire assessing occupational history (jobs held at least 1 yr)	Conditional logistic regression; hospital, age, pack-years of cigarettes, other occupations or industries with increased risks

Reference	Population	Number of Cases	Number of Controls	Relevant Exposures	Exposure Assessment	Analysis; Adjustment for Potential Confounders
McLaughlin et al. 1984	White kidney-cancer cases, 30-64 yr old, diagnosed in Minneapolis-St. Paul metropolitan area in 1974-1979; white controls systematically selected from telephone listings (30-64 yr old) and HCFA listings (65-85 yr old), matched on age ,sex	495 kidney	697	Chemical-petroleum industry; petroleum, tar, pitch products	In-person interview (direct or proxy) with detailed questionnaire assessing occupational history	Adjusted ORs (age, smoking; multivariate logistic regression
McLaughlin et al. 1985	White male kidney cancer cases, 30-64 yr old, diagnosed in Minneapolis-St. Paul metropolitan area in 1974-1979; white controls systematically selected from telephone listings (30-64 yr old) and HCFA listings (65-85 yr old), matched on age, sex	313 kidney	428	Petroleum industry, gasoline-station attendants	In-person interview (direct or proxy) with detailed questionnaire assessing occupational history	Adjusted ORs; age, smoking
Menvielle et al. 2003	Lung-cancer cases, 18 yr old or older, identified through New Caledonia Cancer Registry in France in 1993-1995; population controls randomly selected from electoral rolls, matched on sex and age	228 lung	305	Dockers; transportation-equipment managers; motor-bus, lorry, van drivers; diesel-engine emissions; PAHs	In-person interview (direct or proxy) with standardized and occupation or task-specific questionnaires assessing occupational history (including agents used); job titles coded; industrial hygienist assigned probabilities; frequencies of exposure	Unconditional logistic regression; age, smoking

Reference	Population	Number of Cases	Number of Controls	Relevant Exposures	Exposure Assessment	Analysis; Adjustment for Potential Confounders
Merletti et al. 1991	Male oral- and oropharyngeal-cancer cases, 26-92 yr old, diagnosed in Turin, Italy, in 1982-1984; controls randomly selected from resident files, stratified by age, sex	86 oral, oropharyngeal	373	PAHs	In-person interview with standardized questionnaire assessing lifetime occupational history; job titles coded; industrial hygienists applied JEM to determine exposures to 13 agents	Unconditional logistic regression; age, education, birthplace, tobacco-smoking, alcohol consumption
Mommsen et al. 1982	Consecutive male bladder cancer cases, 42-85 yr old, diagnosed in one hospital in Denmark in 1977-1979; controls selected through National Registry matched on age, sex, region	165 bladder	165	Work with petroleum or asphalt, work with oil or gasoline	In-person interview with standardized questionnaire covering lifetime occupational history and work with chemicals; controls answered mailed questionnaire with follow up survey through telephone or mail	Multivariate logistic regression; nocturia, cigarette smoking, prostatic surgery, cheroot smoker, lowest SES, previous venereal disease, chewing-tobacco use, industrial work, alcohol consumption, symptoms of cystitis, work with chemical materials
Mommsen et al. 1983	Consecutive bladder-cancer cases, 42-85 yr old, diagnosed in one hospital in Denmark in 1977-1980 (through 1979 for males); controls selected through National Registry matched on age, sex, region	212 bladder	259	Work with petroleum or asphalt, work with oil or gasoline	In-person interview with standardized questionnaire covering lifetime occupational history, work with chemicals; controls answered mailed questionnaire with followup survey through telephone or mail	Multivariate logistic regression; cigarette-smoking, cigarillo-smoking, industrial work, chewing-tobacco use, saccharin consumption, previous venereal disease, alcohol use, pipe-smoking, work with chemical materials

Reference	Population	Number of Cases	Number of Controls	Relevant Exposures	Exposure Assessment	Analysis; Adjustment for Potential Confounders
Mommsen and Aagard 1984	Consecutive bladder-cancer cases, 42-85 yr old, diagnosed in one hospital in Denmark in 1977-1980 (through 1979 for males); controls selected through National Registry matched on age, sex, region	212 bladder	259	Work with oil or gasoline, work with kerosene or asphalt	In-person interview with standardized questionnaire covering lifetime occupational history, work with chemicals; controls answered mailed questionnaire with followup survey through telephone or mail	Multivariate logistic regression; Nocturia, cigarette smoking, prostatic surgery, cigarillo-smoking, lowest SES, previous venereal disease, blacksmiths or mechanics, chewing-tobacco use, alcohol consumption symptoms of cystitis, industrial work, work with chemical materials
Morris et al. 1986	MM cases identified through SEER tumor registries in four geographic areas, under 80 yr old, and newly diagnosed in 1977-1981; population controls identified through RDD and population survey of four geographic areas	698 MM	1,683	Aliphatic hydrocarbons (including gas, diesel, kerosene)	Interviews (direct or proxy) with standardized questionnaire to assess occupational history, exposure agents	Mantel-Haenszel ORs; sex, age, race, study area
Nadon et al. 1995	Male cancer cases, 35-70 yr old, diagnosed in 19 large Montreal-area hospitals in 1979-1986 and histologically confirmed for several cancer sites; control series for each cancer type composed of other cancer cases (except lung)	3,726 total cases	Varied depending on size of site under examination	Benzo[a]pyrene, coal, petroleum, wood	In-person interviews with specific questions on details of each job subject had; analyzed and coded by team of chemists, industrial hygienists (about 300 exposures) on semiquantitative scales	Unconditional logistic regression; age, family income, ethnicity, cumulative smoking index

Reference	Population	Number of Cases	Number of Controls	Relevant Exposures	Exposure Assessment	Analysis; Adjustment for Potential Confounders
Najem et al. 1982	White bladder-cancer cases admitted to two community hospitals in northern New Jersey in 1978; nonneoplastic controls selected from same hospitals, matched on age, place of birth, sex, race, current residence	75 bladder	142	Work in petroleum (fuel) industry	In-person interview with standardized questionnaire assessing lifetime occupational history	Mantel-Haenszel OR; smoking
Nisse et al. 2001	Cases of myelodysplastic syndrome diagnosed in hematology department of University of Lille, France, in 1991-1996 with hematologic confirmation; controls randomly selected from electoral registers, matched for sex , age	204 myelodysplastic syndrome	204	PAHs, petrol, oil, exhaust gases	In-person interview with standardized questionnaire assessing lifetime occupational history; exposure to fuels, exhaust determined by team of experts from job titles	Mantel-Haenszel OR; matching variables
Nyberg et al. 2000	Male lung-cancer cases, 40-75 yr old, among stable residents (living outside Sweden no more than 5 years in 1950-1990) identified through Swedish Cancer Registry in 1985-1990; controls randomly selected from population registers, matched on age and year of inclusion	1,042 lung	2,364	Air pollution (NO_2, SO_2)	Mailed questionnaire assessing residence history; geocoding of locations coupled to data from regional emission database provided estimates of air-pollution exposure	Unconditional logistic regression; matching variables, smoking, residential radon level, socioeconomic grouping, other occupations, other combustion products and asbestos

Reference	Population	Number of Cases	Number of Controls	Relevant Exposures	Exposure Assessment	Analysis; Adjustment for Potential Confounders
Parent et al. 2000a	Male cancer cases, 35-70 yr old, diagnosed in 19 large Montreal-area hospital in 1979-1985 and histologically confirmed; control series composed of other cancer cases (except lung), population controls selected through RDD	142 renal-cell carcinoma	2,433 total, 1,900 cancer, 533 population	Jet fuel, aviation gasoline	In-person interviews with specific questions on details of each job subject had; analyzed, coded by team of chemists, industrial hygienists (about 300 exposures) on semiquantitative scales	Mantel-Haenszel OR, logistic regression; respondent status, age, smoking, BMI, occupational confounders
Parent et al. 2000b	Male cases and controls, 35-70 yr old, diagnosed in 19 large Montreal-area hospitals in 1979-1985 and histologically confirmed for one of 19 cancer sites; frequency-matched by approximate age; population-based controls also chosen from electoral lists and with RDD	99 esophageal	2,299 cancer, 533 population	PAHs, gasoline engine emissions, CO, benzo[a]pyrene	In-person interviews with specific question on detail of each job subject had; analyzed, coded by team of chemists and industrial hygienists (about 300 exposures) on semiquantitative scale	Unconditional logistic regression; age, respondent status, birthplace, educational level, beer consumption, spirits consumption, β-carotene index, cigarette-smoking (length, pattern)
Partanen et al. 1991	Cases over 20 yr old, identified through Finnish Cancer Registry in 1977-1978; controls randomly selected from Population Register Centre, matched on year of birth, sex, survival status	408 renal	819	Gasoline, diesel fuel, other distilled fuel oils	Mailed questionnaire or phone interview (direct or proxy) assessing lifetime occupational history; industrial hygienist coded, assigned summary indicators of exposures	Conditional logistic regression; matching variables, smoking, coffee consumption, obesity

Reference	Population	Number of Cases	Number of Controls	Relevant Exposures	Exposure Assessment	Analysis; Adjustment for Potential Confounders
Pesch et al. 2000	Renal-cell cancer cases in large hospitals in five regions in Germany in 1991-1995 with histologic confirmation; controls randomly selected from local residency registries, matched on region, sex, age	935 renal	4,298	Production, use of petroleum products	In-person interviews of lifetime occupational history using questionnaire to assess job-titles and self-reported exposures; exposures ascertained with JEM	Conditional logistic regression; matching variables, smoking
Petralia et al. 1999	Female breast-cancer cases, age 40 yr old or more, identified through major hospitals in two New York counties in 1986-1991 with histological confirmation; controls randomly selected from lists of New York state Department of Motor Vehicles, matched for age, county	301 breast	316	PAHs	In-person interviews assessing lifetime occupational history; occupations, industries coded; assigned potential exposures to PAHs through use of JEM	Unconditional logistic regression; age, years of education, age at first birth, age at menarche, history of benign breast disease, family breast-cancer history, Quetelet index, months of lactation
Pintos et al. 1998	Mouth-, laryngeal-, pharyngeal-cancer cases referred to three surgery services in Brazil in 1987-1989; controls selected among inpatients from same and neighboring hospitals, matched on sex, age, trimester of hospital admission	784	1,568	Use of wood stoves	Interview with standardized questionnaire assessing occupational, environmental exposures	Conditional logistic regression; tobacco and alcohol consumption, race, income, rural residence, schooling

Reference	Population	Number of Cases	Number of Controls	Relevant Exposures	Exposure Assessment	Analysis; Adjustment for Potential Confounders
Rajaraman et al. 2004	Cases of meningioma and acoustic neuroma, 18 yr old or older, diagnosed in one of three US hospitals specializing in brain tumors in 1994-1998; noncancer controls selected from same hospitals, matched on hospital, sex, race, age, proximity of residence to hospital	197 meningioma, 96 acoustic neuroma	799	Gas-station attendants	In-person interviews assessing detailed lifetime occupational history with industrial-hygienist-developed job-specific questions on type, frequency, intensity, and duration of exposure to specific agents	Unconditional logistic regression; matching variables: hospital, sex, race, age, proximity of residence to hospital
Risch et al. 1988	Bladder-cancer cases, 35-79 yr old, identified through combination of cancer-registry reporting and hospital- record review in four cities in Canada in 1979-1982 with histologic confirmation; controls randomly selected from population listings, matched on birth year, sex, residence area	826 bladder	792	Work in petroleum industry	In-person interview with questionnaire assessing specific occupational exposures	Conditional logistic regression; matching variables, lifetime cigarette consumption
Schoenberg et al. 1984	Male bladder-cancer cases, 21-84 yr old, with histologically confirmed diagnosis in New Jersey in 1978-1979; controls identified through RDD (21-64 yr old) HCFA records (65-84 yr old), stratified for age	658 bladder	1,258	Refinery work, garage or gas-station work	In-person interview with questionnaire assessing lifetime occupational history	Logistic regression; age, duration of cigarette-smoking, other occupations

Reference	Population	Number of Cases	Number of Controls	Relevant Exposures	Exposure Assessment	Analysis; Adjustment for Potential Confounders
Sharpe et al. 1989	Cases diagnosed at one of four Montreal-area hospitals in 1982-1986 and one of five other hospitals in 1982-1987; cases histologically confirmed and alive at time of chart review; controls selected from suspected renal-cell carcinoma cases with final diagnosis other than cancer, matched on sex, age, urologist	164 renal	161	Gasoline, kerosene	History of exposure to hydrocarbons obtained through mailed questionnaire, supplemented by telephone interview	Univariate analysis
Siemiatycki et al. 1987	Male cancer cases, 35-70 yr old, diagnosed in 19 large Montreal-area hospitals in 1979-1985 and histologically confirmed for several cancer sites; control series for each cancer type composed of other cancer cases (except lung)	3,726 total cases	Varied, depending on size of site under examination	Automotive and aviation gasoline, kerosene, jet and diesel fuels, heating oils, crude oil	In-person interviews with specific questions on details of each job subject had; analyzed, coded by team of chemists, industrial hygienists (about 300 exposures) on semiquantitative scales	Mantel-Haenszel OR, logistic regression; age, ethnicity, SES, smoking, "dirtiness" index of job

Reference	Population	Number of Cases	Number of Controls	Relevant Exposures	Exposure Assessment	Analysis; Adjustment for Potential Confounders
Siemiatycki et al. 1988	Male cancer cases, 35-70 yr old, diagnosed in 19 large Montreal-area hospitals in 1979-1985 and histologically confirmed for several cancer sites; control series for each cancer type composed of other cancer cases (except lung)	3,726 total cases	Varied, depending on size of site under examination	Exhaust from gasoline, diesel, jet fuel, propane; combustion of propane, natural gas, liquid fuel, wood, coal, coke	In-person interviews with specific questions on details of each job subject had; analyzed, coded by a team of chemists, industrial hygienists (about 300 exposures) on semiquantitative scales	Mantel-Haenszel OR, logistic regression; age, ethnicity, SES, smoking, blue- or white-collar job history
Silverman et al. 1989a	Nonwhite cases, 21-84 years, in 10 US areas in 1977-1978 with histologic confirmation; controls identified through RDD (21-64 yr old) HCFA records (65-84 yr old), matched for age, geographic area	126 bladder	383	Petroleum workers, gasoline service stations	In-person interview with questionnaire assessing job or industry titles; industries and job titles coded by study authors, grouped by potential exposures	Logistic regression; smoking, age
Silverman et al. 1989b	White cases, 21-84 yr old, in 10 US areas in 1977-1978 with histologic confirmation; controls identified through RDD (21-64 yr old) and HCFA records (65-84 yr old), matched for age, geographic area	2,100 bladder	3,874	Petroleum-processing work	In-person interview with questionnaire assessing job or industry titles; industries, job titles coded by study authors, grouped by potential exposures	Logistic regression; smoking, age

Reference	Population	Number of Cases	Number of Controls	Relevant Exposures	Exposure Assessment	Analysis; Adjustment for Potential Confounders
Spiegelman and Wegman 1985	Cases of colon and rectal cancer and cancer controls selected from sample of Third National Cancer Survey of incident cancers in seven US metropolitan areas in 1969-1971	370 colon, 175 rectal, 8 large intestine	1,861 total	Fuel oil	Interviews conducted on primary, secondary occupations, industries, duration; exposure assignment according to NIOSH National Occupational Hazard Survey protocol	Logistic regression; age, race, marital status, region, income group, educational level, body mass, nutritional scores
Steenland et al. 1990	Deceased male lung-cancer cases identified through Central States Teamsters files in 1982-1983; controls selected as every sixth death from files, excluding lung and bladder cancers, motor-vehicle accidents	994 lung	1,085	Diesel or gasoline truck drivers; diesel exposure, nontruck drivers	Interview with next of kin conducted through mail or telephone call assessing occupational history	Unconditional logistic regression; age, smoking, asbestos
Steenland et al. 1998	Deceased, male lung cancer cases identified through the Central States Teamsters files in 1982-1983; controls selected as every sixth death from files, excluding lung and bladder cancers and motor vehicle accidents	994 lung	1,085	Diesel emissions	Interview with next of kin conducted through mail or telephone call assessing occupational history; diesel-emissions exposure calculations based on job history, number of data sources	Logistic regression; age, race, smoking, diet, asbestos
Steineck et al. 1990	Male urothelial-cancer cases, born 1911-1945, diagnosed in Stockholm, Sweden, in 1985-1987; controls randomly selected from population registers	256 urothelial	287	Petrol	Subjects provided occupational histories, specified agents encountered; industrial hygienist used this information to assign exposure status	Logistic regression; age, smoking

Reference	Population	Number of Cases	Number of Controls	Relevant Exposures	Exposure Assessment	Analysis; Adjustment for Potential Confounders
Stemhagen et al. 1983	Liver-cancer cases identified through diagnosis in New Jersey hospitals in 1975-1980 or from death certificates in 1975-1979, all with histologic confirmation; controls selected from hospital records, death certificates, matched for age, race, sex, county of residence	265 liver	530	Gasoline service-station attendants	In-person interview (direct or proxy) to assess occupational history (job titles)	Mantel-Haenszel OR
Swanson et al. 1993	Male lung-cancer cases, 40-84 yr old, identified through the Occupational Cancer Incidence Surveillance Study, diagnosed in Detroit, Michigan, in 1984-1987; cases of colon and rectum cancer, identified in same way, served as control group	3,792 lung	1,966	Drivers of heavy and light trucks, garage and service-station workers	Telephone interview (direct or proxy) assessing lifetime occupational history; job titles coded	Logistic regression; age, pack-years of cigarette-smoking, race
Teschke et al. 1997	Bladder-cancer cases, 19 yr old and older, registered with British Columbia Cancer Agency in 1990-1991 with histologic confirmation; controls selected from provincial voters list matched on age, sex	105 bladder	139	Chemical, petroleum workers	In-person or telephone interview with questionnaire assessing occupational histories and self-reported exposures	Adjusted ORs; sex, age, cigarette smoking

Reference	Population	Number of Cases	Number of Controls	Relevant Exposures	Exposure Assessment	Analysis; Adjustment for Potential Confounders
Viadana et al. 1976	White male cancer cases and nonneoplastic controls admitted to Roswell Park Memorial Institute in 1956-1965, comprising 17 cancer sites, 13 occupations	11,591 total participants		Bus, taxicab, truck drivers; mechanics, repairmen; delivery and route men; locomotive engineers, firemen	Self-reported lifetime occupational histories collected	Relative risk; smoking, age
West et al. 1995	Cases of myelodysplastic syndrome, age 15 yr old or older, from areas of UK; controls selected from outpatient clinics and inpatient wards, matched for age, sex, area of residence, hospital, year of diagnosis	400 myelodysplastic syndrome	400	Petroleum products, diesels or petrols, exhaust gases	In-person interview with questionnaire assessing lifetime occupational, exposure history; duration, intensity of exposure (self-reports)	Matched pairs analysis; matching variables
Williams et al. 1989	Light chain MM cases identified through SEER tumor registries in four geographic areas, under 80 yr old newly diagnosed in 1977-1981; population controls identified through RDD and population survey of four geographic areas	69 light chain MM	1,683	Aliphatic hydrocarbons (including gas, diesel, kerosene)	Interviews (direct or proxy) with standardized questionnaire to assess occupational history, specific exposure agents	Mantel-Haenszel ORs; sex, age, race, study area

Reference	Population	Number of Cases	Number of Controls	Relevant Exposures	Exposure Assessment	Analysis; Adjustment for Potential Confounders
Xu et al. 1996	Lung-cancer cases, 30-70 yr old, diagnosed among residents of Shenyang, China, in 1985-1987; controls randomly selected from population registers and matched on age, sex distribution; subcohort of 610 cases, 959 controls active or retired from Anshan Iron-Steel Complex was analyzed with respect to benzo[a]pyrene exposure	1,249 lung	1,345	Kang, coal, gas, indoor air pollution, Benzo[a]pyrene	Interview with standardized questionnaire assessing cooking habits; indoor air-pollution index generated from questions on cooking fuel, place of cooking, weighted by duration; benzo[a]pyrene exposure assigned to subcohort on basis of indoor, outdoor measurements, person's job history	RR/ORs; age, education, smoking
Yu et al. 1990	Nasopharyngeal-cancer cases, under 50 yr old, identified among residents of Guanzhou City, China, from files of Sun Yat-Sen University Tumor Hospital in 1983-1985; neighborhood controls selected, matched on sex, age	306 nasopharyngeal	306	Combustion products	Interview with standardized questionnaire assessing occupational, dietary factors	Conditional logistic regression; matched pairs, age, sex, dietary factors, birthplace, marital status
Zheng et al. 1992	Oral- and pharyngeal-cancer cases, 20-75 yr old, identified through population-based cancer registry as newly diagnosed in 1988-1990; controls randomly selected from Shanghai Resident Registry, matched on age, sex	204 oral and pharyngeal	414	Petroleum products, kerosene-stove use	In-person interview with standardized questionnaire assessing lifestyle factors	Chi-squared test

Reference	Population	Number of Cases	Number of Controls	Relevant Exposures	Exposure Assessment	Analysis; Adjustment for Potential Confounders
Zheng et al. 1994	Nasopharyngeal-cancer cases diagnosed beginning in 1986 at Wuzhou Cancer Institute or Nasopharyngeal Carcinoma Institute of Zangwu, China, with histologic confirmation; neighborhood controls selected, matched on sex, age, place of residence	88 nasopharyngeal	176	Wood-fuel use	In-person interview with standardized questionnaire assessing lifestyle factors	Conditional logistic regression; matched pairs, sociodemographic score
Zheng et al. 1996	Cases of salivary-gland cancer, 20-75 yr old, identified through the Shanghai cancer registry and diagnosed in 1988-1990; controls randomly selected through Shanghai Resident Registry, matched on sex, age	41 salivary gland	414	Petroleum products, kerosene, coal, gas	In-person interview with standardized questionnaire assessing job history, household exposures, and dietary factors	Mantel-Haenszel OR; sex, age, income
Zheng et al. 2002	Bladder-cancer cases, age 40-85 yr old, identified and histologically confirmed by State Health Registry of Iowa among Iowa residents in 1986-1989; controls randomly selected through driver's license records (under 65 yr old) or HCFA listing (65 yr old and older), matched on sex, age	1,452 bladder	2,434	Petroleum, coal products industry, petroleum-refining industry	Mailed questionnaires obtained lifetime occupational histories of all jobs held 5 yr or more	Unconditional logistic regression; age, lifetime pack-years of cigarette-smoking, family history of bladder cancer

NOTE: HCFA=Health Care Financing Administration; NHL=non-Hodgkin's lymphoma; HD=Hodgkin's disease; JEM= job exposure matrix; MM=multiple myeloma; NIOSH=National Institute for Occupational Safety and Health; OR=odds ratio; RDD=random-digit dialing; RR=relative risk; SES=socioeconomic status; SIR=standardized incidence ratio; SMR=standardized mortality ratio.

REFERENCES

Abbey DE, Nishino N, McDonnell WF, Burchette RJ, Knutsen SF, Beeson WL, Yang JX. 1999. Long-term inhalable particles and other air pollutants related to mortality in nonsmokers. *American Journal of Respiratory and Critical Care Medicine* 159(2):373-382.

Ahrens W, Jockel KH, Patzak W, Elsner G. 1991. Alcohol, smoking, and occupational factors in cancer of the larynx: A case-control study. *American Journal of Industrial Medicine* 20(4):477-493.

Alguacil J, Kauppinen T, Porta M, Partanen T, Malats N, Kogevinas M, Benavides FG, Obiols J, Bernal F, Rifa J, Carrato A. 2000. Risk of pancreatic cancer and occupational exposures in Spain. *Annals of Occupational Hygiene* 44(5):391-403.

Armstrong RW, Imrey PB, Lye MS, Armstrong MJ, Yu MC, Sani S. 2000. Nasopharyngeal carcinoma in Malaysian Chinese: Occupational exposures to particles, formaldehyde and heat. *International Journal of Epidemiology* 29(6):991-998.

Aronson KJ, Siemiatycki J, Dewar R, Gerin M. 1996. Occupational risk factors for prostate cancer: Results from a case-control study in Montreal, Quebec, Canada. *American Journal of Epidemiology* 143(4):363-373.

Asal NR, Geyer JR, Risser DR, Lee ET, Kadamani S, Cherng N. 1988. Risk factors in renal cell carcinoma. II. Medical history, occupation, multivariate analysis, and conclusions. *Cancer Detection and Prevention* 13(3-4):263-279.

Barbone F, Bovenzi M, Cavallieri F, Stanta G. 1995. Air pollution and lung cancer in Trieste, Italy. *American Journal of Epidemiology* 141(12):1161-1169.

Bertazzi PA, Pesatori AC, Zocchetti C, Latocca R. 1989. Mortality study of cancer risk among oil refinery workers. *International Archives of Occupational & Environmental Health* 61(4):261-270.

Boffetta P, Stellman SD, Garfinkel L. 1988. Diesel exhaust exposure and mortality among males in the American Cancer Society prospective study. *American Journal of Industrial Medicine* 14(4):403-415.

Boffetta P, Dosemeci M, Gridley G, Bath H, Moradi T, Silverman D. 2001. Occupational exposure to diesel engine emissions and risk of cancer in Swedish men and women. *Cancer Causes and Control* 12(4):365-374.

Boffetta P, Richiardi L, Berino F, Esteve J, Pisani P, Crosignani P, Raymond L, Zubire L, Del Moral A, Lehmann W, Donato F, Terracini B, Tuyns A, Merletti F. 2003. Occupation and larynx and hypopharynx cancer: An international case-control study in France, Italy, Spain, and Switzerland. *Cancer Causes and Control* 14(3):203-212.

Borgia P, Forastiere F, Rapiti E, Rizzelli R, Magliola ME, Perucci CA, Axelson O. 1994. Mortality among taxi drivers in Rome: A cohort study. *American Journal of Industrial Medicine* 25(4):507-517.

Brown LM, Mason TJ, Williams Pickle L, Stewart PA, Buffler PA, Burau K, Ziegler RG, Fraumeni Jr JF. 1988. Occupational risk factors for laryngeal cancer on the Texas Gulf Coast. *Cancer Research* 48(7):1960-1964.

Bruske-Hohlfeld I, Mohner M, Ahrens W, Pohlabeln H, Heinrich J, Kreuzer M, Jockel KH, Wichmann HE. 1999. Lung cancer risk in male workers occupationally exposed to diesel motor emissions in Germany. *American Journal of Industrial Medicine* 36(4):405-414.

Bruske-Hohlfeld I, Mohner M, Pohlabeln H, Ahrens W, Bolm-Audorff U, Kreienbrock L, Kreuzer M, Jahn I, Wichmann HE, Jockel KH. 2000. Occupational lung cancer risk for men in Germany: Results from a pooled case-control study. *American Journal of Epidemiology* 151(4):384-395.

Carozza SE, Wrensch M, Miike R, Newman B, Olshan AF , Savitz DA, Yost M, Lee M. 2000. Occupation and adult gliomas. *American Journal of Epidemiology* 152(9):838-846.

Chow WH, McLaughlin JK, Malker HS, Weiner JA, Ericsson JL, Stone BJ, Blot WJ. 1994. Occupation and stomach cancer in a cohort of Swedish men. *American Journal of Industrial Medicine* 26(4):511-520.

Chow WH, McLaughlin JK, Malker HS, Linet MS, Weiner JA, Stone BJ. 1995. Esophageal cancer and occupation in a cohort of Swedish men. *American Journal of Industrial Medicine* 27(5):749-757.

Cole P, Hoover R, Friedell GH. 1972. Occupation and cancer of the lower urinary tract. *Cancer* 29(5):1250-1260.

Consonni D, Pesatori AC, Tironi A, Bernucci I, Zocchetti C, Bertazzi PA. 1999. Mortality study in an Italian oil refinery: Extension of the follow-up. *American Journal of Industrial Medicine* 35(3):287-294.

Costantini AS, Miligi L, Kriebel D, Ramazzotti V, Rodella S, Scarpi E, Stagnaro E, Tumino R, Fontana A, Masala G, Vigano C, Vindigni C, Crosignani P, Benvenuti A, Vineis P. 2001. A multicenter case-control study in Italy on hematolymphopoietic neoplasms and occupation. *Epidemiology* 12(1):78-87.

Dai XD, Lin CY, Sun XW, Shi YB, Lin YJ. 1996. The etiology of lung cancer in nonsmoking females in Harbin, China. *Lung Cancer* 14(Suppl 1):S85-S91.

De Stefani E, Boffetta P, Oreggia F, Ronco A, Kogevinas M, Mendilaharsu M. 1998. Occupation and the risk of laryngeal cancer in Uruguay. *American Journal of Industrial Medicine* 33(6):537-542.

Decoufle P, Stanislawczyk K. 1977. *A Retrospective Survey of Cancer in Relation to Occupation*. Cincinnati, OH: Center for Disease Control, National Institute for Occupational Safety and Health.

Demers PA, Vaughan TL, Koepsell TD, Lyon JL, Swanson GM, Greenberg RS, Weiss NS. 1993. A case-control study of multiple myeloma and occupation. *American Journal of Industrial Medicine* 23(4):629-639.

Dietz A, Senneweld E, Maier H. 1995. Indoor air pollution by emissions of fossil fuel single stoves: Possibly a hitherto underrated risk factor in the development of carcinomas in the head and neck. *Otolaryngology - Head & Neck Surgery* 112(2):308-315.

Divine BJ, Barron V, Kaplan SD. 1985. Texaco mortality study. I. Mortality among refinery, petrochemical, and research workers. *Journal of Occupational Medicine* 27(6):445-447.

Divine BJ, Barron V. 1986. Texaco Mortality Study: II. Patterns of mortality among white males by specific job groups. *American Journal of Industrial Medicine* 10(4):371-381.

Divine BJ, Hartman CM, Wendt JK. 1999a. Update of the Texaco mortality study 1947-93: Part I. Analysis of overall patterns of mortality among refining, research, and petrochemical workers. *Occupational & Environmental Medicine* 56(3):167-173.

Divine BJ, Hartman CM, Wendt JK. 1999b. Update of the Texaco mortality study 1947-93: Part II. Analyses of specific causes of death for white men employed in refining, research, and petrochemicals. *Occupational & Environmental Medicine* 56(3):174-180.

Du YX, Cha Q, Chen XW, Chen YZ, Huang LF, Feng ZZ, Wu XF, Wu JM. 1996. An epidemiological study of risk factors for lung cancer in Guangzhou, China. *Lung Cancer* 14(Suppl 1):S9-S37.

Dumas S, Parent ME, Siemiatycki J, Brisson J. 2000. Rectal cancer and occupational risk factors: A hypothesis-generating, exposure-based case-control study. *International Journal of Cancer* 87(6):874-879.

Elci OC, Akpinar-Elci M, Blair A, Dosemeci M. 2003. Risk of laryngeal cancer by occupational chemical exposure in Turkey. *Journal of Occupational & Environmental Medicine* 45(10):1100-1106.

Farrow A, Jacobs A, West RR. 1989. Myelodysplasia, chemical exposure, and other environmental factors. *Leukemia* 3(1):33-35.

Flodin U, Fredriksson M, Persson B. 1987. Multiple myeloma and engine exhausts, fresh wood, and creosote: A case-referent study. *American Journal of Industrial Medicine* 12(5):519-529.

Flodin U, Fredriksson M, Persson B, Axelson O. 1988. Chronic lymphatic leukaemia and engine exhausts, fresh wood, and DDT: A case-referent study. *British Journal of Industrial Medicine* 45(1):33-38.

Fritschi L, Siemiatycki J. 1996. Melanoma and occupation: Results of a case-control study. *Occupational & Environmental Medicine* 53(3):168-173.

Gamble JF, Pearlman ED, Nicolich MJ. 1996. A nested case-control study of kidney cancer among refinery/petrochemical workers. *Environmental Health Perspectives* 104(6):642-650.

Gerhardsson de Verdier MG, Plato N, Steineck G, Peters JM. 1992. Occupational exposures and cancer of the colon and rectum. *American Journal of Industrial Medicine* 22(3):291-303.

Goldberg MS, Parent ME, Siemiatycki J, Desy M, Nadon L, Richardson L, Lakhani R, Latreille B, Valois MF. 2001. A case-control study of the relationship between the risk of colon cancer in men and exposures to occupational agents. *American Journal of Industrial Medicine* 39(6):531-546.

Guberan E, Usel M, Raymond L, Bolay J, Fioretta G, Puissant J. 1992. Increased risk for lung cancer and for cancer of the gastrointestinal tract among Geneva professional drivers. *British Journal of Industrial Medicine* 49(5):337-344.

Gustavsson P, Jakobsson R, Johansson H, Lewin F, Norell S, Rutkvist LE. 1998. Occupational exposures and squamous cell carcinoma of the oral cavity, pharynx, larynx, and oesophagus: A case-control study in Sweden. *Occupational and Environmental Medicine* 55(6):393-400.

Gustavsson P, Jakobsson R, Nyberg F, Pershagen G, Jarup L, Scheele P. 2000. Occupational exposure and lung cancer risk: A population-based case-referent study in Sweden. *American Journal of Epidemiology* 152(1):32-40.

Gustavsson P, Plato N, Lidstrom EB, Hogstedt C. 1990. Lung cancer and exposure to diesel exhaust among bus garage workers. *Scandinavian Journal of Work, Environment & Health* 16(5):348-354.

Hanis NM, Stavraky KM, Fowler JL. 1979. Cancer mortality in oil refinery workers. *Journal of Occupational Medicine* 21(3):167-174.

Hansen ES. 1993. A follow-up study on the mortality of truck drivers. *American Journal of Industrial Medicine* 23(5):811-821.

Hansen J. 2000. Elevated risk for male breast cancer after occupational exposure to gasoline and vehicular combustion products. *American Journal of Industrial Medicine* 37(4):349-352.

Hansen J, Raaschou-Nielsen O, Olsen JH. 1998. Increased risk of lung cancer among different types of professional drivers in Denmark. *Occupational & Environmental Medicine* 55(2):115-118.

Hayes RB, Thomas T, Silverman DT, Vineis P, Blot WJ, Mason TJ, Pickle LW, Correa P, Fontham ETH, Schoenberg JB. 1989. Lung cancer in motor exhaust-related occupations. *American Journal of Industrial Medicine* 16(6):685-695.

Heineman EF, Olsen JH, Pottern LM, Gomez M, Raffn E, Blair A. 1992. Occupational risk factors for multiple myeloma among Danish men. *Cancer Causes and Control* 3(6):555-568.

Hoek G, Brunekreef B, Goldbohm S, Fischer P, Van den Brandt PA. 2002. Association between mortality and indicators of traffic-related air pollution in the Netherlands: A cohort study. *Lancet* 360(9341):1203-1209.

Howe GR, Burch JD, Miller AB, Cook GM, Esteve J, Morrison B, Gordon P, Chambers LW, Fodor G, Winsor GM. 1980. Tobacco use, occupation, coffee, various nutrients, and bladder cancer. *Journal of the National Cancer Institute* 64(4):701-713.

Huebner WW, Schoenberg JB, Kelsey JL, Wilcox HB, McLaughlin JK, Greenberg RS, Preston-Martin S, Austin DF, Stemhagen A, Blot WJ, Winn DM, Fraumeni J Jr. 1992. Oral and pharyngeal cancer and occupation: A case-control study. *Epidemiology* 3(4):300-309.

Huebner WW, Chen VW, Friedlander BR, Wu XC, Jorgensen G, Bhojani FA, Friedmann CH, Schmidt BA, Sales EA, Joy JA, Correa CN. 2000. Incidence of lymphohaematopoietic malignancies in a petrochemical industry cohort: 1983-94 follow up. *Occupational & Environmental Medicine* 57(9):605-614.

Iscovich J, Castelletto R, Esteve J, Munoz N, Colanzi R, Coronel A, Deamezola I, Tassi V, Arslan A. 1987. Tobacco smoking, occupational exposure and bladder cancer in Argentina. *International Journal of Cancer* 40(6):734-740.

Jarvholm B, Silverman D. 2003. Lung cancer in heavy equipment operators and truck drivers with diesel exhaust exposure in the construction industry. *Occupational & Environmental Medicine* 60(7):516-520.

Jarvholm B, Mellblom B, Norrman R, Nilsson R, Nordlinder R. 1997. Cancer incidence of workers in the Swedish petroleum industry. *Occupational & Environmental Medicine* 54(9):686-691.

Jockel KH, Ahrens W, Wichmann HE, Becher H, Bolm-Audorff U, Jahn I, Molik B, Greiser E, Timm J. 1992. Occupational and environmental hazards associated with lung cancer. *International Journal of Epidemiology* 21(2):202-213.

Kadamani S, Asal NR, Nelson RY. 1989. Occupational hydrocarbon exposure and risk of renal cell carcinoma. *American Journal of Industrial Medicine* 15(2):131-141.

Katsouyanni K, Trichopoulos D, Kalandidi A, Tomos P, Riboli E. 1991. A case-control study of air pollution and tobacco smoking in lung cancer among women in Athens. *Preventive Medicine* 20(2):271-278.

Kauppinen T, Partanen T, Degerth R, Ojajarvi A. 1995. Pancreatic cancer and occupational exposures. *Epidemiology* 6(5):498-502.

Kleinerman RA, Wang Z, Wang L, Metayer C, Zhang S, Brenner AV, Zhang S, Xia Y, Shang B, Lubin JH. 2002. Lung cancer and indoor exposure to coal and biomass in rural China. *Journal of Occupational & Environmental Medicine* 44(4):338-344.

Kneller RW, Gao YT, McLaughlin JK, Gao RN, Blot WJ, Liu MH, Sheng JP, Fraumeni JF Jr. 1990. Occupational risk factors for gastric cancer in Shanghai, China. *American Journal of Industrial Medicine* 18(1):69-78.

Kogevinas M, 't Mannetje A, Cordier S, Ranft U, Gonzalez C, Vineis P, Chang-Claude J, Lynge E, Wahrendorf J, Tzonou A, Jockel K, Serra C, Porru S, Hours M, Greiser E, Boffetta P. 2003. Occupation and bladder cancer among men in Western Europe. *Cancer Causes and Control* 14(10):907-914.

Krewski D, Snyder R, Beatty P, Granville G, Meek B, Sonawane B. 2000. Assessing the health risks of benzene: A report on the Benzene State-of-the-Science Workshop. *Journal of Toxicology and Environmental Health-Part A* 61(5-6):307-338.

Lagorio S, Forastiere F, Iavarone I, Rapiti E, Vanacore N, Perucci CA, Carere A. 1994. Mortality of filling station attendants. *Scandinavian Journal of Work, Environment & Health* 20(5):331-338.

Lan Q, Feng Z, Tian D, He X, Rothman N, Tian L, Lu X, Terry MB, Mumford JL. 2001. p53 gene expression in relation to indoor exposure to unvented coal smoke in Xuan Wei, China. *Journal of Occupational and Environmental Medicine* 43(3):226-230.

Lan Q, Chapman RS, Schreinemachers DM, Tian L, He X. 2002. Household stove improvement and risk of lung cancer in Xuanwei, China. *Journal of the National Cancer Institute* 94(11):826-835.

Larkin EK, Smith TJ, Stayner L, Rosner B, Speizer FE, Garshick E. 2000. Diesel exhaust exposure and lung cancer: Adjustment for the effect of smoking in a retrospective cohort study. *American Journal of Industrial Medicine* 38(4):399-409.

Leclerc A, Luce D, Demers PA, Boffetta P, Kogevinas M, Belli S, Bolm-Audorff U, Brinton LA, Colin D, Comba P, Gerin M, Hardell L, Hayes RB, Magnani C, Merler E, Morcet JF, Preston-Martin S, Vaughan TL, Zheng W. 1997. Sinonasal cancer and occupation. Results from the reanalysis of twelve case-control studies. *American Journal of Industrial Medicine* 31(2):153-165.

Lewis RJ, Schnatter AR, Katz AM, Thompson FS, Murray N, Jorgensen G, Theriault G. 2000. Updated mortality among diverse operating segments of a petroleum company. *Occupational & Environmental Medicine* 57(9):595-604.

Lewis RJ, Schnatter AR, Drummond I, Murray N, Thompson FS, Katz AM, Jorgensen G, Nicolich MJ , Dahlman D, Theriault G. 2003. Mortality and cancer morbidity in a cohort of Canadian petroleum workers. *Occupational & Environmental Medicine* 60(12):918-928.

Lindquist R, Nilsson B, Eklund G, Gahrton G. 1991. Acute leukemia in professional drivers exposed to gasoline and diesel. *European Journal of Haematology* 47(2):98-103.

Magnani C, Coggon D, Osmond C, Acheson ED. 1987. Occupation and five cancers: A case-control study using death certificates. *British Journal of Industrial Medicine* 44(11):769-776.

Mandel JS, McLaughlin JK, Schlehofer B, Mellemgaard A, Helmert U, Lindblad P, McCredie M, Adami HO. 1995. International renal-cell cancer study. IV. Occupation. *International Journal of Cancer* 61(5):601-605.

Matos EL, Vilensky M, Mirabelli D, Boffetta P. 2000. Occupational exposures and lung cancer in Buenos Aires, Argentina. *Journal of Occupational & Environmental Medicine* 42(6):653-659.

McLaughlin JK, Blot WJ, Mehl ES, Stewart PA, Venable FS, Fraumeni JF Jr. 1985. Petroleum-related employment and renal cell cancer. *Journal of Occupational Medicine* 27(9):672-674.

McLaughlin JK, Malker HS, Stone BJ, Weiner JA, Malker BK, Ericsson JL, Blot WJ, Fraumeni JF Jr. 1987. Occupational risks for renal cancer in Sweden. *British Journal of Industrial Medicine* 44(2):119-123.

McLaughlin JK, Mandel JS, Blot WJ, Schuman LM, Mehl ES, Fraumeni JF Jr. 1984. A population-based case-control study of renal cell carcinoma. *Journal of the National Cancer Institute* 72(2):275-284.

Menvielle G, Luce D, Fevotte J, Bugel I, Salomon C, Goldberg P, Billon-Galland MA, Goldberg M. 2003. Occupational exposures and lung cancer in New Caledonia. *Occupational & Environmental Medicine* 60(8):584-589.

Merletti F, Boffetta P, Ferro G, Pisani P, Terracini B. 1991. Occupation and cancer of the oral cavity or oropharynx in Turin, Italy. *Scandinavian Journal of Work, Environment and Health* 17(4):248-254.

Mommsen S, Aagard J. 1984. Occupational exposures as risk indicator of male bladder carcinoma in a predominantly rural area. *Acta Radiologica - Oncology* 23(2-3):147-152.

Mommsen S, Aagaard J, Sell A. 1982. An epidemiological case-control study of bladder cancer in males from a predominantly rural district. *European Journal of Cancer and Clinical Oncology* 18(11):1205-1210.

Mommsen S, Aagaard J, Sell A. 1983. An epidemiological study of bladder cancer in a predominantly rural district. *Scandinavian Journal of Urology and Nephrology* 17(3):307-312.

Morris PD, Koepsell TD, Daling JR, Taylor JW, Lyon JL, Swanson GM, Child M, Weiss NS. 1986. Toxic substance exposure and multiple myeloma: A case control-study. *Journal of the National Cancer Institute* 76(6):987-994.

Nadon L, Siemiatycki J, Dewar R, Krewski D, Gerin M. 1995. Cancer risk due to occupational exposure to polycyclic aromatic hydrocarbons. *American Journal of Industrial Medicine* 28(3):303-324.

Nafstad P, Haheim LL, Oftedal B, Gram F, Holme I, Hjermann I, Leren P. 2003. Lung cancer and air pollution: A 27 year follow up of 16,209 Norwegian men. *Thorax* 58(12):1071-1076.

Najem GR, Louria DB, Seebode JJ, et al. 1982. Life time occupation, smoking, caffeine, saccharine, hair dyes and bladder carcinogenesis. *International Journal of Epidemiology* 11(3):212-217.

Nelson NA, Barker DM, Van Peenen PF, Blanchard AG. 1985. Determining exposure categories for a refinery retrospective cohort mortality study. *American Industrial Hygiene Association Journal* 46(11):653-657.

Nelson NA, Van Peenen PF, Blanchard AG. 1987. Mortality in a recent oil refinery cohort. *Journal of Occupational Medicine* 29(7):610-612.

Nisse C, Haguenoer JM, Grandbastien B, Preudhomme C, Fontaine B, Brillet JM, Lejeune R, Fenaux P. 2001. Occupational and environmental risk factors of the myelodysplastic syndromes in the North of France. *British Journal of Haematology* 112(4):927-935.

Nyberg F, Gustavsson P, Jarup L, Bellander T, Berglind N, Jakobsson R, Pershagen G. 2000. Urban air pollution and lung cancer in Stockholm. *Epidemiology* 11(5):487-495.

Parent ME, Hua Y, Siemiatycki J. 2000a. Occupational risk factors for renal cell carcinoma in Montreal. *American Journal of Industrial Medicine* 38(6):609-618.

Parent ME, Siemiatycki J, Fritschi L. 2000b. Workplace exposures and oesophageal cancer. *Occupational & Environmental Medicine* 57(5):325-334.

Partanen T, Heikkila P, Hernberg S, Kauppinen T, Moneta G, Ojajarvi A. 1991. Renal cell cancer and occupational exposure to chemical agents. *Scandinavian Journal of Work, Environment & Health* 17(4):231-239.

Pesch B, Haerting J, Ranft U, Klimpel A, Oeschlagel B, Schill W. 2000. Occupational risk factors for renal cell carcinoma: Agent-specific results from a case-control study in Germany. *International Journal of Epidemiology* 29(6):1014-1024.

Petralia SA, Vena JE, Freudenheim JL, Dosemeci M, Michalek A, Goldberg MS, Brasure J, Graham S. 1999. Risk of premenopausal breast cancer in association with occupational exposure to polycyclic aromatic hydrocarbons and benzene. *Scandinavian Journal of Work, Environment & Health* 25(3):215-221.

Pintos J, Franco EL, Kowalski LP, Oliveira BV, Curado MP. 1998. Use of wood stoves and risk of cancers of the upper aero-digestive tract: A case-control study. *International Journal of Epidemiology* 27(6):936-940.

Poole C, Dreyer NA, Satterfield MH, Levin L, Rothman KJ. 1993. Kidney cancer and hydrocarbon exposures among petroleum refinery workers. *Environmental Health Perspectives* 101(Suppl 6):53-62.

Pope CA 3rd, Burnett RT, Thun MJ, Calle EE, Krewski D, Ito K, Thurston GD. 2002. Lung cancer, cardiopulmonary mortality, and long-term exposure to fine particulate air pollution. *Journal of the American Medical Association* 287(9):1132-1141.

Pope CA 3rd, Thun MJ, Namboodiri MM, Dockery DW, Evans JS, Speizer FE, Heath CW Jr. 1995. Particulate air pollution as a predictor of mortality in a prospective study of U.S. adults. *American Journal of Respiratory and Critical Care Medicine* 151(3 Pt 1):669-674.

Raabe GK, Collingwood KW, Wong O. 1998. An updated mortality study of workers at a petroleum refinery in Beaumont, Texas. *American Journal of Industrial Medicine* 33(1):61-81.

Rafnsson V, Gunaarsdottir H. 1991. Mortality among professional drivers. *Scandinavian Journal of Work, Environment & Health* 17(5):312-317.

Rajaraman P, Roos AJ, Stewart PA, Linet MS, Fine HA, Shapiro WR, Selker RG, Black PM, Inskip PD. 2004. Occupation and risk of meningioma and acoustic neuroma in the United States. *American Journal of Industrial Medicine* 45(5):395-407.

Risch HA, Burch JD, Miller AB, Hill GB, Steele R, Howe GR. 1988. Occupational factors and the incidence of cancer of the bladder in Canada. *British Journal of Industrial Medicine* 45(6):361-367.

Ritz B. 1999. Cancer mortality among workers exposed to chemicals during uranium processing. *Journal of Occupational and Environmental Medicine* 41(7):556-566.

Rosamilia K, Wong O, Raabe GK. 1999. A case-control study of lung cancer among refinery workers. *Journal of Occupational & Environmental Medicine* 41(12):1091-1103.

Saverin R, Braunlich A, Dahmann D, Enderlein G, Heuchert G. 1999. Diesel exhaust and lung cancer mortality in potash mining. *American Journal of Industrial Medicine* 36(4):415-422.

Schnatter AR, Armstrong TW, Nicolich MJ, Thompson FS, Katz AM, Huebner WW, Pearlman ED. 1996. Lymphohaematopoietic malignancies and quantitative estimates of exposure to benzene in Canadian petroleum distribution workers. *Occupational & Environmental Medicine* 53(11):773-781.

Schnatter AR, Katz AM, Nicolich MJ, Theriault G. 1993. A retrospective mortality study among Canadian petroleum marketing and distribution workers. *Environmental Health Perspectives* 101(Suppl 6):85-99.

Schnatter AR, Theriault G, Katz AM, Thompson FS, Donaleski D, Murray N. 1992. A retrospective mortality study within operating segments of a petroleum company. *American Journal of Industrial Medicine* 22(2):209-229.

Schoenberg JB, Stemhagen A, Mogielnicki AP, Altman R, Abe T, Mason TJ. 1984. Case-control study of bladder cancer in New Jersey. I. Occupational exposures in white males. *Journal of the National Cancer Institute* 72(5):973-981.

Sharpe CR, Rochon JE, Adam JM, Suissa S. 1989. Case-control study of hydrocarbon exposures in patients with renal cell carcinoma. *CMAJ Canadian Medical Association Journal* 140(11):1309-1318.

Siemiatycki J, Gerin M, Stewart P, Nadon L, Dewar R, Richardson L. 1988. Associations between several sites of cancer and ten types of exhaust and combustion products. Results from a case-referent study in Montreal. *Scandinavian Journal of Work, Environment & Health* 14(2):79-90.

Siemiatycki J, Wacholder S, Richardson L, Dewar R, Gerin M. 1987. Discovering carcinogens in the occupational environment. Methods of data collection and analysis of a large case-referent monitoring system. *Scandinavian Journal of Work, Environment and Health* 13(6):486-492.

Silverman DT, Levin LI, Hoover RN. 1989a. Occupational risks of bladder cancer in the United States: II Nonwhite men. *Journal of the National Cancer Institute* 81(19):1480-1483.

Silverman DT, Levin LI, Hoover RN, Hartge P. 1989b. Occupational risks of bladder cancer in the United States: I. White men. *Journal of the National Cancer Institute* 81(19):1472-1480.

Soll-Johanning H, Bach E, Jensen SS. 2003. Lung and bladder cancer among Danish urban bus drivers and tramway employees: A nested case-control study. *Occupational Medicine* 53(1):25-33.

Soll-Johanning H, Bach E, Olsen JH, Tuchsen F. 1998. Cancer incidence in urban bus drivers and tramway employees: A retrospective cohort study. *Occupational & Environmental Medicine* 55(9):594-598.

Spiegelman D, Wegman DH. 1985. Occupation-related risks for colorectal cancer. *Journal of the National Cancer Institute* 75(5):813-821.

Steenland K, Deddens J, Stayner L. 1998. Diesel exhaust and lung cancer in the trucking industry: exposure-response analyses and risk assessment. *American Journal of Industrial Medicine* 34(3):220-228.

Steenland NK, Silverman DT, Hornung RW. 1990. Case-control study of lung cancer and truck driving in the Teamsters Union. *American Journal of Public Health* 80(6):670-674.

Steineck G, Plato N, Gerhardsson M, Norell SE, Hogstedt C. 1990. Increased risk of urothelial cancer in Stockholm during 1985-87 after exposure to benzene and exhausts. *International Journal of Cancer* 45(6):1012-1017.

Stemhagen A, Slade J, Altman R, Bill J. 1983. Occupational risk factors and liver cancer. A retrospective case-control study of primary liver cancer in New Jersey. *American Journal of Epidemiology* 117(4):443-454.

Swanson GM, Lin CS, Burns PB. 1993. Diversity in the association between occupation and lung cancer among black and white men. *Cancer Epidemiology, Biomarkers and Prevention* 2(4):313-320.

Teschke K, Morgan MS, Checkoway H, Franklin G, Spinelli JJ, van Belle G, Weiss NS. 1997. Surveillance of nasal and bladder cancer to locate sources of exposure to occupational carcinogens. *Occupational and Environmental Medicine* 54(6):443-451.

van Loon AJ, Kant IJ, Swaen GM, Goldbohm RA, Kremer AM, van den Brandt PA. 1997. Occupational exposure to carcinogens and risk of lung cancer: Results from The Netherlands cohort study. *Occupational & Environmental Medicine* 54(11):817-824.

Vasama-Neuvonen K, Pukkala E, Paakkulainen H, Mutanen P, Weiderpass E, Boffetta P, Shen N, Kauppinen T, Vainio H, Partanen T. 1999. Ovarian cancer and occupational exposures in Finland. *American Journal of Industrial Medicine* 36(1):83-89.

Viadana E, Bross ID, Houten L. 1976. Cancer experience of men exposed to inhalation of chemicals or to combustion products. *Journal of Occupational Medicine* 18(12):787-792.

West RR, Stafford DA, Farrow A, Jacobs A. 1995. Occupational and environmental exposures and myelodysplasia: A case-control study. *Leukemia Research* 19(2):127-139.

Williams AR, Weiss NS, Koepsell TD, Lyon JL, Swanson GM. 1989. Infectious and noninfectious exposures in the etiology of light chain myeloma: A case-control study. *Cancer Research* 49(14):4038-4041.

Wong O, Harris F, Rosamilia K, Raabe GK. 2001. An updated mortality study of workers at a petroleum refinery in Beaumont, Texas, 1945 to 1996. *Journal of Occupational and Environmental Medicine* 43(4):384-401.

Wong O, Trent L, Harris F. 1999. Nested case-control study of leukaemia, multiple myeloma, and kidney cancer in a cohort of petroleum workers exposed to gasoline. *Occupational & Environmental Medicine* 56(4):217-221.

Xu ZY, Brown L, Pan GW, Li G, Feng YP, Guan DX, Liu TF, Liu LM, Chao RM, Sheng JH, Gao GC. 1996. Lifestyle, environmental pollution and lung cancer in cities of Liaoning in northeastern China. *Lung Cancer* 14(Suppl 1):S149-S160.

Yu MC, Garabrant DH, Huang TB, Henderson BE. 1990. Occupational and other non-dietary risk factors for nasopharyngeal carcinoma in Guangzhou, China. *International Journal of Cancer* 45(6):1033-1039.

Zeegers MP, Swaen GM, Kant I, Goldbohm RA, van den Brandt PA. 2001. Occupational risk factors for male bladder cancer: Results from a population based case cohort study in the Netherlands. *Occupational & Environmental Medicine* 58(9):590-596.

Zheng T, Cantor KP, Zhang Y, Lynch CF. 2002. Occupation and bladder cancer: A population-based, case-control study in Iowa. *Journal of Occupational & Environmental Medicine* 44(7):685-691.

Zheng W, Blot WJ, Shu XO, Diamond EL, Gao YT, Ji BT, Fraumeni JF Jr. 1992. Risk factors for oral and pharyngeal cancer in Shanghai, with emphasis on diet. *Cancer Epidemiology, Biomarkers and Prevention* 1(6):441-448.

Zheng W, Shu XO, Ji BT, Gao YT. 1996. Diet and other risk factors for cancer of the salivary glands: A population-based case-control study. *International Journal of Cancer* 67(2):194-198.

Zheng YM, Tuppin P, Hubert A, Jeannel D, Pan YJ, Zeng Y, De The G. 1994. Environmental and dietary risk factors for nasopharyngeal carcinoma: A case-control study in Zangwu County, Guangxi, China. *British Journal of Cancer* 69(3):508-514.

INDEX

R

V

W

X